Maternal Health: Neonatology and Perinatology

Maternal Health: Neonatology and Perinatology

Edited by Talia Atkins

hayle medical

New York

Hayle Medical,
750 Third Avenue, 9th Floor,
New York, NY 10017, USA

Visit us on the World Wide Web at:
www.haylemedical.com

ISBN: 978-1-63241-620-9

The publisher's policy is to use permanent paper from mills that operate a sustainable forestry policy. Furthermore, the publisher ensures that the text paper and cover boards used have met acceptable environmental accreditation standards.

Printed in China.

Cataloging-in-Publication Data

Maternal health : neonatology and perinatology / edited by Talia Atkins.
p. cm.
Includes bibliographical references and index.
ISBN 978-1-63241-620-9
1. Maternal health services. 2. Neonatology. 3. Perinatology. 4. Maternal and infant welfare.
5. Obstetrics. I. Atkins, Talia.
RG940 .M38 2019
618.24--dc23

Table of Contents

Preface

This book aims to highlight the current researches and provides a platform to further the scope of innovations in this area. This book is a product of the combined efforts of many researchers and scientists, after going through thorough studies and analysis from different parts of the world. The objective of this book is to provide the readers with the latest information of the field.

The health of women during pregnancy, childbirth and the postpartum period is known as maternal health. It also includes other dimensions of health care, including prenatal care, postnatal care, preconception and family planning. It aims to reduce maternal morbidity and mortality in women, and facilitate a positive and fulfilling experience for them. The field of medicine dealing with the care of newborn infants is known as neonatology. Neonatal intensive care units (NICUs) are the units of intensive care, which deal with the care of ill or premature newborn. The field of medicine that is focused on the management of the health issues related to the mother and fetus at the time of pregnancy is called perinatology. This book includes some of the vital pieces of work being conducted across the world, on various topics related to maternal health. It attempts to understand the multiple branches that fall under maternal health and how such concepts have practical applications. The extensive content of this book provides the readers with a thorough understanding of the subject.

I would like to express my sincere thanks to the authors for their dedicated efforts in the completion of this book. I acknowledge the efforts of the publisher for providing constant support. Lastly, I would like to thank my family for their support in all academic endeavors.

Editor

1

Persistent pulmonary hypertension of the newborn

Vinay Sharma[1*], Sara Berkelhamer[2] and Satyan Lakshminrusimha[2]

Abstract

Persistent pulmonary hypertension of the newborn (PPHN) is characterized by elevated pulmonary vascular resistance resulting in right-to-left shunting of blood and hypoxemia. PPHN is often secondary to parenchymal lung disease (such as meconium aspiration syndrome, pneumonia or respiratory distress syndrome) or lung hypoplasia (with congenital diaphragmatic hernia or oligohydramnios) but can also be idiopathic. The diagnosis of PPHN is based on clinical evidence of labile hypoxemia often associated with differential cyanosis. The diagnosis is confirmed by the echocardiographic demonstration of – (a) right-to-left or bidirectional shunt at the ductus or foramen ovale and/or, (b) flattening or leftward deviation of the interventricular septum and/or, (c) tricuspid regurgitation, and finally (d) absence of structural heart disease. Management strategies include optimal oxygenation, avoiding respiratory and metabolic acidosis, blood pressure stabilization, sedation and pulmonary vasodilator therapy. Failure of these measures would lead to consideration of extracorporeal membrane oxygenation (ECMO); however decreased need for this rescue therapy has been documented with advances in medical management. While trends also note improved survival, long-term neurodevelopmental disabilities such as deafness and learning disabilities remain a concern in many infants with severe PPHN.

Funded by: 1R01HD072929-0 (SL)

Keywords: Nitric Oxide, Fetal circulation, Pulmonary vascular remodeling, Meconium aspiration, Surfactant, Natriuretic peptide, Meconium aspiration, Prostaglandin E1, Sildenafil, Milrinone

Introduction

Persistent pulmonary hypertension of newborn (PPHN) is secondary to failure of normal circulatory transition at birth. It is a syndrome characterized by elevated pulmonary vascular resistance (PVR) that causes labile hypoxemia due to decreased pulmonary blood flow and right-to-left shunting of blood. Prompt diagnosis and management, including a timely referral to a tertiary care center can dramatically improve outcome. Its incidence has been reported as 1.9 per 1000 live births (0.4–6.8/1000 live births) with mortality rate ranging between 4–33% [1]. This syndrome complicates the course of about 10% of term and preterm infants with respiratory failure and remains a source of considerable morbidity and mortality. This review includes a discussion of fetal circulation and circulatory transition at birth, as well as the pathophysiology, diagnosis, management and long term complications of PPHN.

* Correspondence: vinay.sharma@hcmed.org
[1]Department of Pediatrics (Neonatology), Hennepin County Medical Center, 701 Park Avenue, Shapiro Building, Minneapolis, MN 55415, USA
Full list of author information is available at the end of the article

Findings

Fetal circulation

Pulmonary hypertension with reduced pulmonary blood flow is a normal physiologic state in the fetus. This is because the placenta, not the lung, serves as the organ of gas exchange. Most of the right ventricular output crosses the ductus arteriosus to the aorta (approximately 8-10% of combined ventricular output in an ovine fetus and 13% -21% in human fetuses) [2-4]. Even though pulmonary vascular cross-sectional area increases with fetal lung growth, PVR increases with gestational age when corrected for lung or body weight, suggesting that pulmonary vascular tone increases during late gestation. Multiple pathways appear to be involved in maintaining high pulmonary vascular tone prior to birth. Apart from mechanical factors (fluid-filled lung), hypoxic pulmonary vasoconstriction and circulating vasoconstrictors such as endothelin-1 and products of the prostaglandin pathway (i.e. leukotriene and thromboxane) play a significant role in maintaining high fetal PVR [5].

Serotonin increases fetal PVR [6,7]. The use of selective serotonin reuptake inhibitors (SSRIs) during the last half of pregnancy has been associated with an increased incidence of PPHN in at least three human population studies [8-11]. While the mechanism by which SSRIs induce pulmonary hypertension in newborn is not known, it is speculated that higher drug-induced serotonin levels result in pulmonary vasoconstriction. However, recent studies have questioned the association between maternal SSRI intake and PPHN [12,13]. Furthermore, the severity of PPHN has not been well described and a recent report observed no differences in right pulmonary artery Doppler pulsatility index (PI) in fetuses of mothers exposed to SSRI antidepressants [14]. At present, maternal physical and psychological well-being should be the primary factor guiding antidepressant therapy during pregnancy and postpartum period.

The fetus is in a physiological state of hypoxemia (relative to postnatal standards) with PaO_2 of around 25 mmHg, a level that promotes normal growth and differentiation of pulmonary vascular cells and supports normal branching morphogenesis [15]. However, a normal fetus is not hypoxic and adequate oxygen delivery to the fetal tissues is maintained by multiple mechanisms including high cardiac output *in utero*, high hemoglobin level in the term fetus, and presence of fetal hemoglobin (HbF) with high oxygen affinity (Figure 1).

Transitional circulation

A series of circulatory events take place at birth to ensure a smooth transition from fetal to extra-uterine life. Clamping of the umbilical cord removes the low resistance placental circulation, increasing systemic arterial pressure. Simultaneously, various mechanisms operate to rapidly reduce pulmonary arterial pressure and increase pulmonary blood flow. The most important stimulus to promote pulmonary vasodilation appears to be ventilation of the lungs and an increase in oxygen tension [5]. There is improved oxygenation of the pulmonary vascular bed, further decreasing PVR [16]. An eight-fold increase in pulmonary blood flow occurs, which raises left atrial pressure, closing the foramen ovale. As PVR drops lower than systemic vascular resistance (SVR), there is a reversal of flow across the ductus arteriosus (from aorta to pulmonary artery or left-to-right). The increase in arterial oxygen saturation leads to closure of the ductus arteriosus and ductus venosus. In the final phase of neonatal pulmonary vascular transition, a further decline in PVR is accompanied by rapid structural remodeling of the entire pulmonary bed, from the main pulmonary arteries to the capillaries [17].

Mediators of circulatory transition at birth

Vascular endothelium releases several vasoactive products that play a primary role in pulmonary transition at birth. Pulmonary endothelial nitric oxide (NO) production increases markedly at the time of birth. Oxygen is believed to be an important catalyst for this increased NO production, although the precise mechanism is not clear. It increases oxidative phosphorylation and the release of red blood cell ATP which is a pulmonary vasodilator during fetal life and a potential stimulus for endothelial NO production [18,19]. In intrapulmonary arteries isolated from near-term fetal sheep, both basal and stimulated NO release increase with escalating oxygen tension [20]. The shear stress resulting from increased pulmonary blood flow and increased oxygenation also induce endothelial nitric oxide synthase (eNOS) expression, thus contributing to NO-mediated pulmonary vasodilation after birth [5]. Nitric oxide exerts its action through soluble guanylate cyclase (sGC) and cGMP (Figure 2). The importance of the NO-cGMP pathway in facilitating normal transition has been demonstrated by acute or chronic inhibition of nitric oxide synthase (NOS) in fetal lambs, which produces pulmonary hypertension following delivery [21,22]. Data indicate that eNOS dysfunction induced through increased levels of asymmetric dimethyl arginine (ADMA), a competitive endogenous inhibitor of NOS [23], or by decreased synthesis of the NOS substrate L-arginine [24], may result in pulmonary vasoconstriction.

The arachidonic acid-prostacyclin pathway also plays an important role in the transition at birth. The cyclooxygenase enzyme acts on arachidonic acid to produce prostaglandin endoperoxides. Prostaglandins activate adenylate cyclase to increase cAMP concentrations in vascular smooth muscle cells (Figure 2). Cyclooxygenase-1 in particular is upregulated during late gestation, leading to an increase in prostacyclin production in the third trimester and early postnatal life [25,26]. Inhibition of prostacyclin production by non-steroidal anti-inflammatory drugs (NSAIDs) during late pregnancy has been associated with PPHN although this association has been recently called into question [27].

Finally, atrial natriuretic peptide (ANP), B-type natriuretic peptide (BNP) and C-type natriuretic peptide (CNP) dilate fetal pulmonary vasculature by increasing cGMP through particulate guanylate cyclase (pGC) [28] and may play a role in pulmonary vascular transition at birth (Figure 2).

Pathophysiology of PPHN

Disruption of normal neonatal circulatory transition results in failure to resolve fetal pulmonary hypertension and leads to the persistence of fetal pulmonary

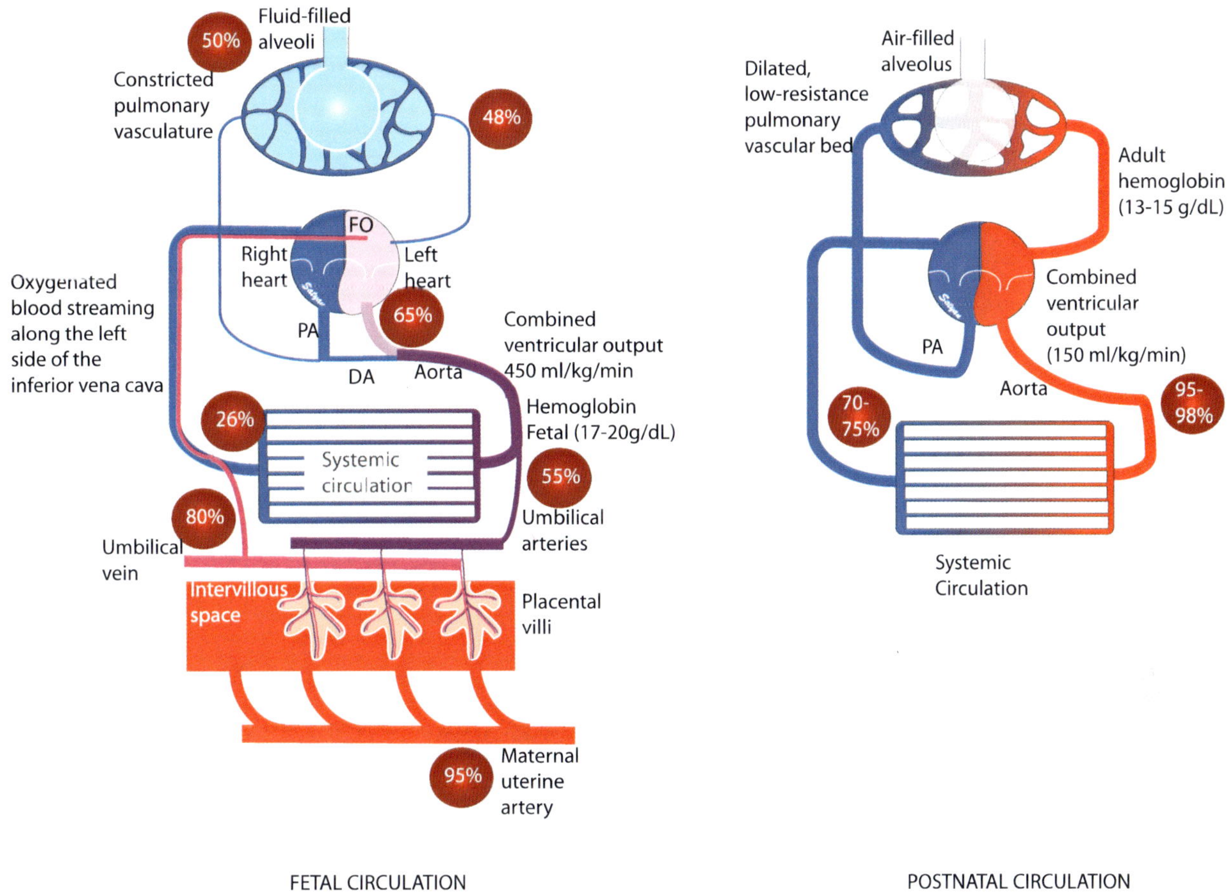

Figure 1 Fetal and postnatal (adult) circulation: in fetuses, placenta is the organ of gas exchange. The umbilical vein carries oxygenated blood from the placenta has the highest fetal oxygen saturation of approximately 80%. Oxygen saturation in various blood vessels is shown in crimson circles. Oxygenated blood is streamed through the ductus venosus and along the left margin of the inferior vena cava. In the heart, oxygenated blood gets shunted across the foramen ovale (FO) to the left heart to supply the cerebral and coronary circulation. Poorly oxygenated blood from the upper half of the body goes to the right side of the heart, the main pulmonary artery and gets shunted through the ductus arteriosus (DA) to the descending aorta. Blood in the descending aorta has a saturation of around 55 %, and this blood flows back to placenta for oxygenation through umbilical arteries. In spite of relative hypoxia, adequate oxygen delivery to the fetal tissues is maintained by (a) high cardiac output, (b) high hemoglobin level in the term fetus and (c) the presence of fetal hemoglobin (HbF) with high oxygen affinity. The saturation gradient across the placenta (85 – 55 = 30%) is similar to the saturation gradient across the lungs in adults (98 – 70% = 28%) but is achieved at a much lower partial pressure of oxygen (PO_2 ~ 32 mmHg in the umbilical vein) in the fetus compared to the adult (PaO_2 ~ 95 mmHg) limiting the fetal risk for oxygen toxicity.

hypertension or PPHN. High pulmonary pressure decreases the blood flow to the lungs. Ventilation-perfusion (VQ) mismatch (Figure 3) and extrapulmonary right-to-left shunting of deoxygenated blood across the patent foramen ovale (PFO) and patent ductus arteriosus (PDA) result in cyanosis. **Differential cyanosis** (saturation in the lower limb is 5-10% lower than right upper limb) occurs due to pulmonary artery to aorta shunt through the PDA (Figure 3). If the PDA is closed and the shunt exclusively is at the PFO level, the degree of cyanosis is similar in both upper and lower limbs. **Labile hypoxemia** (marked change in oxygen saturation with minimal or no change in ventilator settings) is characteristic of PPHN and is due to change in the volume of right-to-left shunt secondary to subtle changes in the delicate balance between PVR and SVR.

Classification

PPHN can be characterized as one of four types:

(1) *Maladaptation*: Secondary to lung parenchymal diseases such as meconium aspiration syndrome (MAS), respiratory distress syndrome (RDS), or pneumonia

(2) *Maldevelopment*: Lung with normal parenchyma and remodeled pulmonary vasculature, also known as idiopathic PPHN

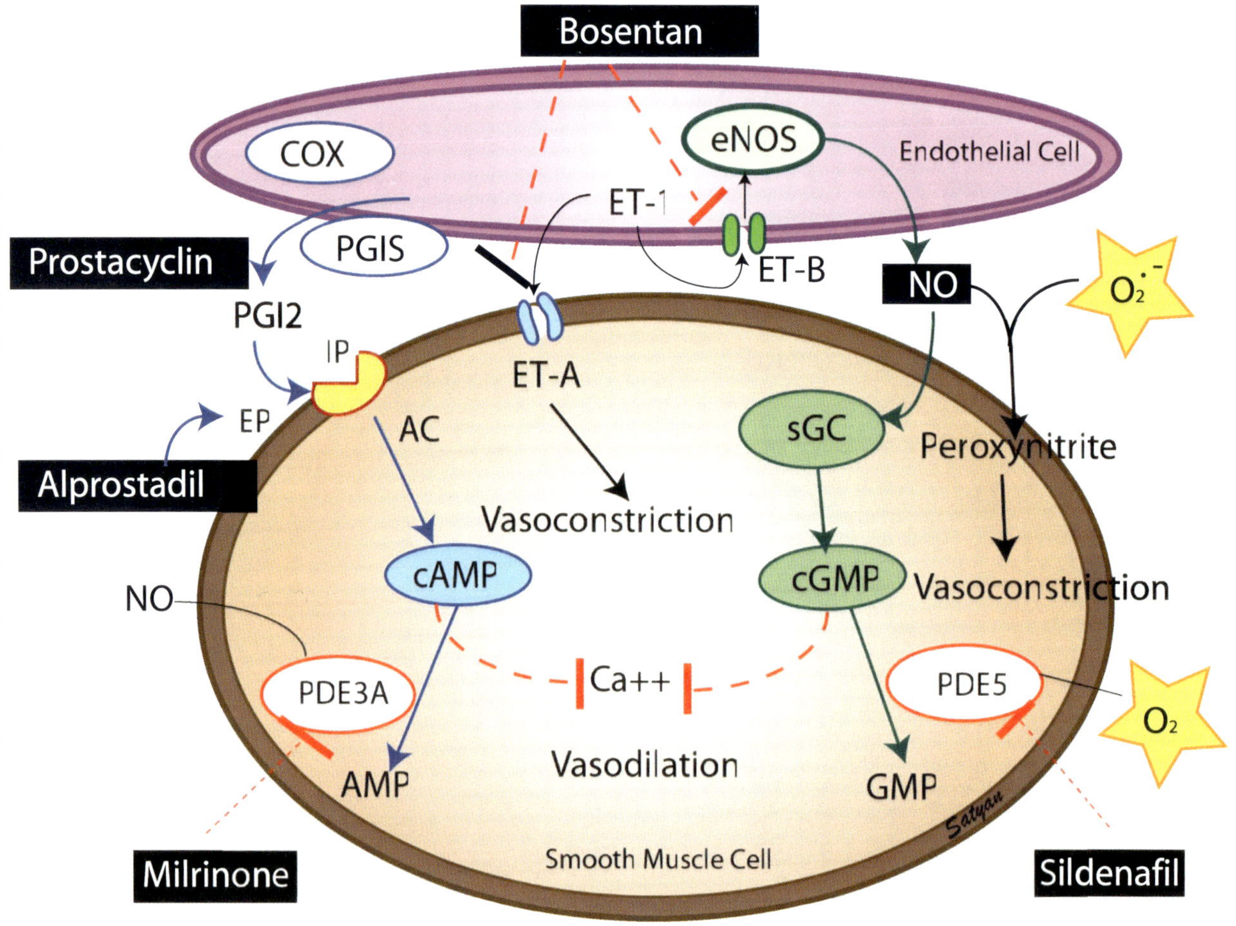

Figure 2 Endothelium derived vasodilators – prostacyclin (PGI_2) and nitric oxide (NO) and vasoconstrictor (endothelin, ET-1). Cyclooxygenase (COX) and prostacyclin synthase (PGIS) are involved in the production of prostacyclin. Prostacyclin acts on its receptor (IP) in the smooth muscle cell and stimulates adenylate cyclase (AC) to produce cyclic adenosine monophosphate (cAMP). Cyclic AMP is broken down by phosphodiesterase 3A (PDE 3A, the enzyme most prevalent in vasculature) in the smooth muscle cell. Milrinone inhibits PDE 3A and increases cAMP levels in arterial smooth muscle cells and cardiac myocytes resulting in pulmonary (and systemic) vasodilation and inotropy. Nitric oxide (NO) stimulates PDE 3A [151,152]. Endothelin is a powerful vasoconstrictor and acts on ET-A receptors in the smooth muscle cell and increases ionic calcium concentration. A second endothelin receptor (ET-B) on the endothelial cell stimulates NO release and vasodilation. Endothelial nitric oxide synthase (eNOS) produces NO which diffuses from the endothelium to the smooth muscle cell and stimulates soluble guanylate cyclase (sGC) enzyme to produce cyclic guanosine monophosphate (cGMP). Cyclic GMP is broken down by PDE5 enzyme in the smooth muscle cell. Sildenafil inhibits PDE5 and increases cGMP levels in pulmonary arterial smooth muscle cells. Natriuretic peptides stimulate particulate guanylate cyclase (pGC) to produce cGMP. Cyclic AMP and cGMP reduce cytosolic ionic calcium concentrations and induce smooth muscle cell relaxation and pulmonary vasodilation. Nitric oxide is a free radical and can avidly combine with superoxide anions to form a toxic vasoconstrictor, peroxynitrite. Hence, the bioavailability of NO in a tissue is determined by the local concentration of superoxide anions. Hyperoxic ventilation with 100% oxygen can increase the risk of formation of superoxide anions in the pulmonary arterial smooth muscle cells and limit the bioavailability of NO and stimulate PDE5 activity [81]. Medications used in PPHN are shown in black boxes.

(3) *Underdevelopment*: Hypoplastic vasculature as seen in CDH and other causes of pulmonary hypoplasia (oligohydramnios secondary to Potter's Syndrome, renal disease or chronic leakage of amniotic fluid)

(4) *Intrinsic obstruction*: high viscosity due to polycythemia resulting in intravascular obstruction and elevated PVR

Maladaption/Parenchymal lung diseases resulting in secondary PPHN

a) *Meconium aspiration syndrome* (MAS) in newborns leads to acute respiratory failure with a mortality of up to 10% [29]. Meconium causes chemical pneumonitis and surfactant inactivation that leads to ventilation-perfusion mismatch. Resulting hypoxemia and hypercarbia cause pulmonary vasoconstriction and PPHN. Structural studies

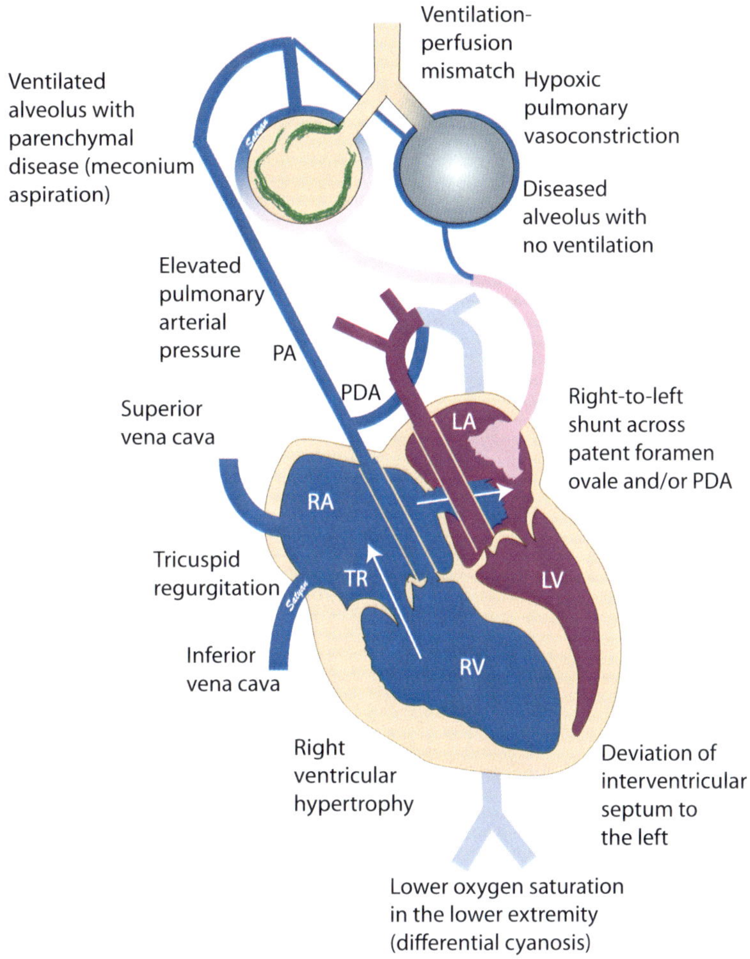

Figure 3 Pathophysiology of PPHN. Parenchymal lung disease and ventilation-perfusion (V/Q) mismatch result in hypoxemia. Increased pulmonary vascular resistance results in reduced pulmona ry blood flow and right to left shunt through PDA and/or PFO. Pulmonary hypertension is often associated with systemic hypotension with deviation of the interventricular septum to the left. The right subclavian artery (and blood flowing to the right upper extremity) is always preductal. The left subclavian artery may be preductal, juxtaductal or postductal. Hence, preductal oxygen saturations should be obtained from the right upper extremity and compared with lower extremity to assess differential cyanosis. PA – pulmonary artery; RV – right ventricle; LV – left ventricle; TR – tricuspid regurgitation; RA – right atrium; LA – left atrium; PDA – patent ductus arteriosus; PFO – patent foramen ovale.

of the lung at postmortem in fatal cases of meconium aspiration suggest that antecedent pulmonary vascular abnormalities exacerbated the postnatal pulmonary hypertension [30]. Decreased eNOS expression has also been reported in umbilical venous endothelial cell cultures from human infants with meconium staining who develop PPHN [31]. Meconium components incite an inflammatory response with release of cytokines and increase the production of vasoconstrictors including endothelin and thromboxane [32]. The incidence of MAS has decreased in developed countries but continues to be prevalent in resource-limited settings often associated with asphyxia [33].

Management of a neonate born through meconium stained amniotic fluid has changed dramatically over the last decade. Amnioinfusion, suctioning at the perineum and tracheal suctioning in vigorous infants did not alter the incidence of MAS in multicenter randomized trials [34-36]. The current guidelines recommend tracheal suctioning only if the infant born through meconium stained amniotic fluid is not vigorous at birth [37]. Recent data from a randomized trial and a translational study have pushed further to question the benefit of tracheal suctioning of meconium at birth even if the newborn is not vigorous [38,39]. Additional studies are required to evaluate the effect of tracheal suctioning in MAS and the incidence and severity of PPHN.

b) Pneumonia and sepsis often present with elevated PVR associated with systemic hypotension and decreased SVR. In addition, some infants with sepsis have myocardial dysfunction resulting in pulmonary venous hypertension due to elevated left atrial pressures [40].

c) Pulmonary hypertension in premature infants: Although PPHN is traditionally considered a disease of term and late preterm infants, it is increasingly being diagnosed in extremely preterm infants [41]. Some preterm infants with RDS present with PPHN in the first few days of life [42] while preterm infants with bronchopulmonary dysplasia (BPD) may be diagnosed with pulmonary hypertension later in the hospital course or after discharge from the Neonatal Intensive Care Unit (NICU). Preterm infants with fetal growth restriction and born after prolonged rupture of membranes are at higher risk for developing pulmonary hypertension [43]. Pulmonary vascular disease significantly increases morbidity and mortality in BPD [44].

Maldevelopment/Idiopathic PPHN ("Black-lung PPHN)

Some cases of PPHN are not secondary to parenchymal lung disease and are referred to as idiopathic or "black-lung" (referring to paucity of pulmonary vascularity and absence of lung disease) PPHN. Idiopathic pulmonary hypertension is secondary to remodeled pulmonary arteries, characterized by smooth muscle hyperplasia and extension of smooth muscle in intra-acinar arteries. The abnormal structural remodeling of the pulmonary circulation as seen in PPHN affects the responsiveness to vasodilator stimuli, and may prevent the access of NO to the vascular smooth muscle cells [45]. Maternal use of NSAIDs during third trimester of pregnancy can lead to premature closure of ductus arteriosus [46] and "black-lung" PPHN. Ovine fetal ligation or constriction of ductus arteriosus can produce similar vascular changes and is widely used to replicate PPHN in newborn lambs, showing the same pulmonary vascular findings as idiopathic pulmonary hypertension [47].

Underdevelopment / Pulmonary hypoplasia

Congenital diaphragmatic hernia (CDH) is developmental defect in the diaphragm separating the thorax and the abdomen and is the most important cause of pulmonary hypoplasia resulting in PPHN. This defect leads to a herniation of the abdominal viscera into the thoracic cavity. CDH occurs in 1/2,500 to 5,000 live births. CDH has a mortality rate of 20-30% and the degree of associated pulmonary hypoplasia and the severity of pulmonary hypertension remain the major determinants of survival [48]. Pulmonary vascular abnormalities in CDH include a decreased number of pulmonary arteries per unit lung volume and peripheral muscularization of small arteries, with medial and adventitial thickening [49]. In spite of marked improvement in survival of PPHN resulting from other causes, the mortality and need for ECMO remain high in infants with CDH.

Pulmonary hypoplasia secondary to renal dysfunction and oligohydramnios or thoracic dystrophy can be associated with pulmonary hypertension [50-52]. Prolonged rupture of membranes is also a risk factor for pulmonary hypertension in preterm infants [53].

Alveolar capillary dysplasia (ACD)

Alveolar capillary dysplasia is generally associated with malalignment of the pulmonary veins (ACD/MPV) and produces respiratory failure early in life and carries a mortality rate that approaches 100% [54]. Recent reports of infants presenting with fulminant symptoms of ACD/MPV well beyond the neonatal period, even as late as 7 months of age, have begun to emerge, challenging the established phenotype and offering the possibility that long-term survivors with milder forms of the disease may exist. [55] FOXF1 transcription factor gene or deletions upstream to FOXF1 were identified in 40% of cases [56]. Blood testing to screen for these defects is now available, but a negative result does not preclude the diagnosis, and histological examination of lung tissue remains the gold standard for diagnosis. A lung biopsy to rule out ACD should be considered for neonates who do not respond to conventional medical management or fail attempts at ECMO decannulation.

Diagnosis

In a term or near-term infant with respiratory distress, the initial evaluation should include simultaneous measurement of pre- and post-ductal oxygen saturation, a chest X-ray and an arterial blood gas. Hypoxemia disproportionate to the severity of parenchymal disease on a chest radiograph should suggest idiopathic PPHN (or cyanotic heart disease). Evidence of the underlying parenchymal disease such as RDS, MAS, or pneumonia may be seen on chest X-ray in secondary PPHN. A complete blood count with differential is often obtained on admission to evaluate for high hematocrit level (polycythemia and increased viscosity contributing to intrinsic vascular obstruction) and to evaluate the risk of underlying infection.

Differentiating PPHN from cyanotic CHD soon after admission is of paramount importance. Preductal and postductal oxygen saturation/PaO_2 measurements are used to differentiate PPHN from structural heart disease. Saturation differences of > 5-10% or PaO_2 differences of 10–20 mmHg between right upper limb and lower limbs are considered significant. In neonates with PPHN and atrial-level right-to-left shunting without a significant ductal shunt, both the right arm and the right leg saturations will be low. Conversely, babies with PDA and coarctation of the aorta might have differential cyanosis. In PPHN, hypoxemia is often labile unlike fixed hypoxemia seen in cyanotic CHD. Hyperoxia test (obtaining an arterial gas after 15 minutes of exposure to 100% oxygen) and/or hyperoxia-hyperventilation (hyperoxia and alkalosis to induce pulmonary vasodilation and improve PaO_2) is no longer widely practiced due to the known adverse effects of hyperoxia and alkalosis. It can be avoided by confirming elevated pulmonary pressures by an early echocardiogram, when available.

Echocardiography is gold standard to confirm the diagnosis, and to monitor the efficacy of specific therapeutic interventions [57]. Measurement of the direction of ductal and foramen ovale shunt, flattening or left-deviation of the interventricular septum and tricuspid regurgitation velocity with simultaneous systemic blood pressure measurement provides an indication of right-sided pressures and hemodynamic physiology.

B-type natriuretic peptide (BNP) concentrations in plasma correspond well with echocardiographic findings of ventricular strain [58]. Reynolds et al. suggested BNP as an early indicator of PPHN in the presence of respiratory illness in neonates without CHD [59]. BNP has been proposed as a biomarker in PPHN, especially to assess efficacy of treatment and to predict rebound PPHN [59,60]. However, its value in the practical management of PPHN is presently unclear. Some centers obtain serial (monthly) echocardiograms with BNP levels to screen for pulmonary hypertension associated with BPD in preterm infants.

Severity of PPHN

Severity of PPHN is commonly assessed by oxygenation index (OI) and Alveolar-arterial oxygen difference ($AaDO_2$). OI is more commonly used during medical management of PPHN since it takes ventilator support into the consideration and is calculated as

$$OI = MAP \times FiO_2 \times 100/PaO_2$$

where MAP is the mean airway pressure in cmH_2O, FiO_2 is the fraction of inspired oxygen, and PaO_2 is partial pressure of oxygen in arterial blood (in mmHg). Hypoxemic respiratory failure can be classified into mild ($OI \leq 15$), moderate ($OI > 15$ to 25), severe (OI 25 to 40) and very severe ($OI > 40$) [61]. Disadvantages of OI include:(a) it can be manipulated by changing FiO_2 or MAP or based on the type of ventilator; (b) it requires arterial access; (c) the value may vary based on the site of arterial access – right radial (preductal) vs. umbilical or posterior tibial (postductal). More recently, oxygen saturation index ($OSI = MAP \times FiO_2 \times 100/\text{Preductal } SpO_2$) has been used in patients without arterial access [62]. If preductal SpO_2 is in the 70-99% range, OSI corresponds to approximately half of OI (OSI of 8 = OI of 16) [63]. More research evaluating the clinical role for this non-invasive index is needed prior to its widespread use.

$AaDO_2$ is the difference between Alveolar partial pressure of oxygen and arterial partial pressure of oxygen and is calculated using the following formula.

$$AaDO_2 = (Patm - P_{H2O}) \times FiO_2 - PaO_2 - PaCO_2/RQ$$

Patm is the atmospheric pressure, which is usually equal to 760 mmHg at sea level but needs to be adjusted in high altitude. P_{H2O} is the pressure of water vapor in one ATM, which is usually considered to be 47 mmHg. RQ is the respiratory quotient and equal to 1 if the energy source is purely carbohydrate or equal to 0.8 when the nutritional source is a combination of carbohydrate, protein, and lipid. The disadvantage of $AaDO_2$ is that it does not take ventilator pressure into account.

Management

The severity of PPHN can range from mild hypoxemia with minimal respiratory distress to severe hypoxemia and cardio-pulmonary instability that requires intensive care support. Infants with PPHN require supportive care tailored to the degree of hypoxemia and physiologic instability. PPHN is often associated with underlying parenchymal lung disease or systemic illness; therapy should target the underlying disease (such as antibiotics for sepsis).

Some hospital based practices such as cesarean sections, induction of labor at late-preterm or early-term gestation, and the use of anesthetics and analgesics delay pulmonary transition at birth. These infants present with "delayed cardiorespiratory adaptation" must be closely monitored and managed with appropriate respiratory support. Respiratory support to recruit the lungs and provide optimal inflation (while avoiding atelectasis and hyperinflation) reduces PVR and is the key step in management of these infants and reduces the risk of PPHN. Many infants with parenchymal lung disease have elevated pulmonary arterial pressures. Premature therapy with early initiation of an inhaled pulmonary vasodilator such as iNO prior to lung recruitment is not beneficial and optimal lung inflation with adequate PEEP and/or surfactant often eliminates the need for specific pulmonary vasodilator therapy.

Mild cases of PPHN with minimal or no respiratory distress can be detected in the newborn nursery either following a desaturation episode or by low postductal oxygen saturation detected on critical congenital heart disease screening [64]. These infants can be managed with supportive care and oxygen supplementation. Close monitoring is important as some of these infants may rapidly deteriorate and require non-invasive ventilation or intubation and mechanical ventilation. Infection should be considered as elevated pulmonary pressures (often associated with systemic hypotension) can be the presenting clinical feature of pneumonia or sepsis.

Supportive care: It is important to maintain normothermia and correct metabolic and hematologic abnormalities such as hypoglycemia, hypocalcaemia, acidosis and polycythemia. Sedation may be necessary to provide comfort and decrease oxygen consumption from agitation in hypoxemic or ventilated patients. Paralysis should be avoided if possible, as it has been associated with increased mortality [1]. The goal of medical management is to selectively reduce pulmonary arterial pressure and to maintain systemic blood pressure.

Hyperventilation and alkali infusions to maintain an alkaline pH were strategies previously in use but should be avoided because of associated concerns of impaired cerebral perfusion and sensorineural deafness with respiratory alkalosis have been raised [65,66]. Similar or improved outcomes with less chronic lung disease were also observed in infants with PPHN maintaining normal PCO_2 (45–60 mmHg) [67,68]. Alkali infusion was associated with increased use of ECMO and need for oxygen at 28 days [1]. Thus, lack of convincing data to support hyperventilation/alkali infusion therapy along with better therapeutic options including inhaled vasodilators have led to decreased use of alkalosis. Most centers avoid acidosis based on animal studies demonstrating exaggerated hypoxic pulmonary vasoconstriction with $pH < 7.25$ [69]. We recommend maintaining $pH > 7.25$, preferably 7.30 to 7.40 during the acute phase of PPHN.

Mechanical ventilation

Given the important contribution of parenchymal lung disease in many cases of PPHN, pharmacologic pulmonary vasodilation alone without lung recruitment would not be expected to cause sustained clinical improvement [70,71]. "Gentle" ventilation strategies with optimal PEEP, relatively low PIP or tidal volume and a degree of permissive hypercapnia are recommended to ensure adequate lung expansion while limiting barotrauma and volutrauma [68,72]. In newborns with severe lung disease, high frequency ventilation is frequently used to optimize lung inflation and minimize lung injury [73]. If a PIP of > 28 cmH_2O or tidal volumes > 6 cc/kg are required to maintain $PaCO_2 < 60$ mmHg on conventional ventilation, we recommend switching to high frequency (jet or oscillator) ventilation. In clinical studies using iNO, the combination of high frequency ventilation and iNO resulted in the greatest improvement in oxygenation in PPHN associated with diffuse parenchymal lung disease such as RDS and pneumonia [74,75].

Oxygen is a specific and potent pulmonary vasodilator and increased oxygen tension is an important mediator of reduction in PVR at birth. Avoiding hypoxemia by mechanical ventilation with high concentrations of oxygen used to be a mainstay of PPHN management. Fetal lamb studies demonstrate that increased fetal oxygen tension augments endogenous NO release [76] and increased pulmonary blood flow induced by rhythmic distention of the lung and oxygen are mediated in part by endogenous NO [77]. However, it has also been shown that brief exposure to 100% oxygen in newborn lambs results in increased contractility of pulmonary arteries [78], reduces response to iNO [79,80] and increases the potential for oxidative stress [81]. Reactive oxygen species (ROS), such as superoxide interact with NO to form a potent oxidant peroxynitrite capable of vasoconstriction and surfactant inactivation [82]. In addition to direct inactivation of NO, ROS can decrease eNOS activity, sGC activity and increase PDE5 activity, resulting in decreased cGMP levels and potentiation of pulmonary vasoconstriction. In the ovine ductal ligation model of PPHN, maintaining oxygen saturations in the 90-97% range results in low PVR [80]. We recommend maintaining preductal oxygen saturations in low to mid-90s with PaO_2 levels between 55 and 80 mmHg during management of infants with PPHN.

Surfactant

Exogenous surfactant therapy improved oxygenation and reduced the need for extracorporeal membrane oxygenation (ECMO) in neonates with PPHN secondary to parenchymal lung disease such as RDS, pneumonia/sepsis or MAS. This multicenter trial also demonstrated that this benefit was greatest for infants with mild to moderate disease, and with an OI of 15–25 [83]. A *post-hoc* analysis of the randomized trial of early nitric oxide use showed that early use of surfactant prior to randomization decreased the risk of death/ECMO especially in infants with parenchymal lung disease [84]. Over the past decade, the use of surfactant in treating secondary PPHN and respiratory failure has increased and might have contributed to improved effectiveness of iNO with reduced need for ECMO. Surfactant inactivation and deficiency are observed in many neonatal respiratory disorders such as pneumonia, RDS and MAS. We recommend that infants with PPHN secondary to parenchymal lung disease receive a dose of surfactant rich in surfactant protein-B (SP-B), such as calfactant - Infasurf® (ONY Inc, Amherst NY) or poractant-α - Curosurf® (Chiesi Farmaceutici, S.p.A, Parma, Italy). Synthetic surfactant (lucinactant, Surfaxin, Discovery laboratories, Inc. Warrington PA) rich in SP-B mimetics has been shown to be resistant to inactivation and effective in animal studies [85,86] and appears to be safe in children with HRF [87] but its efficacy in term infants with hypoxic respiratory failure is not known.

It is not clear if surfactant therapy is beneficial in infants with CDH. Animal studies show benefit [88-90] but a review of the CDH registry did not support the use of surfactant [91]. We recommend administration of surfactant only in the presence of clinical, radiological or biochemical evidence of surfactant deficiency in CDH and administer only 50% of the dose because of pulmonary hypoplasia.

Inhaled Nitric Oxide (iNO)

Nitric Oxide is a potent vasodilator that has also been shown to be an important regulator of vascular tone, growth and remodeling [92]. In the endothelium, NO is produced from the terminal guanidino nitrogen of L-arginine on its conversion to L-citrulline by the enzyme eNOS in a reaction that requires molecular oxygen [92].

As an inhaled vasodilator, iNO selectively dilates the pulmonary circulation without a significant decrease in systemic blood pressure (*selective effect of iNO).* Inhaled NO is also preferentially distributed to the ventilated segments of the lung, resulting in increased perfusion of the ventilated segments, optimizing VQ match (*micro-selective effect of iNO).* Studies have shown that iNO therapy causes marked improvement in oxygenation in term newborns with PPHN [93]. Multicenter randomized clinical studies subsequently confirmed that iNO therapy reduces the need for ECMO in term neonates with hypoxemic respiratory failure [94-96]. Inhaled NO therapy has been approved by the FDA for clinical use in term/near term newborn infants (>34 wks gestation) with hypoxic respiratory failure and PPHN since 2000.

Initiation of iNO: There has been a debate regarding the timing of initiation and optimum starting dose of iNO in PPHN. An OI of 25 is associated with a 50% risk of requiring ECMO or mortality [97] in the absence of specific pulmonary vasodilator therapy. Konduri et al. initially demonstrated that earlier initiation of iNO with an OI of 15–25 did not reduce the need for ECMO but may have a tendency to reduce the risk of progression to severe hypoxemic respiratory failure [98]. *Post-hoc* analysis of the same study suggested that the use of surfactant prior to randomization and enrollment (and use of iNO) at an OI of ≤ 20 was associated with reduced incidence of ECMO/death [84].

Dosing of iNO: Previous clinical trials suggested that the ideal starting dose for iNO is 20 parts per million (ppm) with the effective doses between 5 and 20 ppm [99]. Doses > 20 ppm did not increase the efficacy and were associated with more adverse effects in these infants [95] such as elevated methemoglobin (>7%) and nitrogen dioxide (NO_2) (>3 ppm) [93]. A dose of 5 ppm results in improved oxygenation in PPHN. A dose of 20 ppm results in improved oxygenation *and* results in the most optimal decrease in pulmonary to systemic arterial pressure ratio [100]. To summarize, we recommend initiation of iNO if OI is ~ **20** at a dose of **20** ppm. A complete response to iNO is defined as an increase in PaO_2/ FiO_2 ratio of ≥ **20** mmHg. (20-20-20 rule for initiation of iNO, Figure 4). Methemoglobin levels are monitored at 2 and 8 hours after initiation of iNO and then once a day for the duration of iNO therapy. Some centers stop checking methemoglobin levels after the first couple of days if levels are low (<2%) and iNO dose remains ≤ 20 ppm. High inspired oxygen and high mean iNO dose are risk factors for elevated methemoglobin in term infants [101].

Weaning iNO: Due to rebound vasoconstriction and resultant pulmonary hypertension on abrupt withdrawal, iNO needs to be weaned gradually [102]. Weaning in steps from 20 ppm gradually over a period of time before its discontinuation has been shown to prevent the rebound effect [103]. If there is oxygenation response, inspired oxygen concentration is first weaned below **60%** and then iNO is weaned only if PaO_2 can be maintained ≥ **60** mmHg (or preductal SpO_2 ≥ 90%) for **60** min (60-60-60 rule of weaning iNO). At our center, we wean iNO at a rate of 5 ppm every 4 hours. Once iNO dose is 5 ppm, gradual weaning by 1 ppm q 4 hours is performed (Figure 4). Continuing iNO in the absence of a response or not weaning iNO or extremely slow weaning can potentially lead to suppression of endogenous eNOS [104,105].

Management of iNO-resistant PPHN

In approximately a third of term and near-term infants with PPHN, iNO does not result in sustained improvement in oxygenation [95]. Adequate lung recruitment (with surfactant and/or optimal PEEP/MAP preferably with high frequency ventilation) is crucial to deliver iNO to its target site – the pulmonary vasculature [106]. A repeat echocardiogram to evaluate ventricular function and severity of PPHN (and to rule out cyanotic CHD such as total anomalous pulmonary venous return (TAPVR) that may have been missed on the first echocardiogram [107]) is the next step. Management of systemic hypotension in PPHN is discussed below. If lung recruitment and hemodynamic stability are achieved and iNO is still not effective, patient should be managed in a tertiary center with access to ECMO. Our recommendations for management of iNO-resistant PPHN not responding to iNO in spite of lung recruitment with increased MAP and surfactant are outlined in Figure 5 and summarized here.

(1) Hemodynamic evaluation: A repeat echocardiogram should be performed to evaluate structural heart disease, left ventricular dysfunction, right ventricular dysfunction, and ventricular output For example, if left ventricular dysfunction is associated high left atrial pressures and a left-to-right shunt at the level

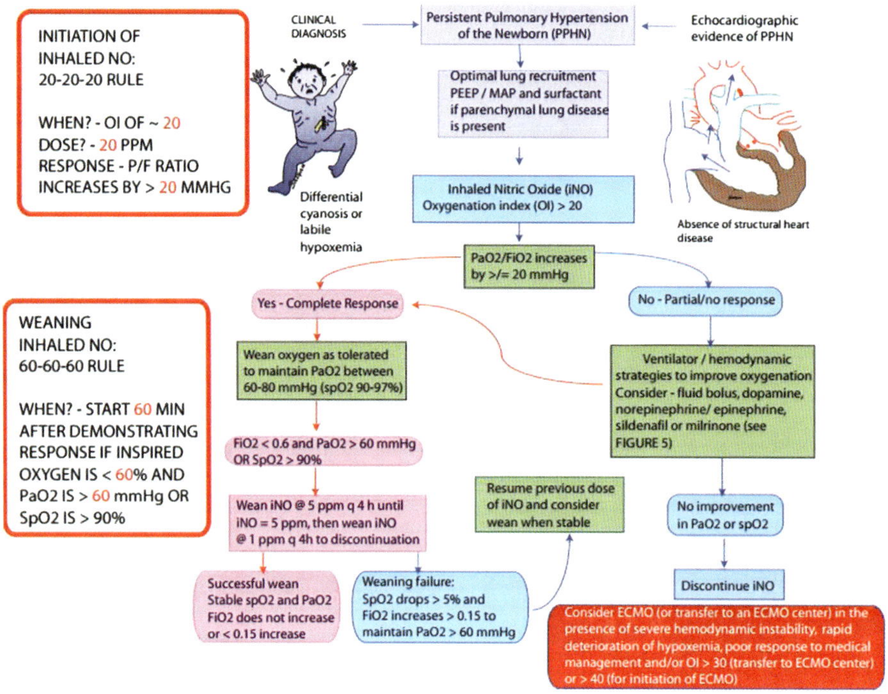

Figure 4 Inhaled Nitric Oxide therapy in neonates with PPHN: The diagnosis of PPHN is based on clinical (labile hypoxemia and differential cyanosis) or echocardiographic findings. Optimal oxygenation and lung recruitment with optimal lung inflation and surfactant in the presence of parenchymal lung disease is the initial step in the management of PPHN. An OI of 20 is a reasonable threshold to initiate iNO. The presence of hemodynamic instability and severe hypoxemia (OI ~ 40 range) is an indication for ECMO. See text for details.

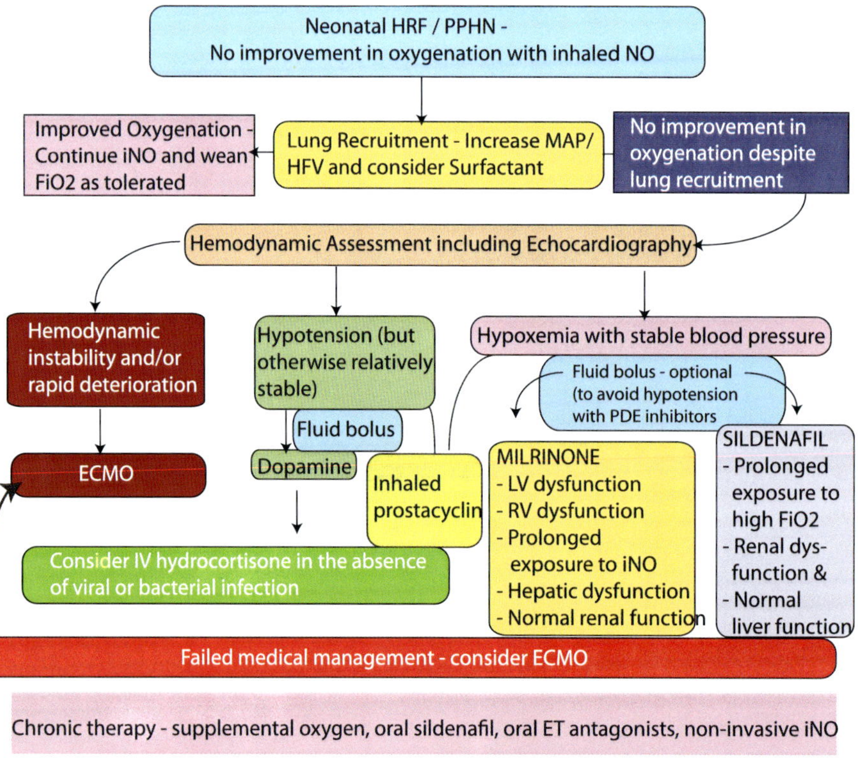

Figure 5 Flow chart showing the author's suggested guidelines for management of iNO resistant PPHN.

of the oval foramen in the presence of a right-to-left shunt at the ductus arteriosus, iNO is contraindicated and an inodilator such as milrinone should be initiated.

(2) Rapid deterioration with hemodynamic instability should necessitate cannulation for ECMO (or immediate transfer to an ECMO center).

(3) In the presence of systemic hypotension, a fluid bolus (10 ml/kg of Lactated Ringers or isotonic saline) followed by dopamine is recommended. Some centers prefer the use of norepinephrine or vasopressin. A cortisol level is drawn in these patients. If the levels are low relative to the infant's stress level and there is no evidence of infection (viral or bacterial), the authors recommend a stress dose of hydrocortisone.

(4) If blood pressure is relatively stable but hypoxemia persists, consider the use of PDE inhibitors. Sildenafil is preferred if normal liver and ventricular function are present and may have added benefit in the context of prolonged hyperoxia. Ventricular dysfunction or hepatic compromise are indications for Milrinone rather than sildenafil as long as normal renal function is present. Chronic therapy (especially in the presence of CDH or BPD) involves PDE 5 inhibitors and endothelin receptor antagonists and non-invasive iNO (Figure 5).

Prostaglandin E1 (PGE1)

Aerosolized prostaglandin E1 (Alprostadil) has been used to treat pulmonary hypertension in adults. In a small pilot phase I-II study, Sood et al. suggested that inhaled PGE1 was a safe and selective pulmonary vasodilator in hypoxemic respiratory failure with or without use of iNO [108]. PGE1 solution for aerosolization is prepared from Alprostadil® (Prostin VR 500, Pfizer, New York NY) and administered as a continuous nebulization through a MiniHeart low flow jet nebulizer (WestMed Inc, Tuczon, AZ) at 150–300 ng/kg/min diluted in saline to provide 4 ml/hr [109].

Intravenous PGE1 has also been used in patients with CDH in combination with iNO to promote pulmonary vasodilation and to maintain ductal patency and reduce right ventricular afterload [110].

Inhaled Prostacyclin (PGI_2)

Prostacyclin administered intravenously is a common therapy in adults with pulmonary arterial hypertension. Inhaled PGI_2 has been used in PPHN resistant to iNO at a dose of 50 ng/kg/min. [111] The intravenous formulation Flolan® (Glaxo-Wellcome, Middlesex, UK) is dissolved in 20 ml of manufacturer's diluent (a glycine buffer, pH ~10). Fresh solution is added to the nebulization chamber every 4 hours [111]. The effect of such alkaline pH on neonatal respiratory tract is not known.

Phosphodiesterase inhibitors

a) Sildenafil (PDE 5 Inhibitor): Studies have shown that cGMP is decreased in response to exogenous NO in animal models of PPHN [112], and increased clearance of cGMP by one or more phosphodiesterases has been proposed as one of the causes [113]. Sildenafil acts by inhibiting cGMP-specific phosphodiesterase type 5 (PDE 5), an enzyme that promotes degradation of cGMP. Studies have shown that oral sildenafil (dose range 1–2 mg/kg every 6 h) improves oxygenation and reduces mortality, in centers limited by non-availability of iNO and ECMO [114,115].

Intravenous sildenafil was shown to be effective in improving oxygenation in patients with PPHN with and without prior exposure to iNO [116]. The use of intravenous sildenafil should be restricted to refractory cases at a center with ECMO back-up, due the potential risk of systemic hypotension [117] and pulmonary hemorrhage, presumably due to sudden reversal of ductal shunt [118]. Based on pharmacokinetic data in neonates with PPHN, intravenous sildenafil is administered as a load of 0.42 mg/kg over 3 hours (0.14 mg/kg/h) followed by 1.6 mg/kg/day as a continuous maintenance infusion (0.07 mg/kg/h).

b) Milrinone (PDE 3 Inhibitor): Milrinone inhibits PDE3 and increases concentration of cAMP in pulmonary and systemic arterial smooth muscle and in cardiac muscle. Milrinone relaxes pulmonary arteries in the fetal lamb model of PPHN [119]. Infants with PPHN refractory to iNO therapy have responded to IV milrinone in 3 case series [120-122] and appears to be particularly useful in the presence of ventricular dysfunction [123,124]. A loading dose (50 mcg/kg over 30–60 min) followed by a maintenance dose (0.33 mcg/kg/min and escalated to 0.66 and then to 1 mcg/kg/min based on response) is commonly used. The loading dose is not recommended in the presence of systemic hypotension and in premature neonates [123]. As with any systemic vasodilator, hypotension is a clinical concern and blood pressure needs to be closely monitored. A fluid bolus (10 ml/kg of Lactated Ringer's solution) prior to loading dose may decrease the risk of hypotension. In addition, one case series described an increased incidence of intracranial hemorrhage with the use of milrinone in PPHN [121]. Milrinone may be the pulmonary vasodilator of choice in the presence of PPHN with left ventricular dysfunction (Figure 5).

Bosentan (Endothelin-1 receptor blocker)

Endothelin receptor antagonists are beneficial and well tolerated in adult patients with pulmonary arterial hypertension [125]. Initial reports suggested that bosentan was an effective drug in the management of PPHN [126]. The results of a multi-center, randomized, double-blind, placebo-controlled exploratory trial of bosentan in PPHN was recently reported. Bosentan (2 mg/kg/dose BID) did not show any additive effect on top of iNO in term neonates with PPHN [127]. However, endothelin receptor antagonists may have a role in the management of chronic pulmonary hypertension associated with BPD or CDH.

Steroids

Antenatal betamethasone attenuated oxidative stress and improved in vitro response to vasodilators in a fetal lamb model of pulmonary hypertension [128]. Glucocorticoids have been found to improve oxygenation and attenuate the pulmonary hypertensive response in animal models of meconium aspiration syndrome, which is a common cause of PPHN [129]. Steroids have been reported to decrease hospital stay and duration of oxygen use in infants with meconium aspiration [130,131]. It is proposed that hydrocortisone attenuates ROS production by induction of superoxide dismutase and normalization of PDE5 activity [132]. Looking at the evidence this far, we do not recommend routine use of steroids in patients with PPHN especially if there is suspicion of viral or bacterial sepsis. Anecdotal use of stress dose hydrocortisone in iNO resistant PPHN associated with systemic hypotension in our unit has resulted in stabilization of systemic blood pressure and improved oxygenation possibly secondary to hemodynamic stability and PDE-5 inhibitory effects [133].

Extracorporeal Membrane Oxygenation (ECMO)

ECMO is a technique of modified cardiopulmonary bypass used over a prolonged period to support heart and lung function. The use of neonatal ECMO has declined from a peak of 1516 cases per year in 1992 to 750–865 cases/year from 2008 to 2012. This decline is likely due to improvements in both perinatal care and availability of advanced therapies for neonatal hypoxemic respiratory failure including high-frequency ventilators, surfactant, and iNO [134]. In newborns with PPHN, mechanical ventilation with oxygen and iNO is the initial treatment, but prolongation of iNO with high oxygen levels may induce chronic lung disease and extend the length of stay in the NICU [135]. On the other hand, initiating ECMO too early may expose newborns to major vessel cannulation and systemic anticoagulation [136]. General accepted criteria to start ECMO is persistent hypoxemia (with an OI of >40 or AaDO2 > 600 in spite of aggressive medical management of PPHN with mechanical ventilation and iNO) and the presence of hemodynamic instability (Figure 5).

Management of systemic hypotension in PPHN

Systemic hypotension is common in infants with PPHN and the causes are outlined in Figure 6. Decreased systemic blood pressure exacerbates right-to-left shunt and worsens hypoxemia in PPHN. The cause of systemic hypotension should be addressed first – administration of volume bolus in hypovolemia, decrease in MAP in the presence of hyperinflation and antibiotics for sepsis. The use of dopamine to increase systemic blood pressure to reduce right-to-left shunt is a common practice. Such a practice is effective in the presence of systemic hypotension. However, increasing systemic pressure to supraphysiologic levels is not recommended. In some patients with PPHN, the presence of a patent ductus arteriosus acts as a pop-off valve, limiting right ventricular preload and dysfunction. Increasing systemic blood pressure limits right-to-left shunt across the PDA and may add to right ventricular strain. In addition, the optimal therapy for reduced pulmonary blood flow is selective pulmonary vasodilation. Instead, if pulmonary blood is forced by higher systemic pressure (by limiting right-to-left shunts) through a constricted pulmonary circuit, endothelial dysfunction due to increased shear stress [47] is likely to exacerbate PPHN. Dopamine (especially at > 10 mcg/kg/min) is not selective to systemic vasculature and can increase pulmonary arterial pressure in PPHN [106]. Norepinephrine infusion is also effective in stabilizing systemic blood pressure and improving oxygenation in neonates with PPHN [137]. Vasopressin may be an effective therapeutic agent with some selectivity to systemic vasoconstriction [138]. As mentioned in the previous paragraph, hydrocortisone may also be effective to stabilize blood pressure in PPHN.

Asphyxia, hypothermia and management of PPHN

Asphyxia is associated with hypoxemia and acidosis. Infants with asphyxia also have evidence of surfactant deficiency and/or meconium aspiration syndrome (Figure 7) [139]. The use of moderate hypothermia (33.5°C for 72 hours) does not result in a significant increase in the incidence of PPHN (25% vs. 22% with conventional management without hypothermia) [140]. However, as compared to moderated hypothermia (33.5°C), deeper whole-body cooling to 32°C is associated with a tendency to increased PPHN (34 vs 25%, p-0.06), increased need for inhaled NO (34 vs 24%, p-0.03) and ECMO (9 vs 4%, p-0.005) [141]. Case reports indicate that patients with hypoxemic respiratory disorders prior to the onset of cooling (especially those that need > 50% inspired oxygen and/or iNO) [142], may experience exacerbation of PPHN with hypothermia and/or rewarming [143]. Mild therapeutic hypothermia by itself is not a cause for PPHN. However, infants predisposed to elevated PVR due to the presence of asphyxia and respiratory disease may not tolerate hypothermia induced pulmonary vasoconstriction [144]. These findings emphasize the need for close monitoring of core temperature, systemic/pulmonary

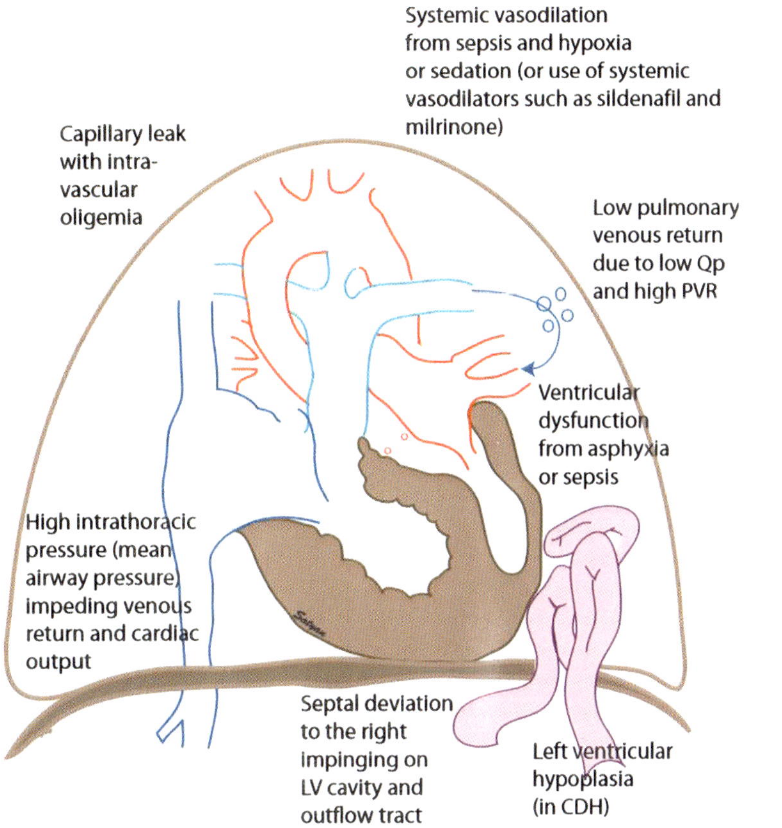

Figure 6 Causes of hypotension in infants with PPHN: Sepsis and hypoxia causes intravascular oligemia due to capillary leak or due to systemic vasodilation. Neonates with PPHN often require high mean airway pressure that impedes venous return to the right side of heart. Increased pulmonary vascular resistance results in less blood flow through pulmonary circulation reducing left ventricular preload. The deviation of the interventricular septum towards left ventricle further impedes left ventricular filling. Neonates with PPHN secondary to sepsis, hypoxia and CDH can also experience systemic hypotension secondary to left ventricular dysfunction.

hemodynamics and oxygenation during hypothermia and rewarming for asphyxia.

In many centers, confusion exists regarding optimal reporting of $PaCO_2$ during whole-body hypothermia. The laboratory may report $PaCO_2$ levels either at baby's temperature (known as the pH-stat method) or corrected for 37°C (alpha-stat method). Decreasing temperature increases the solubility of CO_2 in the blood and decreases $PaCO_2$ and may have implications for PPHN management with potential of overventilation or underventilation. We recommend the pH-stat method and reporting of $PaCO_2$ at actual (and not corrected) body temperature.

Long term outcome of PPHN

PPHN is a syndrome associated with significant long-term morbidity, irrespective of the treatment modality. These infants suffer from long-term consequences such as neurodevelopmental, cognitive and hearing abnormalities [145-147]. Thus, it is essential to provide long-term multidisciplinary follow-up after discharge. Konduri et al. in their long-term follow-up of infants randomized to early iNO in PPHN, noted neurodevelopmental impairment in about 25% of infants and hearing impairment in approximately 23% [145]. Long-term neurodevelopmental outcome at school age for neonates with PPHN critical enough to receive inhaled NO or ECMO is generally encouraging. Rosenberg et al. reported that among 109 school age survivors of PPHN (77 of whom received inhaled NO and 12 that required ECMO), medical, neurodevelopmental and behavioral outcomes did not differ between children treated with iNO, with or without ECMO, and those managed with no exposure to iNO. However, 24% had persistent respiratory problems, 60% had abnormal chest X-rays and 6.4% had some degree of sensorineural hearing loss. Overall, 9.2% of the cohort had a full scale IQ less than 70 and 7.4% had an IQ from 70 to 84 [148]. The UK collaborative trial randomized critically ill neonates into transfer to a regional center for ECMO or continued conventional care at the local NICU. At 7 year follow-up, mortality was significantly lower in the ECMO group

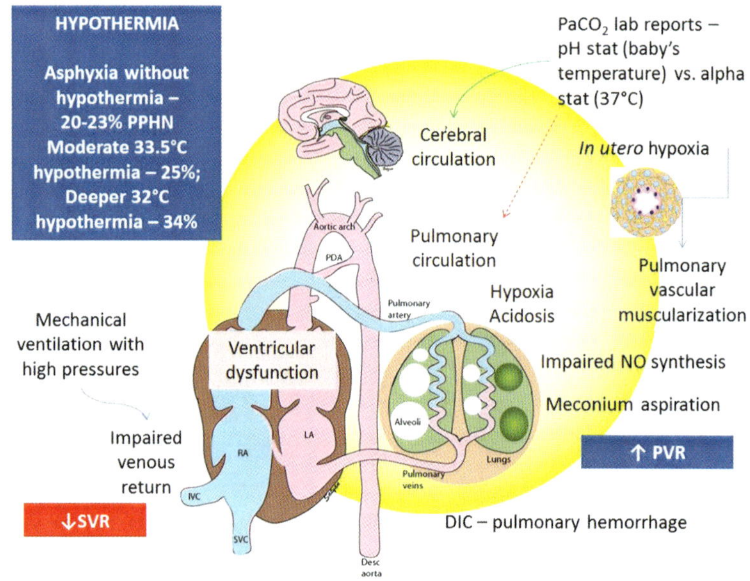

Figure 7 Asphyxia and PPHN: Fetal hypoxia (secondary to *in-utero* asphyxia and meconium aspiration) causes pulmonary vascular remodeling, which down regulates iNO signaling pathways and causes PPHN. In infants with perinatal hypoxia, the combination of hypoxia and acidosis increases the risk of PPHN. Preexisting PPHN may be exacerbated by therapeutic hypothermia. Errors in $PaCO_2$ measurement secondary to body temperature changes may result in fluctuations in PCO_2 leading to changes in cerebral and pulmonary vascular resistance (see text for details).

with no increase in disability [149]. The presence of neurodevelopmental and medical disabilities may reflect the severity of the underlying illnesses experienced by these infants rather than complications of iNO or ECMO. However, therapeutic interventions such as hyperventilation are associated with sensorineural hearing loss and must be avoided [66,150].

Conclusions

Over the last two decades, management of infants with PPHN has included improved with improved ventilation strategies to optimize lung recruitment, provide "gentle" ventilation and minimize oxygen toxicity paired with the therapeutic use of surfactant and iNO. These changes have led to a substantial decrease in the number of neonatal PPHN patients requiring ECMO for respiratory disorders. Animal models have contributed to our understanding of fetal circulation, pulmonary vascular transition at birth and hemodynamic and biochemical abnormalities associate with PPHN. Further clinical research into pulmonary vasodilator therapy, reversal of remodeling of the pulmonary vasculature and right ventricle are crucial. Two challenges which remain in the field of PPHN include management of pulmonary hypoplasia and pulmonary hypertension in CDH and BPD-associated pulmonary hypertension in the premature infant [97]. In addition, asphyxia (with or without MAS and/or therapeutic hypothermia) remains an important cause for PPHN worldwide. Further research to evaluate and develop appropriate strategies to ameliorate pulmonary vascular disease in these conditions are warranted.

Abbreviations

AaDO2: Alveolar-arterial oxygen difference; ACD: Alveolar Capillary Dysplasia; ANP: Atrial Natriuretic Peptide; ATP: Adenosine Triphosphate; BNP: B-type Natriuretic Peptide; BPD: Broncho Pulmonary Dysplasia; CHD: Congenital Heart Disease; CGMP: Cyclic guanosine monophosphate; CNP: C-type Natriuretic Peptide; ECMO: Extracorporeal Membrane Oxygenation; ENOS: Endothelial Nitric oxide synthases; FDA: Food and Drug Administration; FiO2: Fraction of Inspired Oxygen; iNO: Inhaled Nitric Oxide; MAP: Mean Airway Pressure; MAS: Meconium Aspiration Syndrome; NO: Nitric Oxide; NOS: Nitric Oxide Synthase; NSAIDS: Non-Steroidal Anti-Inflammatory Drugs; OI: Oxygenation Index; PDA: Patent Ductus Arteriosus; PDE: Phosphodiesterase; PEEP: Peak End Expiratory Pressure; PFO: Patent Foramen Ovale; PI: Pulsatility Index; PIP: Peak Inspiratory Pressures; PPHN: Persistent Pulmonary Hypertension; PVR: Pulmonary Vascular Resistance; RDS: Respiratory Distress Syndrome; ROS: Reactive Oxygen Species; RQ: Respiratory Quotient; sGC: Soluble Guanylate Cyclase; SP-B: Surfactant Protein-B; SSRI: Selective Serotonin Reuptake Inhibitors; SVR: Systemic Vascular Resistance; VQ: Ventilation-perfusion.

Competing interests

Vinay Sharma (VS) and Sara Berkelhamer(SB) declare that they have no competing interests in published data.
Satyan Lakshminrusimha (SL) was previously a member of the speaker's bureau for Ikaria, manufacturer of inhaled nitric oxide. He also declares that he has no competing interest in published data. He was supported by NICHD HD072929 during the preparation of this manuscript.

Authors' contributions

VS and SL have made substantial contributions to conception and interpretation of data; SB has been involved in drafting the manuscript or revising it critically for important intellectual content; VS, SB and SL have given final approval of the version to be published; and agree to be accountable for all aspects of the work in ensuring that questions related to the accuracy or integrity of any part of the work are appropriately investigated and resolved.

Author details

[1]Department of Pediatrics (Neonatology), Hennepin County Medical Center, 701 Park Avenue, Shapiro Building, Minneapolis, MN 55415, USA.
[2]Department of Pediatrics, Women and Children's Hospital of Buffalo, 219 Bryant St, Buffalo, New York 14222, USA.

References

1. Walsh-Sukys MC, Tyson JE, Wright LL, Bauer CR, Korones SB, Stevenson DK, et al. Persistent pulmonary hypertension of the newborn in the era before nitric oxide: practice variation and outcomes. Pediatrics. 2000;105:14–20.
2. Dawes GS. Pulmonary circulation in the foetus and new-born. Br Med Bull. 1966;22:61–5.
3. Ardran G, Dawes GS, Prichard MM, Reynolds SR, Eyatt DG. The effect of ventilation of the foetal lungs upon the pulmonary circulation. J Physiol. 1952;118:12–22.
4. Rasanen J, Wood DC, Weiner S, Ludomirski A, Huhta JC. Role of the pulmonary circulation in the distribution of human fetal cardiac output during the second half of pregnancy. Circulation. 1996;94:1068–73.
5. Lakshminrusimha S, Steinhorn RH. Pulmonary vascular biology during neonatal transition. Clin Perinatol. 1999;26:601–19.
6. Delaney C, Gien J, Grover TR, Roe G, Abman SH. Pulmonary vascular effects of serotonin and selective serotonin reuptake inhibitors in the late-gestation ovine fetus. Am J Physiol Lung Cell Mol Physiol. 2011;301:L937-44.
7. Delaney C, Gien J, Roe G, Isenberg N, Kailey J, Abman SH. Serotonin contributes to high pulmonary vascular tone in a sheep model of persistent pulmonary hypertension of the newborn. Am J Physiol Lung Cell Mol Physiol. 2013;304:L894-901.
8. Chambers CD, Hernandez-Diaz S, Van Marter LJ, Werler MM, Louik C, Jones KL, et al. Selective serotonin-reuptake inhibitors and risk of persistent pulmonary hypertension of the newborn. N Engl J Med. 2006;354:579–87.
9. Kieler H, Artama M, Engeland A, Ericsson O, Furu K, Gissler M, et al. Selective serotonin reuptake inhibitors during pregnancy and risk of persistent pulmonary hypertension in the newborn: population based cohort study from the five Nordic countries. BMJ. 2012;344:d8012.
10. Reis M, Kallen B. Delivery outcome after maternal use of antidepressant drugs in pregnancy: an update using Swedish data. Psychol Med. 2010;40:1723–33.
11. Grigoriadis S, Vonderporten EH, Mamisashvili L, Tomlinson G, Dennis CL, Koren G, et al. Prenatal exposure to antidepressants and persistent pulmonary hypertension of the newborn: systematic review and meta-analysis. BMJ. 2014;348:f6932.
12. Wilson KL, Zelig CM, Harvey JP, Cunningham BS, Dolinsky BM, Napolitano PG. Persistent pulmonary hypertension of the newborn is associated with mode of delivery and not with maternal use of selective serotonin reuptake inhibitors. Am J Perinatol. 2011;28:19–24.
13. Andrade SE, McPhillips H, Loren D, Raebel MA, Lane K, Livingston J, et al. Antidepressant medication use and risk of persistent pulmonary hypertension of the newborn. Pharmacoepidemiol Drug Saf. 2009;18:246–52.
14. Lim K, Sanders A, Brain U, Riggs W, Oberlander TF, Rurak D. Third trimester fetal pulmonary artery Doppler blood flow velocity characteristics following prenatal selective serotonin reuptake inhibitor (SSRI) exposure. Early Hum Dev. 2012;88:609–15.
15. Gebb SA, Jones PL. Hypoxia and lung branching morphogenesis. Adv Exp Med Biol. 2003;543:117–25.
16. Teitel DF, Iwamoto HS, Rudolph AM. Changes in the pulmonary circulation during birth-related events. Pediatr Res. 1990;27:372–8.
17. Haworth SG, Hislop AA. Adaptation of the pulmonary circulation to extra-uterine life in the pig and its relevance to the human infant. Cardiovasc Res. 1981;15:108–19.
18. Konduri GG, Theodorou AA, Mukhopadhyay A, Deshmukh DR. Adenosine triphosphate and adenosine increase the pulmonary blood flow to postnatal levels in fetal lambs. Pediatr Res. 1992;31:451–7.
19. Steinhorn RH, Morin 3rd FC, Van Wylen DG, Gugino SF, Giese EC, Russell JA. Endothelium-dependent relaxations to adenosine in juvenile rabbit pulmonary arteries and veins. Am J Physiol. 1994;266:H2001–6.
20. Shaul PW, Farrar MA, Zellers TM. Oxygen modulates endothelium-derived relaxing factor production in fetal pulmonary arteries. Am J Physiol. 1992;262:H355–64.
21. Abman SH, Chatfield BA, Hall SL, McMurtry IF. Role of endothelium-derived relaxing factor during transition of pulmonary circulation at birth. Am J Physiol. 1990;259:H1921–7.
22. Fineman JR, Wong J, Morin 3rd FC, Wild LM, Soifer SJ. Chronic nitric oxide inhibition in utero produces persistent pulmonary hypertension in newborn lambs. J Clin Invest. 1994;93:2675–83.
23. Pierce CM, Krywawych S, Petros AJ. Asymmetric dimethyl arginine and symmetric dimethyl arginine levels in infants with persistent pulmonary hypertension of the newborn. Pediatr Crit Care Med. 2004;5:517–20.
24. Pearson DL, Dawling S, Walsh WF, Haines JL, Christman BW, Bazyk A, et al. Neonatal pulmonary hypertension–urea-cycle intermediates, nitric oxide production, and carbamoyl-phosphate synthetase function. N Engl J Med. 2001;344:1832–8.
25. Leffler CW, Hessler JR, Green RS. The onset of breathing at birth stimulates pulmonary vascular prostacyclin synthesis. Pediatr Res. 1984;18:938–42.
26. Brannon TS, North AJ, Wells LB, Shaul PW. Prostacyclin synthesis in ovine pulmonary artery is developmentally regulated by changes in cyclooxygenase-1 gene expression. J Clin Invest. 1994;93:2230–5.
27. Van Marter LJ, Hernandez-Diaz S, Werler MM, Louik C, Mitchell AA. Nonsteroidal antiinflammatory drugs in late pregnancy and persistent pulmonary hypertension of the newborn. Pediatrics. 2013;131:79–87.
28. Lakshminrusimha S, D'Angelis CA, Russell JA, Nielsen LC, Gugino SF, Nickerson PA, et al. C-type natriuretic peptide system in fetal ovine pulmonary vasculature. Am J Physiol Lung Cell Mol Physiol. 2001;281:L361–8.
29. Yoder BA, Kirsch EA, Barth WH, Gordon MC. Changing obstetric practices associated with decreasing incidence of meconium aspiration syndrome. Obstet Gynecol. 2002;99:731–9.
30. Murphy JD, Vawter GF, Reid LM. Pulmonary vascular disease in fatal meconium aspiration. J Pediatr. 1984;104:758–62.
31. Villanueva ME, Zaher FM, Svinarich DM, Konduri GG. Decreased gene expression of endothelial nitric oxide synthase in newborns with persistent pulmonary hypertension. Pediatr Res. 1998;44:338–43.
32. Soukka H, Jalonen J, Kero P, Kaapa P. Endothelin-1, atrial natriuretic peptide and pathophysiology of pulmonary hypertension in porcine meconium aspiration. Acta Paediatr. 1998;87:424–8.
33. Velaphi S, Van Kwawegen A. Meconium aspiration syndrome requiring assisted ventilation: perspective in a setting with limited resources. J Perinatol. 2008;28 Suppl 3:S36–42.
34. Fraser WD, Hofmeyr J, Lede R, Faron G, Alexander S, Goffinet F, et al. Amnioinfusion for the prevention of the meconium aspiration syndrome. N Engl J Med. 2005;353:909–17.
35. Vain NE, Szyld EG, Prudent LM, Wiswell TE, Aguilar AM, Vivas NI. Oropharyngeal and nasopharyngeal suctioning of meconium-stained neonates before delivery of their shoulders: multicentre, randomised controlled trial. Lancet. 2004;364:597–602.
36. Wiswell TE, Gannon CM, Jacob J, Goldsmith L, Szyld E, Weiss K, et al. Delivery room management of the apparently vigorous meconium-stained neonate: results of the multicenter, international collaborative trial. Pediatrics. 2000;105:1–7.
37. Kattwinkel J, Perlman JM, Aziz K, Colby C, Fairchild K, Gallagher J, et al. Part 15: neonatal resuscitation: 2010 American Heart Association Guidelines for Cardiopulmonary Resuscitation and Emergency Cardiovascular Care. Circulation. 2010;122:S909–19.
38. Lakshminrusimha S, Mathew B, Nair J, Gugino SF, Koenigsknecht C, Rawat M, et al. Tracheal suctioning improves gas exchange but not hemodynamics in asphyxiated lambs with meconium aspiration. Pediatr Res. 2014.
39. Nangia S, Sunder SS, Tiwari S, Saili A. Role of endotracheal suction on the occurence of meconium aspiration syndrome in non-vigorous meconium stained neonates - a randomized controlled trial. E-PAS2014: 46801 2014.
40. Sehgal A, Athikarisamy SE, Adamopoulos M. Global myocardial function is compromised in infants with pulmonary hypertension. Acta Paediatr. 2012;101:410–3.
41. Van Meurs KP, Wright LL, Ehrenkranz RA, Lemons JA, Ball MB, Poole WK, et al. Inhaled nitric oxide for premature infants with severe respiratory failure. N Engl J Med. 2005;353:13–22.

42. Kumar VH, Hutchison AA, Lakshminrusimha S, Morin 3rd FC, Wynn RJ, Ryan RM. Characteristics of pulmonary hypertension in preterm neonates. J Perinatol. 2007;27:214–9.
43. Check J, Gotteiner N, Liu X, Su E, Porta N, Steinhorn R, et al. Fetal growth restriction and pulmonary hypertension in premature infants with bronchopulmonary dysplasia. J Perinatol. 2013;33:553–7.
44. Mourani PM, Abman SH. Pulmonary vascular disease in bronchopulmonary dysplasia: pulmonary hypertension and beyond. Curr Opin Pediatr. 2013;25:329–37.
45. Steinhorn RH, Morin 3rd FC, Russell JA. The adventitia may be a barrier specific to nitric oxide in rabbit pulmonary artery. J Clin Invest. 1994;94:1883–8.
46. Levin DL, Mills LJ, Parkey M, Garriott J, Campbell W. Constriction of the fetal ductus arteriosus after administration of indomethacin to the pregnant ewe. J Pediatr. 1979;94:647–50.
47. Wild LM, Nickerson PA, Morin 3rd FC. Ligating the ductus arteriosus before birth remodels the pulmonary vasculature of the lamb. Pediatr Res. 1989;25:251–7.
48. Skari H, Bjornland K, Haugen G, Egeland T, Emblem R. Congenital diaphragmatic hernia: a meta-analysis of mortality factors. J Pediatr Surg. 2000;35:1187–97.
49. Schachtner SK, Wang Y, Scott Baldwin H. Qualitative and quantitative analysis of embryonic pulmonary vessel formation. Am J Respir Cell Mol Biol. 2000;22:157–65.
50. Bizzarro MJ, Copel JA, Pearson HA, Pober B, Bhandari V. Pulmonary hypoplasia and persistent pulmonary hypertension in the newborn with homozygous alpha-thalassemia: a case report and review of the literature. J Matern Fetal Neonatal Med. 2003;14:411–6.
51. Gunthard J, Fliegel C, Ohnacker H, Rutishauser M, Buhler E. Lung hypoplasia and severe pulmonary hypertension in an infant with double heterozygosity for spondyloepiphyseal dysplasia congenita and achondroplasia. Clin Genet. 1995;48:35–40.
52. Semidotskaia Zh D, Bil'chenko OS, Andon'eva NM, Geletko MO. Association of mucopolysaccharidosis with primary pulmonary hypertension and renal hypoplasia. Klin Med (Mosk). 1985;63:126–7.
53. Chock VY, Van Meurs KP, Hintz SR, Ehrenkranz RA, Lemons JA, Kendrick DE, et al. Inhaled nitric oxide for preterm premature rupture of membranes, oligohydramnios, and pulmonary hypoplasia. Am J Perinatol. 2009;26:317–22.
54. Deutsch GH, Young LR, Deterding RR, Fan LL, Dell SD, Bean JA, et al. Diffuse lung disease in young children: application of a novel classification scheme. Am J Respir Crit Care Med. 2007;176:1120–8.
55. Ahmed S, Ackerman V, Faught P, Langston C. Profound hypoxemia and pulmonary hypertension in a 7-month-old infant: late presentation of alveolar capillary dysplasia. Pediatr Crit Care Med. 2008;9:e43–6.
56. Stankiewicz P, Sen P, Bhatt SS, Storer M, Xia Z, Bejjani BA, et al. Genomic and genic deletions of the FOX gene cluster on 16q24.1 and inactivating mutations of FOXF1 cause alveolar capillary dysplasia and other malformations. Am J Hum Genet. 2009;84:780–91.
57. D'Alto M, Romeo E, Argiento P, Di Salvo G, Badagliacca R, Cirillo AP, et al. Pulmonary arterial hypertension: the key role of echocardiography. Echocardiography. 2015;32 Suppl 1:S23–37.
58. Abassi Z, Karram T, Ellaham S, Winaver J, Hoffman A. Implications of the natriuretic peptide system in the pathogenesis of heart failure: diagnostic and therapeutic importance. Pharmacol Ther. 2004;102:223–41.
59. Reynolds EW, Ellington JG, Vranicar M, Bada HS. Brain-type natriuretic peptide in the diagnosis and management of persistent pulmonary hypertension of the newborn. Pediatrics. 2004;114:1297–304.
60. Vijlbrief DC, Benders MJ, Kemperman H, van Bel F, de Vries WB. B-type natriuretic peptide and rebound during treatment for persistent pulmonary hypertension. J Pediatr. 2012;160:111–5.
61. Golombek SG, Young JN. Efficacy of inhaled nitric oxide for hypoxic respiratory failure in term and late preterm infants by baseline severity of illness: a pooled analysis of three clinical trials. Clin Ther. 2010;32:939–48.
62. Thomas NJ, Shaffer ML, Willson DF, Shih MC, Curley MA. Defining acute lung disease in children with the oxygenation saturation index. Pediatr Crit Care Med. 2010;11:12–7.
63. Rawat M, Chandrasekharan PK, Williams A, Gugino S, Koenigsknecht C, Swartz D, et al. Oxygen Saturation Index and Severity of Hypoxic Respiratory Failure. Neonatology. 2015;107:161–6.
64. Manja V, Mathew B, Carrion V, Lakshminrusimha S. Critical congenital heart disease screening by pulse oximetry in a neonatal intensive care unit. J Perinatol. 2015;35(1):67–71.
65. Bifano EM, Pfannenstiel A. Duration of hyperventilation and outcome in infants with persistent pulmonary hypertension. Pediatrics. 1988;81:657–61.
66. Hendricks-Munoz KD, Walton JP. Hearing loss in infants with persistent fetal circulation. Pediatrics. 1988;81:650–6.
67. Dworetz AR, Moya FR, Sabo B, Dworetz AR, Moya FR, Sabo B, et al. Survival of infants with persistent pulmonary hypertension without extracorporeal membrane oxygenation.[comment]. Pediatrics. 1989;84:1–6.
68. Wung JT, James LS, Kilchevsky E, James E. Management of infants with severe respiratory failure and persistence of the fetal circulation, without hyperventilation. Pediatrics. 1985;76:488–94.
69. Rudolph AM, Yuan S. Response of the pulmonary vasculature to hypoxia and H+ ion concentration changes. J Clin Invest. 1966;45:399–411.
70. Kinsella JP, Abman SH. Recent developments in the pathophysiology and treatment of persistent pulmonary hypertension of the newborn. J Pediatr. 1995;126:853–64.
71. Antunes M, Greenspan J, Holt W, Vallieu D, Spitzer A. Assessment of lung-function pre-nitric oxide therapy-a predictor of response. In: Pediatric research. 351 West Camden St, Baltimore: Williams and Wilkins; 1994. p. a212. Md 21201–2436.
72. Gupta A, Rastogi S, Sahni R, Bhutada A, Bateman D, Rastogi D, et al. Inhaled nitric oxide and gentle ventilation in the treatment of pulmonary hypertension of the newborn–a single-center, 5-year experience. J Perinatol. 2002;22:435–41.
73. Kinsella JP, Abman SH. Clinical approaches to the use of high-frequency oscillatory ventilation in neonatal respiratory failure. J Perinatol. 1996;16:S52–5.
74. Kinsella JP, Abman SH. High-frequency oscillatory ventilation augments the response to inhaled nitric oxide in persistent pulmonary hypertension of the newborn: Nitric Oxide Study Group. Chest. 1998;114:100S.
75. Kinsella JP, Truog WE, Walsh WF, Goldberg RN, Bancalari E, Mayock DE. Randomized, multicenter trial of inhaled nitric oxide and high-frequency oscillatory ventilation in severe, persistent pulmonary hypertension of the newborn. J Pediatr. 1997;131:55–62.
76. Tiktinsky MH, Morin 3rd FC. Increasing oxygen tension dilates fetal pulmonary circulation via endothelium-derived relaxing factor. Am J Physiol. 1993;265:H376–80.
77. Cornfield DN, Chatfield BA, McQueston JA, McMurtry IF, Abman SH. Effects of birth-related stimuli on L-arginine-dependent pulmonary vasodilation in ovine fetus. Am J Physiol. 1992;262:H1474–81.
78. Lakshminrusimha S, Russell JA, Steinhorn RH, Ryan RM, Gugino SF, Morin 3rd FC, et al. Pulmonary arterial contractility in neonatal lambs increases with 100% oxygen resuscitation. Pediatr Res. 2006;59:137–41.
79. Lakshminrusimha S, Russell JA, Steinhorn RH, Swartz DD, Ryan RM, Gugino SF, et al. Pulmonary hemodynamics in neonatal lambs resuscitated with 21%, 50%, and 100% oxygen. Pediatr Res. 2007;62:313–8.
80. Lakshminrusimha S, Swartz DD, Gugino SF, Ma CX, Wynn KA, Ryan RM, et al. Oxygen concentration and pulmonary hemodynamics in newborn lambs with pulmonary hypertension. Pediatr Res. 2009;66:539–44.
81. Farrow KN, Groh BS, Schumacker PT, Lakshminrusimha S, Czech L, Gugino SF, et al. Hyperoxia increases phosphodiesterase 5 expression and activity in ovine fetal pulmonary artery smooth muscle cells. Circ Res. 2008;102:226–33.
82. Faraci FM, Didion SP. Vascular protection: superoxide dismutase isoforms in the vessel wall. Arterioscler Thromb Vasc Biol. 2004;24:1367–73.
83. Lotze A, Mitchell BR, Bulas DI, Zola EM, Shalwitz RA, Gunkel JH. Multicenter study of surfactant (beractant) use in the treatment of term infants with severe respiratory failure: Survanta in Term Infants Study Group. J Pediatr. 1998;132:40–7.
84. Konduri GG, Sokol GM, Van Meurs KP, Singer J, Ambalavanan N, Lee T, et al. Impact of early surfactant and inhaled nitric oxide therapies on outcomes in term/late preterm neonates with moderate hypoxic respiratory failure. J Perinatol. 2013;33:944–9.
85. Salvesen B, Curstedt T, Mollnes TE, Saugstad OD. Effects of Natural versus Synthetic Surfactant with SP-B and SP-C Analogs in a Porcine Model of Meconium Aspiration Syndrome. Neonatology. 2014;105:128–35.
86. Wolfson MR, Wu J, Hubert TL, Gregory TJ, Mazela J, Shaffer TH. Lucinactant attenuates pulmonary inflammatory response, preserves lung structure, and improves physiologic outcomes in a preterm lamb model of RDS. Pediatr Res. 2012;72:375–83.

87. Thomas NJ, Guardia CG, Moya FR, Cheifetz IM, Markovitz B, Cruces P, et al. A pilot, randomized, controlled clinical trial of lucinactant, a peptide-containing synthetic surfactant, in infants with acute hypoxemic respiratory failure. Pediatr Crit Care Med. 2012;13:646–53.
88. Davey MG, Biard JM, Robinson L, Tsai J, Schwarz U, Danzer E, et al. Surfactant protein expression is increased in the ipsilateral but not contralateral lungs of fetal sheep with left-sided diaphragmatic hernia. Pediatr Pulmonol. 2005;39:359–67.
89. Davey MG, Danzer E, Schwarz U, Adzick NS, Flake AW, Hedrick HL. Prenatal glucocorticoids and exogenous surfactant therapy improve respiratory function in lambs with severe diaphragmatic hernia following fetal tracheal occlusion. Pediatr Res. 2006;60:131–5.
90. O'Toole SJ, Karamanoukian HL, Morin 3rd FC, Holm BA, Egan EA, Azizkhan RG, et al. Surfactant decreases pulmonary vascular resistance and increases pulmonary blood flow in the fetal lamb model of congenital diaphragmatic hernia. J Pediatr Surg. 1996;31:507–11.
91. Van Meurs K. Congenital Diaphragmatic Hernia Study G: Is surfactant therapy beneficial in the treatment of the term newborn infant with congenital diaphragmatic hernia. J Pediatr. 2004;145:312–6.
92. Moncada S, Palmer RM, Higgs EA. Nitric oxide: physiology, pathophysiology, and pharmacology. Pharmacol Rev. 1991;43:109–42.
93. Davidson D, Barefield ES, Kattwinkel J, Dudell G, Damask M, Straube R, et al. Inhaled nitric oxide for the early treatment of persistent pulmonary hypertension of the term newborn: a randomized, double-masked, placebo-controlled, dose–response, multicenter study. The I-NO/PPHN Study Group. Pediatrics. 1998;101:325–34.
94. Clark RH, Kueser TJ, Walker MW, Southgate WM, Huckaby JL, Perez JA, et al. Keszler M, Kinsella JP: Low-dose nitric oxide therapy for persistent pulmonary hypertension of the newborn. Clinical Inhaled Nitric Oxide Research Group. N Engl J Med. 2000;342:469–74.
95. NINOS. Inhaled nitric oxide in full-term and nearly full-term infants with hypoxic respiratory failure. The Neonatal Inhaled Nitric Oxide Study Group[erratum appears in N Engl J Med 1997 Aug 7;337(6):434]. N Engl J Med. 1997;336:597–604.
96. Roberts Jr JD, Fineman JR, Morin 3rd FC, Shaul PW, Rimar S, Schreiber MD, et al. Inhaled nitric oxide and persistent pulmonary hypertension of the newborn. The Inhaled Nitric Oxide Study Group. N Engl J Med. 1997;336:605–10.
97. Aschner JL, Fike CD. New developments in the pathogenesis and management of neonatal pulmonary hypertension. In The Newborn Lung. Edited by Bancalari E. Philadelphia: Saunders Elsevier; 2008: 241–299.[Polin RA (Series Editor): Neonatology questions and controversies].
98. Konduri GG, Kim UO. Advances in the diagnosis and management of persistent pulmonary hypertension of the newborn. Pediatr Clin North Am. 2009;56:579–600.
99. Konduri GG, Solimano A, Sokol GM, Singer J, Ehrenkranz RA, Singhal N, et al. A randomized trial of early versus standard inhaled nitric oxide therapy in term and near-term newborn infants with hypoxic respiratory failure. Pediatrics. 2004;113:559–64.
100. Tworetzky W, Bristow J, Moore P, Brook MM, Segal MR, Brasch RC, et al. Inhaled nitric oxide in neonates with persistent pulmonary hypertension. Lancet. 2001;357:118–20.
101. Hamon I, Gauthier-Moulinier H, Grelet-Dessioux E, Storme L, Fresson J, Hascoet JM. Methaemoglobinaemia risk factors with inhaled nitric oxide therapy in newborn infants. Acta Paediatr. 2010;99:1467–73.
102. Aly H, Sahni R, Wung JT. Weaning strategy with inhaled nitric oxide treatment in persistent pulmonary hypertension of the newborn. Arch Dis Child Fetal Neonatal Ed. 1997;76:F118–22.
103. Sokol GM, Fineberg NS, Wright LL, Ehrenkranz RA. Changes in arterial oxygen tension when weaning neonates from inhaled nitric oxide. Pediatr Pulmonol. 2001;32:14–9.
104. Sheehy AM, Burson MA, Black SM. Nitric oxide exposure inhibits endothelial NOS activity but not gene expression: a role for superoxide. Am J Physiol. 1998;274:L833–41.
105. Black SM, Heidersbach RS, McMullan DM, Bekker JM, Johengen MJ, Fineman JR. Inhaled nitric oxide inhibits NOS activity in lambs: potential mechanism for rebound pulmonary hypertension. Am J Physiol. 1999;277:H1849–56.
106. Lakshminrusimha S. The pulmonary circulation in neonatal respiratory failure. Clin Perinatol. 2012;39:655–83.
107. Lakshminrusimha S, Wynn RJ, Youssfi M, Pabalan MJ, Bommaraju M, Kirmani K, et al. Use of CT angiography in the diagnosis of total anomalous venous return. J Perinatol. 2009;29:458–61.
108. Sood BG, Delaney-Black V, Aranda JV, Shankaran S. Aerosolized PGE1: a selective pulmonary vasodilator in neonatal hypoxemic respiratory failure results of a Phase I/II open label clinical trial. Pediatr Res. 2004;56:579–85.
109. Sood BG, Keszler M, Garg M, Klein JM, Ohls R, Ambalavanan N, et al. Inhaled PGE1 in neonates with hypoxemic respiratory failure: two pilot feasibility randomized clinical trials. Trials. 2014;15:486.
110. Shiyanagi S, Okazaki T, Shoji H, Shimizu T, Tanaka T, Takeda S, et al. Management of pulmonary hypertension in congenital diaphragmatic hernia: nitric oxide with prostaglandin E1 versus nitric oxide alone. Pediatr Surg Int. 2008;24:1101–4.
111. Kelly LK, Porta NF, Goodman DM, Carroll CL, Steinhorn RH. Inhaled prostacyclin for term infants with persistent pulmonary hypertension refractory to inhaled nitric oxide. J Pediatr. 2002;141:830–2.
112. Steinhorn RH, Russell JA, Morin 3rd FC. Disruption of cGMP production in pulmonary arteries isolated from fetal lambs with pulmonary hypertension. Am J Physiol. 1995;268:H1483–9.
113. Bernus A, Wagner BD, Accurso F, Doran A, Kaess H, Ivy DD. Brain natriuretic peptide levels in managing pediatric patients with pulmonary arterial hypertension. Chest. 2009;135:745–51.
114. Baquero H, Soliz A, Neira F, Venegas ME, Sola A. Oral sildenafil in infants with persistent pulmonary hypertension of the newborn: a pilot randomized blinded study. Pediatrics. 2006;117:1077–83.
115. Vargas-Origel A, Gomez-Rodriguez G, Aldana-Valenzuela C, Vela-Huerta MM, Alarcon-Santos SB, Amador-Licona N. The use of sildenafil in persistent pulmonary hypertension of the newborn. Am J Perinatol. 2010;27:225–30.
116. Steinhorn RH, Kinsella JP, Butrous G, Dilleen M, Oakes M, Wessel DL. Intravenous sildenafil in the treatment of neonates with persistent pulmonary hypertension of the newborn. J Pediatr. 2009. In press.
117. Juliana AE, Abbad FC. Severe persistent pulmonary hypertension of the newborn in a setting where limited resources exclude the use of inhaled nitric oxide: successful treatment with sildenafil. Eur J Pediatr. 2005;164:626–9.
118. Steiner M, Salzer U, Baumgartner S, Waldhoer T, Klebermass-Schrehof K, Wald M, et al. Intravenous sildenafil i.v. as rescue treatment for refractory pulmonary hypertension in extremely preterm infants. Klin Padiatr. 2014;226:211–5.
119. Lakshminrusimha S, Porta NF, Farrow KN, Chen B, Gugino SF, Kumar VH, et al. Milrinone enhances relaxation to prostacyclin and iloprost in pulmonary arteries isolated from lambs with persistent pulmonary hypertension of the newborn. Pediatr Crit Care Med. 2009;10:106–12.
120. McNamara PJ, Shivananda SP, Sahni M, Freeman D, Taddio A. Pharmacology of milrinone in neonates with persistent pulmonary hypertension of the newborn and suboptimal response to inhaled nitric oxide. Pediatr Crit Care Med. 2013;14:74–84.
121. Bassler D, Choong K, McNamara P, Kirpalani H. Neonatal persistent pulmonary hypertension treated with milrinone: four case reports. Biol Neonate. 2006;89:1–5.
122. McNamara PJ, Laique F, Muang-In S, Whyte HE. Milrinone improves oxygenation in neonates with severe persistent pulmonary hypertension of the newborn. J Crit Care. 2006;21:217–22.
123. James AT, Bee C, Corcoran JD, McNamara PJ, Franklin O, El-Khuffash AF. Treatment of premature infants with pulmonary hypertension and right ventricular dysfunction with milrinone: a case series. J Perinatol. 2015;35:268–73.
124. James AT, Corcoran JD, McNamara PJ, Franklin O, El-Khuffash AF. The effect of milrinone on right and left ventricular function when used as a rescue therapy for term infants with pulmonary hypertension. Cardiol Young. 2015:1–10.
125. Rubin LJ, Badesch DB, Barst RJ, Galie N, Black CM, Keogh A, et al. Bosentan therapy for pulmonary arterial hypertension. N Engl J Med. 2002;346:896–903.
126. Mohamed WA, Ismail M. A randomized, double-blind, placebo-controlled, prospective study of bosentan for the treatment of persistent pulmonary hypertension of the newborn. J Perinatol. 2012;32(8):608–13.
127. Steinhorn RH, Fineman J, Kusic-Pajic A, Cornelisse P, Gehin M, Nowbakht P, et al. Bosentan as adjunctive therapy for persistent pulmonary hypertension of the newborn: results of the FUTURE-4 study. Circulation. 2014;130:A13503.

128. Chandrasekar I, Eis A, Konduri GG. Betamethasone attenuates oxidant stress in endothelial cells from fetal lambs with persistent pulmonary hypertension. Pediatr Res. 2008;63:67–72.
129. Soukka H, Halkola L, Aho H, Rautanen M, Kero P, Kaapa P. Methylprednisolone attenuates the pulmonary hypertensive response in porcine meconium aspiration. Pediatr Res. 1997;42:145–50.
130. Tripathi S, Saili A. The effect of steroids on the clinical course and outcome of neonates with meconium aspiration syndrome. J Trop Pediatr. 2007;53:8–12.
131. Ward M, Sinn J. Steroid therapy for meconium aspiration syndrome in newborn infants. The Cochrane database of systematic reviews. 2003(4):Cd003485.
132. Perez M, Wedgwood S, Lakshminrusimha S, Farrow KN, Steinhorn RH. Hydrocortisone normalizes phosphodiesterase-5 activity in pulmonary artery smooth muscle cells from lambs with persistent pulmonary hypertension of the newborn. Pulm Circ. 2014;4:71–81.
133. Perez M, Lakshminrusimha S, Wedgwood S, Czech L, Gugino SF, Russell JA, et al. Hydrocortisone normalizes oxygenation and cGMP regulation in lambs with persistent pulmonary hypertension of the newborn. Am J Physiol Lung Cell Mol Physiol. 2012;302(6):L595–603.
134. Paden ML, Rycus PT, Thiagarajan RR. Update and outcomes in extracorporeal life support. Semin Perinatol. 2014;38:65–70.
135. Gill BS, Neville HL, Khan AM, Cox Jr CS, Lally KP. Delayed institution of extracorporeal membrane oxygenation is associated with increased mortality rate and prolonged hospital stay. J Pediatr Surg. 2002;37:7–10.
136. Bahrami KR, Van Meurs KP. ECMO for neonatal respiratory failure. Semin Perinatol. 2005;29:15–23.
137. Tourneux P, Rakza T, Bouissou A, Krim G, Storme L. Pulmonary circulatory effects of norepinephrine in newborn infants with persistent pulmonary hypertension. J Pediatr. 2008;153:345–9.
138. Mohamed A, Nasef N, Shah V, McNamara PJ. Vasopressin as a rescue therapy for refractory pulmonary hypertension in neonates: case series. Pediatr Crit Care Med. 2014;15:148–54.
139. Lapointe A, Barrington KJ. Pulmonary hypertension and the asphyxiated newborn. J Pediatr. 2011;158:e19–24.
140. Shankaran S, Laptook AR, Ehrenkranz RA, Tyson JE, McDonald SA, Donovan EF, et al. Whole-body hypothermia for neonates with hypoxic-ischemic encephalopathy. N Engl J Med. 2005;353:1574–84.
141. Shankaran S, Laptook AR, Pappas A, McDonald SA, Das A, Tyson JE, et al. Effect of depth and duration of cooling on deaths in the NICU among neonates with hypoxic ischemic encephalopathy: a randomized clinical trial. JAMA. 2014;312:2629–39.
142. Thoresen M, Whitelaw A. Cardiovascular changes during mild therapeutic hypothermia and rewarming in infants with hypoxic-ischemic encephalopathy. Pediatrics. 2000;106:92–9.
143. Shah SK, Khan AM, Cox Jr CS. Pulmonary hypertensive crisis requiring ECMO associated with re-warming from whole body hypothermia for hypoxic ischemic encephalopathy: clinical observations from a case series. Eur J Pediatr Surg. 2010;20:205–6.
144. Benumof JL, Wahrenbrock EA. Dependency of hypoxic pulmonary vasoconstriction on temperature. J Appl Physiol Respir Environ Exerc Physiol. 1977;42:56–8.
145. Konduri GG, Vohr B, Robertson C, Sokol GM, Solimano A, Singer J, et al. Early inhaled nitric oxide therapy for term and near-term newborn infants with hypoxic respiratory failure: neurodevelopmental follow-up. J Pediatr. 2007;150:235–40. 240 e231.
146. Robertson CM, Tyebkhan JM, Hagler ME, Cheung PY, Peliowski A, Etches PC. Late-onset, progressive sensorineural hearing loss after severe neonatal respiratory failure. Otol Neurotol. 2002;23:353–6.
147. Lipkin PH, Davidson D, Spivak L, Straube R, Rhines J, Chang CT. Neurodevelopmental and medical outcomes of persistent pulmonary hypertension in term newborns treated with nitric oxide.[comment]. Pediatr Res. 2002;140:306–10.
148. Rosenberg AA, Lee NR, Vaver KN, Werner D, Fashaw L, Hale K, et al. School-age outcomes of newborns treated for persistent pulmonary hypertension. J Perinatol. 2010;30:127–34.
149. McNally H, Bennett CC, Elbourne D, Field DJ. Group UKCET: United Kingdom collaborative randomized trial of neonatal extracorporeal membrane oxygenation: follow-up to age 7 years. Pediatrics. 2006;117:e845–54.
150. Walton JP, Hendricks-Munoz K. Profile and stability of sensorineural hearing loss in persistent pulmonary hypertension of the newborn. J Speech Hear Res. 1991;34:1362–70.
151. Busch CJ, Graveline AR, Jiramongkolchai K, Liu H, Sanchez LS, Bloch KD. Phosphodiesterase 3A expression is modulated by nitric oxide in rat pulmonary artery smooth muscle cells. J Physiol Pharmacol. 2010;61:663–9.
152. Chen B, Lakshminrusimha S, Czech L, Groh BS, Gugino SF, Russell JA, et al. Regulation of phosphodiesterase 3 in the pulmonary arteries during the perinatal period in sheep. Pediatr Res. 2009;66(6):682–7.

2

Maternal predictors of neonatal outcomes after emergency cesarean section: a retrospective study in three rural district hospitals in Rwanda

Naome Nyirahabimana[1*†], Christine Minani Ufashingabire[2†], Yihan Lin[3,4], Bethany Hedt-Gauthier[1,3], Robert Riviello[3,5], Jackline Odhiambo[6], Joel Mubiligi[1], Martin Macharia[1], Stephen Rulisa[2], Illuminee Uwicyeza[7], Patient Ngamije[7], Fulgence Nkikabahizi[7] and Theoneste Nkurunziza[1]

Abstract

Background: In sub-Saharan Africa, neonatal mortality post-cesarean delivery is higher than the global average. In this region, most emergency cesarean sections are performed at district hospitals. This study assesses maternal predictors for poor neonatal outcomes post-emergency cesarean delivery in three rural district hospitals in Rwanda.

Methods: This retrospective study includes a random sample of 441 neonates from Butaro, Kirehe and Rwinkwavu District Hospitals, born between 01 January and 31 December 2015. We described the demographic and clinical characteristics of the mothers of these neonates using frequencies and proportions. We assessed the association between maternal characteristics with poor neonatal outcomes, defined as death within 24 h or APGAR < 7 at 5 min after birth, using Fisher's exact test. Factors significant at $\alpha = 0.20$ significance level were considered for the multivariate logistic regression model, built using a backwards stepwise process. We stopped when all the factors were significant at the $\alpha = 0.05$ level.

Results: For all 441 neonates included in this study, 40 (9.0%) had poor outcomes. In the final model, three factors were significantly associated with poor neonatal outcomes. Neonates born to mothers who had four or more prior pregnancies were more likely to have poor outcomes (OR = 3.01, 95%CI:1.23,7.35, $p = 0.015$). Neonates whose mothers came from health centers with ambulance travel times of more than 30 min to the district hospital had greater odds of having poor outcomes (for 30–60 min: OR = 3.80, 95%CI:1.07,13.40, $p = 0.012$; for 60+ minutes: OR = 5.82, 95%CI:1.47,23.05, $p = 0.012$). Neonates whose mothers presented with very severe indications for cesarean section had twice odds of having a poor outcome (95% CI: 1.11,4.52, $p = 0.023$).

Conclusions: Longer travel time to the district hospital was a leading predictor of poor neonatal outcomes post cesarean delivery. Improving referral systems, ambulance availability, number of equipped hospitals per district, and road networks may lessen travel delays for women in labor. Boosting the diagnostic capacity of labor conditions at the health center level through facilities and staff training can improve early identification of very severe indications for cesarean delivery for early referral and intervention.

Keywords: Obstetric surgery, Emergency obstetrics, Birth outcomes, Africa

* Correspondence: nnyirahabimana@pih.org
†Equal contributors
[1]Partners In Health, Inshuti Mu Buzima, KigaliP.O. Box: 3432Rwanda
Full list of author information is available at the end of the article

Background

Globally, an estimated 22.9 million cesarean procedures are performed each year, primarily to save the life of either the mother or the infant [1]. However, at 1.77 deaths per 1,000 live births, global neonatal mortality post-cesarean section is three times higher than mortality following vaginal deliveries [2]. In sub-Saharan Africa, 8.8% of all deliveries are through cesarean section [3], falling within the 5–15% range recommended by the World Health Organization [4]. However, intrapartum neonatal mortality in sub-Saharan Africa accounts for 73% of global neonatal intrapartum deaths [5] and neonatal mortality post-cesarean delivery in sub-Saharan Africa is higher than the global average [3].

Poor neonatal outcomes post-cesarean delivery has been defined as mortality, low APGAR scores or admission to the neonatal intensive care unit [6, 7]. A variety of risk factors for poor neonatal outcomes have previously been identified. Shortage of staff, inadequately skilled staff and limited equipment impede timely availability of cesarean sections for women who need it [4]. A study in sub-Saharan Africa found that the majority of countries had limited capacity to provide cesarean sections, with only 20% of hospitals having full time physicians and 47% reporting a lack of anesthetists [8]. In addition, barriers such as the cost of cesarean delivery or delayed referral to the facility providing cesarean section also increase poor neonatal outcomes [4]. Fetal demographic characteristics such as fetal weight, fetal malformations and pre-operative fetal heart rate have also been linked to low APGAR scores [9, 10]. However, data on the effect of maternal factors on neonatal outcomes following cesarean section at district hospitals in Rwanda is limited.

In 2015 in Rwanda, the neonatal mortality rate was 20 per 1000 live births, approximately 30% of which occurred in the first 24 h of life [11]. About 13% of all deliveries are through cesarean section [11]. Of deliveries that need a cesarean section, 45% are performed at district hospitals [12] and at least 60% of all surgeries done at the district hospital are cesarean sections [13]. However, information on the neonatal outcomes immediately after cesarean section at these district hospitals or factors that are linked to poor neonatal outcomes is limited. In this study, we assessed the rates of poor neonatal outcomes and the maternal factors associated with poor neonatal outcomes after emergency cesarean delivery at three rural district hospitals in Rwanda. Identifying maternal predictors of poor neonatal outcomes could inform future interventions to improve neonatal survival post emergency cesarean section at the district hospitals.

Methods

Study setting

We conducted this study at Butaro, Kirehe and Rwinkwavu District Hospitals, three rural facilities that are operated by the Rwandan Ministry of Health with support from Partners In Health, a Boston-based non governmental organization. Rwinkwavu and Kirehe District Hospitals are located in the Eastern Province and Butaro District Hospital is located in the Northern Province of Rwanda. Together, the catchment area of these hospitals includes 46 health centers and serves more than 800,000 people [14]. These districts are in the rural settings where 49% of the population make 30 min travel to get to clean water source, and only 12% have access to electricity. The population in this setting is likely to work in small farming agricultural sector and 77% of poorer households work in agricultural sector compared to 21% of richer ones that work in the same sector [11].

According to Rwanda's protocol on labor and delivery, pregnant women first present to the health center for delivery led by nurses. If the delivery is complicated to be managed at the health center, i.e. nurses trained in emergency obstetric care detect obstetrical emergencies such as mal-presentation, cord prolapse and others, then the mother is referred to the district hospital and transported using a Ministry of Health ambulance. District hospitals are equipped with obstetrical theatres, trained personnel and equipment to perform cesarean delivery, the recommended procedure for high-risk labor. Some health centers have their own ambulance (including 11 out of 46 health centers in the three study districts) and the remaining health centers call to the district hospital for assistance. After being admitted to the district hospital, a midwife or nurse will assess the pregnant woman and determine whether a cesarean section should be considered. A general practitioner makes the final decision for a cesarean section and leads the procedure.

In 2015, there were 7569 deliveries at the three district hospitals. Of all deliveries, 39% were through cesarean section and were considered high risk as they were referred from health centers due to complications or previous complications. More than 90% of deliveries are performed by skilled doctors, nurses and midwives [11]. These hospitals are staffed with 11–20 midwives, 73–90 nurses and 9–14 general practitioners. In the maternity department, two nurses or midwives staff the delivery room during the day or night. One general practitioner is assigned to delivery room during the day, but at night, one general practitioner services the whole of maternity department. Each of the three district hospitals is equipped with at least two operating tables, basic anesthesia equipment and supplies to deliver regional and general anesthesia, four obstetrics tables, thirty ward beds, six incubators and two lamps. A mother who has community-based health insurance is responsible for 10% of the total cost, with the remaining 90% paid by the government. Otherwise, the mother is responsible for all related delivery costs.

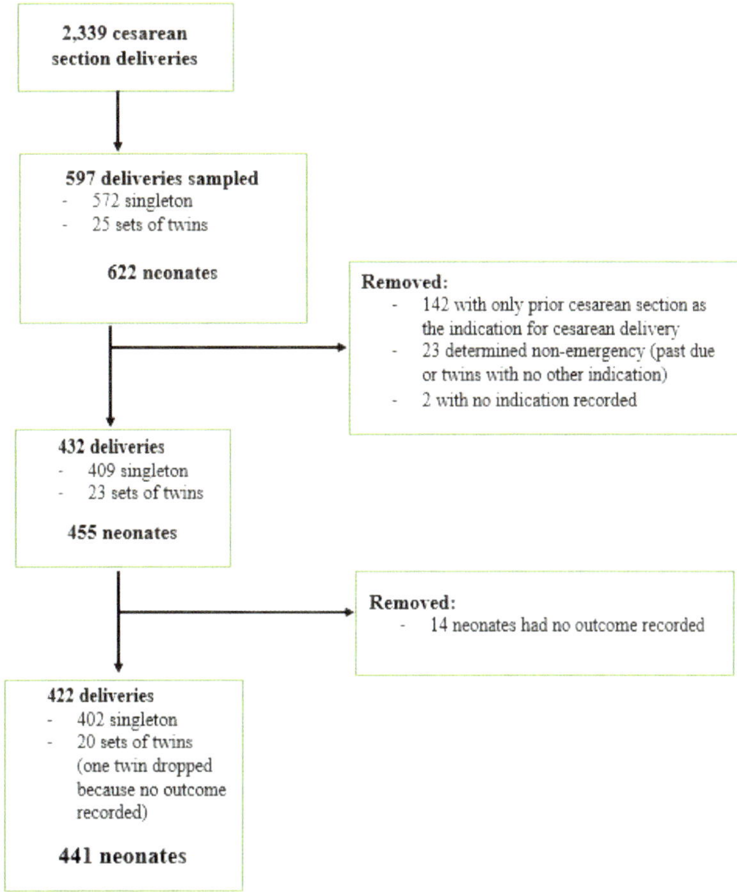

Fig. 1 Flow diagram of chart review

Study design and population

This retrospective cross-sectional study included neonates born to mothers undergoing emergency cesarean section between 01 January and 31 December 2015 at Butaro, Kirehe and Rwinkwavu District Hospitals. Due to the large population of cesarean deliveries at the district hospitals and insufficient resources to collect data on all deliveries, we randomly sampled 200 cesarean deliveries per hospital.

The study's inclusion criterion was emergency cesarean delivery without intrauterine death prior to the decision for cesarean section. Women who received elective cesarean section and those with non-emergent indications for cesarean section were excluded. For sample selection, because the majority of cesarean sections at district hospitals are due to the referral of complicated cases from health centers, we first assumed all cesarean section deliveries were emergency and used segmented sampling to sample 200 women in each hospital. Authors NN and YL led the sampling procedures. All cesarean section charts were grouped by month, a sampling interval determined and charts selected by skipping the interval. During sampling, women who had scheduled or requested for cesarean delivery (charts marked elective) and women with neonatal intrauterine death prior to the decision to conduct the cesarean section were removed and randomly replaced with other women who met inclusion criteria from same month of hospital admission. A total of 597 cesarean deliveries were sampled. During data cleaning, we excluded women with no indication that the cesarean delivery was truly emergent (this included women whose only indication was prior cesarean delivery and women who were post-term or with twins but no other emergent indication). The following diagnoses were considered emergent and included in the study: uterine rupture, fetal distress, cord prolapse, abruption placenta, preeclampsia prolonged rupture of membranes, cephalo-pelvic disproportion, prolonged labor, and mal-presentation.

Data collection and analysis

Demographic and clinical characteristics of mothers and neonates as well as neonatal outcomes were extracted from charts into a pretested data collection form. Data were then transferred into an Access electronic database. Travel time from health center to district hospital was

Table 1 Demographic characteristics of mothers undergoing emergency cesarean section delivery ($N = 441$)

Variable	Number	Percent
District hospital		
Butaro	161	36.5
Kirehe	139	31.5
Rwinkwavu	141	32.0
Mother's age group	$N = 435$	
15–24	176	40.5
25–34	189	43.4
35+	70	16.1
Number of previous pregnancies	$N = 438$	
0	176	40.2
1–3	183	41.8
4+	79	18.0
Mother's marital status	$N = 404$	
Single	32	7.9
Ever married	372	92.1
Mother's weight	$N = 365$	
≤ 50 kg	24	6.6
51–80 kg	329	90.1
> 80 kg	12	3.3
Occupation	$N = 409$	
Farmer	373	91.2
Employed	22	5.4
Unemployed	14	3.4
Insurance	$N = 415$	
Community based health insurance	377	90.8
Private insurance	26	6.3
None	12	2.9
Travel time from health center to the hospital[a]	$N = 356$	
Health center attached to the hospital	91	25.6
30–60 min	200	56.2
> 60 min	65	18.2

[a]Travel time measured as average number of minutes for ambulance to travel from the health center to the district hospital

calculated using an average estimate of the time for an ambulance to travel from the mother's health center of first presentation to the district hospital. We could not obtain an actual measure for a specific mother's travel time as that information is not routinely collected. The severity of the indication for cesarean section was classified into two categories, very severe and severe, based on complication to the fetus and through consultation with a local obstetrician. Very severe indication included uterine rupture, fetal distress, cord prolapse, and abruption placenta and severe indication included preeclampsia, prolonged rupture of membranes, cephalo-pelvic

Table 2 Clinical characteristics of mothers and neonatal outcomes ($N = 441$)

Clinical characteristics	Number	Percent
Number of fetuses		
1	402	91.2
2	39	8.8
Gestational age	$N = 366$	
< 38 weeks	59	16.1
38–42 weeks	284	77.6
> 42 weeks	23	6.3
Duration of contractions prior to admission	$N = 279$	
≤ 12 h	83	29.7
13–24 h	113	40.5
> 24 h	83	29.8
Fetal heart rate at admission (bpm)	$N = 429$	
< 120	59	13.8
120–160	352	82.1
> 160	18	4.2
Maternal blood pressure at admission (SBP/DBP)	$N = 397$	
Hypotensive (<90/<50)	2	0.5
Normal (90–140/50–90)	368	92.7
Hypertensive (>140/>90)	27	6.8
Oxygen saturation on admission	$N = 216$	
Low saturation (≤94%)	7	3.2
Normal saturation (>94%)	209	96.8
Hemoglobin level (grams/deciliter)	$N = 285$	
Low (<12)	48	16.8
Normal (12–16)	231	81.1
Above range (>16)	6	2.1
History of prior cesarean section	$N = 349$	
No	220	63.0
Yes	129	37.0
Indications for cesarean section		
Fetal distress	141	32.0
Prolonged labor	135	30.6
Prior cesarean section	129	29.3
Malpresentation	108	24.5
Cephalopelvic disproportion	69	15.6
Prolonged rupture of membranes	46	7.9
Placenta previa	21	4.8
Intra-uterine rupture	7	1.6
Cord prolapse	6	1.4
Preeclampsia	6	1.4
Abruption placenta	5	1.1
Number of indications per woman		
Single indications	238	54.0
2 indications	179	40.6
3+ indications	24	5.4

Table 2 Clinical characteristics of mothers and neonatal outcomes ($N = 441$) *(Continued)*

Severity of cesarean indication		
Very severe indication[a]	180	40.8
Severe indication[b]	261	59.2
Neonatal clinical outcome		
Alive and APGAR ≥ 7	401	91.0
Died, or APGAR < 7	40	9.0

SBP Systolic blood pressure
DBP Diastolic blood pressure
[a]Very severe indication was defined as intrauterine rupture, fetal distress, cord prolapse, and abruptio placentae
[b]Severe indication was defined as preeclampsia, prolonged rupture of membranes, cephalo-pelvic disproportion, prolonged labor and mal-presentation

disproportion, prolonged labor, and mal-presentation. In the case of more than one indication, we categorized according to the most severe indication. Neonatal outcome was dichotomized into poor neonatal outcome, defined as either death within 24 h or an APGAR score less than 7 at 5 min, or good neonatal outcome, defined as alive with an APGAR greater than or equal to 7 at 5 min.

We described mothers' demographic and clinical characteristics using frequencies and percentages for categorical data. We tested each variable's relationship to neonatal outcome using a Chi-squared test or in the case of small cell counts, a Fisher's exact test. Factors significant at $\alpha = 0.20$ level were retained for consideration in the multivariate logistic regression model. We developed the final model using backward stepwise selection, such that only factors significant at $\alpha = 0.05$ significance level were retained in the final model. We report odds ratios (ORs), 95% confidence intervals (95%CIs) and p-values. For univariate and bivariate analyses, missing data were ignored, but we reported a reduced sample size in the case of missing data. For multivariate analysis, if a variable was missing for 15% or more observations, then we included a missing category in the model. All analyses considered the neonate as the unit of analysis and were completed in Stata v14.0 (College Station, TX: StataCorp LP).

Results

In 2015, a total of 2,339 mothers underwent emergency cesarean section, of which 597 were randomly sampled, corresponding to 622 neonates (Fig. 1). Of these, 422 deliveries, corresponding to 441 neonates, were confirmed to have emergent conditions and had neonatal outcome recorded. For the 435 neonates with mother's ages recorded, 189 (43.4%) were born to mothers between 25–34 years old (Table 1). One hundred and eighty-three neonates (41.8% of 438) were born to women with 1–3 prior pregnancies. Most neonates had mothers with community-based health insurance (377 out of 415, 90.9%). For the 356 neonates with information about travel time from the health center to the district hospital, 91 (25.5%) were from health centers attached to a district hospital, 200 (56.1%) were from health centers between 30–60 min travel time to the district hospital, and 65 (18.2%) were from health centers with over 60 min travel time to get to the district hospital.

Of the 441 neonates, 402 (91.1%) were singleton births (Table 2). For the 336 neonates with gestational age recorded, 59 (16.1%) were less than 38 weeks of gestational age. One hundred and twenty-nine neonates (37.0% of 349) were born to mothers with a history of prior cesarean delivery. The most common indications for cesarean section included fetal distress (32.0%, 141) and prolonged labor (30.6%, 135) and for 203 (46.0%) neonates, their mothers had multiple indications for cesarean delivery. For 180 (40.8%) neonates, the mother presented with a very severe indication for emergency cesarean section and 40 (9.0%) neonates either died or had an APGAR < 7 at 5 min post-delivery.

In the bivariate analysis, five maternal factors were associated with neonatal outcomes (Table 3). These included number of prior pregnancies ($p = 0.057$), mother's weight ($p = 0.060$), travel time from health center to district hospital ($p = 0.022$), number of fetuses ($p = 0.148$), and severity of cesarean section indication ($p = 0.064$). For the multivariate analysis, three of these factors remained significantly associated with neonatal outcomes (Table 4). Neonates born to mothers with four or more prior deliveries had higher odds of having a poor outcome as compared to neonates of mothers with 1–3 prior deliveries (OR = 3.01, 95% CI: 1.23, 7.35, $p = 0.015$). A longer ambulance travel time from health center to hospital was associated with worse neonatal outcomes compared to neonates of mothers coming from health centers attached to the district hospital (OR = 3.80, 95% CI: 1.07, 13.40, $p = 0.038$ for 30–60 min and OR = 5.82, 95% CI: 1.47, 23.05, $p = 0.012$ for 60 min or more). Neonates whose mothers presented with very severe indication had significantly worse outcomes compared to those whose mothers had severe indication (OR = 2.24, 95% CI: 1.11, 4.52, $p = 0.023$).

Discussion

Our study included 441 neonates born via emergency cesarean delivery, of which 9.0% died or had an APGAR score of less than seven at 5 min. This is comparable to outcomes in Africa where a study by the World Health Organization showed an average neonatal death rate of 12.9% after cesarean section [3]. Poor neonatal outcomes were associated with a mother having four or more previous deliveries, longer travel times from the health center to the district hospital, and having a very severe indication for cesarean delivery. The latter result is not surprising, given that the creation of this category was

Table 3 Bivariate analysis of neonatal outcomes

	Alive and APGAR ≥ 7 (*N* = 401)		Died, or APGAR < 7 (*N* = 40)		
	n	%	n	%	*p*-value
District hospital					
Butaro	147	91.3	14	8.7	0.486
Kirehe	128	92.2	10	7.2	
Rwinkwavu	125	88.7	16	11.3	
Mother's age group	(*N* = 395)				
15–24	163	92.6	13	7.4	0.392
25–34	171	90.5	18	9.5	
35+	61	87.1	9	12.9	
Number of prior pregnancies			(*N* = 37)		
0	162	92.1	14	87.9	0.057
1–3	172	94.0	11	6.0	
4+	67	84.8	12	15.2	
History of prior cesarean section	(*N* = 320)		(*N* = 29)		
No	199	90.5	21	9.5	0.320
Yes	121	93.8	8	6.2	
Mother's marital status	(*N* = 371)		(*N* = 33)		
Single	28	87.5	4	12.5	0.317
Ever married	343	92.2	29	7.8	
Mother's weight	(*N* = 333)		(*N* = 32)		
≤ 50 kg	21	87.5	3	12.5	0.060
51–80 kg	303	92.1	31	7.9	
> 80 kg	9	75.0	3	25.0	
Occupation	(*N* = 372)		(*N* = 37)		
Farmer	338	90.6	35	9.3	0.261
Employed	22	100.0	0	0.0	
Unemployed	12	85.7	2	14.3	
Insurance	(*N* = 379)		(*N* = 36)		
Community based health insurance	344	91.2	33	8.8	>0.999
Private insurance	24	92.3	2	7.7	
None	11	91.7	1	8.3	
Travel time from health center to the hospital[c]	(*N* = 321)		(*N* = 37)		
Health center attached to the hospital	88	96.7	5	3.3	0.022
30–60 min	178	89.0	22	11.0	
> 60 min	55	84.6	10	15.4	
Number of fetuses			(*N* = 39)		
1	368	91.5	33	8.5	0.148
2	33	84.6	6	15.4	
Gestational age					
< 38 weeks	54	91.5	5	8.5	0.936
38–42 weeks	262	92.2	22	7.8	
> 42 weeks	85	86.7	13	13.3	

Table 3 Bivariate analysis of neonatal outcomes *(Continued)*

Duration of contractions prior to admission	(*N* = 258)		(*N* = 21)		
≤ 12 h	75	90.4	8	9.6	0.656
13–24 h	106	93.8	7	6.2	
> 24 h	77	92.8	6	7.2	
Maternal blood pressure at admission (SBP/DBP)	(*N* = 365)		(*N* = 32)		
Hypotension (<90/<50)	2	100.0	0	0.0	0.374
Normal (90–140/50–90)	340	92.4	28	7.6	
Hypertension (>140/>90)	23	85.2	4	14.8	
Oxygen saturation on admission	(*N* = 195)		(*N* = 21)		
Low saturation (≤94%)	6	85.7	1	14.3	0.516
Normal saturation (>94%)	189	90.4	20	9.6	
Hemoglobin level (grams/deciliter)	(*N* = 254)		(*N* = 31)		
Low (<12)	42	87.5	6	12.5	0.582
Normal (12–16)	207	89.6	24	10.4	
Above range (>16)	5	83.3	1	16.7	
Severity of cesarean section indication					
Very severe indication[a]	158	87.8	22	12.2	0.064
Severe indication[b]	243	93.1	18	6.9	

SBP Systolic blood pressure
DBP Diastolic blood pressure
[a]Very severe indication included intrauterine rupture, fetal distress, cord prolapse and abruptio placentae
[b]Severe indication was defined as preeclampsia, prolonged rupture of membranes, cephalo-pelvic disproportion, prolonged labor and mal-presentation
[c]Travel time measured as average number of minutes for ambulance to travel from the health center to the district hospital

Table 4 Multivariate analysis of maternal factors as predictors of neonatal outcomes

Variables	OR	95% CI	*p*-value
Number of pregnancies			
0	1.40	[0.60, 3.23]	0.431
1–3	Ref	-	-
4+	3.01	[1.23, 7.35]	0.015
Travel time from the health center to the hospital[c]			
Health center attached to the hospital	Ref	-	-
30–60 min	3.80	[1.07, 13.40]	0.038
> 60 min	5.82	[1.47, 23.05]	0.012
Unknown	2.12	[0.48, 9.35]	0.317
Severity of cesarean section indication			
Very severe indication[a]	2.24	[1.11, 4.52]	0.023
Severe indication[b]	Ref	-	-

[a]Very severe indication included intrauterine rupture, fetal distress, cord prolapse, abruptio placentae
[b]Severe indication was defined as preeclampsia, prolonged rupture of membranes, cephalo-pelvic disproportion, prolonged labor and mal-presentation
[c]Travel time measured as average number of minutes for ambulance to travel from the health center to the district hospital

based on previous knowledge of associated risks for certain complications [15]. However, we recommend continued sensitization and support for health center nurses, for example through the emergency obstetric conditions training [8] or the maternal health mentorship program [16] as well as improving health center diagnostic capacities to quickly identify very severe indications so as to provide timely referral.

Previous studies in sub-Saharan Africa have linked longer travel distance to a main road or to the hospital with higher risks of mortality for neonates and children under five years [17, 18]. Rwandan Ministry of Health's 2014 Health Sector Policy emphasized the decentralization of health facilities with a target to ensure that all people have access to a health center within 5 km of their homes [19]. However, currently health centers lack staff and facilities and are not mandated by Rwanda Ministry of Health to perform cesarean sections and there are only one or two district hospitals in each district, which leads to women having to travel longer distances to seek emergency obstetric care. Moreover, poor and difficult road networks were shown to be associated with delay in reaching health facility where needed level of care is available and contribute to poor neonatal outcome [20]. Thus, the variable considered in this study, travel time from the health center to the district hospital, while not the exact measure of the woman's travel to time to the hospital and likely underestimating the total travel time, is of particular importance in this context, since a pregnant woman must go first to her catchment area health center prior to going to the district hospital. Ambulances should be used to transport emergency patients from health centers to the district hospital, but the availability of ambulances is not always confirmed. Improving road networks would lessen difficulties and travel time to district hospitals for laboring mothers. In the short term, we recommend an improved referral system for emergency obstetric cases as well as ensuring the availability of ambulances at remote health centers to shorten travel times and improve neonatal outcome. In the long run, increasing the number of hospitals per district with facilities and staff to provide emergency obstetric care may reduce travel time and hence the negative effect of longer travels time on neonatal outcome.

Our finding that neonates born to mothers with four or more previous pregnancies were more likely to have bad outcomes is consistent with a study conducted in Nigeria [21]. Although this could reflect the association between increased number of pregnancies and advanced maternal age, which is an established risk factor for poor neonatal outcomes in general [22–24], our analyses that explored mother's age directly did not find an association between maternal age and neonatal outcome. Women who have many pregnancies are often times poorer and less educated [25], and both poverty and low education have been linked to poor neonatal outcomes in sub-Saharan Africa [26]. Finally, previous pregnancies can lead to faster progression of labor [27], and this may lead to precipitated labor that can negatively affect neonatal outcome, if the cesarean section is not immediately available. The link between previous number of deliveries and risk for poor neonatal outcomes among emergency cesarean deliveries should be studied further.

There are several limitations to be considered in this study. Given that this study was retrospective and relied on routinely collected clinical data, some variables such as height of the mother to determine body mass index, income, education levels, nutrition status and tobacco or alcohol use were not available for analysis. Additionally, some of our existing variables had missing data from the chart review. Unfortunately, inadequate documentation is often seen in these settings, and proper documentation should be encouraged for clinical care and future studies. Finally, this study was conducted at district hospitals supported by Partners In Health, whereas other hospitals do not receive this support. However, the population profile and pathways to cesarean delivery are similar to other district hospitals in Rwanda and sub-Saharan Africa and therefore we believe the results are generalizable beyond this population.

Conclusions

Poor neonatal outcomes were linked to longer travel time to district hospitals, mothers having multiple previous pregnancies, and a very severe indication for cesarean delivery. While it is infeasible to provide cesarean sections in health centers in the near future, increasing the number of district hospitals and improving timely access to transport to district hospitals should be considered. Furthermore, it is important to increase the capacity of health centers to diagnose very severe indications for cesarean delivery, and provide regular mentorship to the health center nurses so as to improve time to intervention. Future studies should assess effect of fetal factors and time delays and compare outcomes between cesarean and vaginal deliveries.

Abbreviations

APGAR: Appearance, pulse, grimace, activity, respiration; CI: Confidence interval; IRB: Institutional review board; MOH: Ministry of health; OR: Odds ratio; P: P value; RDHS: Rwanda demographic health survey.

Acknowledgements

We acknowledge Partners In Health/Inshuti Mu Buzima for the support of this work. This study was developed under the Partners In Health/Inshuti Mu Buzima Intermediate Operational Research Training Program, developed and facilitated by Bethany Hedt-Gauthier and Jackline Odhiambo. In addition, Yihan Lin, Theoneste Nkurunziza and Robert Riviello provided direct mentorship to this paper as part of this training. We also acknowledge the contributions of Bahati Ramadhan, Steven Rutegera, Laetitia Uzakunda, Theodette Nyirasabwa, Epimaque Habimana and Alice Bayingana for data collection.

Funding

All data collection and training costs were covered by the Harvard Global Health Initiative Burke Global Health Fellowship grant. Some training facilitators and mentors are Rwanda Human Resources for Health faculty, funded with the support of the Government of Rwanda, the Global Fund to fight AIDS, Tuberculosis and Malaria and Centers for Disease Control and Prevention. BHG received support from the Harvard Medical School Global Health Research Core.

Authors' contributions

NN and CUM led the study design, protocol development, data analysis and manuscript writing. YL, BHG, JO, TN and RR contributed to study design, protocol development and data analysis and results interpretation. NN, YL and JO led and supervised data collection and BHG and YL led data cleaning. JM, MM, SR, IU, FN and PN supported protocol development and reviewed drafts of the manuscript. All authors critically reviewed drafts of the manuscript and will approve the final manuscript for publication.

Competing interests

The authors declare that they have no competing interest.

Author details

[1]Partners In Health, Inshuti Mu Buzima, KigaliP.O. Box: 3432Rwanda. [2]College of Medicine and Health Sciences, University of Rwanda, Kigali, Rwanda. [3]Department of Global Health and Social Medicine, Harvard Medical School, Boston, USA. [4]University of Colorado School of Medicine, Colorado, USA. [5]Brigham and Women's Hospital, Boston, USA. [6]Partners In Health, Boston, USA. [7]Ministry of Health, Kigali, Rwanda.

References

1. Molina G, Weiser TG, Lipsitz SR, Esquivel MM, Uribe-Leitz T, Azad T, et al. Relationship Between Cesarean Delivery Rate and Maternal and Neonatal Mortality. JAMA. 2015;314(21):2263–70.
2. MacDorman MF, Declercq E, Menacker F, Malloy MH. Infant and neonatal mortality for primary cesarean and vaginal births to women with "no indicated risk", United States, 1998–2001 birth cohorts. Birth. 2006;33(3):175–82.
3. Shah A, Fawole BM, Imunya JM, Amokrane F, Nafiou I, Wolomby JJ, et al. Cesarean delivery outcomes from the WHO global survey on maternal and perinatal health in Africa. Int J Gynecol Obstet. 2009;107(3):191–7.
4. Harrison MS, Goldenberg RL. Cesarean section in sub-Saharan Africa. Maternal Health, Neonatology and. Perinatology. 2016;2(1):6.
5. Cavallaro FL, Cresswell JA, França VA, Victora CG, Barros JD. Trends in Caesarean Delivery by Country and Wealth Quintile : Cross-sectional Surveys in Southern Asia and sub-Saharan Africa. Bull World Health Organ. 2013; 91(August 2013):914–22.
6. Yeekian C, Jesadapornchai S, Urairong K, Santibenjakul S, Suksong W, Nuchprayoon C. Comparison of maternal factors and neonatal outcomes between elective cesarean section and spontaneous vaginal delivery. J Med Assoc Thai. 2013;96(4):389–94.
7. Foumane P, Mando E, Mboudou ET, Sama JD, Pisoh WD, Minkande JZ. Outcome of cesarean delivery in women with excessive weight gain during pregnancy. Open J Obstet Gynecol. 2014;4(3):139.
8. Manasyan A, Pasha O, Chomba E, Goudar SS, Mcclure EM, Derman RJ, et al. Assessment of Obstetric and Neonatal Health Services in Developing Country Health Facilities. Am J Perinatol. 2013;30(9):787–94.
9. Abdissa Z, Awoke T, Belayneh T, Tefera Y. Birth outcome after caesarean section among mothers who delivered by caesarean section under general and spinal anesthesia at Gondar University teaching hospital north-west Ethiopia. J Anesth Clin Res. 2013;4(7):4–8.
10. Gori F, Pasqualucci A, Corradetti F, Milli M, Peduto V. Maternal and neonatal outcome after cesarean section: the impact of anesthesia. J Matern Fetal Neonatal Med. 2007;20(1):53–7. doi:10.1080/14767050601134645.
11. National Institute of Statistics of Rwanda (NISR) [Rwanda], Ministry of Health (MOH) [Rwanda], and ICF International. Rwanda Demographic and Health Survey 2014-15. Rockville: NISR, MOH, and ICF International; 2015. http://dhsprogram.com/publications/publication-fr316-dhs-final-reports.cfm. Accessed 12 Jan 2017.
12. Rwanda Ministry of Health. Rwanda Health Statistics Booklet 2011. Rwanda Ministry of Health Annual Health Statistics Booklet, 2012;(August), 37.
13. Petroze RT, Nzayisenga A, Rusanganwa V, Ntakiyiruta G, Calland JF. Comprehensive national analysis of emergency and essential surgical capacity in Rwanda. Br J Surg. 2012;99(3):436–43.
14. National Institute of Statistics of Rwanda (NISR) [Rwanda], Ministry of Health (MOH) [Rwanda], and ICF International. Rwanda Demographic and Health Survey 2010. Calverton: NISR, MOH, and ICF International; 2012. http://dhsprogram.com/publications/publication-fr259-dhs-final-reports.cfm. Accessed 12 Jan 2017.
15. Backes CH, Markham K, Moorehead P, Cordero L, Nankervis C, Giannone PJ. Maternal preeclampsia and neonatal outcomes. J Pregnancy. 2011; 214365. doi: 10.1155/2011/214365.
16. Manzi A, Magge H, Hedt-Gauthie B, Michaelis AP, Cyamatare FR, Nyirazinyoye L, et al. Clinical mentorship to improve pediatric quality of care at the health centers in rural Rwanda: a qualitative study of perceptions and acceptability of health care workers. BMC Health Serv Res. 2014;14(1):275.
17. Kadobera D, Sartorius B, Masanja H, Mathew A, Waiswa P. The effect of distance to formal health facility on childhood mortality in rural Tanzania, 2005-2007. Glob Health Action. 2012;5:1–9.
18. Assefa N, Lakew Y, Belay B, Kedir H, Zelalem D, Baraki N, et al. Neonatal mortality and causes of death in Kersa Health and Demographic Surveillance System (Kersa HDSS), Ethiopia, 2008–2013. Maternal Health, Neonatology and. Perinatology. 2016;2(1):7.
19. Republic of Rwanda, Ministry of Health. Health Sector Policy. 2015. http://www.moh.gov.rw/fileadmin/templates/policies/Health_Sector_Policy___19th_January_2015.pdf. Accessed 12 Jan 2017.
20. Waiswa P, Kallander K, Peterson S, Tomson G, Pariyo GW. Using the three delays model to understand why newborn babies die in eastern Uganda. Trop Med Int Health. 2010;15(8):964–72.
21. Olusanya BO. Perinatal outcomes of multiple births in southwest Nigeria. J Health Popul Nutr. 2011;29(6):639–47.
22. Jacobsson B, Ladfors L, Milsom I. Advanced Maternal Age and Adverse Perinatal Outcome. Obstet Gynecol. 2004;104(4):727–33.
23. Carolan M, Frankowska D. Advanced maternal age and adverse perinatal outcome: A review of the evidence. Midwifery. 2011;27(6):793–801.
24. Laopaiboon M, Lumbiganon P, Intarut N, Mori R, Ganchimeg T, Vogel JP, et al. Advanced maternal age and pregnancy outcomes: a multicountry assessment. BJOG. 2014;121 Suppl:49–56.
25. Uthman OA, Uthman MB, Yahaya I. A population-based study of effect of multiple birth on infant mortality in Nigeria. BMC Pregnancy Childbirth. 2008;8:41.
26. Kinney MV, Kerber KJ, Black RE, Cohen B, Nkrumah F, Coovadia H, et al. Sub-Saharan Africa's mothers, newborns, and children: Where and why do they die? PLoS Med. 2010;7(6):1–9.
27. Zaki MN, Hibbard JU, Kominiarek MA. Contemporary labor patterns and maternal age. Obstet Gynecol. 2013;122(5):1018–24.

3

Maternal diet quality and nutrient intake in the gestational period: results from the delta healthy sprouts comparative impact trial

Lisa M. Tussing-Humphreys[1*], Jessica L. Thomson[2], Melissa H. Goodman[2] and Sarah Olender[1]

Abstract

Background: A woman's diet while pregnant can play an important role in her reproductive health as well as the health of her unborn child. Diet quality and nutrient intake amongst pregnant women residing in the rural Lower Mississippi Delta (LMD) region of the United States is inadequate. The Delta Healthy Sprouts Project was designed to test the comparative impact of two home visiting programs on weight status, dietary intake, and health behaviors of women and their infants residing in the LMD region. This paper reports results pertaining to maternal diet quality and nutrient intake in the gestational period.

Methods: The experimental arm (PATE) received monthly home visits beginning in the second trimester using the Parents as Teachers curriculum enhanced with a nutrition and lifestyle behavior curriculum. The control arm (PAT) received monthly home visits using the Parents as Teachers curriculum only. Maternal diet was assessed via 24-h dietary recall at gestational months (GM) 4 (baseline), 6, and 8. Diet quality was computed using the Healthy Eating Index-2010 (HEI-2010).

Results: Gestational period retention rates for PAT and PATE arms were 77 % (33/43) and 67 % (26/39), respectively. Significant effects were not found for time, treatment, or time by treatment for the HEI-2010 total or component scores, macro- or micronutrient intake or percentage of women meeting recommended nutrient intakes.

Conclusions: Perhaps due to low participant enrollment and higher than expected rates of drop out and noncompliance, we were not able to demonstrate that the enhanced nutrition and lifestyle curriculum (PATE) intervention had a significant effect on diet quality or nutrient intake during pregnancy in this cohort of rural, Southern, primarily African American women.

Keywords: Maternal diet quality, Pregnancy, African American women

Background

A woman's diet throughout pregnancy can play an important role in her reproductive health as well as the health of her unborn child [1]. Modest increases in energy intake in the 2nd and 3rd trimester and greater intake of several micronutrients including iron and folate throughout the gestational period are necessary to support a healthy pregnancy. Sub-optimal maternal nutrition is linked to adverse pregnancy outcomes including excessive maternal weight gain, the development of gestational complications including gestational diabetes mellitus, increased rates of preterm birth, infant growth restriction, and maternal and infant morbidity and mortality [2, 3].

Historically, research examining maternal diet has focused on the adequate intake of single nutrients during the gestational period [4, 5]. Although specific nutrients

* Correspondence: ltussing@uic.edu
[1]Department of Medicine and Cancer Center, University of Illinois at Chicago, 1747 W Roosevelt Road, #416, Chicago, IL 60618, USA
Full list of author information is available at the end of the article

are indeed critical during pregnancy, nutritional research has shifted away from examining single nutrients and has begun to focus on examining the relationship between overall diet, specifically maternal diet quality, and maternal and fetal health [6]. This approach allows for the examination of total diet and the synergy of nutrients eaten together from various foodstuffs [7]. Relatively few studies have examined associations between maternal diet quality and pregnancy related outcomes [5]. However, there is some evidence that consuming a higher quality diet in the gestational period is associated with a reduction in maternal depressive symptoms [8], lower maternal fasting plasma glucose and reduced risk for gestational diabetes mellitus [9], and reduced risk for preeclampsia [10]. A recent summary of the limited but existing evidence suggests that a high-quality maternal diet consumed throughout the gestational period may reduce the risk for preterm birth, infant growth restriction, and fetal anomalies including neural tube defects [5]. Thus, interventions designed to optimize maternal diet during the gestational period have the potential to positively impact both maternal and fetal health.

One method to assess diet quality in pregnancy is to determine a woman's adherence to the Dietary Guidelines for Americans (DGAs) [11] using the Healthy Eating Index (HEI) [12]. The HEI was designed by the United States Department of Agriculture, Center for Nutrition Policy and Promotion, to monitor diet quality in the United States (US) population and is appropriate for monitoring diet quality in at-risk low income subpopulations. The HEI ranges from 0 to 100 points with scores above 80 points indicative of a higher quality diet. In non-pregnant adults, a higher HEI score has been associated with lower total and cause-specific mortality [13] and lower prevalence of metabolic syndrome [14]. The HEI has been used successfully to assess diet quality in pregnancy [15]. However, Pick and colleagues noted that HEI failed to pick up inadequate micronutrient intake in a cohort of pregnant women. This finding suggests that when measuring diet quality in pregnancy, HEI may need to be modified to include key micronutrients (i.e., iron, folate, and calcium) [3, 16] or used in conjunction with more detailed nutrient intake data [17, 18].

The Lower Mississippi Delta (LMD) region of Mississippi is characterized by low education attainment and high rates of both poverty and chronic diseases including hypertension and obesity [19] and constitutes a majority African American population. Reproductive age women residing in this region suffer from some of the highest rates of adverse pregnancy-related outcomes in the US including maternal mortality, infant mortality, preterm birth, and low infant birth weight [20, 21]. Women of lower socioeconomic status, such as those residing in the LMD region, are at risk of being undernourished when they enter pregnancy due to poor diet and shorter intervals between pregnancies which can adversely impact a woman's nutritional state both preconception and during pregnancy [22]. We recently reported that maternal diet quality and nutrient intake in the early 2nd trimester amongst pregnant women residing in the LMD region is strikingly inadequate [23]. Overall, these women had very poor adherence to the 2010 DGAs based on HEI, and only a limited number of women met nutrient intake recommendations for fiber, sodium, calcium or choline. This was largely attributed to their low consumption of greens and beans, fruit, whole grains, and seafood and plant proteins – foods which have relatively high micronutrient and fiber, and low saturated fat and sodium contents. Given that poor maternal nutrition can affect not only the woman but her growing fetus, the diets of these women deserve considerable attention. Clearly, there is a need for interventions in the LMD region that are designed to help women achieve optimal nutrition through improved diet quality and nutrient intake throughout pregnancy.

The Delta Healthy Sprouts Project was designed to test the comparative impact of two maternal, infant, and early childhood home visiting programs on weight status, dietary intake, and health behaviors of women and their infants residing in the rural LMD region of Mississippi [24]. Results of the primary outcome, gestational weight gain, have been previously reported (Thomson, under review). This paper describes and compares the dietary intake outcomes of Delta Healthy Sprouts participants during the gestational period.

Methods

Design and recruitment

This was a longitudinal analysis of the Delta Healthy Sprouts participants' diet behaviors measured at the baseline [enrollment; gestational month (GM) 4] visit and two subsequent gestational (GM 6 and 8) visits. A comprehensive description of the Delta Healthy Sprouts Project has been published elsewhere [24]. Briefly, 82 pregnant women were enrolled in this on-going project conducted in three LMD counties. Inclusion criteria included female gender, at least 18 years of age, less than 19 weeks pregnant with first, second or third child, singleton pregnancy, and resident of Washington, Bolivar, or Humphreys County in Mississippi. Participant enrollment occurred on a rolling basis; hence baseline data were collected between March 2013 and December 2014. The target enrollment was 75 women in each of the two arms (control and experimental) of the project. The sample size of 150 women was based on the following assumptions: 20 % attrition rate, 37 % of control participants with GWG within the Institute of Medicine (IOM) recommendations, and a 22 % difference between treatment arms for GWG within recommendations [24]. However, recruitment was stopped by the study's

Principal Investigator prior to reaching these numbers due to unexpected difficulties recruiting pregnant women meeting study criteria. Recruitment was extended as long as possible, but fiscal issues eventually necessitated the closing of this period. Figure 1 illustrates the CONSORT diagram.

The project was approved by the Institutional Review Board of Delta State University, Cleveland MS (#12-024) and all participants gave written informed consent prior to any study engagement. Delta Healthy Sprouts is registered at clinicaltrials.gov (NCT01746394).

Delta Healthy Sprouts is evaluating the impact of the Parents as Teachers® (PAT) curriculum compared to a nutrition and physical activity enhanced PAT curriculum (PATE) on the primary outcomes of maternal gestational weight gain and postpartum weight control and childhood obesity prevention. Secondary outcomes pertain to maternal diet quality and nutrient intake during the gestational and postpartum periods, maternal physical activity, breast feeding and child feeding practices and other child-health related outcomes. Parents as Teachers is a nationally recognized, evidence based, home visiting program that seeks to increase parental knowledge of child development, improve parenting practices, provide early detection of developmental delays, prevent child abuse, and increase school readiness [25]. Participants were randomly assigned to one of two treatment arms [PAT control ($n = 43$) or PATE experimental ($n = 39$)] and are being followed for 18 months (6 months gestation and 12 months postnatal). At the baseline (GM 4) visit, demographic data and anthropometric measures were collected, 24-h dietary recalls were conducted, and physical activity and other questionnaires were administered.

Intervention

The control arm of the intervention is based on the PAT curriculum that includes one-on-one home visits, developmental screenings, and a resource network for families. Home visitation is the key component of the

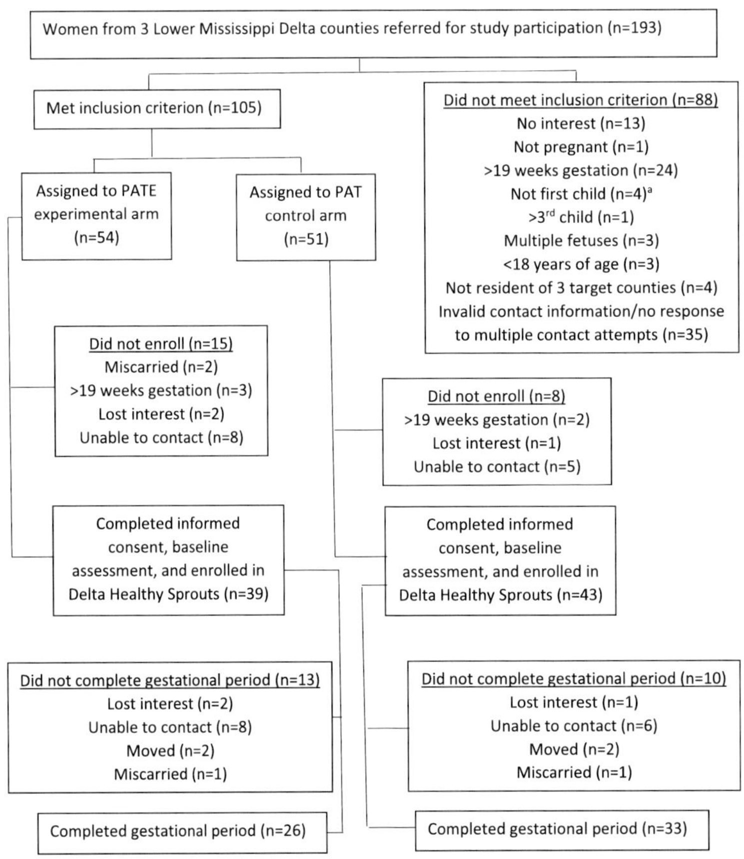

[a] Original exclusion criterion; later changed to pregnant with > 3rd child.

PAT, Parents as Teachers; PATE, Parents as Teachers Enhanced.

Fig. 1 CONSORT diagram of recruitment, assignment, enrollment, and completion of gestational period for Delta Healthy Sprouts Project. [a] Original exclusion criterion; later changed to pregnant with > 3rd child

PAT model where Parent Educators provide parents with research based information and activities. Materials are tailored to the age of the child and are responsive to parental information requests.

The experimental arm of the intervention builds upon the PAT curriculum by adding culturally tailored, maternal weight management and early childhood obesity prevention components. These features are based upon foundational elements from the Diabetes Prevention Program (DPP) and the Infant Feeding Activity and Nutrition Trial (InFANT). Elements based upon the DPP principles included a flexible, culturally sensitive, individualized educational curriculum taught on a one-to-one basis [26]. Elements taken from InFANT included anticipatory guidance and parenting support principles [27]. Anticipatory guidance involves providing practical, developmentally appropriate, child health information to parents in anticipation of significant physical, emotional, and psychological milestones [28]. Parenting support emphasizes children's psychological and behavioral goals, logical and natural consequences, mutual respect, and encouragement techniques [28, 29].

For PATE, emphasis is placed on educating mothers about the ways in which they can facilitate the development of appropriate eating, physical activity, and other health behaviors in their children, including modeling these behaviors themselves. Intervention components of the PATE arm included appropriate weight gain during pregnancy and weight management after pregnancy, nutrition and physical activity in the gestational (mother) and postnatal (mother and infant) periods, breastfeeding, appropriate introduction of solid foods, and parental modeling of positive behaviors. Lessons included hands-on activities, instructional DVDs, and goal setting and reducing barriers for both diet and exercise. At each monthly visit in the gestational period, participants were given weight gain charts that contained reference ranges from the Institute of Medicine gestational weight gain recommendations. Participants' current as well as past weight gain from previous visits was marked on these charts.

Both arms of the intervention were delivered in the home to women beginning in their early second trimester of pregnancy by trained community based Parent Educators. Parent Educators were African American college educated women residing in the target communities. They were trained to deliver the nutrition and physical activity lessons and to collect data from participants, including dietary intake. Home visits occurred monthly and were approximately 60–90 min in length for the PAT lessons, and approximately 90–120 min for the PATE lessons. Additional details regarding Parent Educator training, study methodology and lesson plan outlines have been published elsewhere [24].

Measures

Anthropometric measures obtained on the participants at the baseline visit included height which was measured in duplicate using a portable stadiometer (model seca 217, seca, Birmingham, UK), and weight which was measured using a digital scale (model SR241, SR Instruments, Tonawanda, NY). Both measures were performed without shoes or heavy clothing. Pre-pregnancy weight was self-reported. Body mass index (BMI) was calculated as weight (kg) divided by height (m) squared where height was averaged if the two measurements differed. Weight also was measured at each of the five subsequent gestational visits. Weight gain is examined in another paper (Thomson, under review).

Dietary data were collected from the participants at the baseline, GM 6, and GM 8 visits via multiple pass 24-h dietary recall using Nutrition Data System for Research (NDSR) software. NDSR is a Windows-based dietary analysis program that allows for the calculation of nutrients per ingredient, food, meal, and day in report and analysis formats [30]. The software also includes a dietary supplement assessment module so that nutrient intake from supplemental sources can be captured and quantified [31]. Using the dietary data collected with NDSR, participants' diet quality was calculated using the Healthy Eating Index-2010 (HEI-2010) [12], which measures adherence to the 2010 DGAs. The HEI-2010 includes 12 components that are summed to create a total score ranging from 0 to 100 points. The 12 components include: total vegetables, greens and beans, total fruit, whole fruit, whole grains, dairy, total protein foods, seafood and plant protein foods, fatty acids, refined grains, sodium, and empty calories. For each component, higher scores reflect greater adherence to the 2010 DGAs. An HEI score greater than 80 is representative of a good quality diet; 51 – 80 is consistent with a diet that needs improvement in regard to quality; and a score less than 51 represents a poor quality diet [32]. Additionally, intakes of specific nutrients of interest were determined using the dietary data collected. These nutrients (total and saturated fat, cholesterol, sodium, calcium, fiber, folate, iron, vitamins C and D, and choline) were chosen based on their importance to an overall healthy diet and increased nutrient needs during pregnancy [33–37].

Participants also provided information regarding demographic characteristics (e.g., age, marital status, household size, education, employment, household income, insurance, prenatal care), health history, and current health conditions. Details regarding other measures and questionnaire data that were collected using validated tools, but are not relevant to the current paper, have been published elsewhere [24]. All measures, dietary recalls, and questionnaires were collected or administered by trained research staff (Parent Educators) using laptop computers loaded with relevant software (i.e., NDSR and Snap Surveys).

Statistical analyses

Statistical analyses were performed using SAS® software, version 9.4 (SAS Institute Inc., Cary, NC). Descriptive statistics, including means, standard deviations, frequencies, and percentages, were used to summarize participants' demographic characteristics, anthropometric measures, nutrient intake, and diet quality.

Chi square tests of association or Fisher's exact tests (categorical measures) and two sample t tests (continuous measures) were used to assess differences between PAT and PATE participants' baseline characteristics and between gestational period study completers' and non-completers' baseline characteristics. Study completers were defined as participants who had their GM 9 visit or those who had at least two visits in the gestational period and their post-natal 1 visit. The second definition was used because a substantial proportion of PAT and PATE participants (36 and 42 %) who had their post-natal 1 visit, missed their GM 9 visit due to the early birth of their infant.

Compliance with diet recommendations was determined based on current guidelines set by professional organizations. Participants were classified as compliant with dietary guidelines if they met minimum daily intake for fiber (28 g), calcium (1300 mg for women 18 years of age and 1000 mg for women ≥ 19 years of age), folate (600 mcg), iron (27 mg), vitamin C (80 mg for women 18 years of age and 85 mg for women ≥ 19 years of age), vitamin D (5 mcg), and choline (450 mg) or did not exceed the maximum daily intake for total dietary fat (35 % of total energy), saturated fat (10 % of total energy), cholesterol (300 mg), and sodium (1500 mg for African American women).

Generalized linear mixed models, using maximum likelihood estimation, were used to test for significant treatment, time, and treatment by time (interaction) effects on diet outcomes. Maximum likelihood estimation is an approach for handling missing data in repeated measures. Treatment (PAT vs. PATE) was modeled as a fixed effect and time (GM 4, GM 6, and GM 8 visits) was modeled as a repeated measure using a first-order autoregressive covariance matrix structure. If overdispersion was present, then a multiplicative overdispersion parameter was added to the model. Least squares means with 95 % confidence intervals were computed using these models. Distributions of the diet outcome variables were checked for approximate normality based on both goodness of fit tests (Cramer-von Mises and Anderson-Darling) and visual inspection. If the distribution passed the goodness of fit tests or failed the tests but appeared sufficiently normal for the underlying assumptions of normality to be reasonable for practical purposes of analysis, then the diet outcome (HEI total and component scores; and total fat, sodium, folate, and vitamin D intakes) was modeled using a Gaussian distribution with an identity link function. The remaining variables were checked for approximate gamma, inverse normal, and log normal distributions, again based on goodness of fit tests and visual inspection. Saturated fat and calcium intakes were modeled using a gamma distribution with a log link function. The remaining five diet outcome variables (cholesterol, dietary fiber, iron, vitamin C, and choline) were modeled using quantile regression on the median to test for significant treatment, time and treatment by time effects. Treatment and time were modeled as fixed effects and 95 % confidence intervals for the medians were computed using Markov chain marginal bootstrap resampling. Generalized linear mixed models also were used to test for significant treatment, time, and treatment by time effects on the proportions of participants who met recommended nutrient intakes using a binomial distribution with a logit link function. The significance level of the tests was set at 0.05.

Results

Study retention rates during the gestational period for the PAT and PATE treatment arms were 77 % (33/43) and 67 % (26/39), respectively, and did not differ between arms ($p = 0.310$). Compliance rates for the GM 6 and GM 8 visits were 88 and 84 %, respectively, for PAT participants, and 67 and 51 %, respectively, for PATE participants. Compliance rates for both visits were significantly lower in the PATE arm ($p = 0.018$ and 0.002, respectively). One PAT participant did not provide dietary intake data at the GM 4 (baseline) visit. One PATE participant who missed her GM 6 visit provided dietary intake data during her GM 7 visit. Likewise, two PATE participants who missed their GM 8 visit provided dietary intake data during their GM 9 visit.

Table 1 presents comparisons between treatment arms for baseline characteristics. The majority of both PAT and PATE participants were African American (95 and 97 %), single (91 and 95 %), receiving Medicaid (93 and 90 %), overweight/obese prior to pregnancy (63 and 72 %), and started their prenatal care in their second month of pregnancy (56 % for both). Additionally, PAT and PATE participants were young (mean age = 23 ± 4.6 years and 23 ± 4.7 years) and early in their second trimester of pregnancy (mean gestational age = 17 ± 1.9 weeks and 18 ± 2.4 weeks). There were no significant differences between PAT and PATE participants at baseline. However, women that were retained throughout the gestational period were significantly more likely to have access to a motor vehicle as compared to those not retained (95 % vs. 78 %, $p = 0.036$; data not shown in the table).

Table 1 Delta Healthy Sprouts participant baseline (early second trimester of pregnancy) demographic characteristics by treatment arm

	PAT (*n* = 43)		PATE (*n* = 39)		
Characteristic	n	%	n	%	P
Race					1.000
African American	41	95.3	38	97.4	
White	2	4.7	1	2.6	
Marital status					0.678
Single[a]	39	90.7	37	94.9	
Married	4	9.3	2	5.1	
Education level					0.684
9th–11th grade	7	16.3	7	17.9	
High school/GED	15	34.9	12	30.8	
Some college/technical	17	39.5	13	33.3	
College degree	4	9.3	7	17.9	
Employment status					0.468
Full time/part-time	13	30.2	16	41.0	
Unemployed (looking)	21	48.8	14	35.9	
Homemaker/student	9	20.9	9	23.1	
Household monthly income[b]					0.284
< $500	10	23.3	5	12.8	
$500-$1000	10	23.3	9	23.1	
$1001–$1500	4	9.3	12	30.8	
$1501–$2000	7	16.3	5	12.8	
$2001–$4000	6	14.0	3	7.7	
Don't know/refused	6	14.0	5	12.8	
Smoker in household	12	27.9	12	30.8	0.776
Smoker[c]					0.112
Current	3	7.0	1	2.6	
Stopped before pregnancy	1	2.3	0	0.0	
Stopped after became pregnant	2	4.7	0	0.0	
No	37	86.0	38	97.4	
Medicaid health insurance	40	93.0	35	89.7	0.703
Receiving SNAP	35	81.4	27	69.2	0.200
Receiving WIC	38	88.4	31	79.5	0.271
Own/access to vehicle	39	90.7	35	89.7	1.000
Receiving prenatal care	43	100.0	39	100.0	
Pre-pregnancy weight class[d]					0.386
Underweight (BMI < 18.5)	4	9.3	3	7.7	
Healthy weight (18.5 ≤ BMI < 25)	12	27.9	8	20.5	
Overweight (25 ≤ BMI < 30)	9	20.9	10	25.6	
Obese (BMI ≥ 30)	18	41.9	18	46.2	
	Mean	SD	Mean	SD	P
Age (years)	23.3	4.58	22.7	4.69	0.537
Household size	3.8	1.62	4.1	1.78	0.406
Gestational age[e]	17.4	1.85	17.7	2.43	0.533

PAT Parents as Teachers control treatment; *PATE* Parents as Teachers, Enhanced experimental treatment; *SNAP* Supplemental Nutrition Assistance Program; *WIC* SNAP for Women, Infants, and Children; *BMI* body mass index
[a]Includes 1 participant who indicated she is divorced
[b]Comparison = <$500–$1500 vs. $1501–$4000; don't know/refused excluded
[c]Comparison = no vs. all other responses
[e]Based on self-reported pre-pregnancy weight; comparison = underweight or healthy weight vs. overweight or obese
[e]Based on reported due date; enrollment data collected late for 3 participants

Diet quality and nutrient intake outcomes

Table 2 presents the results of the diet quality analyses by treatment arm and gestational visit. HEI-2010 total diet quality mean scores for PAT participants at GM 4, GM 6, and GM 8 were 41, 41, and 43 points, respectively; corresponding scores for PATE participants were 46, 44, and 45 points, respectively, reflecting overall poor diet quality for all participants at all gestational time points. In particular, HEI-2010 component mean scores were low for greens and beans, whole grains, seafood and plant protein foods, and sodium for both treatment arms. Significant treatment, time and interaction effects were not found for the HEI-2010 total or component scores.

Table 3 presents the results of the nutrient intake analyses by treatment arm and gestational visit. Significant treatment, time and interaction effects were not found for any of the nutrients modeled. However, there was a clinically meaningful reduction in the percentage of total energy from saturated fat in the PATE arm between GM 4 and GM 8 (10.6 to 9.6 %). An unexpected but clinically meaningful reduction in mean calcium intake in the PATE arm between GM 4 and GM 8 (861 mg to 792 mg) also was observed.

Table 4 presents the results of the proportions of participants meeting nutrient intake recommendations by treatment arm and gestational visit. At baseline < 20 % of women met intake recommendations for dietary fiber, sodium, or choline. Whereas, more than half of the women met intake recommendations for cholesterol, folate, iron, vitamin C, and vitamin D at baseline. Significant treatment, time and interaction effects were not found for any of the nutrients modeled. However, clinically meaningful increases in percentages of participants meeting recommendations for saturated fat intake between GM 4 and GM 8 were observed (PAT 30 to 42 %; PATE 47 to 64 %). Likewise, clinically meaningful increases in percentages of PAT participants meeting recommendations for cholesterol and vitamin C intakes between GM 4 and GM 8 were observed (65 to 84 % and 86 to 97 %, respectively). An unanticipated albeit clinically meaningful decrease in percentage of PATE

Table 2 Diet quality scores for Delta Healthy Sprouts participants in the gestational period by treatment arm and visit (time)

		GM 4 (*n* = 43 and 38)[a]			GM 6 (*n* = 39 and 25)			GM 8 (*n* = 36 and 22)[b]			P		
HEI-2010 Component	Arm	LSM	95 % CI		LSM	95 % CI[c]		LSM	95 % CI[c]		Time	Arm	Int
Total vegetables	PAT	2.3	1.8	2.7	1.8	1.3	2.2	2.1	1.6	2.5	0.877	0.237	0.367
(Range 0-5)	PATE	1.7	1.3	2.2	1.9	1.4	2.5	1.8	1.2	2.4			
Greens & beans	PAT	0.6	0.1	1.0	0.8	0.3	1.3	0.5	0.0	1.0	0.243	0.820	0.797
(Range 0-5)	PATE	0.6	0.1	1.1	0.8	0.2	1.5	0.2	0.0	0.9			
Total fruit	PAT	1.3	0.7	1.9	2.2	1.5	2.8	1.5	0.8	2.1	0.713	0.860	0.086
(Range 0–5)	PATE	1.8	1.1	2.4	1.4	0.6	2.2	1.9	1.1	2.8			
Whole fruit	PAT	1.1	0.4	1.7	1.8	1.1	2.4	1.2	0.5	1.8	0.248	0.214	0.539
(Range 0–5)	PATE	1.6	0.9	2.2	1.8	1.0	2.6	1.9	1.1	2.8			
Whole grains	PAT	2.4	1.4	3.4	1.8	0.7	2.8	2.1	1.1	3.2	0.818	0.388	0.375
(Range 0–10)	PATE	2.5	1.4	3.5	3.1	1.8	4.4	2.1	0.7	3.5			
Dairy	PAT	4.4	3.5	5.2	3.6	2.7	4.5	4.0	3.1	4.9	0.311	0.086	0.543
(Range 0–10)	PATE	3.7	2.7	4.6	3.4	2.3	4.5	2.7	1.5	3.9			
Total protein foods	PAT	4.4	4.0	4.8	4.3	3.9	4.7	4.2	3.8	4.6	0.960	0.561	0.548
(Range 0–5)	PATE	4.3	3.9	4.7	4.5	4.0	4.9	4.6	4.0	5.1			
Seafood & plant proteins	PAT	0.7	0.1	1.3	1.0	0.4	1.6	0.8	0.2	1.4	0.960	0.813	0.362
(Range 0–5)	PATE	1.2	0.6	1.8	0.7	0.0	1.4	0.9	0.1	1.7			
Fatty acids	PAT	5.2	4.1	6.2	5.2	4.2	6.3	6.4	5.2	7.5	0.397	0.060	0.576
(Range 0–10)	PATE	6.8	5.7	7.9	6.3	5.0	7.7	6.8	5.3	8.2			
Sodium	PAT	2.4	1.4	3.3	2.9	2.0	3.9	2.9	1.9	3.9	0.780	0.118	0.653
(Range 0–10)	PATE	3.5	2.5	4.5	3.1	1.9	4.4	3.7	2.4	5.0			
Refined grains	PAT	5.8	4.8	6.9	4.5	3.4	5.6	5.3	4.2	6.5	0.054	0.104	0.554
(Range 0–10)	PATE	6.2	5.1	7.3	5.0	3.6	6.4	7.0	5.5	8.5			
Empty calories	PAT	10.5	8.8	12.2	10.7	9.0	12.5	12.2	10.4	14.1	0.759	0.450	0.519
(Range 0–20)	PATE	11.9	10.1	13.7	11.9	9.7	14.1	11.5	9.2	13.9			
Total	PAT	40.9	37.1	44.8	40.6	36.5	44.6	43.2	39.0	47.5	0.696	0.100	0.813
(Range 0–100)	PATE	45.6	41.5	49.7	43.9	38.9	49.0	45.1	39.7	50.5			

GM gestational month; *HEI-2010* Healthy Eating Index-2010; *LSM* least squares mean; *CI* confidence interval; *Int* interaction (time x arm); *PAT* Parents as Teachers control treatment; *PATE* Parents as Teachers Enhanced experimental treatment

[a]Missed dietary recall for 1 PATE participant

[b]Excluded dietary recall for 1 PATE participant (in hospital and consumed ice only)

[c]Negative lower limits are not feasible and were changed to 0

participants meeting recommendations for calcium intake between GM 4 and GM 8 also was observed (29 to 13 %).

Discussion

In this paper, we describe and compare the gestational dietary intake outcomes of rural, Southern, primarily African American pregnant women participating in the Delta Healthy Sprouts randomized, comparative impact trial. Overall, our results suggest that the PAT curriculum and the more complex PATE intervention, were not effective at improving maternal diet quality or the adequacy of intake for several nutrients including dietary fiber, calcium and choline during the gestational period.

Other lifestyle interventions conducted in the gestational period have been successful at improving maternal diet quality and nutrient intake. The UPBEAT trial [38], conducted in the United Kingdom with a largely Caucasian population, was effective at improving diet quality in pregnant women with obesity. This one-on-one intervention was delivered in an antenatal clinic once weekly for 8 weeks with a health educator beginning between 16 and 19 weeks gestation. The intervention was successful at reducing maternal glycemic load and total and saturated fat intake and increasing dietary fiber. The LIMIT trial [18], a randomized prenatal dietary and lifestyle intervention conducted in a cohort of pregnant overweight and obese, predominately Caucasian, high SES, Australian women, was effective at improving maternal diet quality, measured by HEI, and intake of dietary fiber and saturated fat compared to standard care [18]. This intervention included six sessions implemented on

Table 3 Nutrient intakes for Delta Healthy Sprouts participants in the gestational period by treatment arm and visit (time)

		GM 4 ($n = 43$ and 38)[a]			GM 6 ($n = 39$ and 25)			GM 8 ($n = 36$ and 22)[b]			P		
Nutrient	Arm	LSM	95 % CI		LSM	95 % CI		LSM	95 % CI		Time	Arm	Int
Total fat (% energy)	PAT	35.7	33.4	38.0	32.8	30.5	35.2	34.6	32.1	37.1	0.175	0.990	0.233
RDI ≤ 35 %	PATE	35.6	33.2	38.1	34.9	32.0	37.8	32.7	29.5	35.8			
Saturated fat (% energy)	PAT	11.4	10.4	12.5	10.7	9.7	11.7	10.5	9.5	11.6	0.204	0.178	0.780
RDI ≤ 10 %	PATE	10.6	9.6	11.6	10.4	9.3	11.7	9.6	8.5	10.8			
Cholesterol (mg)[c]	PAT	203	141	266	193	130	256	165	102	227	0.211	0.151	0.143
RDI ≤ 300 mg	PATE	179	116	242	248	185	311	228	166	291			
Fiber (g)[c]	PAT	10.7	8.4	13.1	11.7	9.4	14.0	11.3	9.0	13.6	0.881	0.607	0.869
RDI ≥ 28 g	PATE	10.2	7.9	12.5	11.3	9.0	13.6	10.4	8.1	12.7			
Sodium (mg)	PAT	3770	3332	4208	3839	3379	4298	3725	3246	4203	0.700	0.334	0.900
RDI ≤ 1500 mg	PATE	3624	3158	4090	3718	3144	4293	3378	2766	3990			
Calcium (mg)[d]	PAT	960	842	1094	939	818	1078	966	837	1115	0.305	0.281	0.151
RDI = 1000 mg	PATE	861	749	990	1015	855	1205	792	659	951			
Folate (mcg)	PAT	1246	1071	1421	1275	1092	1459	1252	1061	1444	0.904	0.278	0.990
RDI = 600 mcg	PATE	1142	956	1329	1200	970	1429	1157	912	1401			
Iron (mg)[c]	PAT	41.2	36.3	46.2	41.6	36.7	46.5	41.9	37.0	46.9	0.710	0.555	0.917
RDI = 27 mg	PATE	39.2	34.2	44.1	43.0	38.1	47.9	40.3	35.4	45.2			
Vitamin C (mg)[c,e]	PAT	162	117	207	197	152	241	183	139	228	0.690	0.471	0.947
RDI = 85 mg	PATE	153	109	198	179	134	224	163	118	208			
Vitamin D (mcg)	PAT	12.4	10.7	14.2	11.6	9.8	13.4	12.3	10.5	14.2	0.907	0.380	0.559
RDI = 5 mcg	PATE	10.9	9.1	12.8	11.3	9.2	13.4	11.0	8.8	13.2			
Choline (mg)[c]	PAT	240	181	299	248	189	307	206	147	265	0.745	0.392	0.403
RDI = 450 mg	PATE	223	164	282	280	221	339	239	180	298			

GM gestational month; *HEI-2010* Healthy Eating Index-2010; *LSM* least squares mean; *CI* confidence interval; *Int* interaction (time x arm); *PAT* Parents as Teachers control treatment; *PATE* Parents as Teachers Enhanced experimental treatment

[a]Missed dietary recall for 1 PATE participant

[b]Excluded dietary recall for 1 PATE participant (in hospital and consumed ice only)

[c]Values are medians and associated 95 % confidence intervals from quantile regression

[d]RDI = 1300 mg for participants 18 years of age

[e]RDI = 80 mg for participants 18 years of age

an individual basis both in person and over the phone by a registered dietitian and trained research assistants. While our one-on-one intervention was implemented monthly between GM 4 and 9 in the participant's home by a trained lay parent educator, only three of the five lessons (GM 5, 6 and 7) were delivered prior to the final gestational diet intake assessment at GM 8. It may be that the dose of our intervention was too low to foster or the timing of our final diet intake was not optimal for detecting positive dietary changes. Lifestyle changes, including dietary changes, involve the adoption of new positive behaviors [39] and research suggests that lifestyle habits can take anywhere from 66 to 254 days to form [40]. Thus, the short duration of our gestational intervention may not have allowed for the time needed to develop and adopt positive dietary behaviors [39]. Given that our intervention spans into the postpartum period, future analyses will assess the adoption of positive diet behaviors in this cohort of women over a longer period of time.

The UPBEAT [38] and LIMIT [18] prenatal lifestyle intervention trials focused their messaging solely on maternal gestational weight gain, diet, and lifestyle behaviors. The Delta Healthy Sprouts Project was built on the framework of the evidence-based PAT curriculum which covers topics related to parental knowledge of child development, positive parenting practices, early detection of developmental delays, preventing child abuse, and school readiness. Thus, combining the PATE diet and lifestyle curriculum with the existing PAT program may have diluted the diet and lifestyle messaging. Further, some studies suggest that multi-component dietary advice such as USDA MyPlate, which was used as the framework for the PATE dietary messaging, can be overwhelming to some individuals due to the knowledge required to comprehend the complex recommendations [41]. The considerable and diverse number of messages provided in the PATE curriculum may have overwhelmed the women randomized to this arm of the

Table 4 Percentages of Delta Healthy Sprouts participants meeting recommended nutrient intakes in the gestational period by treatment arm and visit (time)

		GM 4 (*n* = 43 and 38)[a]			GM 6 (*n* = 39 and 25)			GM 8 (*n* = 36 and 22)[b]			P		
Nutrient[c]	Arm	LSM	95 % CI		LSM	95 % CI		LSM	95 % CI		Time	Arm	Int
Total fat (% energy)	PAT	48.8	34.1	63.8	53.9	38.0	69.0	49.7	33.6	65.9	0.650	0.467	0.684
RDA ≤ 35 %	PATE	50.0	34.2	65.8	55.4	35.8	73.6	64.5	42.6	81.6			
Saturated fat (% energy)	PAT	30.2	18.2	45.8	43.8	29.0	59.9	41.6	26.5	58.4	0.285	0.063	0.570
RDA ≤ 10 %	PATE	47.4	31.9	63.4	48.2	29.5	67.5	63.5	41.7	80.9			
Cholesterol (mg)	PAT	65.1	49.5	78.1	64.3	47.9	77.9	83.7	67.5	92.7	0.414	0.607	0.304
RDA ≤ 300 mg	PATE	68.4	51.8	81.4	69.1	48.5	84.2	67.1	45.1	83.6			
Fiber (g)	PAT	0.0	NC	NC	0.0	NC	NC	0.0	NC	NC	NC	NC	NC
RDA ≥ 28 g	PATE	7.9	NC	NC	0.0	NC	NC	9.1	NC	NC			
Sodium (mg)	PAT	0.0	NC	NC	2.6	NC	NC	5.6	NC	NC	NC	NC	NC
RDA ≤ 1500 mg	PATE	15.8	NC	NC	0.0	NC	NC	0.0	NC	NC			
Calcium (mg)[d]	PAT	41.9	27.9	57.3	40.7	26.3	57.0	44.3	28.8	61.0	0.245	0.054	0.130
RDA = 1000 mg	PATE	28.9	16.5	45.6	41.8	24.2	61.8	13.4	4.2	35.2			
Folate (mcg)	PAT	90.7	77.4	96.5	91.4	77.6	97.0	88.7	73.8	95.6	0.929	0.486	0.871
RDA = 600 mcg	PATE	86.8	71.8	94.5	85.1	66.9	94.1	85.7	65.5	95.0			
Iron (mg)	PAT	90.7	77.4	96.5	91.1	77.5	96.8	88.4	73.8	95.4	0.975	0.260	0.486
RDA = 27 mg	PATE	81.6	65.8	91.1	79.2	61.4	90.2	84.9	65.7	94.3			
Vitamin C (mg)[e]	PAT	86.0	71.8	93.7	89.4	74.9	96.0	97.3	82.3	99.6	0.267	0.184	0.495
RDA = 85 mg	PATE	84.2	68.6	92.9	81.4	61.6	92.3	87.0	65.6	95.9			
Vitamin D (mcg)	PAT	83.7	69.3	92.2	85.0	70.2	93.2	82.6	66.8	91.8	0.949	0.699	0.790
RDA = 5 mcg	PATE	78.9	62.9	89.3	79.9	61.4	90.9	83.4	63.2	93.6			
Choline (mg)	PAT	14.0	6.2	28.3	15.7	7.2	31.1	8.1	2.5	23.2	0.525	0.992	0.349
RDA = 450 mg	PATE	18.4	8.8	34.5	7.5	1.8	26.7	13.0	4.0	34.7			

GM gestational month; *HEI-2010* Healthy Eating Index-2010; *LSM* least squares mean; *CI*, confidence interval; *Int* interaction (time x arm); *PAT* Parents as Teachers control treatment; *PATE* Parents as Teachers Enhanced experimental treatment; *NC*, not computed since model failed to converge due to time points with zero and close to zero percentages

[a]Missed dietary recall for 1 PATE participant

[b]Excluded dietary recall for 1 PATE participant (in hospital and consumed ice only)

[c]Based on food and supplements combined

[d]RDA = 1300 mg for participants 18 years of age

[e]RDA = 80 mg for participants 18 years of age

study. The higher attrition and lower compliance with home visits during the gestational period, despite no other notable participant characteristic differences, suggests some level of displeasure with the PATE lessons. The standard PAT curriculum provides some simple maternal dietary advice including importance of taking prenatal vitamins, safe and healthy fish options during pregnancy, and consuming more calories during the 2nd and 3rd trimester. The three point increase in total HEI-2010 score and improvements in saturated fat, cholesterol and vitamin C intake in the PAT arm suggests that simple nutrition messaging, when presented in the context of a more global maternal and child health curriculum, may promote positive maternal dietary behaviors in the gestational period. Further research is needed to better understand the impact of simple vs. complex nutrition messaging on maternal diet in rural, disadvantaged pregnant women.

Women are bombarded with information during pregnancy [39]. All of the women in our study were receiving prenatal care at baseline and more than 80 % of our participants were enrolled in the Women Infants and Children (WIC) supplemental nutrition program. Further, 88 and 83 %, respectively, of our PAT and PATE participants indicated they had received advice about healthy eating from their prenatal care provider. Thus, it is probable that participants were overwhelmed by a vast amount of health and lifestyle-related information and possible that our diet advice conflicted with advice received from their clinician or WIC counselor. Research suggests that pregnant women tend to place the most importance on recommendations made by their doctor/

clinical provider [42, 43]. Whereas women tend to be somewhat dismissive of health recommendations that were not addressed by their health care provider. Therefore, women in the PATE arm may have been less likely to follow our diet recommendations if similar advice was not also encouraged by their provider [39]. Future interventions should consider involving obstetrical healthcare providers to allow for consistent messaging around gestational lifestyle behaviors.

Our study was implemented in the largely rural, socioeconomically disadvantaged LMD region. Studies suggest that socioeconomic status (SES) is positively associated with diet quality [44]. There are several hypothesized explanations for this relationship. Research suggests that low SES individuals may experience greater reward from food given their limited access to non-food related rewards due to cost or access [45]. Further, low SES neighborhoods and regions, like the LMD, have fewer large supermarkets and more convenience stores and fast-food outlets that offer relatively low cost, nutrient poor, energy dense foods [46]. Research has shown that living in low SES areas is associated with less consumption of fruits and vegetables and a tendency to select foods that are more readily accessible [47, 48]. Epstein and colleagues [45] suggest that even when access to healthier food is improved through participation in food assistance programs, low SES individuals will continue to choose foods of low nutritive value that provide greater food reinforcement. Epstein hypothesizes that reducing access to low quality foods through policy-related changes and increasing the availability of low-cost, non-food reinforcement, may encourage the selection of healthier food choices in low SES populations.

Several strengths of the Delta Healthy Sprouts Project deserve consideration. Participants were visited in their homes, thus alleviating the burden of travel for these rural residents. Although the study's sample size is relatively small, no other studies were found which focused on the diet, including nutrient intake and diet quality, of this population of pregnant women. Dietary intake was measured three times in the gestational period (vs. the more typical pre/post measurement schedule). Despite the strengths of this study, there are some limitations that bear mentioning. The potential for socially desirable responses for survey questions and dietary recalls cannot be discounted. To reduce this bias potential, parent educators were trained to not ask leading questions and to maintain neutral facial expressions, particularly when conducting dietary recalls. Data collection was not blinded and therefore a potential source of bias. However, because the data was collected in the participants' homes, it was not practically, logistically, or financially feasible to have a second set of blinded research staff whose purpose was solely to collect data. Stopping recruitment before target enrollment numbers were reached likely limited our ability to detect statistically significant differences between treatment arms, especially given the low compliance rates with visits observed in the PATE arm (Thomson JL, under review). A post hoc power and sample size analysis revealed that the actual sample sizes of 33 PAT and 26 PATE participants were sufficient to detect a statistically significant difference of 9.9 points in change in total HEI-2010 scores between treatment arms with 80 % power and a type 1 error rate of 0.05. Given the relatively short duration of the intervention in the gestational period, achieving such a large effect was unlikely. Finally, the high attrition rate may limit generalizability of these study results.

Conclusion

In conclusion, designing effective interventions that enable women to improve their dietary intake during pregnancy remains a challenge as evidenced by the lack of impact on maternal diet quality observed in the current study. Future interventions designed for rural, low income, minority populations of pregnant women might consider recruiting women earlier in their pregnancy (e.g., first trimester), increasing the treatment dosage, and involving prenatal care providers to ensure reinforcement and consistency in health behavior messaging. Given the importance of optimum maternal nutrition for positive maternal and fetal health outcomes, research efforts need to remain focused on populations at risk for poor pregnancy and birth outcomes, including residents of the LMD region.

Abbreviations

BMI, body mass index; DGAs, dietary guidelines for Americans; DPP, Diabetes Prevention Program; GM, gestational month; HEI, healthy eating index; InFANT, Infant Feeding and Nutrition Trial; LMD, Lower Mississippi Delta; NDSR, nutrition data system for research; PAT, parents as teachers; PATE, Parents as Teachers enhanced curriculum; US, United States; USDA, United States Department of Agriculture; WIC, Women, infants, and children

Acknowledgements

We thank Debra Johnson, Shakari Moore, and Donna Ransome for their research support, and the mothers who participated in this study. The views expressed are solely those of the authors and do not reflect the official policy or position of the US government.

Funding

This research is supported by the United States Department of Agriculture, Agricultural Research Service Project 6001-53000-001-00D (Thomson), and in kind support from the Delta Health Alliance.

Authors' contributions

LMT-H contributed to the study design, data analysis and interpretation, and drafted the manuscript. JLT contributed to the study design; data acquisition, analysis, and interpretation. MHG contributed to the data acquisition, analysis, and interpretation. SO contributed to the data acquisition, analysis, and interpretation. All authors participated in the drafting and revising of the manuscript. All authors read and approved the final manuscript.

Authors' information

No additional information to disclose.

Competing interests

The authors declare that they have no competing interests

Author details

[1]Department of Medicine and Cancer Center, University of Illinois at Chicago, 1747 W Roosevelt Road, #416, Chicago, IL 60618, USA. [2]United States Department of Agriculture, Agricultural Research Service, 141 Experiment Station Road, Stoneville, MS 38776, USA.

References

1. Ramakrishnan U, Grant F, Goldenberg T, Zongrone A, Martorell R. Effect of women's nutrition before and during early pregnancy on maternal and infant outcomes: a systematic review. Paediatr Perinat Epidemiol. 2012;26 Suppl 1:285–301.
2. King JC. The risk of maternal nutritional depletion and poor outcomes increases in early or closely spaced pregnancies. J Nutr. 2003;133(5 Suppl 2): 1732S–6S.
3. Rifas-Shiman SL, Rich-Edwards JW, Kleinman KP, Oken E, Gillman MW. Dietary quality during pregnancy varies by maternal characteristics in Project Viva: a US cohort. J Am Diet Assoc. 2009;109(6):1004–11. Pubmed Central PMCID: 4098830.
4. Poon AK, Yeung E, Boghossian N, Albert PS, Zhang C. Maternal Dietary Patterns during Third Trimester in Association with Birthweight Characteristics and Early Infant Growth. Scientifica. 2013;2013:786409. Pubmed Central PMCID: 3893866.
5. Rodriguez-Bernal CL, Rebagliato M, Chatzi L, Carbinell CC, Martos C, Ballester F. Maternal Diet Quality and Pregnancy Outcomes In: Preedy VR, Lan-Anh H, Patel V, B., editors. Diet Quality 1. 1 ed. New York, NY: Humana Press; 2013. p. 65-79.
6. Martin CL, Sotres-Alvarez D, Siega-Riz AM. Maternal Dietary Patterns during the Second Trimester Are Associated with Preterm Birth. J Nutr. 2015;145(8): 1857–64. Pubmed Central PMCID: 4516771.
7. Hu F. Dietary Pattern Analysis: A New Direction in Nutritional Epidemiology. Current Opinion in Lipidology 132002. 2002. p. 3-9.
8. Baskin R, Hill B, Jacka FN, O'Neil A, Skouteris H. Antenatal dietary patterns and depressive symptoms during pregnancy and early post-partum. Matern Child Nutr. 2016. doi:10.1111/mcn.12218. [Epub ahead of print].
9. Shin MK, Kim YS, Kim JH, Kim SH, Kim Y. Dietary Patterns and Their Associations with the Diet Quality Index-International (DQI-I) in Korean Women with Gestational Diabetes Mellitus. Clin Nutr Res. 2015;4(4):216–24. Pubmed Central PMCID: 4641983.
10. Brantsaeter AL, Haugen M, Samuelsen SO, Torjusen H, Trogstad L, Alexander J, et al. A dietary pattern characterized by high intake of vegetables, fruits, and vegetable oils is associated with reduced risk of preeclampsia in nulliparous pregnant Norwegian women. J Nutr. 2009;139(6):1162–8. Pubmed Central PMCID: 2682988.
11. USDA. Dietary Guidelines for Americans, 2010. In: Services HaH, editor. 7 ed. Washington, DC: U.S. Government Printing Office 2010.
12. Guenther PM, Casavale KO, Reedy J, Kirkpatrick SI, Hiza HAB, Kuczynski KJ, et al. Update of the Healthy Eating Index: HEI-2010. J Acad Nutr Diet. 2013; 113(4):569–80. PubMed PMID: WOS:000317257300013.
13. Yu DX, Sonderman J, Buchowski MS, McLaughlin JK, Shu XO, Steinwandel M, et al. Healthy Eating and Risks of Total and Cause-Specific Death among Low-Income Populations of African-Americans and Other Adults in the Southeastern United States: A Prospective Cohort Study. Plos Med. 2015;12(5). PubMed PMID: WOS:000355304100008.
14. Fogli-Cawley JJ, Dwyer JT, Saltzman E, McCullough ML, Troy LM, Meigs JB, et al. The 2005 Dietary Guidelines for Americans and risk of the metabolic syndrome. Am J Clin Nutr. 2007;86(4):1193–201. PubMed PMID: WOS: 000250134600042.
15. Pick ME, Edwards M, Moreau D, Ryan EA. Assessment of diet quality in pregnant women using the healthy eating index. J Am Diet Assoc. 2005; 105(2):240–6. PubMed PMID: WOS:000226733100015.
16. Melere C, Hoffmann JF, Nunes MAA, Drehmer M, Buss C, Ozcariz SGI, et al. Healthy eating index for pregnancy: adaptation for use in pregnant women in Brazil. Rev Saude Publ. 2013;47(1):20–8. PubMed PMID: WOS:000320026700004.
17. Moran LJ, Sui Z, Cramp CS, Dodd JM. A decrease in diet quality occurs during pregnancy in overweight and obese women which is maintained post-partum. Int J Obesity. 2013;37(5):704–11. PubMed PMID: WOS:000318772400012.
18. Dodd JM, Cramp C, Sui ZX, Yelland LN, Deussen AR, Grivell RM, et al. The effects of antenatal dietary and lifestyle advice for women who are overweight or obese on maternal diet and physical activity: the LIMIT randomised trial. Bmc Med. 2014;13:12. PubMed PMID: WOS:000344122400001.
19. Robert Wood Johnson Foundation. County Health Rankings and Roadmaps, 2016 July 16, 2016. Available from: http://www.countyhealthrankings.org. Accessed 16 July 2016.
20. Mississippi State Department of Health. Vital Statistics Mississippi 2012 July 16, 2016. Available from: http://msdh.ms.gov/phs/2012/Bulletin/vr2012.pdf. Accessed 16 July 2016.
21. Smith BL, Sandlin AT, Bird TM, Steelman SC, Magann EF. Maternal mortality in the Mississippi delta region. South Med J. 2014;107(5):275–9. doi:10.1097/ SMJ.0000000000000102.
22. Bhutta ZA, Das JK, Rizvi A. The Lancet Nutrition Interventions Review Group, and the Maternal and Child Nutrition Study Group. Evidence-based interventions for improvement of maternal and child nutrition: what can be done and at what cost? Lancet. 2013;382(9890):396. PubMed PMID: WOS:000322638500029.
23. Thomson JL, Tussing-Humphreys LM, Goodman MH, Olender S. Baseline Demographic. Psychosocial, and Behavioral Characteristics of Rural, Southern Women in Early Pregnancy. Maternal and child health journal: Anthropometric; 2016.
24. Thomson JL, Tussing-Humphreys LM, Goodman MH. Delta Healthy Sprouts: A randomized comparative effectiveness trial to promote maternal weight control and reduce childhood obesity in the Mississippi Delta. Contemp Clin Trials. 2014;38(1):82–91. PubMed PMID: WOS:000337203900009.
25. PAT. Parents as Teachers National Center Inc. [January 25, 2016]. Available from: http://www.parentsasteachers.org. Accessed 16 July 2016.
26. Knowler WC, Barrett-Connor E, Fowler SE, Hamman RF, Lachin JM, Walker EA, et al. Reduction in the incidence of type 2 diabetes with lifestyle intervention or metformin. N Engl J Med. 2002;346(6):393–403. Pubmed Central PMCID: 1370926.
27. Campbell KJ, Lioret S, McNaughton SA, Crawford DA, Salmon J, Ball K, et al. A parent-focused intervention to reduce infant obesity risk behaviors: a randomized trial. Pediatrics. 2013;131(4):652–60.
28. Nowak AJ, Casamassimo PS. Using anticipatory guidance to provide early dental intervention. J Am Dent Assoc. 1995;126(8):1156–63.
29. Mullis RL, Hill EW, Readdick CA. Attachment and social support among adolescents. J Genet Psychol. 1999;160(4):500–2.
30. Feskanich D, Sielaff BH, Chong K, Buzzard IM. Computerized collection and analysis of dietary intake information. Comput Methods Prog Biomed. 1989;30(1):47–57.
31. Harnack L, Stevens M, Van Heel N, Schakel S, Dwyer JT, Himes J. A computer-based approach for assessing dietary supplement use in conjunction with dietary recalls. J Food Composition Anal. 2008; 21(Suppliment 1):S78–82. Pubmed Central PMCID: 2151738.
32. Basiotis PP, Carlson A, Gerrior SA, Juan WY, Lino W. The Healthy Eating Index: 1999 - 2000. In: U.S. Department of Agriculture CfNPaP, editor. 2002.
33. Hacker AN, Fung EB, King JC. Role of calcium during pregnancy: maternal and fetal needs. Nutr Rev. 2012;70(7):397–409.
34. Jiang X, West AA, Caudill MA. Maternal choline supplementation: a nutritional approach for improving offspring health? Trends Endocrinol Metab. 2014;25(5):263–73.

35. Qiu C, Coughlin KB, Frederick IO, Sorensen TK, Williams MA. Dietary fiber intake in early pregnancy and risk of subsequent preeclampsia. Am J Hypertens. 2008;21(8):903–9.
36. Reynolds CM, Vickers MH, Harrison CJ, Segovia SA, Gray C. High fat and/or high salt intake during pregnancy alters maternal meta-inflammation and offspring growth and metabolic profiles. Physiol Rep. 2014;1:2(8). Pubmed Central PMCID: 4246600.
37. IOM. Dietary Reference Intakes Tables and Applications 2013 November 16, 2015. Available from: https://fnic.nal.usda.gov/dietary-guidance/dietary-reference-intakes/dri-tables-and-application-reports. Accessed 16 July 2016.
38. Poston L, Bell R, Croker H, Flynn AC, Godfrey KM, Goff L, et al. Effect of a behavioural intervention in obese pregnant women (the UPBEAT study): a multicentre, randomised controlled trial. Lancet Diab Endocrinol. 2015;3(10): 767–77.
39. Skouteris H, McPhie S, Hill B, McCabe M, Milgrom J, Kent B, et al. Health coaching to prevent excessive gestational weight gain: A randomized-controlled trial. Br J Health Psychol. 2016;21(1):31–51.
40. Lally P, Chipperfield A, Wardle J. Healthy habits: efficacy of simple advice on weight control based on a habit-formation model. Int J Obes (Lond). 2008;32(4):700–7.
41. Merriam PA, Ma Y, Olendzki BC, Schneider KL, Li W, Ockene IS, et al. Design and methods for testing a simple dietary message to improve weight loss and dietary quality. BMC Med Res Methodol. 2009;9:87. Pubmed Central PMCID: 2811706.
42. Olander EK, Atkinson L, Edmunds JK, French DP. The views of pre- and post-natal women and health professionals regarding gestational weight gain: An exploratory study. Sex Reprod Healthcare. 2011;2(1):43–8.
43. Whitaker KM, Wilcox S, Liu J, Blair SN, Pate RR. Pregnant women's perceptions of weight gain, physical activity, and nutrition using Theory of Planned Behavior constructs. J Behav Med. 2016;39(1):41–54. Pubmed Central PMCID: 4753045.
44. Darmon N, Drewnowski A. Does social class predict diet quality? Am J Clin Nutr. 2008;87(5):1107–17.
45. Lin H, Carr KA, Fletcher KD, Epstein LH. Food reinforcement partially mediates the effect of socioeconomic status on body mass index. Obesity. 2013;21(7):1307–12. Pubmed Central PMCID: 3742692.
46. Baker EA, Schootman M, Barnidge E, Kelly C. The role of race and poverty in access to foods that enable individuals to adhere to dietary guidelines. Prev Chronic Dis. 2006;3(3):A76. Pubmed Central PMCID: 1636719.
47. Diez-Roux AV, Nieto FJ, Caulfield L, Tyroler HA, Watson RL, Szklo M. Neighbourhood differences in diet: the Atherosclerosis Risk in Communities (ARIC) Study. J Epidemiol Community Health. 1999;53(1):55–63. Pubmed Central PMCID: 1756776.
48. Morland K, Wing S, Diez RA. The contextual effect of the local food environment on residents' diets: the atherosclerosis risk in communities study. Am J Public Health. 2002;92(11):1761–7. Pubmed Central PMCID: 1447325.

4

Timing and cause of perinatal mortality for small-for-gestational-age babies in South Africa: critical periods and challenges with detection

Tina Lavin[1*], David B. Preen[1] and Robert Pattinson[2]

Abstract

Background: Little information exists on timing and cause of death for small-for-gestational-age (SGA) babies in low-and-middle-income-countries (LMICs), despite evidence from high-income countries suggesting critical periods for SGA babies. This study explored the timing and cause of stillbirth and early neonatal mortality (END, <7 days) by small-for-gestational age in three provinces in South Africa. In South Africa, the largest category of perinatal deaths is unexplained stillbirth, of which up to one-quarter have intra-uterine growth restriction.

Methods: Secondary analysis of the South African Perinatal Problems Identification Program (PPIP) database allowed for the analysis of gestational age at death and clinically confirmed diagnosis of stillbirth and early neonatal death (END) (>1000 g and >28 weeks) across gestation. Comparisons by province, size-for-gestational-age, gestational age groups, and maternal condition at death were performed. The provinces investigated were: Western Cape (fortnightly antenatal care visits from 32 to 38 weeks), Limpopo and Mpumalanga (no antenatal care visits between 32 to 38 weeks).

Results: There were 528,727 births in the study period and 8111 stillbirths and 5792 early neonatal deaths. Similar timing of deaths across gestation was seen for the three provinces with the greatest proportion of deaths for SGA babies at 33–37 weeks (stillbirths 52.9 %; END 43.3 %; $p < 0.05$). SGA babies had a greater proportion of deaths due to hypertension (SGA22.9 %; AGA 18.6 %; LGA 18.6 %; $p < 0.05$) and intrauterine growth restriction (SGA 6.8 %; AGA 1.7 %; LGA 1.4 %; $p < 0.05$). No increase was seen in poor maternal condition for SGA babies and 54.9 % of deaths had a healthy mother. Of mothers that were healthy the greatest proportion of SGA stillbirths were due to unexplained intrauterine death (53.9 %).

Conclusion: There was a peak in stillbirths for SGA babies 33–37 weeks in all provinces. Detecting SGA is further complicated as in most cases the mother is healthy. Further research into Umbiflow Doppler velocimetry use in low-risk populations is warranted and may be a viable strategy to increase current detection of SGA babies at risk of mortality in LMICs.

Keywords: Small-for-gestational-age, Intrauterine growth restriction, Perinatal mortality, South Africa, Low-and-middle-income countries, Doppler

* Correspondence: tina.lavin@uwa.edu.au
[1]Centre for Health Services Research, School of Population Health, The University of Western Australia (M431), 35 Stirling Highway, Crawley, WA 6009, Australia
Full list of author information is available at the end of the article

Background

Approximately 25 % of children born in low-and-middle-income countries (LMICs) are small-for-gestational-age (SGA) [1]. Babies who are SGA are at increased risk of mortality and neonatal morbidity [2, 3], making the detection and clinical management of such infants crucial. The condition may constitute a small but healthy fetus or be due to pathological growth failure (intrauterine growth restriction (IUGR)) [4]. The purpose of identifying SGA fetuses, defined as a birth weight in the lowest decile on standard growth curves [5], is to recognise those most at risk of poor outcomes [3].

Studies to date have indicated that there may be a critical period for increased mortality for SGA babies [3, 5, 6]. A UK study found that stillbirths between 28 and 36 weeks were increased for SGA babies [5]. Other studies have found that SGA babies are at increased risk of stillbirth compared to non-SGA babies at all gestational ages [3], and that the risk of stillbirth for SGA babies increases with advancing gestational age [6].

In South Africa, the largest category of perinatal deaths is unexplained stillbirth, of which up to one-quarter have IUGR [7]. Early recognition can prevent some of these deaths. Early antenatal detection of SGA babies remains a challenge in LMICs, but is important as most deaths occur in the late preterm or term period, where survival of live born infants in well-resourced units is high [8]. As detection of SGA at the population level is challenging due to resource constraints, identifying critical periods and causes of mortality across gestation may elucidate the best approach.

This study explores the gestational age at death and cause of stillbirth and early neonatal mortality (up to 7 days neonatal life) by size-for-gestational age in three South African provinces.

Methods

Secondary analysis of the South African Perinatal Problems Identification Program (PPIP) database allowed for the analysis of gestational age at death and clinically confirmed diagnosis of stillbirth and early neonatal death (END) across gestation. The program also allowed for comparisons between SGA, appropriate-for-gestational-age (AGA) and large-for-gestational-age (LGA) babies from 1 October and 2013 and 31 August 2015 and between three provinces: Western Cape, Limpopo and Mpumalanga. Western Cape has fortnightly antenatal care visits between 32 and 38 weeks, while Limpopo and Mpumalanga do not have visits between 32 and 38 weeks, preventing the opportunity for detection of SGA at these gestations. These provinces were chosen (from nine available) as they have the greatest PPIP coverage, auditing >90 % of perinatal deaths. PPIP is a perinatal quality audit system that has been described in detail elsewhere [7, 9]. Briefly, at each clinical site ($n = 292$) across the three provinces the clinical team perform a review shortly after a death has occurred. The primary obstetric cause of death was defined by the PPIP technical team as the main obstetric event or pregnancy occurrence which was integral in the pathway to perinatal death, as described in other published studies [7]. IUGR was also identified at the time of death through clinical evaluation. Maternal condition at the time of death was also recorded. Categories for the primary obstetric cause of stillbirth and early neonatal death were as follows: antepartum haemorrhage, spontaneous preterm labour (intrapartum stillbirth), unexplained intrauterine death, fetal abnormality, hypertensive disorders, infections, intrapartum asphyxia, intrauterine growth restriction, maternal disease, miscellaneous (rhesus isoimmunisation, twin-to-twin transfusion, extra-uterine pregnancy and other cause of death not described), no obstetric cause and trauma. The maternal condition is defined as either healthy (where the clinician examining her could not find any clinical problems) or the occurrence of a recognised medical or obstetric complication (eg. cardiac, endocrine, respiratory disease or other disease that are an indirect cause of morbidity), categorised as coincidental conditions, medical and surgical disorders, non-pregnancy related infections, extra-uterine pregnancy, pregnancy-related sepsis, obstetric haemorrhage, hypertension, anaesthetic complications, embolism, and acute collapse (cause unknown).

Gestational age was calculated based on date of last menstrual period, ultrasound or clinical examination and cases were excluded if the gestation age was unknown or if the estimated age was considered 'uncertain'. There was no hierarchy employed based on method of gestational age estimation. Detailed data were extracted on all stillbirths >1000 g and 28–42 weeks gestation and early neonatal deaths less than 7 days of neonatal life. Data were only included up to 42 weeks gestation as Theron weight distribution curves are not considered reliable for growth measurements after 42 weeks gestation [10, 11]. Only women who had reported receiving antenatal care were included as SGA can be detected antenatally. Data extracted from the three provinces represent 58.6 % of all deaths in South Africa that met the study criteria. Birth weight for gestation was obtained from Theron charts. SGA was defined as neonates with <10th centile for gestational age based on South African specific growth charts [10, 11].

Statistical analysis

Stillbirth and early neonatal death cumulative incidence were calculated for each province using the number of reported births (all births for stillbirth, live births for neonatal death rate) as the denominator. The frequencies of deaths occurring across gestation were compared between SGA, AGA and LGA babies as well as between provinces. Comparisons between the proportion of primary cause of deaths were made by size-for-gestational-age, gestational age at death and in relation to maternal conditions. Gestational age was grouped into three categories for analysis: 28–32 weeks, 33–37 weeks and 38–42 weeks. Frequency distributions were performed and Pearson's chi-squared test or Fisher's exact test (where $n < 5$) were used to determine crude differences between proportions for the key comparisons made (i.e. size-for-gestational-age, gestational age at death, maternal condition and between provinces). Independent t-tests were used to compare means between key groups. A p-value <0.05 was accepted as statically significant.

The PPIP program has ethical approval from the Faculty of Heath Sciences Ethics Committee at the University of Pretoria. The data are collected with permission from the South African Department of Health. This secondary analysis was approved by the PPIP technical task team and UWA Human Ethics Committee.

Results

There were 528,727 births >1000 g in the study period (Mpumalanga = 145,362; Western Cape = 173,597; Limpopo = 209,768), of which 8111 (1.5 %) were stillbirths (Mpumalanga =2501; Limpopo = 3808; Western Cape = 1802) and 3792 (0.7 %) died in the early neonatal period (<7 days) (Mpumalanga =1163; Limpopo = 2124; Western Cape = 505). The cumulative incidence of stillbirth for the study period was highest in Limpopo (18.2 per 1000 births) and Mpumalanga (17.2/1000) compared to Western Cape (10.4/1000). The cumulative incidence of early neonatal death was highest in Limpopo at 10.3 per 1000 live births, followed by Mpumalanga (8.1 per 1000) and Western Cape (3.0 per 1000). After exclusion of deaths prior to 28 weeks (and after 42 weeks), deaths with unknown or uncertain gestation and women who had not received ANC, the number of deaths used for analysis was 6133 (Mpumalanga $n = 2198$; Limpopo $n = 3032$; Western Cape $n = 903$). The greatest proportion of babies in the study were AGA (61.5 %), followed by SGA (22.6 %) and LGA (12.3 %).

Gestational age at death

There were no differences between provinces in terms of representation and timing of stillbirths between SGA, AGA, LGA, therefore data from the three provinces were combined and presented as means and standard errors. Stillbirths who were AGA or LGA occurred across gestation without any significant increases or decreases. A larger proportion of SBs occurred for SGA babies in the 33–37 week period in all provinces (Fig. 1). When considering macerated and fresh stillbirths a peak at 33–37 weeks was also seen for SGA babies (Fig. 1). A similar pattern was seen for early neonatal deaths (END) with a peak at 33–37 weeks for SGA babies. The timing of END for AGA and LGA babies increased during the 38–42 week period but remained low at 28–32w and 33–37w.

Primary causes of death

Stillbirths by size-for-gestational-age

The primary cause of stillbirth across the sample was unexplained intrauterine death (33.1 %), followed by intrapartum asphyxia (17.2 %) and hypertensive disorders (19.7 %) (Table 1). Some primary causes of death were more frequent in the SGA group, such as fetal abnormality (37.8 %) and intrauterine growth restriction (59.8 %) which represented up to half of all deaths despite only representing 26.2 % of the total sample ($p < 0.05$). Intrapartum asphyxia for SGA babies was indicated in 13.3 % of deaths due to intrapartum asphyxia across gestation ($p < 0.05$).

Early neonatal deaths by size-for-gestational-age

The primary cause of early neonatal death (<7 days) was intrapartum asphyxia (42.1 %), followed by spontaneous preterm labour (18.7 %), fetal abnormality (11.4 %) and hypertensive disorders (7.3 %) (Table 2). Cause of death in SGA babies were intrauterine growth restriction (91.3 %), hypertensive disorders (37.0 %), fetal abnormality (33.3 %), and spontaneous preterm labour (36.0 %) which represented a large proportion of all deaths by cause despite representing only 23.7 % of the sample.

Stillbirths across gestational age groups (28–32, 33–37, and 38–42 weeks)

The main causes of stillbirth at 28–32 weeks and 33–37 weeks for babies of all gestations were unexplained intrauterine death (34.5 %; 33.4 %, respectively), hypertensive disorders (27.7 %; 20.2 %) and antepartum haemorrhage (18.2 %;17.9 %). For stillbirths during the 38–42 week period the main causes were unexplained intrauterine death (33 %), intrapartum asphyxia (31.1 %) and hypertensive disorders (13.5 %) (Table 3). Mortality was highest in the 33–37 week period with death due to unexplained intrauterine death (31.5 %), hypertension (25.5 %), antepartum haemorrhage (17.0 %). Most deaths for SGA babies from spontaneous preterm labour (70.4 %), antepartum haemorrhage (64.8 %) and hypertensive disorders (57.8 %) occurred during the 33–37 week period ($p < 0.05$). Most SGA deaths from intrapartum asphyxia occurred during the 38–42 week period ($p < 0.05$).

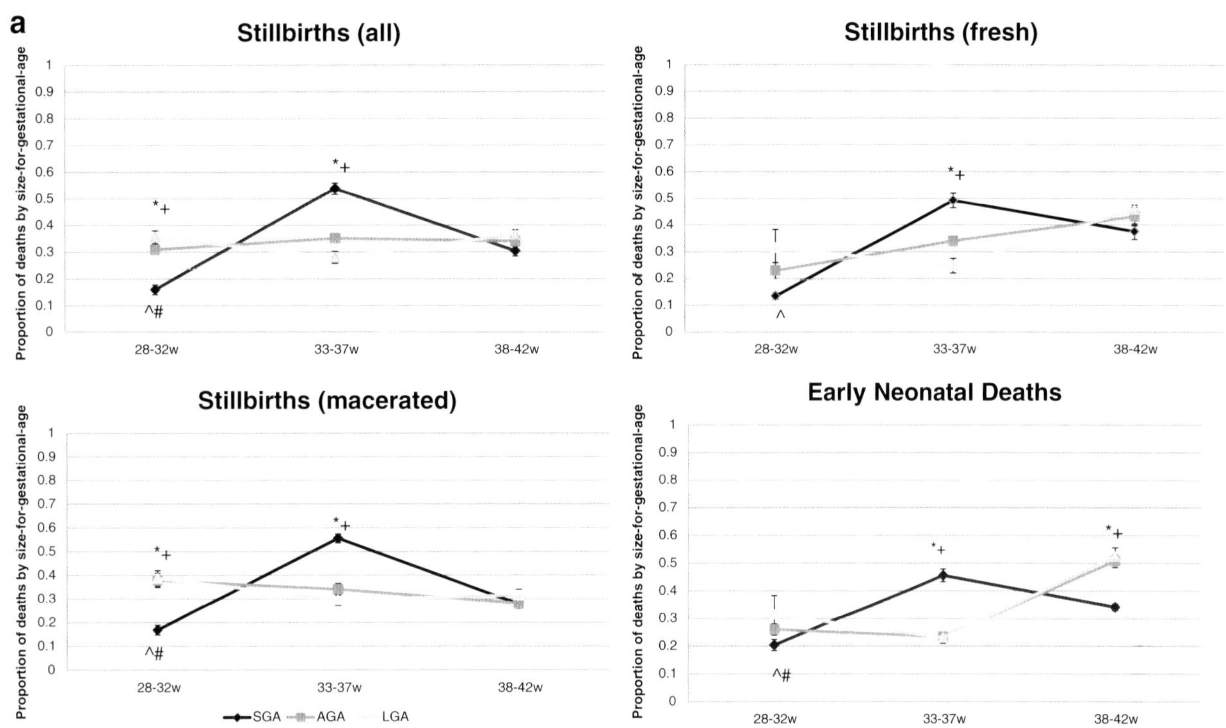

Fig. 1 Proportion of deaths (standard error for provinces combined) across gestation by size-for-gestational-age. *$p < 0.05$ with AGA; +$p < 0.05$ with LGA. ^SGA significantly increased at 33–37w compared to 28–32w; #SGA significantly increased at 33–37w compared to 38–42 weeks. Legend: SGA (*black line*); AGA (*gray line*); LGA (*light gray line*)

Table 1 Primary cause of stillbirth by size-for-gestation (Western Cape, Limpopo and Mpumalanga combined); $n = 4059$

Primary cause of stillbirth	SGA	AGA	LGA	
	n (%)	*n* (%)	*n* (%)	All %
APH	145 (13.6)	399 (16.0)	51 (10.2)	14.7
Unexplained Intrauterine death	367 (34.5)	812 (32.5)	164 (32.8)	33.1
Fetal abnormality	54 (5.1)*	67 (2.7)	22 (4.4)	3.5
Hypertensive disorders	244 (22.9)*^	463 (18.6)	93 (18.6)	19.7
Infections	26 (2.4)	42 (1.7)	7 (1.4)	1.8
Intrapartum asphyxia	93 (8.7)*^	512 (20.5)	93 (18.6)	17.2
Intrauterine growth restriction	73 (6.8)*^	42 (1.7)	7 (1.4)	3.0
Maternal disease	12 (1.1)*^	56 (2.2)	41 (8.2)	2.7
Misc.	22 (2.1)	27 (1.1)	6 (1.2)	1.4
No obstetric cause	1 (0.1)	2 (0.1)	1 (0.2)	0.1
Spont. Preterm labour	27 (2.5)	65 (2.6)	12 (2.4)	2.6
Trauma	1 (0.1)	8 (0.3)	2 (0.4)	0.3
All	1065	2495	499	100.0

*$p < 0.05$ with AGA; ^$p < 0.05$ with LGA; Pearson chi-sq tests, Fisher's exact where cell count <5

Table 2 Primary cause of early neonatal death (<7 days) by size-for-gestational age (provinces combined); $n = 1742$

Primary cause death (END)	SGA	AGA	LGA	
	n (%)	*n* (%)	*n* (%)	All %
APH	18 (44)	59 (5.1)	3 (1.6)	4.6
Unexplained Intrauterine death	1 (0.2)	2 (0.2)	0 (0.0)	0.2
Fetal abnormality	66 (16.0)*	112 (9.8)	20 (10.9)	11.4
Hypertensive disorders	47 (11.4)*	68 (5.9)	12 (6.5)	7.3
Infections	11 (2.7)	26 (2.3)	5 (2.7)	2.4
Intrapartum asphyxia	103 (25.0)*^	619 (54.0)	11 (62.0)	42.1
Intrauterine growth restriction	21 (5.1)*^	2 (0.2)	0 (0.0)	1.3
Maternal disease	1 (0.2)	7 (0.6)	2 (1.1)	0.6
Misc.	7 (1.7)	17 (1.5)	5 (2.7)	1.7
No obstetric cause	20 (4.9)	44 (3.8)	5 (2.7)	4.0
Spont. Preterm labour	117 (28.4)*^	190 (16.6)	18 (9.8)	18.7
Trauma	0 (0.0)	0 (0.0)	0 (0.0)	0.0
All	412	1146	184	100.0

*$p < 0.05$ with AGA; ^$p < 0.05$ with LGA; Pearson chi-sq tests, Fisher's exact where cell count <5

Table 3 Primary cause of stillbirth for SGA babies across GA; $n = 1042$

Primary cause death	28–32w	33–37w	38–42w	All
	n (%)	*n* (%)	*n* (%)	*n* (%)
APH	23 (13.5)	94 (17.0)	28 (8.8)	145 (13.9)
Unexplained Intrauterine death	63 (37.1)	174 (31.5)^	130 (40.6)	367 (35.2)
Fetal abnormality	9 (5.3)	30 (5.4)	15 (4.7)	54 (5.2)
Hypertensive disorders	52 (30.6)	141 (25.5)^	51 (15.9)	244 (23.4)
Infections	3 (1.8)	9 (1.6)^	14 (4.4)	26 (2.5)
Intrapartum asphyxia	7 (4.1)	36 (6.5)^	50 (15.6)	93 (8.9)
Intrauterine growth restriction	7 (4.1)	42 (7.6)	24 (7.5)	73 (7)
Maternal disease	1 (0.6)	6 (1.1)	5 (1.6)	12 (1.2)
Spont. Preterm labour	5 (2.9)	19 (3.4)^	3 (0.9)	27 (2.6)
Trauma	0 (0.0)	1 (0.2)	0 (0)	1 (0.1)
All	170 (100.0)	552 (100.0)	320 (100.0)	1042 (100.0)

^with 38–42 week age group; Pearson chi-sq tests, Fisher's exact where cell count <5

Table 4 Primary cause of ENND for SGA babies at each gestation, $n = 385$

Primary cause death	28–32w	33–37w	38–42w	All
	n (%)	*n* (%)	*n* (%)	*n* (%)
APH	8 (9.2)	5 (3.0)	5 (3.5)	18 (1.1)
Unexplained Intrauterine death	0 (0.0)	1 (0.6)	0 (0.0)	1 (0.1)
Fetal abnormality	7 (8.0)	31 (18.6)*	28 (21.4)	66 (4.0)
Hypertensive disorders	17 (19.5)	23 (13.8)^	7 (5.3)	47 (2.9)
Infections	1 (1.1)	5 (3.0)	5 (3.8)	11 (0.7)
Intrapartum asphyxia	2 (2.3)	31 (18.6)*^	70 (53.4)	103 (6.3)
Intrauterine growth restriction	2 (2.3)	10 (6.0)	9 (6.9)	21 (1.3)
Maternal disease	1 (1.1)	0 (0.0)	0 (0.0)	1 (0.1)
Spont. Preterm labour	49 (56.3)	61 (36.5)*^	7 (5.3)	117 (7.1)
Trauma	0 (0.0)	0 (0)	0 (0)	0 (0.0)
All	87 (100.0)	167 (100.0)	131 (100.0)	385 (100.0)

*$p < 0.05$ with 28–32w age group; ^ with 38–42 week age group; Pearson chi-sq tests, Fisher's exact where cell count <5

Early neonatal deaths across gestational age groups (28–32, 33–37, and 38–42 weeks)

The main causes of early neonatal death at 28–32 weeks were spontaneous preterm labour (57.4 %), hypertensive disorders (14.8 %) and antepartum haemorrhage (10.2 %). For deaths between 33 and 37 weeks the main causes of death were intrapartum asphyxia (47.3 %), fetal abnormality (17.7 %), spontaneous preterm labour (16 %) and hypertensive disorders (9.2 %). At 38–42 weeks intrapartum asphyxia was the main cause of death (77.1 %), followed by fetal abnormality (11.5 %) (Table 4). The largest causes of death during the 33–37 week period, when SGA deaths peaked, were for spontaneous preterm labour (36.5 %), fetal abnormality (18.6 %) and intrapartum asphyxia (18.6 %) (Table 4). Most deaths from intrapartum asphyxia for SGA babies occurred during the 38–42 week period (68 %), while most deaths from hypertensive disorders (48.9 %) and fetal abnormality (47 %) occurred during the 33–37 week period ($p < 0.05$).

Maternal condition

There were no significant differences in the proportion of deaths to healthy mothers by size-for-gestational-age (SGA $n = 605$, 54.9 %; AGA $n = 1394$, 55.4 %; LGA $n = 279$, 53.8 %). Of mothers who were healthy, the greatest proportion of stillbirths was seen for unexplained intrauterine death (all sizes-for-gestation 50.6 %; SGA 53.9 %). More mothers of SGA babies were hypertensive compared to AGA and LGA babies (SGA 26.3 %; AGA 21.6 %; LGA 21.2 %; $p < 0.05$), however fewer mothers of SGA babies had medical and surgical complications compared to LGA babies (SGA 5.1 %; LGA 11 %; $p < 0.05$).

Causes of stillbirth and condition of mother for SGA babies across gestational groups are presented in Table 5. Causes of early neonatal death and condition of mother for small-for-gestational age babies across gestational groups are presented in Table 6.

Discussion

Our findings indicate that there are specific characteristics unique to SGA babies in terms of gestational age at death and causes of perinatal morality.

Timing of perinatal deaths across gestation

The same pattern of timing of stillbirth across gestation was seen for the three provinces with the greatest proportion of deaths for SGA babies during the 33–37 week period. This was in contrast to AGA and LGA babies where no peaks in the proportion of stillbirths across gestation were seen. This is consistent with observations in high-income countries where peaks have been observed between 34–37 weeks and 32–36 weeks [3, 5]. In the current study a greater proportion of ENDs for SGA babies also occurred during the 33–37 week period, suggesting that this is a critical time for both antepartum and postpartum mortality. It is also well-established that there is increased neonatal mortality for SGA preterm babies compared to AGA preterm babies [1], stressing the vulnerability of SGA babies in particular.

Table 5 Cause of stillbirth and condition of mother for small-for-gestational age babies, $n = 1227$

	Healthy mother			Medical surgical			Hypertension			Other maternal condition		
	28–32w	33–37w	38–42w	28–32w	33–37w	38–42w	28–32w	33–37w	38–42w	28–32w	33–37w	38–42w
Antepartum haemorrhage	10 (4.8)	20 (6.9)	8 (3.5)	2 (25.0)	4 (12.5)	0 (0.0)	3 (5.5)	16 (9.4)	4 (6.2)	19 (76.0)	62 (68.1)^	16 (42.1)
Unexplained Intrauterine death	97 (46.2)	151 (51.9)	117 (51.8)	3 (37.5)	8 (25.0)	3 (18.8)	0 (0.0)	1 (0.6)^	6 (9.2)	1 (4.0)	10 (11.0)	9 (23.7)
Fetal abnormality	21 (10.0)	24 (8.2)	14 (6.2)	0 (0.0)	3 (9.4)	0 (0.0)	2 (3.6)	7 (4.1)	1 (1.5)	0 (0.0)	1 (1.1)	0 (0.0)
Hypertensive disorders	6 (2.9)	11 (3.8)	5 (2.2)	1 (12.5)	5 (15.6)	1 (6.3)	46 (83.6)*	124 (72.9)	47 (72.3)	2 (8.0)	7 (7.7)	4 (10.5)
Infections	6 (2.9)	1 (0.3)*^	7 (3.1)	0 (0.0)	2 (6.3)	2 (12.5)	0 (0.0)	1 (0.6)	0 (0.0)	1 (4.0)	5 (5.5)	6 (15.8)
Intrapartum asphyxia	12 (5.7)	24 (8.2)	42 (18.6)	0 (0.0)	3 (9.4)	4 (25.0)	1 (1.8)	8 (4.7)	2 (3.1)	1 (4.0)	2 (2.2)	2 (5.3)
Intrauterine growth restriction	47 (22.4)	36 (12.4)*	21 (9.3)	1 (12.5)	0 (0.0)	0 (0.0)	3 (5.5)	5 (2.9)	3 (4.6)	0 (0.0)	1 (1.1)	0 (0.0)
Spont. Preterm labour	9 (4.3)	17 (5.8)^	2 (0.9)	0 (0.0)	0 (0.0)	1 (6.3)	0 (0.0)	0 (0.0)	1 (1.5)	0 (0.0)	2 (2.2)	0 (0.0)
All	210 (100)	291 (100)	226 (100)	8 (100)	32 (100)	16 (100)	55 (100)	170 (100)	65 (100)	25 (100)	91 (100)	38 (100.0)

*$p < 0.05$ with 28–32week group; ^$p < 0.05$ with 38–42 weeks group. Pearson's chi-sq or Fishers exact where cell count <5

Current antenatal care timing differs between the provinces, with Western Cape, the most well-resourced province, continuing fortnightly antenatal care visits between 32 and 38 weeks, while Limpopo and Mpumalanga cease antenatal care visits between 32 and 38 weeks. Previous work has shown that stillbirth risk is increased during periods without antenatal care [12]. The peak in stillbirths for SGA babies seen in all provinces between 33 and 37 weeks gestation suggests that the current detection and management of SGA is not adequate even in Western Cape where frequent antenatal care visits occur.

Causes of death/mother's condition

Growth restriction may not necessarily play a principle role in the cause of death for all SGA babies, as SGA may also be due to slow growth of an otherwise healthy baby [4, 13]. In our study a greater proportion of SGA babies had deaths due to hypertension which is known to have placental pathology [13], indicating that growth restriction played a role in these deaths. It is important to consider that all the babies in the current cohort were considered viable (i.e. >1000 g and >28 weeks) and that very severe cases of placental insufficiency and congenital abnormalities could have died as late miscarriages.

Table 6 Cause of Early neonatal death and condition of mother for small-for-gestational age babies, $n = 388$

	Healthy mother			Medical surgical			Hypertension			Other maternal condition		
	28–32w	33–37w	38–42w	28–32w	33–37w	38–42w	28–32w	33–37w	38–42w	28–32w	33–37w	38–42w
APH	1 (1.9)	3 (2.5)	3 (2.9)	0 (0.0)	0 (0.0)	0 (0.0)	0 (0.0)	1 (2.9)	0 (0.0)	8 (50.0)	1 (8.3)*	2 (25.0)
Unexplained Intrauterine death	0 (0.0)	1 (0.8)	0 (0.0)	0 (0.0)	0 (0.0)	0 (0.0)	0 (0.0)	0 (0.0)	0 (0.0)	0 (0.0)	0 (0.0)	0 (0.0)
Fetal abnormality	6 (11.5)	19 (16.1)	24 (23.1)	0 (0.0)	0 (0.0)	3 (50.0)	1 (5.6)	4 (11.4)	2 (13.3)	0 (0.0)	1 (8.3)	1 (12.5)
Hypertensive disorders	1 (1.9)	9 (7.6)^	1 (1.0)	0 (0.0)	0 (0.0)	1 (16.7)	16 (88.9)	21 (60.0)	5 (33.3)	0 (0.0)	1 (8.3)	0 (0.0)
Infections	0 (0.0)	3 (2.5)	3 (2.9)	0 (0.0)	0 (0.0)	1 (16.7)	0 (0.0)	0 (0.0)	0 (0.0)	1 (6.2)	2 (16.7)	2 (25.0)
Intrapartum asphyxia	2 (3.8)	24 (20.3)*	58 (55.8)	0 (0.0)	1 (33.3)	1 (16.7)	0 (0.0)	4 (11.4)^	7 (46.7)	0 (0.0)	2 (16.7)	3 (37.5)
Intrauterine growth restriction	1 (1.9)	7 (5.9)	8 (7.7)	0 (0.0)	0 (0.0)	0 (0.0)	1 (5.6)	2 (5.7)	1 (6.7)	0 (0.0)	1 (8.3)	0 (0.0)
Spont. Preterm labour	41 (78.8)	52 (44.1)	7 (6.7)	1 (100.0)	2 (66.7)	0 (0.0)	0 (0.0)	3 (8.6)	0 (0.0)	7 (43.8)	4 (33.3)	0 (0.0)
All	52 (100.0)	118 (100.0)	104 (100.0)	1 (100.0)	3 (100.0)	6 (100.0)	18 (100.0)	35 (100.0)	15 (100.0)	16 (100.0)	12 (100.0)	8 (100.0)

*$p < 0.05$ with 28–32week group; ^$p < 0.05$ with 38–42 weeks group. Pearson's chi-sq or Fishers exact where cell count <5

Therefore the deaths in the current study could have been potentially avoided if at risk fetuses were detected early.

Detecting SGA is complicated as in most cases the mother is healthy. In the current study there was no increase in poor maternal condition for SGA babies and more than half of all deaths had a healthy mother. Of mothers that were healthy the greatest proportion of SGA stillbirths were due to unexplained intrauterine death. Earlier detection of fetuses at risk antenatally may reduce the number of unexplained intrauterine deaths.

Challenges with detection

Better detection of SGA babies is needed in South Africa and LMICs. Palpation and symphysis fundal height are commonly used in LMICs due to limited alternative resources, despite the limited evidence to support this as an effective method to predict growth restriction [14]. Clinical trials in high-income countries estimate that up to 76 % of SGA cases can be detected antenatally [15]. The use of Doppler velocimetry to measure altered umbilical artery blood flow in high risk women has enhanced the ability to detect fetuses with pathological growth restriction [16], reducing perinatal mortality [17]. However, challenges with Doppler measurement in South Africa are present as there are a large number of perinatal deaths to low-risk healthy mothers [7] and who would therefore not be referred for screening. Studies in South Africa have explored the use of a continuous wave Doppler analyser using a PC (Umbiflow), a simpler alternative to umbilical artery Doppler, which can be operated by nurses and midwives at the primary health care centre level [18, 19]. The Umbiflow is able to detect fetuses at risk of stillbirth based on abnormal umbilical artery blood flow. While meta-analyses in high-income countries found Doppler use in low-risk pregnancies to be ineffective to reduce perinatal mortality and morbidity [20], there may be potential benefit of Doppler or Umbiflow use in low risk populations in LMICs where stillbirth rates are higher. However, once a fetus at risk of stillbirth is detected, quality clinical care must also be provided to increase the risk of survival.

Challenges with clinical management

Once SGA has been detected there are challenges in the clinical management of such babies. Currently there are no effective approaches for the reversal or improvement of the growth pattern of a fetus [21], therefore prenatal clinical management is focused on identifying the optimal timing of delivery. The gestational age of the fetus is a critical component of the decision-making process, as fetal mortality is lower than neonatal mortality prior to 31 weeks [22], and delivery after 39 weeks results in increased perinatal mortality [23]. While it is known that the neonatal mortality risk is higher for preterm SGA babies compared to term SGA babies [1], it unclear how much size-for-gestational age impacts the risk of neonatal mortality in the preterm compared to late preterm infant [24, 25]. It has recently been suggested that the delivery of SGA babies around 37 weeks is optimal to avoid increased risk of stillbirth occurring after week 37 [26]. Causes of death for SGA babies in other studies have shown different patterns across gestation with a greater proportion of deaths due to congenital abnormality (32–42 weeks) and intrapartum asphyxia (37–42 weeks) at older gestations [5]. We observed similar findings in our data with SGA deaths from intrapartum asphyxia and fetal abnormality occurring more frequently at older gestations. Standard guidelines for managing labour in South African include partogram and monitoring of fetal heart rate with a fetal stethoscope or doptone in Community Health Centres and electronically at district hospitals and above. However it is estimated that in 44 % of deaths these guidelines are not adhered to due to limited resources and staff [27]. Caesarean delivery is not readily accessible in some districts, and long transport times exist between Community Health Centres to facilities that are able to perform caesarean section deliveries. It is likely these factors play a role in the high proportion of deaths due to fetal asphyxia observed in the current study. It is also important to note that spontaneous preterm labour is an underlying cause of early neonatal death where the maternal condition contributes to increased risk of death from disorders associated with prematurity. Early neonatal deaths for preterm neonates reflect access and quality of care after birth for preterm infants. The final cause of death for a preterm neonate could be due to a causes such as hyaline membrane disease, hypoxic ischaemic encephalopathy and meconium aspiration. Doppler measurements in combination with growth charts can be used to inform the management of SGA pregnancies [17]. This has been shown to decrease the induction of labour and hospital admissions in high-income countries [17].

Limitations

There are some limitations to the current study. First, there is likely some ambiguity in the assignment of gestational age from the perinatal audit data. Last menstrual period or ultrasound estimates for gestational age may not be accurate and the SGA category may erroneously capture appropriately sized infants who measure small for their misassigned gestational age. We sought to reduce this issue by using only data where gestational age estimates were considered 'certain'. Second, macerated SGA babies are likely to be overestimated as death may have occurred up to 2 weeks prior [28] thus the fetus may have been appropriate-for-gestational age at the time of death. Third, as we had access to aggregated data at a centre level, and data for the number of live births for SGA, AGA and LGA were unavailable we were unable to calculate stillbirth risk, relative risks between live and stillborn babies or perform individual unit analysis using multivariable regression. Fourth, both multiple and single gestations were included in the current study. These were not separated due to limited statistical power and therefore any differences in patterns of mortality between multiple and single gestations are not presented in the current study. Deaths directly related to multiple gestation such as twin-to-twin transfusion only represented 0.3 % of all deaths in the current study, therefore it is unlikely that the inclusion of multiple gestations introduced significant bias.

Conclusion

Mortality from SGA in South Africa accounts for a considerable number of deaths, yet there is little research on the timing, causes and detection of SGA in low-resource settings. The detection and management of SGA is important as most deaths occur in late preterm or term infants, where the chance of survival is high when adequate care can be delivered. If SGA infants can be detected antenatally and managed effectively there is an opportunity to significantly reduce the burden of perinatal mortality in LMICs. Further studies on the relationship between antenatal detection and outcome of SGA are needed, especially in LMICs.

Abbreviations

AGA: Appropriate-for-gestational-age; END: Early neonatal death (up to 7 days neonatal life); IUGR: Intrauterine growth restriction; LGA: Large-for-gestational-age; LMIC: Low-and-middle-income-countries; PPIP: Perinatal Problems Identification Program; SGA: Small-for-gestational-age

Acknowledgments

We are grateful for the funding provided through the University of Western Australia Research Collaboration Award to the support this research.

Funding

University of Western Australia, Research Collaboration Award.

Authors' contributions

TL and RP conceptualized the manuscript. TL performed data analysis; TL, DP and RP interpreted findings, TL drafted manuscript. DP and RP reviewed the manuscript and approved the final version. All authors read and approved the final manuscript.

Competing interests

The authors declare they have no competing interests.

Author details

[1]Centre for Health Services Research, School of Population Health, The University of Western Australia (M431), 35 Stirling Highway, Crawley, WA 6009, Australia. [2]SAMRC Maternal and Infant Health Care Strategies, Department of Obstetrics and Gynaecology, University of Pretoria, Pretoria, South Africa.

References

1. Katz J, Lee AC, Kozuki N, Lawn JE, Cousens S, Blencowe H, Ezzati M, Bhutta ZA, Marchant T, Willey BA, et al. Mortality risk in preterm and small-for-gestational-age infants in low-income and middle-income countries: a pooled country analysis. Lancet. 2013;382(9890):417–25.
2. Chiswick ML. Intrauterine growth-retardation. Brit Med J. 1985;291(6499):845–8.
3. Pilliod RA, Cheng YW, Snowden JM, Doss AE, Caughey AB. The risk of intrauterine fetal death in the small-for-gestational-age fetus. Am J Obstet Gynecol. 2012;207(4):318.e1-6.
4. Gardosi J, Mul T, Mongelli M, Fagan D. Analysis of birthweight and gestational age in antepartum stillbirths. Br J Obstet Gynaecol. 1998;105(5):524–30.
5. Decourcywheeler RHB, Wolfe CDA, Warburton F, Goodman J, Reynolds F, Gamsu H. The association between small-size for gestational-age and perinatal and neonatal death in a UK-regional-health-authority. Paediatr Perinat Ep. 1995;9(4):431–40.
6. Williams RL, Creasy RK, Cunningham GC, Hawes WE, Norris FD, Tashiro M. Fetal growth and perinatal viability in California. Obstet Gynecol. 1982;59(5):624–32.
7. Allanson ER, Muller M, Pattinson RC. Causes of perinatal mortality and associated maternal complications in a South African province: challenges in predicting poor outcomes. BMC Pregnancy and Childbirth. 2015;15:37.
8. Velaphi SC, Mokhachane M, Mphahlele RM, Beckh-Arnold E, Kuwanda ML, Cooper PA. Survival of very-low-birth-weight infants according to birth weight and gestational age in a public hospital. S Afr Med J. 2005; 95(7):504–9.
9. Allanson ER, Pattinson RC. Quality-of-care audit and perinatal mortality in South Africa. B World Health Organ. 2015;93:424–8.
10. Theron GB, Geerts L, Thompson ML, Theron AM. A centile chart for fetal weight for gestational ages 24–27 weeks. S Afr Med J. 2008;98(4):270–1.
11. Theron GB, Thompson ML. A centile chart for birth weight for an urban population of the Western Cape. S Afr Med J. 1995;85(12):1289–92.
12. Vogel JP, Habib NA, Souza JP, Gulmezoglu AM, Dowswell T, Carroli G, Baaqeel HS, Lumbiganon P, Piaggio G, Oladapo OT. Antenatal care packages with reduced visits and perinatal mortality: a secondary analysis of the WHO Antenatal Care Trial. Reprod Health. 2013;10:19.
13 Gruenwald P. Chronic fetal distress and placental insufficiency. Biol Neonatorum. 1963;5(3-4):215.
14 Peter JR, Ho JJ, Valliapan J, Sivasangari S. Symphysial fundal height (SFH) measurement in pregnancy for detecting abnormal fetal growth. Bjog-Int J Obstet Gy. 2012;119:78.
15 Pearce JM, Campbell S. A comparison of symphysis-fundal height and ultrasound as screening-tests for light-for-gestational age infants. Brit J Obstet Gynaec. 1987;94(2):100–4.
16 Reuwer PJ, Bruinse HW, Stoutenbeek P, Haspels AA. Doppler assessment of the fetoplacental circulation in normal and growth-retarded fetuses. Eur J Obstet Gynecol Reprod Biol. 1984;18(4):199–205.
17 Neilson JP, Alfirevic Z. Doppler ultrasound for fetal assessment in high risk pregnancies. Cochrane Database Syst Rev. 2000;2:CD000073.
18 Hugo EJC, Odendaal HJ, Grove D. Evaluation of the use of umbilical artery Doppler flow studies and outcome of pregnancies at a secondary hospital. J Matern-Fetal Neo M. 2007;20(3):233–9.
19 Theron GB, Theron AM, Odendaal HJ, Bunn AE. Comparison between a newly developed PC-based Doppler umbilical artery waveform analyser and a commercial unit. Samj S Afr Med J. 2005;95(1):62–4.
20 Alfirevic Z, Stampalija T, Medley N. Fetal and umbilical Doppler ultrasound in normal pregnancy. Cochrane Database Syst Rev. 2015;4:CD001450.
21 Gulmezoglu M, de Onis M, Villar J. Effectiveness of interventions to prevent or treat impaired fetal growth. Obstet Gynecol Surv. 1997;52(2):139–49.
22 Seeds JW, Peng T. Impaired growth and risk of fetal death: is the tenth percentile the appropriate standard? Am J Obstet Gynecol. 1998;178(4): 658–69.

5

Congenital Diaphragmatic hernia – a review

Praveen Kumar Chandrasekharan[1*], Munmun Rawat[1], Rajeshwari Madappa[2], David H. Rothstein[3] and Satyan Lakshminrusimha[1]

Abstract

Congenital Diaphragmatic hernia (CDH) is a condition characterized by a defect in the diaphragm leading to protrusion of abdominal contents into the thoracic cavity interfering with normal development of the lungs. The defect may range from a small aperture in the posterior muscle rim to complete absence of diaphragm. The pathophysiology of CDH is a combination of lung hypoplasia and immaturity associated with persistent pulmonary hypertension of newborn (PPHN) and cardiac dysfunction. Prenatal assessment of lung to head ratio (LHR) and position of the liver by ultrasound are used to diagnose and predict outcomes. Delivery of infants with CDH is recommended close to term gestation. Immediate management at birth includes bowel decompression, avoidance of mask ventilation and endotracheal tube placement if required. The main focus of management includes gentle ventilation, hemodynamic monitoring and treatment of pulmonary hypertension followed by surgery. Although inhaled nitric oxide is not approved by FDA for the treatment of PPHN induced by CDH, it is commonly used.

Extracorporeal membrane oxygenation (ECMO) is typically considered after failure of conventional medical management for infants ≥ 34 weeks' gestation or with weight >2 kg with CDH and no associated major lethal anomalies. Multiple factors such as prematurity, associated abnormalities, severity of PPHN, type of repair and need for ECMO can affect the survival of an infant with CDH. With advances in the management of CDH, the overall survival has improved and has been reported to be 70-90% in non-ECMO infants and up to 50% in infants who undergo ECMO.

Keywords: Lung Hypoplasia, Pulmonary Hypertension, Extracorporeal membrane oxygenation

Background

Congenital Diaphragmatic hernia (CDH) is characterized by a defect in the diaphragm leading to the protrusion of abdominal contents into the thoracic cavity affecting the normal development of the lungs. The condition may present as an isolated lesion or as part of a syndrome. The incidence of CDH based on the available literature ranges from approximately 0.8 - 5/10,000 births and varies across the population [1–4]. There is slightly higher male predominance and a lower risk of isolated CDH reported among African-Americans [3, 5]. In spite of advances made in the medical and surgical management of CDH, the mortality and morbidity remain high [6–8]. CDH infants also have a prolonged length of stay in the hospital requiring multi-disciplinary approach for their management and follow-up after hospital discharge.

* Correspondence: pkchandr@buffalo.edu
[1]Department of Pediatrics, Women and Children's Hospital of Buffalo, Buffalo, NY, USA
Full list of author information is available at the end of the article

Review

Etiology

The etiology of CDH largely remains unclear and currently is thought to be multifactorial. The majority of the cases have an isolated diaphragmatic defect presenting with pulmonary hypoplasia and persistent pulmonary hypertension of newborn (PPHN). CDH can be associated with cardiac, gastrointestinal, genitourinary anomalies or with chromosomal aneuploidy such as trisomies. Multiple genetic factors along with environmental exposures and nutritional deficiencies have been proposed to be the possible etiologies for CDH [9–11]. Studies in rodent models have pointed towards a disturbance in Vitamin A pathway [12]. Nitrofen, a herbicide, when administered to pregnant rodents, results in CDH in the majority of offspring [13, 14]. Similar effects were seen in WT1 and COUP-TFII mutant mouse models. Studies in neonates with CDH have shown low retinol and retinol-binding protein levels from cord blood samples [9, 15].

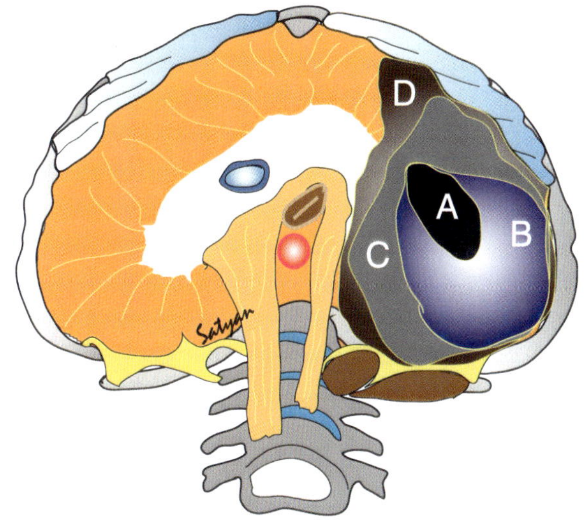

Fig. 2 Size of the defect – The size of the defect may vary between small (A) to diaphragmatic agenesis (D). Defects B & C are considered moderate to large (Tsao et al. 2008).

Pathology

Location (Fig. 1): Postero-lateral hernias also known as Bochdalek hernias are the most common type (70–75%) with the majority occurring on the left side (85%) and less frequently on the right side (13%) or bilateral (2%). Anterior defects or Morgagni hernias (23–28%) and central hernias (2–7%) are the other types [16, 17].

Size (Fig. 2): The diaphragm begins to develop at approximately 4 weeks of gestation and is fully formed by 12 weeks [18]. The defect may range from a small opening of the posterior muscle rim to complete absence of diaphragm.

The embryologic basis of CDH remains controversial. It was thought initially that the defect happened secondary to failure of different parts of the diaphragm to fuse resulting in a patent pleuroperitoneal canal [19, 20]. Rat models have shown a defect in the primordial diaphragm called the pleuroperitoneal fold [16]. This, in turn, allows the gut to enter the thoracic cavity when it returns from the extraembryonic coelom of the umbilicus. Another speculation is that lung hypoplasia may be the primary causal factor in the pathophysiology of diaphragmatic hernia [21]. If the development of lung bud is disturbed, there is an impaired development of a post hepatic mesenchymal plate (PHMP) that is closely related to the development of lung, resulting in a defective diaphragm [21]. Evidence from electron microscopy in a rat model [22] of CDH further supports the fact that when the development of the PHMP is impaired, a diaphragmatic defect occurs.

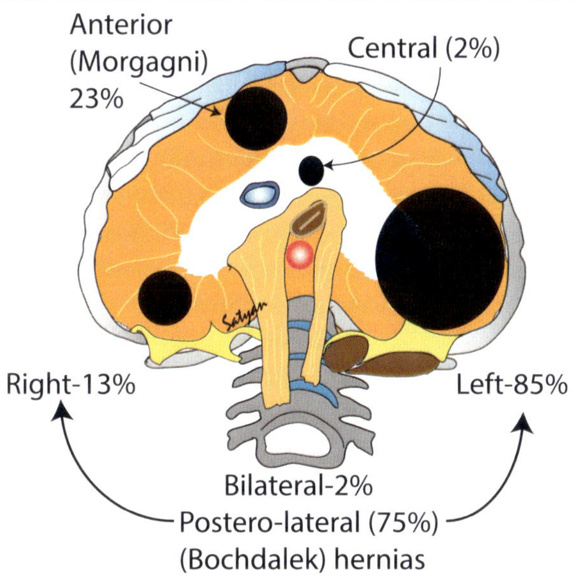

Fig. 1 Classification of CDH based on location of the diaphragmatic hernias: Most common type of hernias are the posterior lateral hernias (70–75%) also known as Bochdalek hernias, with majority occurring on the left side (85%) and less frequently on the right side (13%) or bilateral (2%). Other types of hernias are the anterior defects or Morgagni hernias (23–28%) followed by the rare central hernias (2–7%).

A weakness in the diaphragm can cause diaphragmatic eventration and may be mistaken for a diaphragmatic hernia. Diaphragmatic eventration is more common on the right side and is not associated with severe lung hypoplasia. While a complete absence of the diaphragm may occur resulting in diaphragmatic agenesis and severe lung hypoplasia. Irrespective of the basis, a defect in the diaphragm causes the abdominal viscera to herniate into the thoracic cavity resulting in abnormal lung development. The defect also leads to abnormal fetal breathing movements resulting in the void of stretch-induced lung maturation [16]. Thus the major underlying pathophysiology of CDH appears to be a combination of lung immaturity and hypoplasia that leads to PPHN. This may be further aggravated by left ventricular underdevelopment and right ventricular hypertrophy resulting in ventricular dysfunction [23–26].

Lung hypoplasia/immaturity

Lung hypoplasia occurs on the ipsilateral side of herniation, with the contralateral side being affected to a variable extent (Fig. 3). Hypoplasia was initially thought to be secondary to physical compression of the lung by abdominal contents arresting lung development. Recently, a two-hit hypothesis has been proposed based on rat model explaining the lung injury in CDH [27] (Fig. 4). According to this hypothesis, the initial insult occurs during the stages of organogenesis resulting in bilateral hypoplasia, followed by compression of the ipsilateral lung secondary to the herniation of the abdominal viscera at later stages. This theory explains the variability of lung hypoplasia on the contralateral side. The interference results in decreased branching of the bronchioles and pulmonary vessels leading to acinar hypoplasia [28, 29]. The terminal bronchioles are decreased with thickening of alveolar septa. The lung is relatively immature [28] and hypoplasia of pulmonary vasculature leads to PPHN.

Pulmonary hypertension in CDH

In CDH, the total pulmonary vascular bed is reduced with decreased number of vessels per unit of lung. In addition, pulmonary vascular remodeling with medial hyperplasia and peripheral extension of the muscle layer into small arterioles is evident [30–32]. The paucity of pulmonary vasculature and remodeling of the vessels contribute to the 'fixed' or irreversible component of PPHN in CDH [33, 34]. Altered vasoreactivity possibly due to an imbalance of autonomic innervation (increased sympathetic and decreased parasympathetic) [35], and/or impaired endothelium-dependent relaxation of pulmonary arteries [36, 37] or an imbalance between vasoconstrictor and vasodilator mediators may contribute to the reversible component of PPHN [35, 38]. Following birth, a combination of pulmonary arterial hypertension, right ventricular hypertrophy and/or failure, and left ventricular hypoplasia with pulmonary venous hypertension results in severe PPHN unresponsive to conventional management [39].

Ventricular dysfunction

Ventricular dysfunction is observed in some patients with severe PPHN due to CDH. During fetal life, the ductus arteriosus serves as a pop-off value and limits right ventricular strain. After birth, remodeled pulmonary vasculature in CDH results in pulmonary hypertension and leads to right ventricle (RV) dysfunction. This is more pronounced after birth when there is excessive strain on the right ventricle. Abnormalities of the left ventricle (LV) have been reported in infants with CDH [26, 40]. When compared to neonates with other causes of PPHN, infants with left sided CDH had significantly lower left ventricular mass assessed by echocardiography. Reduced left ventricular output has been documented in left sided and right sided CDH [41]. The reduced left ventricular mass contributes to functional LV hypoplasia and may result in increased left atrial pressure and pulmonary venous hypertension (Fig. 5) [42].

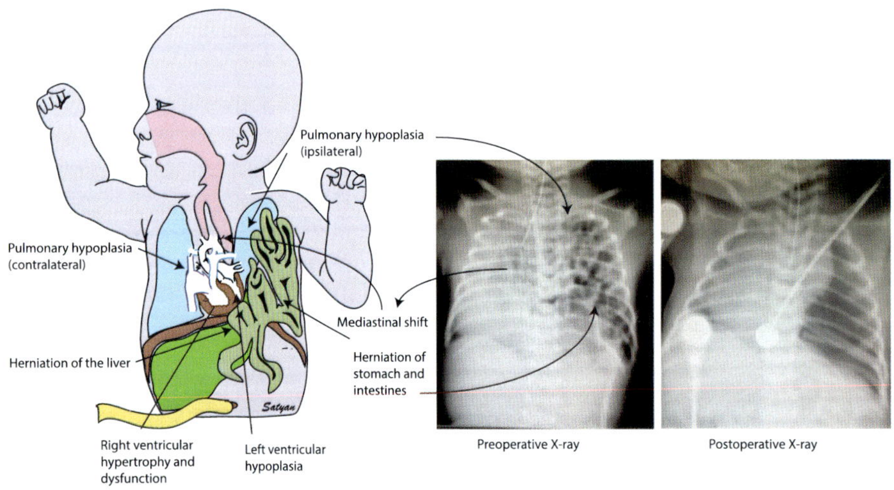

Fig. 3 Anatomical and radiological features of CDH – A defect in the diaphragm causes the abdominal viscera to herniate into the thoracic cavity. Left sided hernias are common (85%) which results in herniation of both small and large intestines along with solid intra-abdominal organs. Herniation of viscera into the thoracic cavity results in abnormal lung development on the ipsilateral side with variable effect on the contralateral side. The effect of abnormal lung development on the contralateral side depends on the extent of herniation and the effect on mediastinal shift. Pulmonary hypoplasia results in abnormal pulmonary vasculature resulting in persistent pulmonary hypertension leading to right ventricular dysfunction. This is more pronounced after transitioning from fetal circulation. Left ventricular dysfunction can be secondary to direct compression in left sided hernia and secondary to low ventricular volumes in right sided hernias. Pre-operative chest and abdomen x-ray shows the air and fluid filled loops of bowels on the left side of the thorax with the endotracheal tube above the thoracic vertebra level 4 pushed towards the right side signifying mediastinal shift.

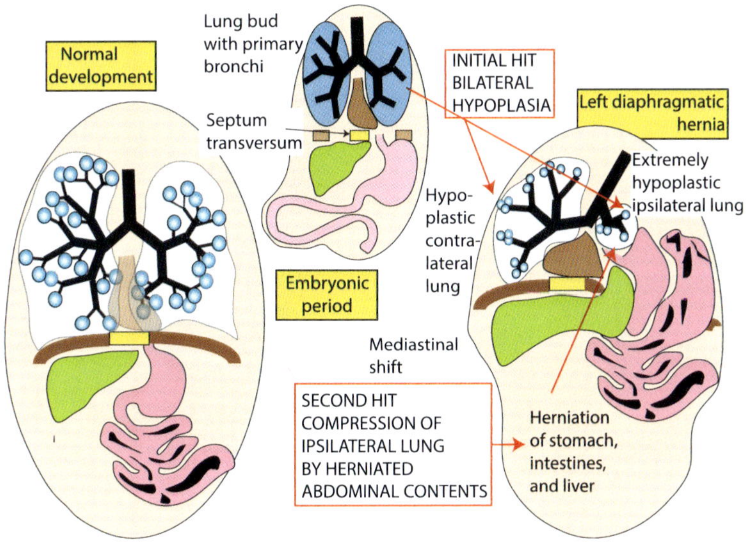

Fig. 4 Two-hit hypothesis for CDH

Diagnosis

Prenatal diagnosis by ultrasound detects more than 50% of CDH cases at a mean gestational age of 24 weeks [43]. Three-dimensional ultrasound imaging, fetal echocardiography and fetal magnetic resonance imaging (MRI) are other prenatal diagnostic modalities used in assessing the severity and outcome of CDH. Left sided CDH may be characterized by the presence of heterogeneous mass which may be stomach filled with fluid or intestines. In contrast, isolated right-sided CDH is extremely difficult to diagnose by ultrasound if the liver is the only organ that has herniated. Indirect signs such as a shift in cardiac axis, identifying the gall bladder and vasculature in the liver using Doppler may aide in the diagnosis [44]. MRI has been found to be useful in detecting fetal anomalies and can be a valuable adjunct to evaluate the position of the liver and estimating lung volume [45, 46]. Associated cardiac and neural tube defects may affect the outcome of infants with CDH [47].

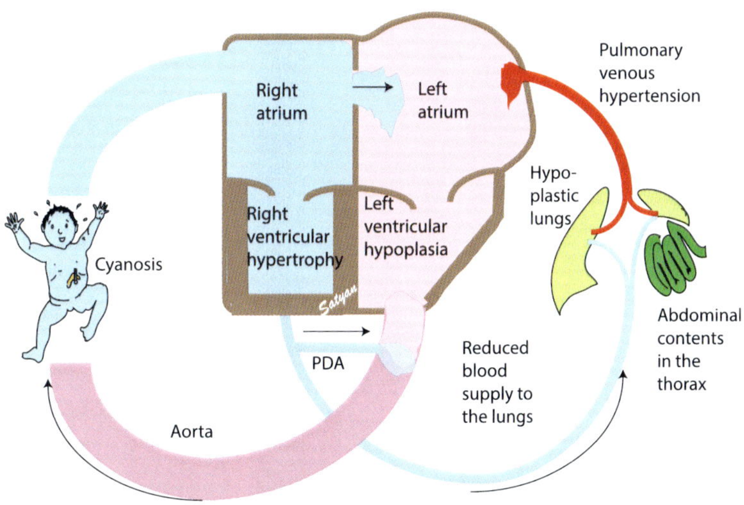

Fig. 5 Cardiovascular effects of CDH – Hypoplastic lungs secondary to herniation of abdominal viscera leads to concomitant hypoplasia of the pulmonary vessels. This results in reduced blood supply to the hypoplastic alveolar-capillary unit. Once the infant transitions from fetal circulation, this effect is more pronounced resulting in pulmonary hypertension which leads to right ventricular dysfunction. Secondary to pulmonary hypertension, there is shunting of blood from right to left across the patent foramen ovale and the patent ductus arteriosus. Left ventricular dysfunction along with left atrial dysfunction results in pulmonary venous hypertension and worsening of pulmonary arterial hypertension. This presents clinically in a wide spectrum of labile pre & postductal saturations to profound cyanosis.

Associated syndromes and anomalies requiring genetic work up

Most common associated chromosomal abnormalities are the trisomies 18, 13 and 21 [48]. Chromosomal aneuploidies such as monosomy X, tetrasomy 12 p, tetraploidy 21 have also been associated with CDH [43, 48]. CDH is the most common finding in Fryns syndrome [49]. CDH can also be part of Pentalogy of Cantrell, Apert, Brachmann-Cornelia De Lange, Beckwith-Wiedemann, CHARGE, Coffin-Siris, Goldenhar sequence, Simpson-Golabi-Behmel, Stickler, Pierre Robin sequence and VACTERL [48, 50].

Once diagnosed, the patient should be referred to a tertiary care center for further prenatal workup and management. A multi-disciplinary prenatal consult involving the obstetrics, neonatology, pediatric surgery, genetics at a center that has expertise in managing infants with CDH and extracorporeal membrane oxygenation (ECMO) are imperative. In addition, if an MRI was done, radiology is also involved in the multi-disciplinary prenatal consult.

Fetal predictors of outcomes

Major determinants of the outcomes in CDH are i) the presence of associated anomalies especially heart disease and ii) extent of lung hypoplasia and (iii) position of the liver [43].

The prognosis of isolated CDH is generally better than CDH complicated by multiple anomalies. Population-based studies report higher survival for isolated CDH compared to CDH with anomalies [4, 51]. Metkus et al. reported higher survival for CDH detected after 25 weeks by ultrasound [52]. This has not been validated and in the true sense, herniation that occurs before 25 weeks tends to have severe lung hypoplasia compared to herniation after 25 weeks [53].

Liver herniation (liver-up) is associated with worse prognosis. Earlier studies have reported 100% survival without liver herniation (liver-down) as compared to 56% with liver herniation [52]. The survival decreased from 74 to 45% with liver herniation as reported by a meta-analysis [54]. In another study, liver herniation was highly predictive of ECMO (80% - liver-up vs. 25% - liver-down) and survival (45% - liver-up vs. 93% liver-down) [55].

Metkus et al. [52] used the ratio of the contralateral lung size compared with the head circumference to come up with the lung-to-head ratio (LHR, Fig. 6) to assess the severity of pulmonary hypoplasia and to predict postnatal outcome in fetuses with CDH [52, 55, 56]. Since these measurements differed by gestational age and were not found to be consistent across centers [57, 58], observed to expected lung-to–head ratio (O/E LHR) was studied which was independent of gestational age [59]. LHR ratio

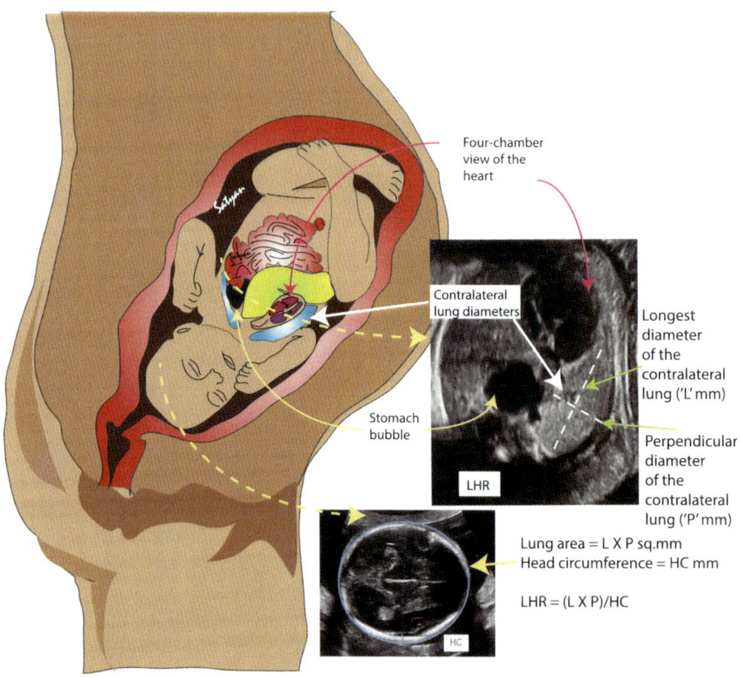

Fig. 6 Lung to head ratio (LHR) measurement – Obstetric ultrasound technique is used to measure the lung to head ratio known as LHR to assess the severity of CDH. The head circumference is measured as shown. The contralateral lung area is calculated as a product of the longest and perpendicular diameter of the contralateral lung. The ratio of this area to the head circumference gives the LHR. A LHR of <0.6 has been associated with poor outcome while a ratio of >1.35 has been associated with survival. Alternatively, an observed to expected LHR measurement is used in order to overcome bias secondary to gestational age.

is often used along with liver herniation to predict outcome (see Table 1 below)

Management

Antenatal Management – Medical

Antenatal corticosteroids are administered to mothers in some centers to improve lung maturation in neonates with CDH. While some animal results are promising [60], no significant advantages are reported in human infants [61]. It may be prudent to administer antenatal corticosteroids prior to delivery of preterm infants with CDH based on their premature gestation.

Pregnant rats with nitrofen induced CDH demonstrated significant improvement in lung structure, increased pulmonary vessel density, reduced right ventricular hypertrophy following antenatal therapy with high-dose sildenafil [36]. To our knowledge there are no human trials evaluating the role of antenatal phosphodiesterase inhibitors in CDH.

Antenatal Management - Surgical

Tracheal occlusion: In the surgically induced lamb model of CDH with hypoplastic lungs, occlusion of the fetal trachea led to an acceleration of lung growth. Harrison et al. at the University of California in San Francisco (UCSF) reported the first randomized controlled trial of open hysterotomy-guided fetal endoscopic tracheal occlusion. No improvement in survival was observed when compared with conventional postnatal care. Junior et al. reported a meta-analysis of various fetoscopic tracheal occlusion studies. Fetoscopic tracheal occlusion procedure increased neonatal survival at 30 days and 6 months among patients with severe CDH. However, it was associated with higher rate of premature rupture of membranes and decreased gestational age at delivery by 2 weeks [62]. A new minimally invasive operation termed percutaneous fetal endoluminal tracheal occlusion (FETO) is being subjected to randomized clinical trials with ongoing recruitment. More information about FETO can be found at http://www.chop.edu/centers-programs/center-fetal-diagnosis-and-treatment/fetoscopic-endoluminal-tracheal-occlusion-feto or http://childrens.memorialhermann.org/FETO-trial/.

Table 1 Antenatal ultrasound predictors of survival in CDH

A. LHR is calculated by dividing fetal lung area (mm^2) by fetal head circumference (mm). Fetal lung area is usually measured at the level of the four-chamber view of the heart by multiplying the longest diameter of the contralateral lung by its longest perpendicular diameter. Alternatively, some obstetricians trace the lung margin and measure the lung area. The fetal head circumference is measured by its longest electronic ellipse.
- a. LHR > 1.35 associated with 100% survival
- b. LHR 1.35 to 0.6 associated with 61% survival
- c. LHR < 0.6 – no survival

B. Observed to expected LHR (O/E LHR) is calculated by dividing the observed LHR by the expected ratio for gestational age
- a. The fetal lung area increases 16-fold compared to 4-fold increase in the head circumference between 12 and 32 weeks' gestation
- b. O/E LHR < 25% is considered severe CDH (survival 10% with liver up and 25% with liver down)
- c. O/E LHR < 15% with liver up – 100% mortality

C. Position of liver (or presence of liver herniation)
- a. Liver herniation with LHR < 1.0 – 60% mortality
- b. Liver in the thorax – 56% survival;

The timing of delivery

The optimal timing of delivery of an infant with CDH is controversial. Stevens et al. initially reported that among infants delivered by elective cesarean section, early term birth (at 37–38 weeks gestation) was associated with less use of ECMO (22 vs. 35.5%) compared to term delivery (at 39–41 weeks) [63]. However, more recent analysis suggested decreased mortality with advancing gestation [64]. Among 928 infants with CDH in this review, neonatal and infant mortality decreased from 25 and 36% respectively at 37 weeks gestation to 17 and 20% at 40 weeks gestation. We recommend delivery after completion of 39 weeks of gestation to avoid complications associated with prematurity and early term delivery [65].

Postnatal Management – Medical (Fig. 7)

Delivery room (DR) Deliveries should be conducted at centers with capabilities of managing an infant with CDH and associated complications. Resuscitation in the DR is based on neonatal resuscitation program (NRP) guidelines [66]. All infants with CDH or suspected CDH need an orogastric/nasogastric tube with suction to decompress the bowel. Bag-mask ventilation should be avoided. The majority of these infants (especially with a prenatal diagnosis of CDH) require intubation in the delivery room. A pre-ductal pulse oximeter is placed on the right upper extremity as soon as possible. Ventilation using a T-piece resuscitator is preferred to avoid high airway pressures. Peak inspiratory pressure (PIP) should be preferably below 25 cm H_2O to avoid damage to the hypoplastic/immature lung. Oxygen can be titrated to maintain preductal saturations recommended by NRP. In some institutions, preductal saturations > 70% are accepted for the first 1–2 h if pH and arterial carbon dioxide for $PaCO_2$ are within normal limits.

Stabilization Central or peripheral venous access is obtained for administering fluids and medications. An arterial line for monitoring blood pressure and to draw blood gases is needed. Although it has been traditional to place an umbilical arterial line, it may be preferable to obtain a preductal arterial line in the right radial or ulnar artery. Umbilical artery line values reflect postductal arterial oxygen tension (PaO_2) and lead to increased fraction of inspired oxygen (FIO_2). Systemic blood pressures are maintained at normal values for gestational age

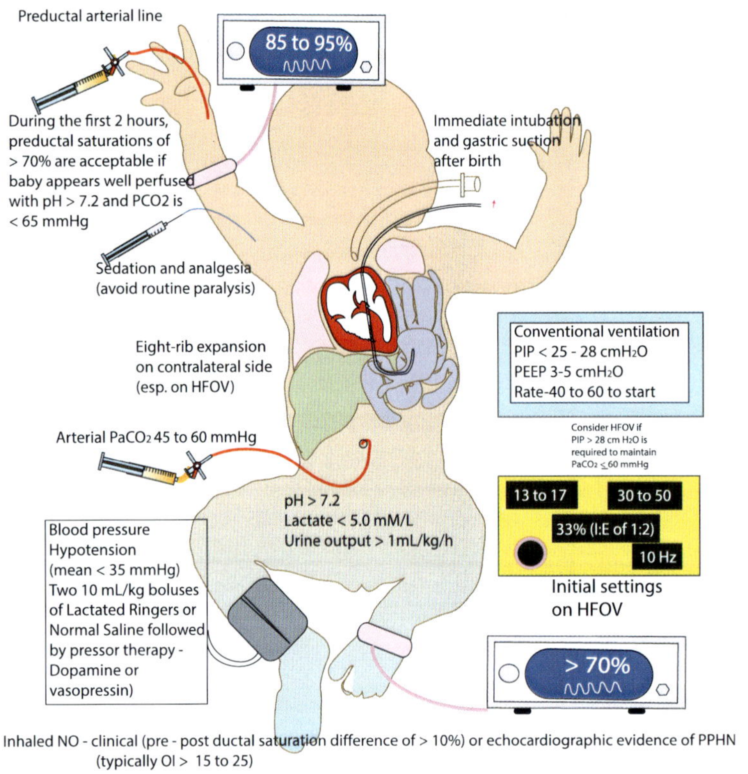

Fig. 7 Management of CDH – At birth infants with CDH or suspected CDH should have an orogastric/nasogastric tube with suction to attain bowel decompression. Bag-mask ventilation should be avoided. The majority of these infants (especially with prenatal diagnosis of CDH) require intubation in the delivery room. A pre-ductal pulse oximeter is placed on the right upper extremity as soon as possible. Oxygen saturation targets are based on NRP guidelines. Ventilation using a T-piece resuscitator is preferred to avoid high airway pressures. Ventilator parameters are as shown in the figure. Preductal blood gases and invasive blood pressure monitoring are preferred. Inhaled nitric oxide is often used for the management of PPHN. For blood pressure management, fluid boluses and vasopressor agents are used based on the parameters in the figure.

[67]. Pre-ductal saturations are maintained between 85–95%. A chest x-ray is obtained to assess the initial condition of the lung and herniated content.

Mechanical Ventilation The optimal ventilation mode for infants with CDH and hypoplastic lungs is not known. Many centers initiate conventional mechanical ventilation (CMV) for respiratory support and optimize ventilation by adjusting PIP and respiratory rate. The recently concluded VICI (Ventilation in infants with congenital diaphragmatic hernia) trial compared CMV and high-frequency oscillatory ventilation (HFOV) as the initial mode of ventilation in CDH. There was no statistically significant difference in the combined outcome of mortality or bronchopulmonary dysplasia (BPD) [68]. In this study, 91 (53.2%) patients initially received CMV and 80 (46.8%) HFOV. Forty-one patients (45.1%) randomized to CMV died/had BPD compared with 43 patients (53.8%) in the HFOV group. An odds ratio of 0.62 [95% confidence interval (95% CI) 0.25–1.55] ($P = 0.31$) for death/BPD for CMV vs HFOV was demonstrated, after adjustment for center, LHR, side of the defect, and liver position. Patients initially ventilated by CMV were ventilated for fewer days ($P = 0.03$), less often needed ECMO support ($P = 0.007$), inhaled nitric oxide (iNO, $P = 0.045$), sildenafil ($P = 0.004$), had a shorter duration of vasoactive drugs ($P = 0.02$), and less often failed treatment ($P = 0.01$) as compared with infants initially ventilated by HFOV. It is important to note that guidelines for initial settings for CMV in this study included low positive end-expiratory pressure (PEEP) (3 to 5 cm H_2O) and PIP (20 to 25 cm H_2O). These findings suggest that an initial attempt at CMV is reasonable for patients with CDH.

A review of autopsies of 68 infants with CDH showed significant pulmonary injury (alveolar damage, hyaline membrane formation, pneumothoraces in 2/3 of autopsies) secondary to mechanical ventilation where 53 infants were switched to HFOV in a median time of 15 h from birth [69]. In view of preventing volutrauma and barotrauma, a gentler approach to ventilation is preferred in infants with CDH. CMV mode [70, 71] with

PIP usually below 25 cm H_2O and PEEP ≤ 5 cm H_2O targeting preductal saturations of >85%, post-ductal saturations of >70% and $PaCO_2$ of 45–60 mmHg are used to initiate ventilation. Many centers switch to HFOV or jet ventilation as a rescue therapy if the ventilator targets cannot be achieved on CMV. The settings on HFOV are not well defined. Mean airway pressure (MAP) is usually adjusted to maintain adequate inflation of the contralateral lung to 8 ribs in a range of 13–17 cm H_2O [71–73].

The role of surfactant Although animal studies strongly suggest the presence of an immature lung with surfactant deficiency, a retrospective analysis failed to support any beneficial effect of surfactant replacement therapy in term infants with CDH [74]. Its use in preterm infant was also associated with lower survival rate [75]. However, this trial by its retrospective nature may be biased as sicker patients may have received surfactant Although there are no increasing trends in use of surfactant, it is still being used in preterm infants with CDH across centers [76]. Prospective trials are needed to evaluate the benefits of surfactant in infants with CDH. The beneficial effect of surfactant cannot be ruled out in a premature lung and it is unclear if there is a direct causal association between surfactant administration and mortality in infants with CDH.

Hemodynamic monitoring and management Invasive blood pressure (BP) monitoring is preferred over non-invasive monitoring. Pre and post-ductal saturations and heart rate should be continuously monitored. Optimal end-organ perfusion is the goal to hemodynamic monitoring in infants with CDH. Signs of adequate perfusion include normal range of heart rate for gestational age, normal capillary refill, a urine output >1.0 ml/kg/h, arterial pH >7.2 and lactate levels of <3-5 mmol/L [71]. If there are signs suggestive of poor perfusion, volume resuscitation and vasopressor therapy should be considered. The treatment should be streamlined based on cardiac function assessed by echocardiogram and volume requirement. In case of hypovolemia, a bolus with an isotonic solution like 0.9% normal saline or lactated Ringer's solution, 10 ml/kg intravenously can be given. Volume resuscitation is usually followed by vasopressor/inotropic therapy.

Vasopressor/inotropic therapy (Table 2)

Dopamine is the most commonly used cardiovascular medication in NICU and is given as an infusion [77] aiming to maintain systemic BP appropriate for gestational age. Dobutamine is preferred in infants with poor myocardial contractility. Norepinephrine and epinephrine may be used as first line agents in some institutions secondary to their potent vasoconstrictor activity. Epinephrine infusion can falsely increase the lactate levels and can interfere with management [77]. Low-dose hydrocortisone is beneficial in vasopressor-resistant hypotension in the immediate postnatal period [78]. Vasopressin was reported to be effective in stabilizing systemic hemodynamics in a retrospective chart review with decreased pulmonary/systemic pressure ratio, in patients with CDH [79].

Management of pulmonary hypertension (Fig. 8) PPHN in CDH infants is secondary to hypoplastic lungs and pruned, remodeled vasculature [39, 80]. Pulmonary arterial hypertension along with left ventricular hypoplasia and right ventricular hypertrophy and/or failure complicated by pulmonary venous hypertension results in severe PPHN not responsive to conventional therapy. Due to right to left shunting, pre and postductal saturation difference may be observed. The absence of a difference does not rule out pulmonary hypertension. In some patients with CDH the immediate postnatal phase, there is a short period of better oxygenation referred to as "honeymoon" period [39]. However, progressive deterioration in oxygenation is commonly observed with deteriorating PPHN. An echocardiogram is the best non-invasive test to assess cardiac function and pulmonary pressures in an infant with CDH and is usually done within the first 24 h and followed up as needed [81].

If preductal saturations decreases below 85%, ventilation adjustments and hemodynamic management take precedence prior to initiating any therapy. Measures to increase systemic blood pressure may minimize the right-to-left shunting. However, there is no need to increase blood pressure to supranormal values if preductal saturation remains above 80%. Catecholamines, especially dopamine, besides increasing systemic vascular resistance also increases pulmonary vascular resistance [30, 82]. The CDH consortium recommends maintaining arterial blood pressure at normal levels for gestational age if preductal saturations are between 80 to 95% [83].

Inhaled Nitric Oxide (iNO) is the first agent of choice for treatment of pulmonary hypertension in infants >34 weeks' gestation. It is a selective pulmonary vasodilator and relaxes pulmonary vascular smooth muscle cells. The criteria for initiating iNO is based on the severity of PPHN as assessed by the oxygenation index (OI). (Note: oxygenation index (OI), = Mean airway pressure x FiO_2 x 100 ÷ PaO_2). Oxygen saturation index (OSI) is a non-invasive means of estimating oxygenation status and can be used in the absence of an arterial blood gas but requires further validation [84, 85]. It is calculated using the following formula: Oxygen saturation index (OSI) = Mean airway pressure x FiO_2 x 100 ÷ preductal SpO_2). Studies in the past have reported a mean OI of 25±9 as the cut off for initiation of iNO [86]. Currently, in neonates with PPHN not due to

Table 2 Vasoactive medications commonly used in CDH: Typical doses, route of administration of inotropic and vasodilator medications in the management of CDH

Drug	Route	Units	Initial dose	Maintenance Dose range
DOPAmine	IV	μg/kg/min	1 to 5	1 to 50 (usually 2.5 to 20)
DOBUTamine	IV	μg/kg/min	1 to 5	1 to 40 (usually 2.5 to 20)
EPInephrine	IV	μg/kg/min	0.05 to 0.1	0.1 to 1
NOREPInephrine	IV	μg/kg/min	0.05 to 0.1	0.05 to 2
PGE1 – Alprostadil	IV	μg/kg/min	0.05 to 0.1	0.01 to 4
PGE1 – Alprostadil	Inhaled	μg/kg/min	0.15 to 0.3	0.15 to 0.3
Milrinone	IV	μg/kg/min	0.25 to 0.75 (some units use a load of 50 μg/kg)	0.25 to 1
Dexamethasone	IV	mg/kg/dose	0.05 to 0.6	0.05 to 0.6
Hydrocortisone	IV	mg/kg/dose	1 to 5	0.5 to 5
Nitric oxide (NO)	Inhaled	Ppm	5 to 20	1 to 80
Vasopressin	IV	Units/kg/min	0.0001 to 0.002	0.0001 to 0.008
Prostacyclin (Epoprostenol - Flolan)	IV	ng/kg/min	1 to 3	50 to 80
Prostacyclin (Epoprostenol - Flolan)	Inhaled	ng/kg/min	50	25 to 50
Prostacyclin (Treprostinil – Remodulin)	SQ or IV	ng/kg/min	1.25 to 2	50 to 80
Prostacyclin (Treprostinil – Remodulin)	Inhaled	μg/breath	6	
Prostacyclin (Iloprost)	Inhaled	μg/breath	2.5 or 5	
Prostacyclin (Beraprost)	PO	μg	80	80 to 120 (adult dose)
Sildenafil	IV	mg/kg/h	0.14 for 3 h	0.07
Bosentan	PO	mg/kg/dose	1 to 2	1 to 2

CDH, it is acceptable to start iNO with an OI of ≥20 and evidence of right-to-left shunting by clinical exam (a pre - postductal saturation difference of ≥10%) [71] [87] [80] and/or echocardiographic evidence of extrapulmonary right to left shunting [88]. The typical initial dose is 20 parts per million (ppm) [89] although variable dosing has been mentioned in the literature. A complete response to iNO is considered to be an increase in the ratio of arterial oxygen tension (PaO_2) to fraction of inspired oxygen (FiO_2) by ≥20 mmHg post iNO therapy [80].

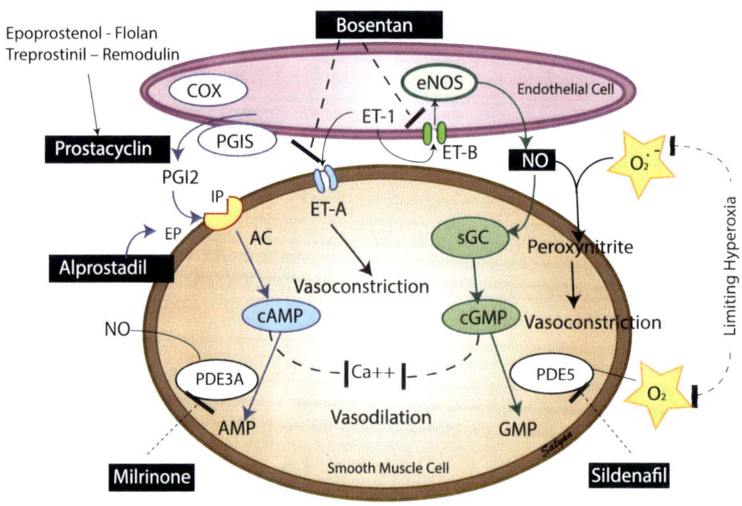

Fig. 8 Management of pulmonary hypertension in CDH: pulmonary vasodilators and nitric oxide – prostacyclin – endothelin pathways. AC – acetylcholine, Ca- calcium, cAMP - cyclic adenosine monophosphate, cGMP – cyclic guanosine monophosphate, COX – cycloxygenase, eNOS – endothelial nitric oxide synthase, ET – endothelin, EP – prostaglandin E receptor, IP – prostacyclin I receptor, NO – nitric oxide, PGI – prostaglandin I, sGC - soluble guanylyl cyclase, PDE – phosphodiesterase inhibitor

In contrast to PPHN from conditions other than CDH, iNO did not reduce the need for ECMO or death in a prospective, randomized trial in infants with CDH [90]. The ventilation approach, choice of ventilator and the OI at enrollment in this study were different from current practice [33]. In spite of this negative study, iNO continues to be used in US tertiary centers in the management of infants with CDH without a change in ECMO utilization or mortality [91]. If there is no response to iNO after optimizing ventilation and hemodynamic status, iNO is gradually weaned. Some patients decompensate and become hypoxemic with discontinuation of iNO. In these instances, iNO is weaned to a low dose for a few hours and then discontinued.

The rationale for continuing vs. weaning off iNO when there is no response is unclear. Continuing iNO with high oxygen could be detrimental. Nitric oxide is a free radical and can combine with superoxide anions to form peroxynitrite, which is a toxic vasoconstrictor. Thus, continuing iNO therapy in the absence of response remains controversial.

Infants with corrected CDH are at risk for late pulmonary hypertension. Inhaled nitric oxide may play an important role in treating exacerbations of pulmonary hypertension in these patients [88] [92, 93].

Prostaglandin (PGE1) intravenous (IV) PGE1 has been used in infants with CDH especially in the setting of right heart failure [94]. A trial of PGE1 to reopen the ductus may reduce the load on the right ventricle. Some groups have suggested starting PGE1 infusion when the duration of right-to-left shunting through the ductus arteriosus was longer than left to right shunting [95]. In patients with ductal-dependent critical congenital heart disease associated with CDH, IV PGE1 is necessary to maintain ductal patency. Inhalational PGE1 is also used as an alternative agent in treating PPHN in infants with CDH [96]. These are non-FDA approved therapies and lack evidence.

Prostacyclin (PGI_2) is commonly used in adults may be useful in the management of late pulmonary hypertension in infants post CDH repair. Currently, there is no evidence to support this therapy but some centers use it as a second-line pulmonary vasodilator. Prostacyclin can be used as an inhaled agent or an intravenous agent. Three forms of prostacyclin are used in the management of pulmonary hypertension (Table 2). Epoprostenol (Flolan), Treprostinil (Remodulin) and inhaled Iloprost (Ventavis - inhaled prostacyclin analog) are approved for adults with pulmonary arterial hypertension.

Sildenafil is a phosphodiesterase (PDE) 5 inhibitor that inhibits cyclic guanosine monophosphate (cGMP) degradation leading to vasodilation. Oral sildenafil improves oxygenation and reduces mortality in PPHN in centers limited by non-availability of iNO and ECMO [97, 98]. IV sildenafil was shown to be effective in improving oxygenation in patients with PPHN with and without prior exposure to iNO [99]. There are no trials to support its use in infants with CDH. A chronic sildenafil trial was planned in CDH infants but is currently terminated and not recruiting patients (NCT00133679). As per FDA, high mortality is associated with its use in pediatric patients (1–17 y of age) with pulmonary arterial hypertension [100]. Parents should be informed about the benefits and side-effects of sildenafil prior to initiation for chronic use in CDH.

Milrinone is a PDE 3 inhibitor which increases cyclic adenosine monophosphate (cAMP) concentration in smooth muscle and myocardium. It has both lusitropic and inotropic properties. In a fetal lamb model of PPHN, milrinone relaxed pulmonary arteries [101] and reduced pulmonary arterial pressure. The benefits of milrinone in children following surgery for congenital heart disease have been well established [102]. Multiple case series have shown IV milrinone to be effective in treating infants with iNO resistant PPHN [103, 104–106]. Milrinone therapy has been used in the management of iNO resistant PPHN in infants with CDH. Hypotension is a clinical concern and the infants should be monitored closely. Despite lack of evidence, the use of milrinone in the management of infants with CDH has increased [76]. A loading dose (50 µg/kg for 30–60 min) followed by a maintenance dose (0.33 µg/kg per minute and escalation to 0.66 and then to 1 µg/kg per minute based on response) are commonly used. The loading dose of milrinone will increase the risk of hypotension but may achieve steady state plasma levels sooner [107]. Hence, the loading dose is not recommended in the presence of systemic hypotension in patients with CDH [108]. Some clinicians administer a volume bolus prior to the loading dose of milrinone to avoid systemic hypotension.

A multicenter trial investigating the use of milrinone in infants with CDH has been proposed by the NICHD Neonatal Research Network and will begin enrollment shortly (NCT02951130).

Bosentan is a blocker of endothelin receptors and is occasionally used as an oral agent in the management of chronic pulmonary hypertension in CDH. There is limited experience with its use in neonates [109]. Liver function tests should be closely followed during its use.

Extracorporeal membranous oxygenation (ECMO) is considered as the last lifesaving option for infants ≥ 34 weeks' gestation or with weight >2 kg with CDH and no associated major lethal anomalies after conventional medical management has failed. Strong evidence for ECMO is lacking although the number of infants with CDH who undergo ECMO treatment has not decreased. Selection criteria for ECMO varies across centers and remains controversial. The Euro consortium experts have published criteria [71] for ECMO. There is considerable institutional variability but the following approach seems reasonable – (a) Inability to maintain preductal saturations >85% or postductal saturations >70% along with (b) increased $PaCO_2$ and respiratory acidosis with pH <7.15 despite optimal ventilator management, (c) PIP of >28 cm H_2O or MAP >17 cm H_2O to achieve saturations >85%, (d) inadequate oxygen delivery with metabolic acidosis, (e) systemic hypotension resistant to fluid and pressor therapy resulting in urine output <0.5 ml/kg/h for a 12–24 h period and (f) consistently elevated OI ≥ 40.

Venoarterial (VA) ECMO is preferred in the presence of cardiovascular compromise. There is a shift towards increased use of venovenous (VV) ECMO in patients with CDH and has comparable mortality rates [110, 111]. Functionally VA ECMO has the advantage of decreasing the load on the right side of the heart. However, VV ECMO allows oxygenated blood to flow through pulmonary circulation resulting in enhanced pulmonary vasodilation while preserving the carotid arteries. In addition, maintaining pulsatile flow with oxygenated blood may improve coronary perfusion and cardiac function with VV ECMO. Failure of VV ECMO and a switch to VA ECMO may be required in some patients.

Duration of treatment on ECMO is a subject of debate. Congenital Diaphragmatic Hernia Study Group retrospective data from 1995–2004 showed increased survival in infants treated for 9 days compared to 14 days [112]. A single institution 19-year retrospective review concluded that in patients with severe CDH, improvement in pulmonary function sufficient to wean from ECMO can take 4 weeks or longer and might need a second ECMO run [113]. The study reported survival rates based on the duration of ECMO run as 56% for 2 weeks, 46% for 3 weeks, 43% for 4 weeks after which the survival dropped to 15%. 44% (7/16) of infants who were treated on the second run of ECMO survived. ELSO registry data [112] shows an increase in mortality for ECMO duration > 2 weeks. Prolonged duration of ECMO is a predictor of mortality [112, 114].

Postnatal management - Surgical

When considering repair of the CDH, the surgeon faces three questions: a) what is the benefit; b) when is the optimal time; and c) what is the best approach? The first question, although philosophical, is critical. Our understanding of the benefits of repair are incomplete, but most literature supports the idea that reduction of the herniated visceral contents from the thoracic cavity and closure of the diaphragmatic defect are important in the long-term but provide little immediate benefit to the patient [115]. Reducing herniated contents back to the abdomen to permit expansion of the compressed lungs does not result in immediate improvement in PPHN and hypoxemia. Pulmonary hypertension is, however, the "rate-limiting" disease process in CDH and rarely does hernia reduction/repair significantly improve outcome by itself. This is particularly important as the surgical stress of operation is often severe enough to induce pulmonary hypertensive crises in the sicker patients, and if undertaken in a patient while on ECMO, can lead to severe hemorrhagic complications.

Optimal timing of CDH repair can be difficult to determine, particularly in patients who require ECMO. For those patients not requiring ECMO, repair is usually offered no sooner than 48–72 h after birth, with the assumption that these patients' pulmonary vasculature is not so compromised as to pose a significant risk of peri- or postoperative decompensation. Once a patient requires ECMO, the decision process becomes more difficult. There are generally three approaches: early repair, immediately after ECMO initiation (typically <72 h); delayed repair, often done as a last-hope operation in the setting of inability to wean off ECMO; and repair after decannulation [116]. The data on the influence of timing of repair on outcomes are hampered by limited numbers, retrospective design, patient group heterogeneity, and thus do not serve well to inform the decision in a generalizable and reliable manner. In broad strokes, best outcomes appear to be in patients repaired after decannulation (technically, these may be repaired the day prior to anticipated decannulation, but in a patient who has improved while on ECMO). Following this, those patients repaired shortly after cannulation do better than those repaired after several weeks on ECMO. Improvements in the medical treatment and prevention of bleeding diatheses while on ECMO, and improved ECMO circuits, have helped to mitigate some of the lethal bleeding complications of repair on ECMO.

Surgical approach

Repair of the CDH may be accomplished through a thoracic or abdominal approach, and may be performed in an open or minimally invasive manner. Long-term outcomes depend, perhaps most importantly, on the characteristics of the diaphragmatic defect. Patients with a small muscular defect that is easily approximated primarily should have negligible recurrence rates and complications. There has been an increasing trend toward thoracoscopic repairs, which are thought to minimize post-operative pain and scarring and hasten recovery. Several series have demonstrated higher recurrences rates through the thoracoscopic approach, although these may have been biased by higher rates of unfavorable anatomy and an inherent learning curve [117]. Patients at the other end of the spectrum, with diaphragmatic agenesis, uniformly require placement of a patch to close the diaphragmatic defect (Fig. 9a & b). These are typically made of synthetic

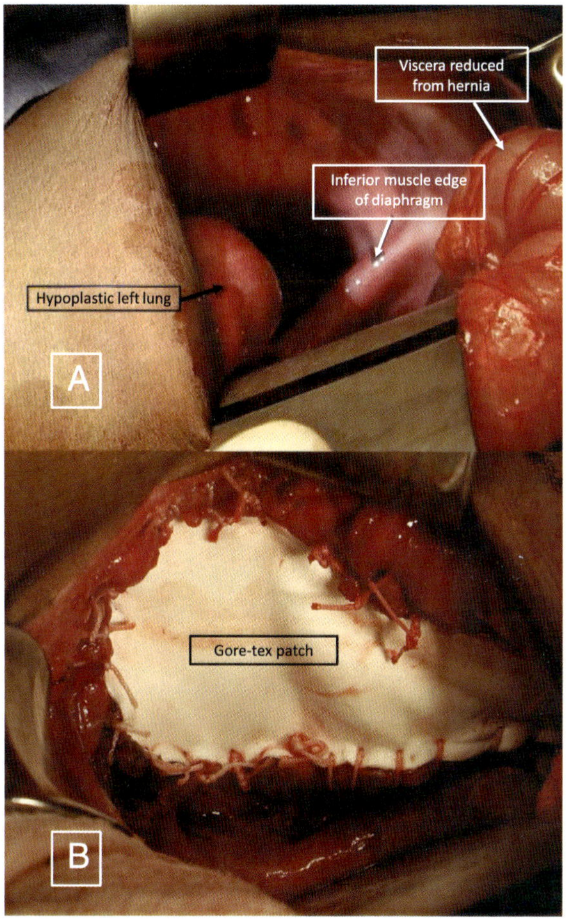

Fig. 9 a Left sided diaphragmatic hernia showing the hypoplastic left lung, inferior muscle edge of the diaphragm and reduced viscera. **b** Prosthetic patch – Gore-Tex patch used to close the defect

materials (Goretex® is most popular) but there has been growing recent interest in combining synthetic materials with additional biologic layers in an effort to buttress the repair and promote native tissue ingrowth for long-term stability [118]. Lastly, several groups have lauded the benefits of autologous, muscle flap closure of the defect [119].

Follow-up and outcomes

Infants with CDH face considerable long-term respiratory issues, nutritional problems, neurodevelopmental delays, hernia recurrence and orthopedic deformities [120]. The American Academy of Pediatrics (AAP) came out with guidelines for follow-up of infants who are discharged with CDH [120]. A multidisciplinary approach with long-term follow-up is required for these infants.

Respiratory morbidities include chronic lung disease, rebound pulmonary hypertension, obstructive pulmonary disease and infection. Treatment with ECMO and patch repair were associated with more significant pulmonary morbidity [121] with decreased inspiratory muscle strength. Adolescent survivors often-faced mild to moderate obstructive disease requiring bronchodilator therapy along with weak inspiratory muscle strength [122]. Nutritional problems include gastro esophageal reflux [123, 124] aversion to oral feeds, gastrostomy tube feeding and failure to thrive. Neurological and development problems range from physical disability to neurocognitive and functional delays. Hearing loss is common in these infants [125, 126]. Orthopedic deformities such as pectus and scoliosis are seen in patients post CDH repair [122, 127].

Conclusion

Despite the unclear etiology of CDH and management of PPHN, over the past few decades, reports have suggested increasing trends of survival in infants with CDH [76]. With the medical and surgical advances in the management of CDH, the reported overall survival is 70-90% [7, 76, 128]. With ECMO, the survival is around 50% [112–114] with different centers reporting different criteria and outcomes. Multiple factors such as prematurity, ECMO, associated abnormalities especially cardiac, need for transport, severity of PPHN, type of repair can affect the outcome and survival of an infant with CDH [51, 114, 128, 129].

Abbreviations

CDH: Congenital Diaphragmatic hernia; CMV: Conventional mechanical ventilation; ECMO: Extracorporeal Membrane Oxygenation;
ELSO: Extracorporeal Life Support Organization; HFOV: High-frequency oscillatory ventilation; iNO: Inhaled nitric oxide; LHR: Lung to head ratio; PPHN: Persistent pulmonary hypertension of newborn

Acknowledgements

Not applicable

Funding

Praveen Chandrasekharan – Salary support from University at Buffalo - Dr. Henry C. and Bertha H. Buswell Fellowship.
Satyan Lakshminrusimha - grant 1R01HD072929-0 (SL) and Women and Children's Hospital of Buffalo Foundation.

Authors' contributions

PKC: concept, collection of data, writing the manuscript, critique and revision. MR: concept, collection of data, writing the manuscript, critique and revision. RM: Contributed to management, critique and revision. DR: Wrote the surgical management section, contributed to ECMO management, revised and critiqued. Surgical correction with Goretex patch copyrighted to DR. SL: mentor, concept, collection of data, writing the manuscript, critique and responsible for all illustration/figures. Illustrations copyrighted to SL. All authors read and approved the final manuscript.

Authors information

Praveen Kumar Chandrasekharan, Attending – Neonatology, Research Assistant Professor.
Department of Pediatrics, Women and Children's Hospital of Buffalo, Buffalo, NY.
Munmun Rawat, Attending – Neonatology, Research Assistant Professor.
Department of Pediatrics, Women and Children's Hospital of Buffalo, Buffalo, NY.
Rajeshwari Madappa, Pediatrician.
SIGMA Hospital, Mysore, India.
David H. Rothstein, Pediatric Surgeon, Associate Professor.

Department of Pediatric Surgery, Women and Children's Hospital of Buffalo, Buffalo, NY.
Satyan Lakshminrusimha, Chief of Neonatology, Vice Chair and Professor of Pediatrics.
Department of Pediatrics, Women and Children's Hospital of Buffalo, Buffalo, NY.

Competing interests

The authors declare that they have no competing interests.

Author details

[1]Department of Pediatrics, Women and Children's Hospital of Buffalo, Buffalo, NY, USA. [2]SIGMA Hospital, Mysore, India. [3]Department of Pediatric Surgery, Women and Children's Hospital of Buffalo, Buffalo, NY, USA.

References

1. Colvin J, Bower C, Dickinson JE, Sokol J. Outcomes of congenital diaphragmatic hernia: a population-based study in Western Australia. Pediatrics. 2005;116(3):e356–363.
2. Gallot D, Boda C, Ughetto S, Perthus I, Robert-Gnansia E, Francannet C, Laurichesse-Delmas H, Jani J, Coste K, Deprest J, et al. Prenatal detection and outcome of congenital diaphragmatic hernia: a French registry-based study. Ultrasound Obstet Gynecol. 2007;29(3):276–83.
3. Yang W, Carmichael SL, Harris JA, Shaw GM. Epidemiologic characteristics of congenital diaphragmatic hernia among 2.5 million California births, 1989–1997. Birth Defects Res A Clin Mol Teratol. 2006;76(3):170–4.
4. McGivern MR, Best KE, Rankin J, Wellesley D, Greenlees R, Addor MC, Arriola L, de Walle H, Barisic I, Beres J, et al. Epidemiology of congenital diaphragmatic hernia in Europe: a register-based study. Arch Dis Child Fetal Neonatal Ed. 2015;100(2):F137–144.
5. Tennant PW, Samarasekera SD, Pless-Mulloli T, Rankin J. Sex differences in the prevalence of congenital anomalies: a population-based study. Birth Defects Res A Clin Mol Teratol. 2011;91(10):894–901.
6. Brownlee EM, Howatson AG, Davis CF, Sabharwal AJ. The hidden mortality of congenital diaphragmatic hernia: a 20-year review. J Pediatr Surg. 2009; 44(2):317–20.
7. Mah VK, Zamakhshary M, Mah DY, Cameron B, Bass J, Bohn D, Scott L, Himidan S, Walker M, Kim PC. Absolute vs relative improvements in congenital diaphragmatic hernia survival: what happened to "hidden mortality". J Pediatr Surg. 2009;44(5):877–82.
8. Stege G, Fenton A, Jaffray B. Nihilism in the 1990s: the true mortality of congenital diaphragmatic hernia. Pediatrics. 2003;112(3 Pt 1):532–5.
9. Beurskens LW, Tibboel D, Lindemans J, Duvekot JJ, Cohen-Overbeek TE, Veenma DC, de Klein A, Greer JJ, Steegers-Theunissen RP. Retinol status of newborn infants is associated with congenital diaphragmatic hernia. Pediatrics. 2010;126(4):712–20.
10. Beurskens LW, Tibboel D, Steegers-Theunissen RP. Role of nutrition, lifestyle factors, and genes in the pathogenesis of congenital diaphragmatic hernia: human and animal studies. Nutr Rev. 2009;67(12):719–30.
11. Wat MJ, Veenma D, Hogue J, Holder AM, Yu Z, Wat JJ, Hanchard N, Shchelochkov OA, Fernandes CJ, Johnson A, et al. Genomic alterations that contribute to the development of isolated and non-isolated congenital diaphragmatic hernia. J Med Genet. 2011;48(5):299–307.
12. Anderson D. Incidence of congenital diaphragmatic hernia in the young of rats bred on a diet deficient in Vitamin A. Am J Dis Child. 1941;62:888–9.
13. Tenbrinck R, Tibboel D, Gaillard JL, Kluth D, Bos AP, Lachmann B, Molenaar JC. Experimentally induced congenital diaphragmatic hernia in rats. J Pediatr Surg. 1990;25(4):426–9.
14. Tenbrinck R, Gaillard JL, Tibboel D, Kluth D, Lachmann B, Molenaar JC. Pulmonary vascular abnormalities in experimentally induced congenital diaphragmatic hernia in rats. J Pediatr Surg. 1992;27(7):862–5.
15. Major D, Cadenas M, Fournier L, Leclerc S, Lefebvre M, Cloutier R. Retinol status of newborn infants with congenital diaphragmatic hernia. Pediatr Surg Int. 1998;13(8):547–9.
16. Greer JJ. Current concepts on the pathogenesis and etiology of congenital diaphragmatic hernia. Respir Physiol Neurobiol. 2013;189(2):232–40.
17. Veenma DC, de Klein A, Tibboel D. Developmental and genetic aspects of congenital diaphragmatic hernia. Pediatr Pulmonol. 2012;47(6):534–45.
18. Moore KL, Persaud TV, Torchia MG. The developing human: clinically oriented embryology. 2011.
19. Wells LJ. Development of the human diaphragm and pleural sacs. Contrib Embryol Carnegie Ins. 1954;35:107–34.
20. Harrison MR. The fetus with a diaphragmatic hernia: pathophysiology, natural history, and surgical management. In: The unborn patient fetal diagnosis and treatment. 2nd ed. Philadelphia: W.B. Saunders; 1990. p. 259–319.
21. Iritani I. Experimental study on embryogenesis of congenital diaphragmatic hernia. Anat Embryol (Berl). 1984;169(2):133–9.
22. Mayer S, Metzger R, Kluth D. The embryology of the diaphragm. Semin Pediatr Surg. 2011;20(3):161–9.
23. Aggarwal S, Stockman PT, Klein MD, Natarajan G. The right ventricular systolic to diastolic duration ratio: a simple prognostic marker in congenital diaphragmatic hernia? Acta Paediatr. 2011;100(10):1315–8.
24. Irish MS, Karamanoukian HL, O'Toole SJ, Glick PL. You gotta have heart. J Pediatr. 1996;129(1):175–6. author reply 176–177.
25. Menon SC, Tani LY, Weng HY, Lally PA, Lally KP, Yoder BA, Congenital Diaphragmatic Hernia Study G. Clinical characteristics and outcomes of patients with cardiac defects and congenital diaphragmatic hernia. J Pediatr. 2012;162:114–9.
26. Schwartz SM, Vermilion RP, Hirschl RB. Evaluation of left ventricular mass in children with left-sided congenital diaphragmatic hernia. J Pediatr. 1994; 125(3):447–51.
27. Keijzer R, Liu J, Deimling J, Tibboel D, Post M. Dual-hit hypothesis explains pulmonary hypoplasia in the nitrofen model of congenital diaphragmatic hernia. Am J Pathol. 2000;156(4):1299–306.
28. George DK, Cooney TP, Chiu BK, Thurlbeck WM. Hypoplasia and immaturity of the terminal lung unit (acinus) in congenital diaphragmatic hernia. Am Rev Respir Dis. 1987;136(4):947–50.
29. DiFiore JW, Fauza DO, Slavin R, Wilson JM. Experimental fetal tracheal ligation and congenital diaphragmatic hernia: a pulmonary vascular morphometric analysis. J Pediatr Surg. 1995;30(7):917–23. discussion 923–914.
30. Lakshminrusimha S. The pulmonary circulation in neonatal respiratory failure. Clin Perinatol. 2012;39(3):655–83.
31. Kitagawa M, Hislop A, Boyden EA, Reid L. Lung hypoplasia in congenital diaphragmatic hernia. A quantitative study of airway, artery, and alveolar development. Br J Surg. 1971;58(5):342–6.
32. Shehata SM, Mooi WJ, Okazaki T, El-Banna I, Sharma HS, Tibboel D. Enhanced expression of vascular endothelial growth factor in lungs of newborn infants with congenital diaphragmatic hernia and pulmonary hypertension. Thorax. 1999;54(5):427–31.
33. Pierro M, Thebaud B. Understanding and treating pulmonary hypertension in congenital diaphragmatic hernia. Semin Fetal Neonatal Med. 2014;19(6): 357–63.
34. Sluiter I, van der Horst I, van der Voorn P, Boerema-de Munck A, Buscop-van Kempen M, de Krijger R, Tibboel D, Reiss I, Rottier RJ. Premature differentiation of vascular smooth muscle cells in human congenital diaphragmatic hernia. Exp Mol Pathol. 2013;94(1):195–202.
35. Lath NR, Galambos C, Rocha AB, Malek M, Gittes GK, Potoka DA. Defective pulmonary innervation and autonomic imbalance in congenital diaphragmatic hernia. Am J Physiol Lung Cell Mol Physiol. 2012;302(4):L390–398.
36. Luong C, Rey-Perra J, Vadivel A, Gilmour G, Sauve Y, Koonen D, Walker D, Todd KG, Gressens P, Kassiri Z, et al. Antenatal sildenafil treatment attenuates pulmonary hypertension in experimental congenital diaphragmatic hernia. Circulation. 2011;123(19):2120–31.
37. Schmidt AF, Rojas-Moscoso JA, Goncalves FL, Gallindo RM, Monica FZ, Antunes E, Figueira RL, Sbragia L. Increased contractility and impaired relaxation of the left pulmonary artery in a rabbit model of congenital diaphragmatic hernia. Pediatr Surg Int. 2013;29(5):489–94.
38. Shinkai T, Shima H, Solari V, Puri P. Expression of vasoactive mediators during mechanical ventilation in nitrofen-induced diaphragmatic hernia in rats. Pediatr Surg Int. 2005;21(3):143–7.
39. Nair J, Lakshminrusimha S. Update on PPHN: mechanisms and treatment. Semin Perinatol. 2014;38(2):78–91.

40. Siebert JR, Haas JE, Beckwith JB. Left ventricular hypoplasia in congenital diaphragmatic hernia. J Pediatr Surg. 1984;19(5):567–71.
41. Byrne FA, Keller RL, Meadows J, Miniati D, Brook MM, Silverman NH, Moon-Grady AJ. Severe left diaphragmatic hernia limits size of fetal left heart more than right diaphragmatic hernia. Ultrasound Obstet Gynecol. 2015;46:688–94.
42. Kinsella JP, Ivy DD, Abman SH. Pulmonary vasodilator therapy in congenital diaphragmatic hernia: acute, late, and chronic pulmonary hypertension. Semin Perinatol. 2005;29(2):123–8.
43. Graham G, Devine PC. Antenatal diagnosis of congenital diaphragmatic hernia. Semin Perinatol. 2005;29(2):69–76.
44. Garne E, Haeusler M, Barisic I, Gjergja R, Stoll C, Clementi M, Euroscan Study G. Congenital diaphragmatic hernia: evaluation of prenatal diagnosis in 20 european regions. Ultrasound Obstet Gynecol. 2002;19(4):329–33.
45. Quinn TM, Hubbard AM, Adzick NS. Prenatal magnetic resonance imaging enhances fetal diagnosis. J Pediatr Surg. 1998;33(4):553–8.
46. Worley KC, Dashe JS, Barber RG, Megison SM, McIntire DD, Twickler DM. Fetal magnetic resonance imaging in isolated diaphragmatic hernia: volume of herniated liver and neonatal outcome. Am J Obstet Gynecol. 2009;200(3): 318 e311–316.
47. Sweed Y, Puri P. Congenital diaphragmatic hernia: influence of associated malformations on survival. Arch Dis Child. 1993;69(1 Spec No):68–70.
48. Pober BR, Lin A, Russell M, Ackerman KG, Chakravorty S, Strauss B, Westgate MN, Wilson J, Donahoe PK, Holmes LB. Infants with bochdalek diaphragmatic hernia: sibling precurrence and monozygotic twin discordance in a hospital-based malformation surveillance program. Am J Med Genet A. 2005;138A(2):81–8.
49. Slavotinek AM. Fryns syndrome: a review of the phenotype and diagnostic guidelines. Am J Med Genet A. 2004;124A(4):427–33.
50. Deprest J, Brady P, Nicolaides K, Benachi A, Berg C, Vermeesch J, Gardener G, Gratacos E. Prenatal management of the fetus with isolated congenital diaphragmatic hernia in the era of the TOTAL trial. Semin Fetal Neonatal Med. 2014;19(6):338–48.
51. Tennant PW, Pearce MS, Bythell M, Rankin J. 20-year survival of children born with congenital anomalies: a population-based study. Lancet. 2010; 375(9715):649–56.
52. Metkus AP, Filly RA, Stringer MD, Harrison MR, Adzick NS. Sonographic predictors of survival in fetal diaphragmatic hernia. J Pediatr Surg. 1996; 31(1):148–51. discussion 151–142.
53. Singh SJ, Cummins GE, Cohen RC, Cass D, Harvey JG, Martin HC, Pitkin J, Shun A, Glasson MJ. Adverse outcome of congenital diaphragmatic hernia is determined by diaphragmatic agenesis, not by antenatal diagnosis. J Pediatr Surg. 1999;34(11):1740–2.
54. Mullassery D, Ba'ath ME, Jesudason EC, Losty PD. Value of liver herniation in prediction of outcome in fetal congenital diaphragmatic hernia: a systematic review and meta-analysis. Ultrasound Obstet Gynecol. 2010;35(5):609–14.
55. Hedrick HL, Danzer E, Merchant A, Bebbington MW, Zhao H, Flake AW, Johnson MP, Liechty KW, Howell LJ, Wilson RD, et al. Liver position and lung-to-head ratio for prediction of extracorporeal membrane oxygenation and survival in isolated left congenital diaphragmatic hernia. Am J Obstet Gynecol. 2007;197(4):422 e421–424.
56. Lipshutz GS, Albanese CT, Feldstein VA, Jennings RW, Housley HT, Beech R, Farrell JA, Harrison MR. Prospective analysis of lung-to-head ratio predicts survival for patients with prenatally diagnosed congenital diaphragmatic hernia. J Pediatr Surg. 1997;32(11):1634–6.
57. Peralta CF, Cavoretto P, Csapo B, Vandecruys H, Nicolaides KH. Assessment of lung area in normal fetuses at 12–32 weeks. Ultrasound Obstet Gynecol. 2005;26(7):718–24.
58. Ba'ath ME, Jesudason EC, Losty PD. How useful is the lung-to-head ratio in predicting outcome in the fetus with congenital diaphragmatic hernia? a systematic review and meta-analysis. Ultrasound Obstet Gynecol. 2007;30(6): 897–906.
59. Jani J, Nicolaides KH, Keller RL, Benachi A, Peralta CF, Favre R, Moreno O, Tibboel D, Lipitz S, Eggink A, et al. Observed to expected lung area to head circumference ratio in the prediction of survival in fetuses with isolated diaphragmatic hernia. Ultrasound Obstet Gynecol. 2007;30(1):67–71.
60. Kapur P, Holm BA, Irish MS, Sokolowski J, Patel A, Glick PL. Lung physiological and metabolic changes in lambs with congenital diaphragmatic hernia after administration of prenatal maternal corticosteroids. J Pediatr Surg. 1999;34(2):354–6.
61. Lally KP, Bagolan P, Hosie S, Lally PA, Stewart M, Cotten CM, Van Meurs KP, Alexander G, Congenital Diaphragmatic Hernia Study G. Corticosteroids for fetuses with congenital diaphragmatic hernia: can we show benefit? J Pediatr Surg. 2006;41(4):668–74. discussion 668–674.
62. Junior EA, Tonni G, Martins WP, Ruano R. Procedure-Related Complications and Survival Following Fetoscopic Endotracheal Occlusion (FETO) for Severe Congenital Diaphragmatic Hernia: Systematic Review and Meta-Analysis in the FETO Era. Eur J Pediatr Surg. 2016. doi:10.1055/s-0036-1587331.
63. Stevens TP, van Wijngaarden E, Ackerman KG, Lally PA, Lally KP. Timing of delivery and survival rates for infants with prenatal diagnoses of congenital diaphragmatic hernia. Pediatrics. 2009;123(2):494–502.
64. Hutcheon JA, Butler B, Lisonkova S, Marquette GP, Mayer C, Skoll A, Joseph KS. Timing of delivery for pregnancies with congenital diaphragmatic hernia. BJOG. 2010;117(13):1658–62.
65. Sengupta S, Carrion V, Shelton J, Wynn RJ, Ryan RM, Singhal K, Lakshminrusimha S. Adverse neonatal outcomes associated with early-term birth. JAMA Pediatr. 2013;167(11):1053–9.
66. Kattwinkel J, Perlman JM, Aziz K, Colby C, Fairchild K, Gallagher J, Hazinski MF, Halamek LP, Kumar P, Little G, et al. Part 15: neonatal resuscitation: 2010 american heart association guidelines for cardiopulmonary resuscitation and emergency cardiovascular care. Circulation. 2010;122(18 Suppl 3):S909–919.
67. Gien J, Kinsella JP. Differences in preductal and postductal arterial blood gas measurements in infants with severe congenital diaphragmatic hernia. Arch Dis Child Fetal Neonatal Ed. 2016;101(4):F314–318.
68. Snoek KG, Capolupo I, van Rosmalen J, Hout Lde J, Vijfhuize S, Greenough A, Wijnen RM, Tibboel D, Reiss IK, Consortium CE. Conventional mechanical ventilation versus high-frequency oscillatory ventilation for congenital Diaphragmatic hernia: a randomized clinical trial (the VICI-trial). Ann Surg. 2016;263(5):867–74.
69. Sakurai Y, Azarow K, Cutz E, Messineo A, Pearl R, Bohn D. Pulmonary barotrauma in congenital Diaphragmatic hernia: a clinicopathological correlation. J Pediatr Surg. 1999;34(12):1813–7.
70. Wung JT, Sahni R, Moffitt ST, Lipsitz E, Stolar CJ. Congenital diaphragmatic hernia: survival treated with very delayed surgery, spontaneous respiration, and no chest tube. J Pediatr Surg. 1995;30(3):406–9.
71. Reiss I, Schaible T, van den Hout L, Capolupo I, Allegaert K, van Heijst A, Gorett Silva M, Greenough A, Tibboel D, Consortium CE. Standardized postnatal management of infants with congenital diaphragmatic hernia in Europe: the CDH EURO consortium consensus. Neonatology. 2010;98(4): 354–64.
72. Habib RH, Pyon KH, Courtney SE. Optimal high-frequency oscillatory ventilation settings by nonlinear lung mechanics analysis. Am J Respir Crit Care Med. 2002;166(7):950–3.
73. van den Hout L, Tibboel D, Vijfhuize S, te Beest H, Hop W, Reiss I, Consortium C-E. The VICI-trial: high frequency oscillation versus conventional mechanical ventilation in newborns with congenital diaphragmatic hernia: an international multicentre randomized controlled trial. BMC Pediatr. 2011;11:98.
74. Van Meurs K, Congenital Diaphragmatic Hernia Study G. Is surfactant therapy beneficial in the treatment of the term newborn infant with congenital diaphragmatic hernia? J Pediatr. 2004;145(3):312–6.
75. Lally KP, Lally PA, Langham MR, Hirschl R, Moya FR, Tibboel D, Van Meurs K, Congenital Diaphragmatic Hernia Study G. Surfactant does not improve survival rate in preterm infants with congenital diaphragmatic hernia. J Pediatr Surg. 2004;39(6):829–33.
76. Hagadorn JI, Brownell EA, Herbst KW, Trzaski JM, Neffs S, Campbell BT. Trends in treatment and in-hospital mortality for neonates with congenital diaphragmatic hernia. J Perinatol. 2015;35:748–54.
77. Noori S, Seri I. Neonatal blood pressure support: the use of inotropes, lusitropes, and other vasopressor agents. Clin Perinatol. 2012;39(1):221–38.
78. Seri I, Tan R, Evans J. Cardiovascular effects of hydrocortisone in preterm infants with pressor-resistant hypotension. Pediatrics. 2001;107(5):1070–4.
79. Acker SN, Kinsella JP, Abman SH, Gien J. Vasopressin improves hemodynamic status in infants with congenital diaphragmatic hernia. J Pediatr. 2014;165(1):53–8. e51.
80. Sharma V, Berkelhamer S, Lakshminrusimha S. Persistent pulmonary hypertension of the newborn. Maternal Health, Neonatology Perinatol. 2015;1(1):14.
81. Suda K, Bigras JL, Bohn D, Hornberger LK, McCrindle BW. Echocardiographic predictors of outcome in newborns with congenital diaphragmatic hernia. Pediatrics. 2000;105(5):1106–9.
82. Tourneux P, Rakza T, Bouissou A, Krim G, Storme L. Pulmonary circulatory effects of norepinephrine in newborn infants with persistent pulmonary hypertension. J Pediatr. 2008;153(3):345–9.

83. Snoek KG, Reiss IK, Greenough A, Capolupo I, Urlesberger B, Wessel L, Storme L, Deprest J, Schaible T, van Heijst A, et al. Standardized postnatal management of infants with congenital diaphragmatic hernia in Europe: the CDH EURO consortium consensus - 2015 update. Neonatology. 2016; 110(1):66–74.
84. Rawat M, Chandrasekharan PK, Williams A, Gugino S, Koenigsknecht C, Swartz D, Ma CX, Mathew B, Nair J, Lakshminrusimha S. Oxygen saturation index and severity of hypoxic respiratory failure. Neonatology. 2015;107(3): 161–6.
85. Thomas NJ, Shaffer ML, Willson DF, Shih MC, Curley MA. Defining acute lung disease in children with the oxygenation saturation index. Pediatr Crit Care Med. 2010;11(1):12–7.
86. Davidson D, Barefield ES, Kattwinkel J, Dudell G, Damask M, Straube R, Rhines J, Chang CT. Inhaled nitric oxide for the early treatment of persistent pulmonary hypertension of the term newborn: a randomized, double-masked, placebo-controlled, dose–response, multicenter study. The I-NO/PPHN study group. Pediatrics. 1998;101(3 Pt 1):325–34.
87. Konduri GG, Kim UO. Advances in the diagnosis and management of persistent pulmonary hypertension of the newborn. Pediatr Clin North Am. 2009;56(3):579–600. Table of Contents.
88. Kinsella JP. Inhaled nitric oxide in the term newborn. Early Hum Dev. 2008; 84(11):709–16.
89. Konduri GG, Solimano A, Sokol GM, Singer J, Ehrenkranz RA, Singhal N, Wright LL, Van Meurs K, Stork E, Kirpalani H, et al. A randomized trial of early versus standard inhaled nitric oxide therapy in term and near-term newborn infants with hypoxic respiratory failure. Pediatrics. 2004;113(3 Pt 1):559–64.
90. Neonatal Inhaled Nitric Oxide Study Group. Inhaled nitric oxide and hypoxic respiratory failure in infants with congenital diaphragmatic hernia. The neonatal inhaled nitric oxide study group (NINOS). Pediatrics. 1997;99(6): 838–45.
91. Campbell BT, Herbst KW, Briden KE, Neff S, Ruscher KA, Hagadorn JI. Inhaled nitric oxide use in neonates with congenital diaphragmatic hernia. Pediatrics. 2014;134(2):e420–426.
92. Iocono JA, Cilley RE, Mauger DT, Krummel TM, Dillon PW. Postnatal pulmonary hypertension after repair of congenital diaphragmatic hernia: predicting risk and outcome. J Pediatr Surg. 1999;34(2):349–53.
93. Schwartz IP, Bernbaum JC, Rychik J, Grunstein M, D'Agostino J, Polin RA. Pulmonary hypertension in children following extracorporeal membrane oxygenation therapy and repair of congenital diaphragmatic hernia. J Perinatol. 1999;19(3):220–6.
94. Mohseni-Bod H, Bohn D. Pulmonary hypertension in congenital diaphragmatic hernia. Semin Pediatr Surg. 2007;16(2):126–33.
95. Inamura N, Kubota A, Nakajima T, Kayatani F, Okuyama H, Oue T, Kawahara H. A proposal of new therapeutic strategy for antenatally diagnosed congenital diaphragmatic hernia. J Pediatr Surg. 2005;40(8):1315–9.
96. Shiyanagi S, Okazaki T, Shoji H, Shimizu T, Tanaka T, Takeda S, Kawashima K, Lane GJ, Yamataka A. Management of pulmonary hypertension in congenital diaphragmatic hernia: nitric oxide with prostaglandin-E1 versus nitric oxide alone. Pediatr Surg Int. 2008;24(10):1101–4.
97. Baquero H, Soliz A, Neira F, Venegas ME, Sola A. Oral sildenafil in infants with persistent pulmonary hypertension of the newborn: a pilot randomized blinded study. Pediatrics. 2006;117(4):1077–83.
98. Vargas-Origel A, Gomez-Rodriguez G, Aldana-Valenzuela C, Vela-Huerta MM, Alarcon-Santos SB, Amador-Licona N. The use of sildenafil in persistent pulmonary hypertension of the newborn. Am J Perinatol. 2010;27(3):225–30.
99. Steinhorn RH, Kinsella JP, Pierce C, Butrous G, Dilleen M, Oakes M, Wessel DL. Intravenous sildenafil in the treatment of neonates with persistent pulmonary hypertension. J Pediatr. 2009;155(6):841–7. e841.
100. Abman SH, Kinsella JP, Rosenzweig EB, Krishnan U, Kulik T, Mullen M, Wessel DL, Steinhorn R, Adatia I, Hanna B, et al. Implications of the U.S. Food and drug administration warning against the use of sildenafil for the treatment of pediatric pulmonary hypertension. Am J Respir Crit Care Med. 2013; 187(6):572–5.
101. Lakshminrusimha S, Porta NF, Farrow KN, Chen B, Gugino SF, Kumar VH, Russell JA, Steinhorn RH. Milrinone enhances relaxation to prostacyclin and Iloprost in pulmonary arteries isolated from lambs with persistent pulmonary hypertension of the newborn. Pediatr Crit Care Med. 2009; 10(1):106–12.
102. Hoffman TM, Wernovsky G, Atz AM, Bailey JM, Akbary A, Kocsis JF, Nelson DP, Chang AC, Kulik TJ, Spray TL, et al. Prophylactic intravenous use of milrinone after cardiac operation in pediatrics (PRIMACORP) study. Prophylactic intravenous use of milrinone after cardiac operation in pediatrics. Am Heart J. 2002;143(1):15–21.
103. Patel N. Use of milrinone to treat cardiac dysfunction in infants with pulmonary hypertension secondary to congenital diaphragmatic hernia: a review of six patients. Neonatology. 2012;102(2):130–6.
104. Bassler D, Choong K, McNamara P, Kirpalani H. Neonatal persistent pulmonary hypertension treated with milrinone: four case reports. Biol Neonate. 2006;89(1):1–5.
105. McNamara PJ, Laique F, Muang-In S, Whyte HE. Milrinone improves oxygenation in neonates with severe persistent pulmonary hypertension of the newborn. J Crit Care. 2006;21(2):217–22.
106. McNamara PJ, Shivananda SP, Sahni M, Freeman D, Taddio A. Pharmacology of milrinone in neonates with persistent pulmonary hypertension of the newborn and suboptimal response to inhaled nitric oxide. Pediatr Crit Care Med. 2013;14(1):74–84.
107. Bailey JM, Hoffman TM, Wessel DL, Nelson DP, Atz AM, Chang AC, Kulik TJ, Spray TL, Akbary A, Miller RP, et al. A population pharmacokinetic analysis of milrinone in pediatric patients after cardiac surgery. J Pharmacokinet Pharmacodyn. 2004;31(1):43–59.
108. Lakshminrusimha S, Keszler M. Persistent Pulmonary Hypertension of the Newborn. Neoreviews. 2015;16(12):e680–92.
109. Steinhorn RH, Fineman J, Kusic-Pajic A, Cornelisse P, Gehin M, Nowbakht P, Pierce CM, Beghetti M, investigators F-s. Bosentan as adjunctive therapy for persistent pulmonary hypertension of the newborn: results of the randomized multicenter placebo-controlled exploratory trial. J Pediatr. 2016; 177:90–6. e93.
110. Dimmitt RA, Moss RL, Rhine WD, Benitz WE, Henry MC, Vanmeurs KP. Venoarterial versus venovenous extracorporeal membrane oxygenation in congenital diaphragmatic hernia: the extracorporeal life support organization registry, 1990–1999. J Pediatr Surg. 2001;36(8):1199–204.
111. Guner YS, Khemani RG, Qureshi FG, Wee CP, Austin MT, Dorey F, Rycus PT, Ford HR, Friedlich P, Stein JE. Outcome analysis of neonates with congenital diaphragmatic hernia treated with venovenous vs venoarterial extracorporeal membrane oxygenation. J Pediatr Surg. 2009;44(9):1691–701.
112. Haricharan RN, Barnhart DC, Cheng H, Delzell E. Identifying neonates at a very high risk for mortality among children with congenital diaphragmatic hernia managed with extracorporeal membrane oxygenation. J Pediatr Surg. 2009;44(1):87–93.
113. Kays DW, Islam S, Richards DS, Larson SD, Perkins JM, Talbert JL. Extracorporeal life support in patients with congenital diaphragmatic hernia: how long should we treat? J Am Coll Surg. 2014;218(4):808–17.
114. Seetharamaiah R, Younger JG, Bartlett RH, Hirschl RB, Congenital Diaphragmatic Hernia Study G. Factors associated with survival in infants with congenital diaphragmatic hernia requiring extracorporeal membrane oxygenation: a report from the congenital diaphragmatic hernia study group. J Pediatr Surg. 2009;44(7):1315–21.
115. Tsao K, Lally KP. Surgical management of the newborn with congenital diaphragmatic hernia. Fetal Diagn Ther. 2011;29(1):46–54.
116. Desai AA, Ostlie DJ, Juang D. Optimal timing of congenital diaphragmatic hernia repair in infants on extracorporeal membrane oxygenation. Semin Pediatr Surg. 2015;24(1):17–9.
117. Gander JW, Fisher JC, Gross ER, Reichstein AR, Cowles RA, Aspelund G, Stolar CJ, Kuenzler KA. Early recurrence of congenital diaphragmatic hernia is higher after thoracoscopic than open repair: a single institutional study. J Pediatr Surg. 2011;46(7):1303–8.
118. Grethel EJ, Cortes RA, Wagner AJ, Clifton MS, Lee H, Farmer DL, Harrison MR, Keller RL, Nobuhara KK. Prosthetic patches for congenital diaphragmatic hernia repair: surgisis vs gore-Tex. J Pediatr Surg. 2006;41(1):29–33. discussion 29–33.
119. Brant-Zawadzki PB, Fenton SJ, Nichol PF, Matlak ME, Scaife ER. The split abdominal wall muscle flap repair for large congenital diaphragmatic hernias on extracorporeal membrane oxygenation. J Pediatr Surg. 2007; 42(6):1047–50. discussion 1051.
120. Lally KP, Engle W, American Academy of Pediatrics Section on S, American Academy of Pediatrics Committee on F, Newborn. Postdischarge follow-up of infants with congenital diaphragmatic hernia. Pediatrics. 2008;121(3):627–32.
121. Muratore CS, Kharasch V, Lund DP, Sheils C, Friedman S, Brown C, Utter S, Jaksic T, Wilson JM. Pulmonary morbidity in 100 survivors of congenital diaphragmatic hernia monitored in a multidisciplinary clinic. J Pediatr Surg. 2001;36(1):133–40.

122. Trachsel D, Selvadurai H, Bohn D, Langer JC, Coates AL. Long-term pulmonary morbidity in survivors of congenital diaphragmatic hernia. Pediatr Pulmonol. 2005;39(5):433–9.
123. Peetsold MG, Kneepkens CM, Heij HA, IJsselstijn H, Tibboel D, Gemke RJ. Congenital diaphragmatic hernia: long-term risk of gastroesophageal reflux disease. J Pediatr Gastroenterol Nutr. 2010;51(4):448–53.
124. Morandi A, Macchini F, Zanini A, Pasqua N, Farris G, Canazza L, Gentilino V, Di Cesare A, Leva E. Endoscopic surveillance for congenital diaphragmatic hernia: unexpected prevalence of silent esophagitis. Eur J Pediatr Surg. 2015;26:291–5.
125. Morini F, Capolupo I, Masi R, Ronchetti MP, Locatelli M, Corchia C, Bagolan P. Hearing impairment in congenital diaphragmatic hernia: the inaudible and noiseless foot of time. J Pediatr Surg. 2008;43(2):380–4.
126. Partridge EA, Bridge C, Donaher JG, Herkert LM, Grill E, Danzer E, Gerdes M, Hoffman CH, D'Agostino JA, Bernbaum JC, et al. Incidence and factors associated with sensorineural and conductive hearing loss among survivors of congenital diaphragmatic hernia. J Pediatr Surg. 2014;49(6):890–4. discussion 894.
127. Russell KW, Barnhart DC, Rollins MD, Hedlund G, Scaife ER. Musculoskeletal deformities following repair of large congenital diaphragmatic hernias. J Pediatr Surg. 2014;49(6):886–9.
128. Tsao K, Lally KP. The congenital diaphragmatic hernia study group: a voluntary international registry. Semin Pediatr Surg. 2008;17(2):90–7.
129. Wynn J, Krishnan U, Aspelund G, Zhang Y, Duong J, Stolar CJ, Hahn E, Pietsch J, Chung D, Moore D, et al. Outcomes of congenital diaphragmatic hernia in the modern era of management. J Pediatr. 2013;163(1):114–9. e111.

6

Oral hypoglycemic agents: do the ends justify the means?

Oded Langer

Abstract

Background: Glyburide has replaced insulin as the first line of therapy in the treatment of gestational diabetes in the United States. Glyburide and metformin therapies were reported to be comparable to insulin yet also cost-effective, patient-friendly, and potentially compliance-enhancing. Recently, the efficacy of the use of these oral hypoglycemic drugs has been questioned. In this review, the questionable concerns will be addressed: Which diabetic drug(s) cross the placenta? What is the quality of evidence and the data source validity? Which treatment modalities are most effective in reducing the primary outcome in GDM? Which drug is most effective in improving secondary outcomes?

Findings: This review documents the methodological issues in study design that have impacted the results for the provision of health care interventions in GDM. The review summarizes the contents of the articles qualitatively and assesses the theoretical and empirical evidence. Multiple types of studies exist and every study design serves a specific purpose. Different study designs addressing the same question can yield varying results. The risk of presenting uncertain results without categorically knowing the direction and magnitude of the effect holds true for both randomized and nonrandomized controlled trials. The review further emphasizes the importance of achieving the targeted levels of glycemic control.

Conclusion: The implications of this review are critical to addressing the current gaps in the literature on the efficacy of the use of oral hypoglycemic agents in GDM. The emphasis needs to be placed on patient treatment in order to manage hyperglycemia to reduce fetal and maternal morbidity. In this regard, we need to delineate proper outcome criteria that will reflect disease severity and treat using appropriate pharmacological therapy.

Keywords: Gestational diabetes, Glyburide, Metformin, Health research design

Introduction

The time has come to place the emphasis on patient treatment of gestational diabetes mellitus (GDM) in order to manage hyperglycemia to reduce fetal and maternal morbidity rather than debating the diagnostic criteria. We need to clearly define outcome criteria that reflect the severity of the disease and the appropriate pharmacological therapy to treat it. Then, randomized and/or other well-designed studies should be performed to demonstrate improvement in perinatal outcome with justified cost of care.

The current American Diabetes Association and European Association for the Study of Diabetes recommendations state that achieving specific glycemic goals can substantially reduce morbidity. Thus, effective treatment of hyperglycemia has become a top priority [1]. Approximately 35-70 % of GDM women will require pharmacological treatment during pregnancy to achieve glycemic goals [2].

Historically, insulin has been the recommended treatment for GDM in the U.S. when dietary and lifestyle measures have failed. Today, randomized controlled trials support the efficacy and short-term safety of glyburide (pregnancy category B) and metformin (pregnancy category B) in the treatment of GDM [3, 4]. The stress free use and low cost of these oral hypoglycemic agents are advantages in comparison to insulin use. These demonstrated advantages have led to a change in clinical practice. Several guideline bodies, including the American College of Obstetrics and Gynecology [5], the UK National Institute for Health and Care Excellence, [6] and the Canadian Diabetes Association [7] endorsed the use of glyburide. Insulin, metformin, and glyburide today

Correspondence: odlanger@gmail.com
Columbia University, New York, USA

are widely used to treat GDM. In general, however, common sense and good clinical judgment should prevail with adjustments for individual preferences, comorbidities, and other patient factors.

In the United States, glyburide use increased from 7.4 % of pharmacological treatment to 64.5 %, superseding insulin as the most common treatment in 2007. Glyburide has replaced insulin as the more common pharmacotherapy for GDM over the past decade [8]. Therefore, it is remarkable that recent studies of glyburide have questioned its use. These studies reported that fetal plasma glyburide concentrations in humans were approximately 70 % of maternal plasma levels [9, 10]. Moreover, 2 observational studies [11, 12] posted warnings about safety issues with the use of glyburide. In this review, several research gaps will be addressed:

1. Which diabetic drug(s) cross the placenta?
2. What is the quality of evidence and data source validity?
3. Which treatment modalities are most effective in reducing the primary outcome in GDM?
4. Which drug is most effective in improving secondary outcomes?

Findings

Which diabetic drug(s) cross the placenta?

It is important to note that when measuring placental transfer, one needs to understand the limitations of the measurement system and the unit of measure. 1 mg = 1,000 microgram (μg); 1 μg = 1,000 nanograms (ng); therefore, 1 mg = 1,000,000 ng. Two systems were used to measure placental drug concentration. One is high-performance liquid chromatographic analysis (HPLC-UV) and the mass spectrometry (LC-MS/MS). Comparison of glyburide concentration measured by each system revealed a strong association ($y = 0.9321x + 6.9427$, $r^2 = 0.9597$). However, the level of sensitivity for detection is different in each system.

The majority of drugs used in pregnancy cross the placenta although very few will cause adverse fetal outcome. Transfer of drugs across the placenta is affected by: molecular weight, protein kinase A (pKa), lipid solubility, placental blood flow, blood protein binding, elimination half-life and the specific placental transport system that affects the ability of drugs to enter the fetal compartment.

In glyburide, protein binding is greater than 99 %; it has a short elimination half-life time (6–8 hrs.); the pKa of 5.3 makes glyburide ionize in plasma making it transportable; transport against the concentration gradient from fetus to mother provides a concentration ratio 0.92 ± 0.23; and finally, effluxing glyburide by specific placental transporters. These mechanisms suggest minimal to no transfer of glyburide to the fetal compartment [2].

The recirculating single-cotyledon human placental model is widely used to characterize the transport and metabolism of numerous drugs and nutrients. It has been recognized as an in vitro surrogate for human placental transfer. It facilitates the study of intact human placenta independent of fetal metabolism. Finally, each experiment can be validated with the addition of antipyrine as a reference point for the level of transfer.

Our group [3] demonstrated, using HPLC/UV, that in cord blood samples, minimal glyburide levels (<14 ng/mL) were detectable despite maternal plasma levels of 50-150 ng/ml. Even with increased concentration of glyburide to 100 times the therapeutic level, transport was not appreciably altered. The finding of similar cord-serum insulin concentrations in our two treatment groups also indicates that little, if any, glyburide reached the fetuses. This result confirms in vitro studies [13, 14] in which no maternal-fetal or fetal-maternal transfer of glyburide was detected in full-term placentas perfused immediately after delivery. In addition, glyburide has no effect on the placental transport and uptake of glucose. Furthermore, maternal hyperglycemia does not alter glyburide transfer in vitro. In summary, there was virtually no significant transport of glyburide in either maternal-to-fetal or fetal-to-maternal directions with an average transport of 0.26 % at 2 h. Our findings of negligible glyburide transfer across the placenta were reconfirmed by multiple studies using the single cotyledon model [2].

Two recent studies of glyburide placental transport *in vivo* have caused a furor in the literature [9, 10]. Hebert et al. used LC-MS/MS for the determination of glyburide levels below 10 ng/ml. Maternal blood concentrations ranged from non-detectable to 32.7 ng/ml. The umbilical venous concentrations ranged from non-detectable to12.5 ng/ml. with a mean of approximately 1 ng/ml. Her findings confirmed our original studies of negligible glyburide levels in the fetal compartment.

Hebert et al. [9] reported that the mean maternal-fetal concentration ratio of glyburide was 0.7 ± 0.4. However, concentration is time dependent. Fetal-maternal ratio is the result of a given concentration at a single point in time. Thus, the drug concentration and the ratio are affected by the time of obtaining the sample and the sampling technique used. In our study, [3] the time from administration to obtaining the fetal sample was 8 ± 4 hours with a maternal concentration 50–150 ng. In Hebert's study [9], the time was up to 13 hours with maternal concentration 0.13-32.7 ng. In Schwartz et al. [10], the time was 13.3 ± 6.5 hours with maternal concentration 15.4 ± 20.8 ng with a range of 0.93-70.71.

Schwartz et al., [10] using LC-MS/MS, found in 15 of the 19 umbilical samples that glyburide concentration was <10 ng/ml. Seven of the 19 umbilical samples showed a higher glyburide concentration than the maternal sample, but only one of these seven measured greater than 10 ng/mL. The overall cord glyburide mean was 7.56 ± 8.2, with a median of 3.7. In summary, all three studies reported negligible levels of glyburide in the fetal compartment. However, the time of sampling differed in each study resulting in different maternal concentrations which, in turn, affects the glyburide concentration ratio between the mother and fetus.

Does metformin cross the placenta?

Vanky, et al. [15] demonstrated that metformin passes freely across the placenta and fetal serum levels are comparable with maternal values in polycystic ovary (PCO) patients. Tertti, et al. [16] examined in vivo placental transfer of metformin in 217 GDM patients randomized to metformin or insulin. Metformin concentration was determined in maternal serum at 36 weeks gestational age and at delivery. Umbilical cord blood was also obtained at birth. The median umbilical cord/maternal serum metformin concentration ratio was 0.73. Since metformin is a polar positively charged compound, an effort was made to characterize its permeability across the human placenta using the ex vivo placental perfusion model. It was found that metformin permeability across the placenta is mediated by a carrier that transports cationic compounds bi-directionally, with a higher transfer rate from the fetal to the maternal side [17, 18].

And what about Insulin?

Despite existing dogma that insulin does not cross the placenta, already in the early 80s, it was demonstrated that beef-pork-insulin (antibody) crosses the placenta probably by changing the formation (size) of the antibody insulin complex [19]. More than two decades later, Lindsay et al. [20] reported that insulin antibodies were detected in the cord blood of 95 % of offspring at birth. McCance et al. [21] evaluated the presence of insulin antibodies and their effect on placental transfer with insulin aspart and human insulin. They concluded that insulin antibodies do not develop during pregnancy with the use of aspart in type 1 diabetes and that 1-5 % of human insulin concentration was transferred to the fetal circulation. Boskovic et al. [22] found that no placental transfer could be detected during the perfusion of insulin lispro with 100 and 200 micro U/ml. In contrast, concentration-dependent transfer to the fetus was shown at 580 micro U/ml and higher. Maternal serum level of ≥ 580 U/ml is equal to approximately 75 units of insulin. The authors concluded that insulin lispro is unlikely to cross the placenta at a single standard dose and is also unlikely to reach or harm the unborn baby. Their conclusion was based on the assumption that type 2 and GDM women will probably not receive this amount of insulin. However, this is an erroneous conclusion. GDM and type 2 patients are often overweight and obese, many morbidly obese, characterized by insulin resistance and, therefore, require much larger insulin doses (1–2 units/kg).

In a study of long-acting insulin analogs, the authors suggested that glargine probably does not cross the placenta [23]. Pollex et al. [24] added insulin glargine to the maternal compartment. Experiments were carried out at therapeutic levels 150, 225, and 300 mmol/l. Concentrations of 150pmol/l showed no detectable insulin levels in the fetal compartment. However, after perfusion with concentrations of 150, 225 and 300 nmol/l, the rate of transfer remained low. Thus, transfer begins when the glargine dose is >0.3 unit/kg. The authors concluded that insulin glargine, when used at the therapeutic concentrations, is not likely to cross the placenta. Again, these are flawed conclusions. They are based on the assumption that their designated therapeutic level is universal; it is not. We must all acknowledge that therapeutic levels will be different in different centers related to policy, rate of patients that achieve targeted glycemic goals, obesity, etc.

The view that the placenta is an absolute barrier to drugs is completely inaccurate. The fetus is to some extent exposed to all drugs taken by the mother. There is, however, sufficient evidence to suggest that the placenta is capable of limiting fetal exposure to the drug especially in the case of glyburide. What is important for all drugs, be it oral to insulin, is not which cross the placenta and to which extent, but rather which ones may adversely affect the fetus. To date, thousands of patients have been treated with glyburide, metformin and insulin during pregnancy with no teratogenic effects on the fetus. Patients should not be denied the better treatment option and benefits provided by these drugs; at the same time, future investigations should continue to determine their safety just as they would for any other drug in pregnancy.

What is the quality of the evidence and data source validity?

Validity is one of the main concerns in research because it applies to both design and methodology. Most errors of validity can be traced to problems with data collection. Therefore, the basic question remains, does the research really measure what it claims to be measuring? Grimes, et al. addressed this major concern in 2 thought-provoking articles [25, 26].

Sources of data abstracted from administrative databases or birth certificates have become expedient and trendy for the potential researcher. However, they are not epidemiologic research data. They are solely the bureaucratic foundation for claims made for services by health care providers and institutions. They are, in fact, billing systems. Actual documentation of events is often related to the probability of reimbursement. These databases were never intended as sources for epidemiologic research because they contain only basic demographic and medical information. They have considerable limitations that must be taken into consideration and should be used solely to abstract information for which they were intended, i.e., billing [8].

For example, an administrative database will rarely, if at all, specify a particular drug (glyburide, metformin, acarbose, etc.) to which the patient was prescribed or exposed but rather will indicate that the patient was prescribed, "an oral agent." It has been shown that only 59 % of diagnoses in administrative databases were confirmed by actual chart review [27].

Two examples of studies whose data were abstracted from administrative databases demonstrated some of the above limitations. In the study by Castillo, et al. [11], the authors could not ascertain the severity of GDM because of missing data from glucose tolerance tests. The omission of race/ethnicity as well as gestational age in the database precluded the possibility to determine large or small for gestational age infants as potential confounders. They were also limited to the ascertainment of obesity through the use of the International Classification of Diseases (Ninth revision clinical modification) [ICD-9-CM] diagnosis code and could not, therefore, rule out the possibility of the effect of obesity on choice of treatment. In addition, there was failure to provide information on drug dosage. It has become the standard of care that achieving targeted levels of glycemic control is paramount for treatment of GDM women. But, no glucose data during pregnancy was available. A priori, an inability to evaluate the impact of the level of glycemic control during pregnancy should disqualify any study addressing outcome of diabetes in pregnancy Table 1.

Cheng's, et al. study [12] further exposed the limitations of the administrative database. The authors conducted a retrospective cohort study of women diagnosed with GDM who required pharmaceutical therapy. They were enrolled in the Sweet Success California Diabetes and Pregnancy Program between 2001 and 2004, a California state-wide program. Although they sought to compare insulin and glyburide treated women, the database did not include a variable for a glyburide recipient. Rather, the variable was indicated as "oral agent." Thus, the authors speculated that all oral agents prescribed were glyburide. The second major limitation of the study was the lack of glucose data throughout pregnancy. Information on neonatal metabolic, respiratory, previous macrosomia or birth trauma data was also not reported Table 1.

The use of administrative databases results in very large sample sizes which, in turn, can lead to spurious statistical associations ("mass significance"). Although the sample size can demonstrate statistical significance, the results may not always be clinically significant. A large sample size, containing confounders, can be challenging when there are weak associations. Risk levels of 1 and 2 should be considered questionable because they may represent potential bias. They are more of a commotion than a signal to consider clinical changes. In general, unless relative risk (RR) in cohort studies exceed 2 to 3 or odds ratios (OR) in case–control studies exceed 3 or 4, associations in observational research findings should not be considered credible. [25, 26, 28] Table 1.

Which treatment modalities are most effective in reducing primary outcome in GDM?

It has been generally acknowledged that abnormal levels of glycemia result in adverse pregnancy outcome in GDM. Therefore, the achievement of targeted levels of

Table 1 Comparison of Administrative Database Studies

	Castillo et al. [11]			Cheng et al. [12]		
	Glyburide	Insulin	R.R 95 % C.I.	Glyburide	Insulin	O.R. 95 % C.I.
	N = 4982	N = 4191		N = 2073	N = 8604	
LGA	4.7 %	3.2 %	1.43 (1.16-1.76)	17.6 %	19.0 %	1.03 (0.83-1.20)
Macrosomia	n.a.	n.a.	—	13.4 %	13.1 %	1.29 (1.03-1.64)
Hypoglycemia	1.9 %	1.3 %	1.40 (1.00-1.95)	n.a.	n.a.	—
Jaundice	0.3 %	0.4 %	0.96 (0.48-1.91)	n.a.	n.a.	—
Neonatal RDS	2.9 %	1.7 %	1.63 (1.23-2.15)	n.a.	n.a.	—
Preterm	9.5 %	8.9 %	1.06 (0.93-1.00)	n.a.	n.a.	—
NICU admission	10.2 %	7.2 %	1.41 (1.23-1.62)	8.1 %	6.5 %	1.32 (1.07-2.00)
Birth injury	2.2 %	1.6 %	1.35 (1.00-1.82	n.a.	n.a	—
Cesarean delivery	50.6 %	52.5 %	0.97 (0.93-1.00)	38.8 %	44.9 %	0.77 (0.65-0.91)

n.a. = not available, LGA = large for gestational age, NICU = neonatal intensive care unit glycemic control is the cornerstone of treatment [1, 29]. Moreover, the majority of studies evaluating the efficacy of glyburide in comparison to insulin used success of achieving glycemic control as the primary outcome variable. Table 2 Appropriately designed randomized controlled trials, or prospective and retrospective studies, with the correct sample size and clear definitions of well and poor glycemic control will maximize production of accurate data [28].

As a rule of thumb, the ability of studies to duplicate a finding is the gold standard of science. Reproducibility of a study is often a rare occurrence. However, regardless of the research design, the majority of studies have consistently demonstrated that insulin and oral agent treated patients (glyburide and/or metformin) achieved the desired level of glycemic control Table 2.

What we don't yet definitely know is whether metformin or glyburide is the more effective oral hypoglycemic agent. Silva et al., [30, 31] in 2 randomized clinical trials (RCTs) comparing metformin to glyburide, concluded that the achieved levels of glycemia were comparable for both drugs. In addition, there was no difference in perinatal results: cesarean section (C/S), large for gestational age (LGA), neonatal hypoglycemia, or rate of neonatal intensive care unit (NICU) admission [31].

In contrast, Moore et al. [32] in a randomized study showed that the failure rate to achieve the glycemic target was 34.7 % for metformin and 16.2 % for glyburide. In a recent randomized clinical trial (RCT) study, Zohar et al., [33] found that metformin vs. glyburide failed to achieve targeted glycemic levels 29 % vs. 22 %, $p = 0.41$, respectively. The obstetrical and neonatal outcomes were comparable including anthropometric measures, cord blood insulin and C-peptide. In addition a meta-analysis demonstrated that both metformin and glyburide are as effective as insulin in the management of GDM [34]. The above studies demonstrated comparable success rates and in one a higher failure rate with metformin. However, it is remarkable to note that a meta-analysis [35] reported in favor of metformin for maternal weight gain (mean difference −2.06 kg (−3.98 to −0.14), birth weight (mean difference −209 g (−314 to −104), macrosomia (risk ratio 0.33 (0.13 to 0.81), and large for gestational age newborns (risk ratio 0.44 (0.21 to 0.92), even when treatment failure was higher with metformin. If studies cited are at best inconclusive, meta-analysis simply magnifies the impact of poor quality data.

Disease severity is another factor that influences the success rate in the achievement of targeted glucose levels. The greater the disease severity as reflected by the fasting plasma glucose, success rates to achieve adequate levels of glucose decrease. However, the rates of success remain comparable for glyburide and insulin treated patients at all severity levels [36]. The question remains, how successful are those who failed to achieve glycemic control with either glyburide or metformin after transfer to insulin. The rate of success for achieving glycemic control in metformin treated patients ranged from 54-79 %. The success

Table 2 Achievement of Glycemic Control by Study Design and Treatment Modality

	Design	Patient No. Oral/Insulin	Oral type	Well control Oral / Insulin	Comparison of control
Langer'00 [3]	RCT	201 / 203	glyburide	82 % vs. 88 %	similar
Lain'09 [50]	RCT	41 / 41	glyburide	91 % vs. 97 %	similar
Bertini'05 [51]	RCT	24 / 27	glyburide	79 %	similar
Ogunyemi'07 [52]	RCT	48 / 49	glyburide	93 %	similar
Tempe'13 [53]	RCT	32 / 32	glyburide	91 % vs. 94 %	similar
Silva'07 [54]	RCT	36 / 36	glyburide	—	similar
Rowen'09 [4]	RCT	363 / 370	metformin	54 %	for Metformin
Moore'07 [32]	RCT	31 / 32	metformin	MBG	similar
Spaulonci,'13 [55]	RCT	47 / 47	metformin	74 %	similar
Tertti'13 [16]	RCT	110 / 107	metformin	79 %	similar
Niromanesh'12 [56]	RCT	80 / 80	metformin	86 %	similar
Ijas'11 [57]	RCT	50 / 50	metformin	68 %	similar
Ramos'07 [43]	Retrospective	122	glyburide	84 %	for glyburide
Jacobson'05 [58]	Retrospective	236 /268	glyburide	86 % vs. 63 %	dissimilar
Conway'04 [37]	Retrospective	75	glyburide	84 %	similar
Yogev'10 [38]	Retrospective	124	glyburide	75 %	similar
Rochon'06 [39]	Retrospective	101	glyburide	81 %	similar
Kahn'06 [40]	Retrospective	95	glyburide	81 %	similar

rate after transfer to insulin was not reported [37–40]. To date, there is no reported data for success of metformin patients transferred to insulin.

The success rate for achieving glycemic control with glyburide ranged from 75-84 %. Transfer failure from glyburide to insulin ranged from 54-67 %. In a logistic regression evaluating predictors of glyburide failure, the main predictor was glyburide dose (O.R. 3.73 95 %, C.I. 2.15-6.48). In addition, there was a weak association (potential bias) for disease severity (O.R. 1.58) and no association to body mass index (BMI), previous GDM, and ethnicity.

Given the approximate doubling in glyburide clearance during pregnancy, should we increase the starting and maximal dose during pregnancy? [9] From the scientific perspective, it is important to understand the pharmacokinetic and pharmacodynamic considerations. However, in the clinical, real world environment, drug management decisions need to be determined based on patient's diet, weight and ethnicity. In our study, 31 % of GDM subjects achieved targeted levels of glycemic control with a 2.5 mg dose. Twenty-seven percent required 5 mg; 21 % - 10 mg; 9 % - 15 mg; and, only 12 % required the maximal dose of 20 mg [36]. Thus, approximately 2/3 s of the patients achieved targeted levels of glycemic control with less than 50 % of the maximal dose. The amount and frequency of drug administration will both determine the optimal therapeutic effect. The lower limit for glycemic benefits of glyburide are nearly fully realized at half-maximal dose and higher doses should generally be avoided. The upper limit of the range is such that no more than 5-10 % of subjects will experience a toxic effect is a major consideration [41]. In light of this clinical data, it is possible that combination therapy with a lower dose of each medication should be considered in order to successfully maximize glucose control. The goal is to provide drug efficacy without unacceptable toxicity.

Which drug is most effective in improving secondary outcomes?

A well planned and executed RCT is the gold standard in study design. However, the outcome results that are measured in a single specific trial cannot be regarded as absolute proof. Ioannidis concluded, "Controversies are most common with highly cited nonrandomized studies, but even the most highly cited randomized trials may be challenged and refuted over time, especially small ones" [28].

Different study designs that address the same research question will yield varying results. There is risk of presenting uncertain results for both nonrandomized and randomized controlled trials when there is questionable knowledge if the direction and magnitude of the effect holds true [42]. The majority of maternal and neonatal complications are the result of maternal hyperglycemia that in turn causes fetal hyperinsulinemia. In our RCT we showed that neonatal cord insulin (μU) was similar in glyburide and insulin treated patients (14 ± 4 vs. 15 ± 2.3 respectively) [3]. Ramos et al., in a retrospective study compared glyburide vs. insulin treated GDMs. Neonatal hypoglycemia was defined as <45 mg/dl within 1 h of birth. There was no difference between glyburide and insulin, 23 % vs. 27 %, p = 0.58 [43]. Finally, 2 meta-analyses concluded that neonatal hypoglycemia is not associated with glyburide therapy [44, 45].

How does glyburide affect the mother?

Yogev et al., [46] using continuous glucose monitoring (CGM) found asymptomatic hypoglycemic episodes in 63 % of insulin and 28 % of glyburide treated subjects. Brustman et al. [47] with a large sample size studied the effect of glyburide therapy on the number of episodes of maternal hypoglycemia in patients using self monitoring blood glucose (mean of 310 ± 190 samples/patient). When hypoglycemia was defined between 40–50 mg/dL, 65 % of subjects had no episodes. When the maternal hypoglycemia definition was <40, over 90 % had no episodes of hypoglycemia. Overall, only 2–3 episodes were found in a minority of patients (~2-4 %).

Several outcome variables are used as secondary outcome measures in the majority, if not all studies, addressing diabetes in pregnancy. These variables are associated with maternal hyperglycemia which in turn causes fetal hyperinsulinemia. Fetal hyperinsulinemia has been shown to be associated with metabolic complications (hyperbilirubinemia, hypoglycemia, respiratory complications, and polycythemia) and the resultant macrosomia/LGA and shoulder dystocia. However, it should be noted that these complications are mainly the result of abnormal glucose levels. In addition, different secondary outcome variables have different weighted importance since some are transitory while others have long term impact on the neonate.

The secondary outcomes in the largest randomized and retrospective studies are compared in Table 3. Within each of the three studies, no significant difference was found in any of the secondary outcome variables. In contrast, the rate of several outcome variables among the three studies was significantly different, (e.g. LGA, macrosomia) probably due to failure to achieve targeted levels of glycemic control. Again, this comparison reemphasizes that the cornerstone for the successful treatment of GDM is the control of the level of glycemia and not the pharmacological treatment modality.

Systematic reviews and meta-analyses have become increasingly important in health care. Clinicians read them to keep up to date in their field and they are often used as a starting point for developing clinical practice guidelines.

Table 3 Summary of Secondary Outcome Results

	Rowen et al. [4] Randomized		Langer et al. [3] Randomized		Jacobson et al. [58] Retrospective	
	Metformin n = 363	Insulin n = 370	Glyburide n = 201	Insulin n = 203	Glyburide n = 236	Insulin n = 268
LGA	19.3 %	18.6 %	12.0 %	13.0 %	25.0 %	24.0 %
Ponderal Index >2.85	—	—	9.0 %	12.0 %	—	—
Macrosomia	22.9 %	21.4 %	7.2 %	4.7 %	25.0 %	24.0 %
Hypoglycemia	15.2 %	18.6 %	9.0 %	6.0 %	31.0 %	27.0 %
Hyperbilirubinemia	8.0 %	8.4 %	6.0 %	4.0 %	25.0 %	22.0 %
Phototherapy	—	—	—	—	9.0 %	5.0 %
Polycythemia	—	—	2.0 %	3.0 %	—	—
RDS	3.3 %	4.3 %	2.0 %	3.0 %	—	—
5 min Apgar	0.8 %	0.3 %	3.1 %	4.2 %	—	—
NICU admission	12.7 %	12.2 %	6.0 %	7.0 %	15.0 %	24.0 %
Shoulder dystocia	—	—	1.5 %	1.6 %	—	—
Preeclampsia	8.3 %	6.8 %	6.0 %	6.0 %	12.0 %	6.0 %
Chronic hypertension	8.5 %	7.3 %	6.0 %	9.1 %	—	—
Cesarean delivery	22.9 %	21.4 %	23.0 %	24.0 %	39.0 %	35.0 %

Granting agencies may require a systematic review to ensure there is justification for further research. As with all research, the value of a systematic review depends on what was done, what was found, and the clarity of the reported results [48].

Meta-analysis [25, 26, 42] was originally designed for low prevalence conditions to produce hypotheses for future studies. Moreover, including observational studies, in addition to randomized trials, is at best controversial [44, 45]. Several meta-analyses of randomized controlled trials addressing oral agents have been published. However, verification of the methodology and the statistical analysis used in each study are not feasible because the raw data are not available. However, the chance for error(s) is much less in a single study than in a systematic review or meta-analysis. Different designs addressing the same question often yield differences in the results.

For example, in the meta-analysis comparing glyburide to insulin, the largest study contained 404 subjects [3] while each of the other seven studies had fewer than 100 participants for a total of 384 patients Tables 2 and 4. Most of the individual studies were not statistically powered to examine the less common neonatal complications that can be associated with hyperglycemia, such as macrosomia or hypoglycemia. This is of even greater significance when not all seven studies were included in the analysis for each complication. Jiang et al. [34] used 2 studies for the evaluation of cesarean section, and 5 for macrosomia. Zeng et al. [49] reevaluated the rate of neonatal hypoglycemia when only 3 RCTs were included. Euclid, the father of geometry, taught us that the whole is equal to the sum of its parts. However, in meta-analysis, not all parts are equal and very often they are not necessarily included in the whole. A meta-analysis can be no better than its component parts.

Table 4 compares 6 meta-analyses with their component studies. The similarities between the studies suggest that there will be comparable results from each meta-analysis. Table 5 compares the outcome in each meta-analysis demonstrating similarity on the one hand and differences on the other. The combination of dissimilar studies can devalue the relevance of any meta-analysis.

Outcome definitions and vigorous ascertainment of results were not always provided in the studies. In some outcomes such as preterm birth, caesarean section, birth weight, and Apgar score, there is agreed consensus on definitions. In contrast, in those variables where definitions and detection protocols are less universal, greater differences, i.e., neonatal hypoglycemia, respiratory distress, jaundice, and admission to the neonatal intensive care unit, will result in varying rates in each individual study. For neonatal hypoglycemia, different definitions have been used in the studies with criteria ranging from 45 to less than 25 mg/dl and using from 1–9 blood determinations. In addition, in some studies, administration of I.V. glucose to neonates will classify them as hypoglycemic regardless of the actual blood glucose reading [Tables 4 and 5].

Table 4 Individual Studies Included in the Various Meta-Analyses

	Dhulkotia [45]	Poolsup [59]	Balsells [35]	Zeng [49]	Jiang [34]	Gui [60]
Metformin studies						
Moore [32]	+	+	+	—	+	+
Rowan [4]	+	+	+	—	+	+
Niromanesh [56]	—	+	+	—	+	+
Ijas [57]	—	+	+	—	+	+
Spaulonci [55]	—	+	+	—	+	—
Tertti [16]	—	+	+	—	+	+
Silva [31]	—	—	—	—	—	—
Hassan [61]	—	—	—	—	+	—
Hague [62]	—	—	—	—	+	—
Therapy efficacy	n.a.	similar	similar	n.a.	similar	similar
Glyburide studies						
Silva [54]	+	+	+	+	+	—
Tempe [53]	—	+	+	+	+	—
Bertini [51]	—	—	—	+	+	—
Ogunyemi [52]	+	+	—	+	+	—
Langer [3]	+	+	+	+	+	—
Lain [50]	—	—	+	+	+	—
Mukhopad-hyay [63]	—	+	+	+	—	—
Therapy efficacy	similar	dissimilar	dissimilar	similar	suitable	n.a.

Summary

The introduction of glyburide and metformin in the treatment of gestational diabetes has profoundly altered the management approach with comparable outcomes to insulin therapy. These therapies are cost-effective, patient-friendly, and potentially compliance-enhancing. Therefore, there may be greater risk to the fetus in withholding these medications than in prescribing them.

The outcome of a clinical debate depends on the adequacy of the respective accounts of existing data. Some types of counter explanations to a concept lack consistency and predictability very often because of faults in validity, i.e. the methodology did not measure what should have been measured. Nevertheless, despite occasional vague explanations, science is better off being tolerant of second-guessers. Science should have both a conservative bias – which prevents rapid and bewildering

Table 5 Results of 6 Meta-Analyses Comparing Glyburide to Insulin Therapy

	Dhulkotia 2010 [45]	Poolsup 2014 [59]	Balsells 2015 [35]	Zeng 2014 [49]	Jiang 2015 [34]	Moretti 2008 [44]
Therapy efficacy Glyburide vs. Insulin	similar	dissimilar	dissimilar	similar	suitable	similar
Macrosomia	similar	Increase O.R. 2.34	Increase R.R. 2.62	Increase R.R. 2.22	Increase O.R 3,09	similar
LGA	similar	similar	similar	similar	n.a.	similar
Neonatal hypoglycemia	similar	Increase O.R. 2.06	Increase R.R.2.04	Increase O.R. 1.98	Increase R.R. 2.64	similar
Neonatal hyperbilirubinemia.	n.a.	similar	similar	n.a.	n.a.	n.a
Preterm	n.a.	similar	similar	similar	similar	n.a.
NICU admission	n.a.	similar	similar	similar	similar	similar
Preeclampsia	n.a.	similar	similar	—	similar	n.a.
Cesarean delivery	similar	similar	similar	similar	similar	n.a.

n.a. = not available
In Moretti and Dhulkotia, the meta-analyses included observational and RCT studies in addition to insulin and metformin studies

shifts of views – and eventually openness, such that persistent innovators can ultimately triumph if their claims actually merit consideration. In the words of T.S. Elliot, "Where is the wisdom we have lost in knowledge? Where is the knowledge we have lost in information?"

Competing interests

The author declares that he has no competing interests.

References

1. Position statement of the American Diabetes Association (ADA) and the European Association for the Study of Diabetes (EASD). Diabetes Care 2012,35:1364–1379.
2. Langer O. The diabetes in pregnancy dilemma: leading change with proven solutions. 2nd ed. Shelton, CT: People's Medical Publishing House; 2015.
3. Langer O, Conway DL, Berkus MD, Xenakis EM-J, Gonzales O. A comparison of glyburide and insulin in women with gestational diabetes mellitus. N Engl J Med. 2000;343:1134–8.
4. Rowan JA, Hague WM, Gao W, Battin MR, Moore MP, MiG Trial Investigators. Metformin versus insulin for the treatment of gestational diabetes. N Engl J Med. 2008;358:2003–15.
5. Committee on Practice Bulletins–Obstetrics. Practice bulletin No. 137. Gestational diabetes mellitus. Obstet Gynecol. 2013;122:406–16.
6. National Collaborating Centre for Women's and Children's Health. Diabetes in pregnancy: Management of diabetes and its complications from preconception to the postnatal period. London: RCOG Press; 2008.
7. Berger H, Feig D, Gagnon R, Kader T, Keely E, Kozak S, et al. Can J Diabetes. 2013;37:S168–83.
8. Castillo CW, Boggess K, Stürmer T, Brookhart MA, Benjamin Jr DK, Jonsson Funk M. Trends in glyburide compared with insulin use for gestational diabetes treatment in the United States, 2000–2011. Obstet Gynecol. 2014;123(6):1177–84.
9. Hebert MF, Ma X, Naraharisetti SB, Krudys KM, Umans JG, Hankins GDV, et al. Are we optimizing gestational diabetes treatment with glyburide? The pharmacologic basis for better clinical practice. Clin Pharmacol Ther. 2009;85(6):607–14.
10. Schwartz RA, Rosenn B, Aleksa K, Koren G. Glyburide transport across the human placenta. Obstet Gynecol. 2015;125(3):583–8.
11. Castillo CW, Boggess K, Stürmer T, Brookhart MA, Benjamin DK Jr, Jonsson Funk M: Association of adverse pregnancy outcomes with glyburide vs. insulin in women with gestational diabetes. [published online March 30, 2015]. JAMA Pediatr. doi:10.1001/jamapediatrics.2015.74.
12. Cheng YW, Chung JH, Block-Kurbisch I, Inturrisi M, Caughey AB. Treatment of gestational diabetes mellitus: glyburide compared to subcutaneous insulin therapy and associated perinatal outcomes. J Matern Fetal Neonatal Med. 2012;25(4):379–84.
13. Elliott BD, Langer O, Schenker S, Johnson RF. Insignificant transfer of glyburide occurs across the human placenta. Am J Obstet Gynecol. 1991;165:807–12.
14. Elliott BD, Schenker S, Langer O, Johnson R, Prihoda T. Comparative placental transport of oral hypoglycemic agents in humans: a model of human placental drug transfer. Am J Obstet Gynecol. 1994;171:653–60.
15. Vanky E, Zahisen K, Spigset O, Carlsen SM. Placental passage of metformin in women with polycystic ovary syndrome. Fertil Steril. 2005;83(5):1575–8.
16. Tertti K, Laine K, Ekblad U, Rinne V, Ronnemaa T. The degree of fetal metformin exposure does not influence fetal outcome in gestational diabetes mellitus. Acta Diabet. 2014;51(5):731–8.
17. Kovo M, Kogman N, Ovadia O, Nakash I, Golan A, Hoffman A. Carrier-mediated transport of metformin across the human placenta determined by using the ex vivo perfusion of the placental cotyledon model. Prenat Diagn. 2008;28(6):544–8. doi:10.1002/pd.2026.
18. Nanovskaya TN, Nekhayeva IA, Patrikeeva SL, Hankins GD, Ahmed MS. Transfer of metformin across the dually perfused human placental lobule. Am J Obstet Gynecol. 2006;195(4):1081–5. Epub 2006 Jul 5.
19. Bauman W, Yalow R. Transplacental passage of insulin complexed to antibody. Proc Natl Acad Sci. 1981;78(7):4588–90.
20. Lindsay RS, Ziegler AG, Hamilton BA, Calder AA, Johnstone FD, Walker JD, et al. Type 1 diabetes-related antibodies in the fetal circulation: prevalence and influence on cord inulin and birth weight in offspring of mothers with type 1 diabetes. J Clin Endocrinol Metab. 2004;89:3436–9.
21. McCance DR, Damm P, Mathiesen ER, Hod M, Kaaja R, Dunne F, et al. Evaluation of insulin antibodies and placental transfer of insulin aspart in pregnant women with type 1 diabetes mellitus. Diabetologia. 2008;51(11):2141–3. doi:10.1007/s00125-008-1120-y. Epub 2008 Aug 23.
22. Boskovic R, Feig D, Derewlany L, Knie B, Portnoi G, Koren G. Transfer of insulin lispro across the human placenta: in vitro perfusion studies. Diabetes Care. 2003;26:1390–4.
23. Kovo M, Wainstein J, Matas Z, Haroutiumiam S, Hoffman A, Golan A. Placental transfer of the insulin analog glargine in the ex vivo perfused placental cotyledon model. Endocr Res. 2011;36(1):19–24.
24. Pollex E, Feig D, Lubetsky A, Yip PM, Koren G. Insulin glargine safety in pregnancy: a transplacental transfer study. Diabetes Care. 2010;33(1):29–33.
25. Grimes DA, Schulz KF. False Alarms and pseudo-epidemics: The limitations of observational epidemiology. Obstet Gynecol. 2012;120(4):920–7.
26. Grimes DA. Epidemiologic research using administrative databases. Obstet Gynecol. 2010;116(5):1018–19.
27. Severinsen MT, Kristensen SR, Overvad K, Dethlefsen C, Tjønneland A, Johnsen SP. Venous thromboembolism discharge diagnoses in the Danish National Patient Registry should be used with caution. J Clin Epidemiol. 2010;63(2):223–8. doi:10.1016/j.jclinepi.2009.03.018.
28. Ioannidis JP. Contradicted and initially stronger effects in highly cited clinical research. JAMA. 2005;294:218–28.
29. Langer O. Glycemic targets for the optimal treatment of GDM. Clin Obstet Gynecol. 2013;56(4):788–802. doi:10.1097/GRF.0b013e3182a8e07d.
30. Silva JC, Pacheco C, Bizato J, deSouza BV, Ribeiro TE, Bertini AM. Metformin compared with glyburide for the management of gestational diabetes. Int J Gynaecol Obstet. 2010;111:37–40.
31. Silva JC, Fachin DR, Coral ML, Bertini AM. Perinatal impact of the use of metformin and glyburide for the treatment of gestational diabetes mellitus. J Perinat Med. 2012;40(3):225–8.
32. Moore LE, Clokey D, Rappaport VJ, Curet LB. Metformin compared with glyburide in gestational diabetes: a randomized controlled trial. Obstet Gynecol. 2010;115(1):55–9.
33. Zohar N, Zafran N, Salim R, Hissin N, Hasanein J, Letova Y, et al. A comparison between two oral hypoglycemic: glyburide and metformin and their combination for the treatment of gestational diabetes mellitus – a prospective randomized controlled study. Am J Obst & Gynecol Supplement. 2015;212:S23.
34. Yun-fa Jiang, Xue-yan Chen, Tao Ding, Xiao-feng Wang, Zhong-ning Zhu, Su-wen Su: Comparative efficacy and safety of oral antidiabetic drugs in management of gestational diabetes: network meta-analysis of randomized controlled trials. J Clin Endocrinol Metab 2015:1–11; doi:10.1210/jc.2014-4403.
35. Balsells M, García-Patterson A, Solà I, Roqué M, Gich I, Corcoy R. Glibenclamide, metformin, and insulin for the treatment of gestational diabetes: a systematic review and meta-analysis. BMJ. 2015;350:h102. doi:10.1136/bmj.h102.
36. Langer O, Yogev Y, Xenakis EM, Rosenn B. Insulin and glyburide therapy: dosage, severity level of gestational diabetes, and pregnancy outcome. Am J Obstet Gynecol. 2005;192(1):134–9.
37. Conway DL, Gonzales O, Skiver D. Use of glyburide for the treatment of gestational diabetes: the San Antonio experience. J Matern Fetal Neonatal Med. 2004;15(1):51–5. PMID: 15101612.
38. Yogev Y, Melamed N, Chen R, Nassie D, Pardo J, Hod M. Glyburide in gestational diabetes–prediction of treatment failure. J Matern Fetal Neonatal Med. 2011;24(6):842–6. doi:10.3109/14767058.2010.531323. Epub 2010 Nov 10.
39. Rochon M, Rand L, Roth L, Gaddipati S. Glyburide for the management of gestational diabetes: Risk factors predictive of failure and associated pregnancy outcomes. Obstet Gynecol. 2006;195:1090–4.
40. Khan BF, Davies JK, Lynch AM, Reynolds RM, Barbour LA. Predictors of glyburide in the treatment of gestational diabetes. Obstet Gynecol. 2006;107(6):1303–9.
41. Iain L, Buxton O, Benet LZ. Pharmokinetics: The dynamics of drug absorption, distribution, metabolism, and elimination. In: Brunton LL, Chabner B, Knollman B, editors. Goodman and Gilman, The pharmacological basis of therapeutics. Twelfthth ed. New York: McGraw-Hill; 2010. p. 17–40.
42. Peinemann F, Tushabe DA, Kleijnen J. Using Multiple Types of Studies in Systematic Reviews of Health Care Interventions – A Systematic Review. PLoS One. 2013;8(12):e85035. doi:10.1371/journal.pone.0085035.

43. Ramos GA, Jacobson GF, Kirby RS, Ching JY, Ferrara A, Field DR. Comparison of glyburide and insulin for the management of gestational diabetics with markedly elevated oral glucose challenge test and fasting hyperglycemia. J Perinatol. 2007;27(5):262–7. Epub 2007 Mar 15.
44. Moretti ME, Rezvani M, Koren G. Safety of glyburide for gestational diabetes: a meta-analysis of pregnancy outcomes. Ann Pharmacother. 2008;42:483–90.
45. Dhulkotia JS, Ola B, Fraser R, Farrell T. Oral hypoglycemic agents vs insulin in management of gestational diabetes: a systematic review and meta-analysis. Am J Obstet Gynecol. 2010;203(5):457.e1–9. doi:10.1016/j.ajog.2010.06.044. Epub 2010 Aug 24.
46. Yogev Y, Ben-Haroush A, Chen R, Rosenn B, Hod M, Langer O. Undiagnosed asymptomatic hypoglycemia: diet, insulin, and glyburide for gestational diabetic pregnancy. Obstet Gynecol. 2004;104(1):88–93.
47. Brustman L, Langer O, Scarpelli S, El Daouk M, Fuchs A, Rosenn B. Hypoglycemia in glyburide-treated gestational diabetes: is it dose-dependent? Obstet Gynecol. 2011;117(2 Pt 1):349–53. doi:10.1097/AOG.0b013e318207782a.
48. Moher D, Liberati A, Tetzlaff J, Altman DG, the PRISMA Group Preferred Reporting Items for Systematic Reviews and Meta-Analyses. The PRISMA Statement. Ann Intern Med. 2009;151:264–9.
49. Zeng YC, Li MJ, Chen Y, Jiang L, Wang SM, Mo XL, et al. The use of glyburide in the management of gestational diabetes mellitus: a meta-analysis. Adv Med Sci. 2014;59(1):95–101. doi:10.1016/j.advms.2014.03.001. Epub 2014 Mar 22.
50. Lain KY, Garabedian MJ, Daftary A, Jeyabalan A. Neonatal adiposity following maternal treatment of gestational diabetes with glyburide compared with insulin. Am J Obstet Gynecol. 2009;200:501. e501-506.
51. Bertini AM, Silva JC, Taborda W, Becker F, Lemos Bebber FR, Zucco Viesi JM, et al. Perinatal outcomes and the use of oral hypoglycemic agents. J Perinat Med. 2005;33(6):519–23.
52. Ogunyemi D, Jesse M, Davidson M. Comparison of glyburide versus insulin in management of gestational diabetes mellitus. Endocr Pract. 2007;13:427–8.
53. Tempe A, Mayanglambam RD. Glyburide as treatment option for gestational diabetes mellitus. J Obstet Gynaecol Res. 2013;39(6):1147–52.
54. Silva JC, Bertini AM, Taborda W, Becker F, Bebber FR, Aquim GM, et al. Glibenclamide in the treatment for gestational diabetes mellitus in a compared study to insulin. Arq Bras Endocrinol Metab. 2007;51:541–6.
55. Spaulonci CP, Bernardes LS, Trindade TC, Zugaib M, Francisco RP. Randomized trial of metformin vs insulin in the management of gestational diabetes. Am J Obstet Gynecol. 2013;209(1):34.e1–7. doi:10.1016/j.ajog.2013.03.022. Epub 2013 Mar 21.
56. Niromanesh S, Alavi A, Sharbaf FR, Amjadi N, Moosavi S, Akbari S. Metformin compared with insulin in the management of gestational diabetes mellitus: a randomized clinical trial. Diabetes Res Clin Pract. 2012;98(3):422–9. doi:10.1016/j.diabres.2012.09.031. Epub 2012 Oct 12.
57. Ijas H, Vaarasmaki M, Morin-Papunen L, Keravuo R, Ebeling T, Saarela T, et al. Metformin should be considered in the treatment of gestational diabetes: a prospective randomized study. BJOG. 2011;118:880–5.
58. Jacobson GF, Ramos GA, Ching JY, Kirby RS, Ferrara A, Field DR. Comparison of glyburide and insulin for the management of gestational diabetes in a large managed care organization. Am J Obstet Gynecol. 2005;193(1):118–24.
59. Poolsup N, Suksomboon N, Amin M. Efficacy and safety of oral antidiabetic drugs in comparison to insulin in treating gestational diabetes mellitus: a meta-analysis. PLoS One. 2014;9(10):e109985. doi:10.1371/journal.pone.0109985. PMID: 25302493.
60. Gui J, Liu Q, Feng L. Metformin vs insulin in the management of gestational diabetes: a meta-analysis. PLoS One. 2013;8(5):e64585. doi:10.1371/journal.pone.0064585.
61. Hassan JA, Karim N, Sheikh Z. Metformin prevents macrosomia and neonatal morbidity in gestational diabetes. Pak J Med Sci. 2012;28:384–9.
62. Hague WM, Davoren PM, Oliver J, Rowan J. Contraindications to use of metformin. Metformin may be useful in gestational diabetes. BMJ. 2003;326(7392):762.
63. Mukhopadhyay P, Bag TS, Kyal A, Saha DP, Khalid N. Oral hypoglycemic glibenclamide: can it be a substitute to insulin in the management of gestational diabetes mellitus? A comparative study. J SAFOG. 2012;4:28–31.

7

A retrospective review of the Pediatric Development Clinic implementation: a model to improve medical, nutritional and developmental outcomes of at-risk under-five children in rural Rwanda

Eric Ngabireyimana[1†], Christine Mutaganzwa[2,7*†], Catherine M. Kirk[2], Ann C. Miller[5], Kim Wilson[4,5], Evodia Dushimimana[6], Olivier Bigirumwami[1], Evelyne S. Mukakabano[1], Fulgence Nkikabahizi[1] and Hema Magge[2,3,4]

Abstract

Background: As more high-risk newborns survive the neonatal period, they remain at significant medical, nutritional, and developmental risk. However, no follow-up system for early intervention exists in most developing countries. In 2014, a novel Pediatric Development Clinic (PDC) was implemented to provide comprehensive follow-up to at-risk under-five children, led by nurses and social workers in a district hospital and surrounding health centers in rural Rwanda.

Methods: At each PDC visit, children undergo clinical/nutritional assessment and caregivers participate in counseling sessions. Social assessments identify families needing additional social support. Developmental assessment is completed using Ages and Stages Questionnaires. A retrospective medical record review was conducted to evaluate the first 24 months of PDC implementation for patients enrolled between April 2014–December 2015 in rural Rwanda. Demographic and clinical characteristics of patients and their caregivers were described using frequencies and proportions. Completion of different core components of PDC visits were compared overtime using Fisher's Exact test and *p*-values calculated using trend analysis.

Results: 426 patients enrolled at 5 PDC sites. 54% were female, 44% were neonates and 35% were under 6 months at enrollment. Most frequent referral reasons were prematurity/low birth weight (63%) and hypoxic-ischemic encephalopathy (34%). In 24 months, 2787 PDC visits were conducted. Nurses consistently completed anthropometric measurements (age, weight, height) at all visits. Some visit components were inconsistently recorded, including adjusted age ($p = 0.003$), interval growth, danger sign assessment, and feeding difficulties ($p < 0.001$). Completion of other visit components, such as child development counseling and play/stimulation activities, were low but improved with time ($p < 0.001$).

(Continued on next page)

* Correspondence: mutaganzwa@gmail.com
[†]Equal contributors
[2]Department of Pediatrics, Partners In Health/Inshuti Mu Buzima, Rwinkwavu, Rwanda
[7]P.O. Box 3432, Kigali, Rwanda
Full list of author information is available at the end of the article

(Continued from previous page)

Conclusions: It is feasible to implement PDCs with non-specialized providers in rural settings as we were able to enroll a diverse group of high-risk infants. We are seeing an improvement in services offered at PDCs over time and continuous quality improvement efforts are underway to strengthen current gaps. Future studies looking at the outcomes of the children benefiting from the PDC program are underway.

Keywords: High-risk newborns, survival, early childhood development, primary care, sub-Saharan Africa

Background

Global advances have been made over the past decade to improve neonatal care and the burden of neonatal mortality and morbidity in low and middle-income countries [1] with prematurity as the leading cause of death among children under 5 years of age [2]. Ongoing efforts to eliminate preventable neonatal deaths globally must also be accompanied by efforts to ensure children not only survive but also thrive [3]. The first 3 years of life are a critical period of brain development [4]; interventions during this early period can improve growth and development [5] which impact long-term outcomes including educational attainment and productivity later in life [6, 7]. Certain populations of children are at increased risk of developmental delay and growth faltering, such as those born preterm and low birth weight, or with hypoxic-ischemic encephalopathy (HIE), congenital malformations, genetic syndromes, or birth injuries. It is known that these high-risk infants can have a range of challenges such as vision and hearing impairment, speech and motor delays, and poor nutrition, among others [8–11]. In high-income countries, longitudinal follow-up of these children is integrated into routine pediatric care and is typically conducted by specialists [12]. In sub-Saharan Africa, there are very few interventions to support early childhood development and the majority are generalized, community-based programs [13, 14] that do not meet the unique needs of high-risk infants. The use of an intensive home-visiting model has shown promise for improving the development of children with HIE in low and middle income countries [15]. However, to our knowledge there are no early childhood development interventions integrated into routine primary care for at-risk children in low-income countries without access to pediatricians and subspecialists, especially in sub-Saharan Africa.

Rwanda has made tremendous improvements in reducing under-five mortality [16], and expanded access to neonatal care through neonatal units at district hospitals and essential neonatal care at health centers. However, there is no formal follow-up system for children after being discharged from hospital neonatal units, especially in rural areas where there are no specialists; these children remain at increased risk for mortality and morbidities into childhood [17]. "A follow-up of preterm and low birth weight children discharged from Rwinkwavu District Hospital neonatal unit between October 2011 and October 2013 showed rates of chronic and acute malnutrition that were double and triple national prevalence rates, respectively, and that caregivers frequently reported feeding difficulties. Furthermore, two-thirds of the children had an abnormal developmental screening (Kirk, et al., unpublished data)".

In Rwanda, screening for malnutrition in infants and young children is conducted at the community level by community health workers [18] and early childhood development programs have been piloted in selected communities [19, 20]. As in many other sub-Saharan African countries, a barrier to delivering specialized follow-up is the limited availability of pediatricians outside of higher-level referral facilities [21], and other specialists such as developmental pediatricians, neurologists, and physical, speech and occupational therapists. Task-shifting has been used as an approach across low-resource settings to overcome the gap between the availability of specialized providers and service needs [22]. However, this approach has not been explored for pediatric follow-up care among high-risk infants.

Since April 2014 the Ministry of Health, in collaboration with Partners In Health/Inshuti Mu Buzima and UNICEF, has been implementing the Pediatric Development Clinic (PDC) to serve neonates discharged from a rural hospital neonatal unit and other high-risk children under-five in need of follow-up. The PDC provides medical, nutritional and developmentally supportive programs to allow for early identification of complications and intervention to support children to reach their full potential. We hope that this study will provide a pragmatic approach to implementing a feasible clinic model for comprehensive medical, nutritional, developmental support for high-risk infants until age 5 years in resource-limited settings without access to complex care services and medical specialists.

Methods

Study aim and design

This study aims to provide a description of the PDC intervention's first 2 years of implementation using a retrospective electronic medical record review of routinely-collected data. The study population includes all children referred into PDC from April 2014–December 2015. In order to ensure all referred children completed at least one visit following their referral date, we analyzed all of the visits for these children in the first 2 years of clinic implementation (April 2014–March 2016). We hypothesize that as the program matures, over time we will see greater adherence to clinic procedures and increase in documentation of appropriate clinical and developmental assessment and follow-up.

Study intervention

This study was conducted in the Rwinkwavu District Hospital catchment area in Southern Kayonza District in rural Rwanda. Rwinkwavu District Hospital is a public Ministry of Health facility supported by Partners In Health/Inshuti Mu Buzima since 2005. Southern Kayonza serves a population of approximately 188,363 [23] with one district hospital and eight health centers. Rwinkwavu District Hospital has provided neonatal care since 2010 and was among the first district hospitals to initiate specialized neonatal care services [24]. The first PDC was opened in April 2014 at Rwinkwavu District Hospital to provide medical, nutritional and developmental follow-up for high-risk children discharged from the neonatal unit (see Fig. 1). Four months later, in August 2014, PDC was expanded to two health centers and thereafter to two more in June 2015.

The PDC serves children with prematurity, birth weight under 2000 g, HIE, hydrocephalus, cleft lip and palate, trisomy 21, or other developmental delays. In April 2015, additional referral criteria – post-central nervous system infections (meningitis and cerebral malaria) – were added, and in February 2016 (after the inclusion period for this study), children diagnosed with severe acute malnutrition requiring hospitalization began being referred to PDC after discharge from the hospital. Children are referred to PDC using standardized referral criteria and a form completed from Rwinkwavu District Hospital neonatal unit, maternity ward, pediatric ward or emergency department when a child meeting referral

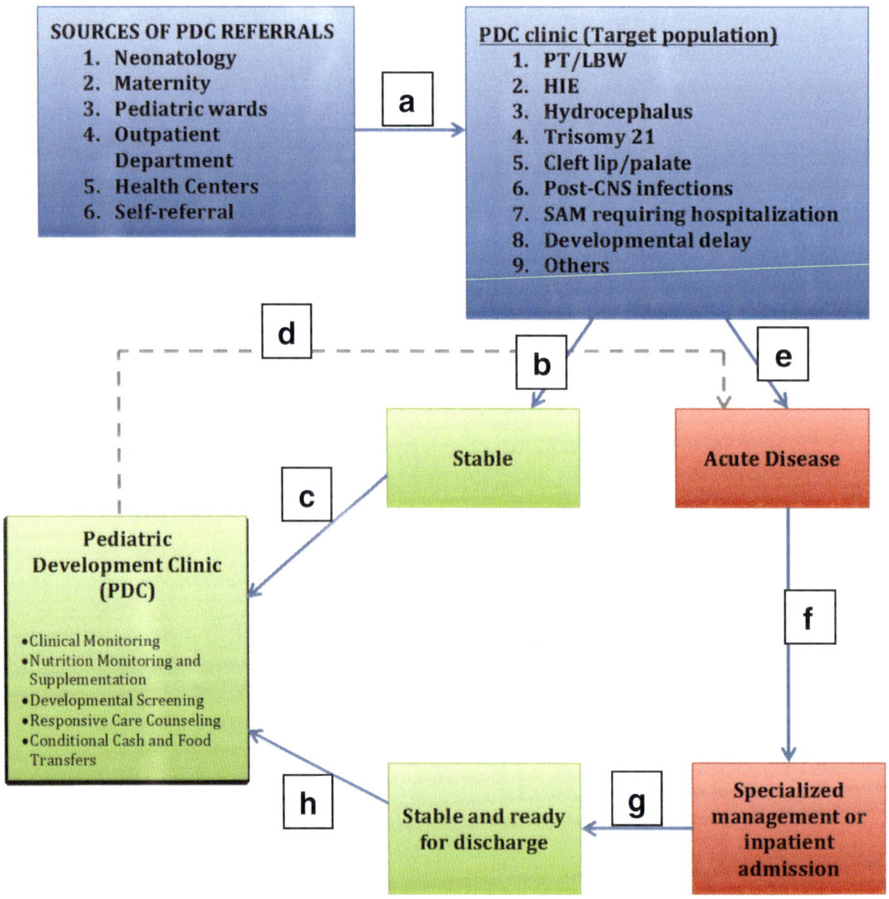

Fig. 1 Pediatric Development Clinic (PDC) Referral and Clinic Flow. Routine Clinic Flow: Different health facilities and services (**a**) refer all stable under-five children meeting referral criteria (**b**) to PDC for enrolment (**c**). At any PDC visit assessment, if an acute illness is identified, an immediately referral (**d**) for acute care is issued (**e**) followed by specialized care (**f**) if needed. When the child has been stabilized and preparing for hospital discharge (**g**), a referral back to continue PDC follow-up (**h**) is completed

criteria is identified. The goal is to identify at-risk infants as young as possible for early enrollment. Children may additionally be referred informally from outpatient clinics at health centers and Rwinkwavu District Hospital, health center maternity wards or via self-referral from the community.

The clinic was designed to be integrated into the public system with as minimal additional external resources as possible to maximize the potential for scalability. Building on an existing platform for chronic care services, the PDCs were integrated into the non-communicable disease (NCD) clinics in the public health system. Only one additional staff member was hired at the district hospital clinic due to the addition of patients to an already high-volume NCD clinic. The PDC is operated at each site on a weekly basis. The PDC team is led by a general practitioner based at the Rwinkwavu District Hospital PDC with routine clinic visits conducted by a nurse and social worker. Each clinic is equipped with a child-friendly space for group counseling and play, and a consultation room with basic furnishings, medical equipment for assessing growth and vitals, as well as structured medical record forms for monitoring patients. Health center teams receive mentorship and supervision from the district hospital team, and the hospital team receives mentorship from additional technical advisors as needed (including a pediatrician and a nutritionist). Prior to initiation of PDC, each team was trained on the PDC protocol and completion of medical record forms for each specific condition. When a health center clinic is first opened, the district hospital doctor, nurse and social worker provide weekly mentorship to provide intensive support following the initial training. After approximately two to 3 months of weekly mentorship (and depending on assessed level of skill and comfort of the providers) mentorship de-intensifies to at least one visit per month. The supervision team meets monthly to discuss strengths and weaknesses of implementation at each clinic, address specific challenges, and create future plans for the clinic.

On a visit day, children's clinical, nutritional and developmental status are assessed by the nurse. According to the protocol, the following are documented for all children: age, weight, height, interval growth for infants up to 6 months, head circumference for infants up to 18 months, immunization status, and vital signs. The child's anthropometric measurements are plotted on World Health Organization growth charts [25, 26] and counseling provided accordingly. Also, a condition-specific protocol of additional screening is completed based on the reason for referral. For preterm infants – the primary referral base – this includes Kangaroo Mother Care (KMC) follow-up, micronutrient supplementation, and vision/hearing screening among other standard follow-up measures. Developmental screening using an Ages and Stages Questionnaire (ASQ-3) [27] is conducted at ages 6, 12, 24, 36, 48 and 60 months; the ASQ-3 was previously adapted and translated into the local language, Kinyarwanda, for use in Rwanda [19].

In addition, the children's primary caretakers participate in group education led by the social worker on different topics depending on the age of their children such as KMC, hygiene, nutrition, family planning, breastfeeding, and the importance of play and early stimulation. A structured social assessment is performed for further individual counseling and to identify families who qualify for conditional food or cash transfers, or additional counseling and home visits according to pre-determined clinical and social criteria. Rwanda's community-based poverty categorizations, known as *Ubudehe*, were used to establish social need [28]; *Ubudehe* is a government mechanism to help communities identify the most vulnerable households so that government-provided social support to achieve poverty reduction can be targeted to these households. Home visits are conducted weekly by social workers with nurses to provide support to families identified during clinic and social assessments as needing additional or home-based support.

Data collection

Data were extracted from electronic medical records (EMR) and paper-based patient charts by trained data collectors. The EMR undergoes routine data quality checks, and discrepancies for key indicators between paper-based charts and the EMR were addressed during data collection.

Measures

Demographic characteristics for children and their primary caretakers were extracted from patients' referral and intake forms. Children's age was categorized as neonates less than 1 month, infants 1 to 5 months, 6 to 11 months and children 12 months and above. Gestational age in weeks was categorized according to WHO classification as "extremely preterm" or less than 28 weeks, "very preterm" from 28 to less than 32 weeks, "moderate to late preterm" from 32 to less than 37 weeks and "term" as 37 weeks and above. Birth weight in grams was categorized as "extremely low birth weight" (less than 1000 g), "very low birth weight" (from 1000 to 1499 g), "low birth weight" (1500 to 1999 g) and birth weight above 2000 g. Mother's age was categorized in intervals from 15 to less than 20, from 20 to 24, 25 to 34 and 35 to 44 years and 45 years and above. Caretakers' socio-economic status was categorized using Rwanda's *Ubudehe* classification based on households that qualify for automatic government support or those who do not qualify. The number of other dependents in a household was categorized as "none" if the child attending PDC was the only child in the home, or "1–3", "4 to 5", or "6 and above".

Based on visit forms that were completed at each patient visit, we assessed whether the nurse had conducted the required assessments at each patient visit according to the PDC protocol. To assess changes in clinic implementation over time, patient visits were grouped into 6 months intervals: April to Sept 2014, October 2014 to March 2015, April to September 2015 and October 2015 to March 2016.

Analysis

We described patient demographic and clinical characteristics, and programmatic process using frequencies and proportions for categorical variables. We compared percent of different aspects of PDC protocol completed at each visit across 6 months intervals using a non-parametric test for trend [29] to determine if there were significant differences in protocol adherence over time.

Ethics

The Rwanda National Ethics Committee (RNEC) No.882/RNEC/2016 and Ministry of Health approved this study. Additionally, the institutional review board at Boston Children's Hospital (Boston, Massachusetts) exempted this study from review.

Results

From April 2014 to December 2015, 426 children enrolled in the PDC. Table 1 describes characteristics of the participants and their caregivers. Of 417 children with gender recorded, more than half were female (54.2%, n = 225/417). Most were neonates (43.7%, n = 172/394) or less than 6 months old (35.0%, n = 138/394) at the time of enrollment. Most enrollees (56.7%, n = 160/282) were preterm. The clinic also enrolled children with a birth weight under 2000 g, with 53.5% (n = 124/334) of those with available birth weight data in the low, very low or extremely low birthweight categories. Most enrolled children were born at Rwinkwavu District Hospital (64.7%, n = 247/382) and were referred into PDC from hospital departments. Two-thirds of children (64.3%, n = 214/333) were living in households with one to three other dependents.

Almost all children were brought to the PDC by their mothers (98.1%, n = 306/312). The majority of caregivers were between 25 and 34 years of age (41.1%, n = 120/292), and were married or cohabitating (88%, n = 337/383), and had some primary school education (41.4%, n = 142/343). Nearly all patients were living in Rwinkwavu catchment area (92.7%, n = 383/413) with some patients coming from neighboring hospital catchment areas. Of caregivers, 6.3% (n = 23/367) were known to be living with HIV. The most common mode of transport to the clinic was walking (43.4%, n = 177/408) or motorcycle taxis (36.5%, n = 149/408). Of those with *Ubudehe* status recorded, 71.4% (n = 202/282) percent did not qualify for automatic government support.

The most frequent diagnosis of PDC clinic patients was prematurity and/or low birth weight (62.9%, n = 266/423) followed by HIE (33.7%, n = 142/422, Table 2). Less common diagnoses included hydrocephalus (1.3%, n = 5/390), trisomy 21 (2.3%, n = 9/390), and cleft lip and/or palate (1.8%, n = 7/390). Fifty-six children had more than one diagnosis (13.2%).

We assessed whether families had received social support and developmental screening with the ASQ-3 according to protocol (Table 3). Of 364 participants with social support data available, almost every mother received transport fees at one or more visits during PDC (96.7%, n = 352) and 43.7% received food packages (n = 159). Additionally, more than one-third of children with available data (36.3%, n = 132) received infant formula for some period of time as part of a treatment plan for insufficient maternal breastmilk supply or other difficulties with breastfeeding to achieve adequate growth. Developmental screening using the ASQ-3 was completed for more than the half of children in the clinic who were 6 months or older (56.4%, n = 184/326 eligible children 6 months or older).

The proportion of visits over time with clinical, nutritional and developmental screening and counseling completed according to protocol are shown in Table 4. Overall, age, weight, height/length, and head circumference were measured consistently at visits (98.3%, n = 2486/2529; 98.9%, n = 2755/2787; 98.2%, n = 2736/2787 and 95.8%, n = 2366/2431 respectively). Vaccination status was assessed at 88.1% (n = 2138/2529) of visits and feeding difficulties were assessed at 84.5% (n = 2138/2529) of visits. Danger signs were assessed at 70.1% (n = 1953/2787) of visits and interval growth for children under 6 months was assessed at 70.4% (n = 1168/2431) of visits. Child development activities were assessed less frequently; general child development counseling was provided 52.1% of the time and availability of playthings for stimulation in the home was assessed at 6.6% of visits. Adjusted age for preterm infants was assessed 21.6% (n = 232/1074) of the time for those children under age 24 months with a documented gestational age recorded.

Significant, steady improvements in assessment over time were documented in development counseling – from 21.8% (n = 64/2675) in the first 6 months to 65.6% (n = 554/2675) in the most recent 6 months of clinic implementation ($p < 0.001$) as well as evaluation of home stimulation activities from 2.5% (n = 7/2529) to 8.5% (n = 69/2529, p = 0.001). Danger signs assessment

Table 1 Demographic characteristics of children enrolled in PDCs from April 2014 to March 2016 and their caretakers

Child characteristics	Total $N = 426$	
	n	%
Gender ($N = 415$)		
Male	190	45.8
Female	225	54.2
Age at first visit ($N = 394$)		
Neonate (< 1 month)	172	43.7
1–5 months	138	35.0
6–11 months	26	6.6
12 months and above	58	14.7
Gestational age in weeks ($N = 282$)		
Extremely preterm (<28 weeks)	13	4.6
Very preterm (29 to <32 weeks)	38	13.5
Moderate to late preterm (32 to <37 weeks)	109	38.7
Term (37 + weeks)	122	43.3
Birth weight categories (grams) ($N = 334$)		
Extremely low, < 1000 g	4	1.2
Very low, 1000–1499 g	61	18.3
Low, 1500–1999 g	114	34.1
2000 g or more	155	46.4
Site of birth ($N = 382$)		
District Hospital	247	64.7
Health Center	97	25.4
Home	26	6.8
En route	8	2.1
National Referral Hospital	4	1.1
Referral site ($N = 355$)		
District Hospital	310	87.3
Health Center	24	6.8
Other	21	5.9
Caretaker characteristics	n	%
Relationship with the child ($N = 312$)		
Mother	306	98.1
Father	2	0.6
Grandmother	3	1.0
Other relative	1	0.3
Mother's age ($N = 292$)		
15–19 years	17	5.8
20–24 years	98	33.6
25–34 years	120	41.1
35–44 years	52	17.8
45 years and above	5	1.7
Marital status ($N = 383$)		
Married or cohabitating	337	88.0
Not currently married/ cohabitating	46	12.0
HIV status ($N = 367$)		
Positive	23	6.3
Negative	344	93.7
Caretaker education level ($N = 343$)		
No formal education	57	16.6
Some primary	142	41.4
Primary completed	128	37.3
Secondary or higher completed	16	4.7
Ubudehe classification ($N = 282$)		
Does not qualify for government support	202	71.4
Qualifies for government support	80	28.3
Household lives within Rwinkwavu catchment area ($n = 413$)		
Yes	383	92.7
No	30	7.3
Transport means to the health facility ($N = 408$)		
Walking	177	43.4
Bicycle	4	1.0
Motorbike	149	36.5
Mini bus	54	13.2
Other	24	5.9
Number of dependents in a household ($N = 333$)		
No other children	23	6.9
1 to 3	214	64.3
4 to 5	66	19.8
6 and above	30	9.0

improved substantially between the first and second 6 months from 43.2% ($n = 136/2787$) to 72.2% ($n = 625/2787$), then stabilized ($p < 0.001$). Feeding difficulty and vaccination status assessments were more varied across time: feeding difficulty fluctuated from 88.1% ($n = 244/2529$) in the first 6 months to 78.6% ($n = 496/2529$) then 82.2% ($n = 664/2529$) and up to 90.3% ($n = 734/2529$) in the most recent 6 months of implementation ($p < 0.001$). Vaccination status also varied, with some declines from 93.5% ($n = 259/2529$) in the first 6 months of implementation to 87.6% ($n = 553/2529$), then 86.1% ($n = 696/2529$) and 88.7% ($n = 721/2529$, $p = 0.171$). Proportion of interval growth assessment dropped significantly in the last 6 months from 74.5% ($n = 196/1659$) to 57.3% ($n = 236/1659$, $p < 0.001$).

Discussion

We report the successful implementation of the novel PDC in a rural African setting during its first 24 months of operation. Our findings show relative completeness of follow-up visits according to PDC protocol for 2 years in

Table 2 Medical diagnoses of PDC patients at enrollment in Rwinkwavu catchment area

Medical conditions	n	%
Children with any diagnosis on record		
Diagnosed as preterm/LBW (*N* = 423)	266	62.9
Diagnosed with HIE (*N* = 422)	142	33.7
Diagnosed with Hydrocephalus (*N* = 390)	5	1.3
Diagnosed with Trisomy 21 (*N* = 390)	9	2.3
Diagnosed with Cleft lip and/or palate (*N* = 390)	7	1.8
Diagnosed with other development delays (*N* = 390)	22	5.6
Diagnosed with other condition (*N* = 390)	22	5.6
Child has multiple diagnoses (*N* = 423)	56	13.2

this population of previously underserved high-risk children. In a setting with very few specialists, the program was designed to tackle a health worker shortage based on a task shifting model that relies primarily on nurses and social workers to deliver care with general practitioner oversight. Our findings show this task shifted model is feasible for delivering follow-up care for the early identification of complications among a population of children at risk of medical, nutritional, and developmental impairments. This builds on the large body of evidence demonstrating successes of task shifting in other domains, especially in HIV care [30].

The PDC is reaching a diverse population of at-risk children under-5 years of age, many of whom were previously not reached at all [31]. By providing services for these high-risk children, PDC has the potential to empower caretakers who face stigma and high levels of stress when looking after children experiencing developmental problems [32]. The targeted population of PDC was focused on those infants born with perinatal risk whose long-term outcomes could benefit significantly with early assessment and intervention to catch up with their non-medically vulnerable peers– namely, those born preterm and/or low birth weight and significant HIE, as well as other less common perinatal conditions requiring medical and nutritional follow-up. The majority of children were less than 6 months at the time of enrollment, which is critical for ensuring services are provided as early as possible. By enrolling children in their first few months of life and routinely screening these children for medical, nutritional and developmental concerns, the PDC has created a platform for early identification and intervention rather than the default system of waiting until children are sick and present to care before care is provided [33]. Additionally, creating a comprehensive platform rather than a vertical program targeted solely at one population, such as preterm infants for KMC, optimizes the impact of investing in a chronic care operational delivery model.

Table 3 Developmental screening and social support provided to PDC patients at enrolment

	n	%
Socioeconomic assistance ever received (*N* = 364)		
Transport fees	352	96.7
Infant formula	132	36.3
Food package	159	43.7
ASQ assessment completed if child is 6+ months old (*N* = 326)		
Yes	184	56.4
No	142	43.6

Most caretakers were mothers and were married or cohabiting. Caretakers play an enormous role in the development of young children and the very rare involvement of father's in the program is an aspect that the clinic is trying to address. Involving fathers in children's care can mean not only that when mothers are not available, they can step in and avoid missing appointments, but more importantly, that fathers are also involved in early stimulation activities at home [34] which can improve children's developmental outcome [35]. Additionally, supporting older siblings who may serve as caretakers is an area for consideration in future programming. Further, almost half of caretakers were less than 25 years of age, with several adolescent mothers, which has been shown to be associated with social and medical vulnerability and a barrier to adherence to care [36]. This unique population of mothers can benefit from services promoting positive parenting and stimulation [37] to empower them to create a nurturing home environment for optimal development.

In serving this unique and vulnerable population of patients, the provision of conditional food and cash transfers aims to break barriers to adherence to chronic care and ensure adequacy of access to at least minimum nutritional needs. As the PDC patients' families were primarily not eligible for government support, social support is an integral component of the PDC program. The majority of patients in the program benefit from some form of conditional food and cash transfers, particularly transport fees to reduce financial barriers to accessing the PDC. Future research to assess PDC impact on patient outcomes is needed, which, in combination with a costing analysis – that takes into consideration required start-up costs for equipment and staff training, staff time, social supports, medications, supplies, operational costs, as well as costs of mentorship and supervision for both health center and hospital teams – will be important to assessing potential for scale-up.

Although there was significant variability in the proportion of visit assessments completed over time,

Table 4 Progress of Pediatric Development Clinics services in the first 24 months of implementation

Time periods	0–6 months		7–12 months		13–18 months		19–24 months		
	n	%	n	%	n	%	n	%	*P* value*
Total number of visits during period	315	11.3	716	25.7	890	31.9	866	31.1	
Visit location (*N* = 2787)									
Rwinkwavu District Hospital	250	79.4	363	50.7	391	43.9	444	51.3	<0.001
Decentralized Health Center	65	20.6	353	49.3	499	56.1	422	48.7	
Danger signs assessed at visit (*N* = 2787)									
Yes	136	43.2	508	71.0	684	76.9	625	72.2	<0.001
No	179	56.8	208	29.1	206	23.2	241	27.8	
Age recorded at visit (*N* = 2529)									
Yes	272	98.2	617	97.8	795	98.4	802	98.7	0.302
No	5	1.8	14	2.2	13	1.6	11	1.4	
Adjusted age for preterm babies ≤24 months (*N* = 1074)									
Yes	27	20.8	91	31.1	64	18.2	50	16.7	0.003
No	103	79.2	202	68.9	288	81.8	249	83.3	
Weight recorded at visit (*N* = 2787)									
Yes	312	99.1	708	98.9	876	98.4	859	99.2	0.790
No	3	1.0	8	1.1	14	1.6	7	0.8	
Height recorded at visit (*N* = 2787)									
Yes	308	97.8	695	97.1	877	98.5	856	98.9	0.021
No	7	2.2	21	2.9	13	1.5	10	1.2	
Head circumference recorded at visit if ≤18 months (*N* = 2431)									
Yes	284	96.3	607	92.1	779	97.4	696	97.3	<0.001
No	11	3.7	52	7.9	21	2.6	19	2.7	
Interval growth calculated at visit if ≤6 months (*N* = 1659)									
Yes	196	74.5	385	76.4	351	73.1	236	57.3	<0.001
No	67	25.5	119	23.6	129	26.9	176	42.7	
Vaccination status recorded (*N* = 2529)									
Yes	259	93.5	553	87.6	696	86.1	721	88.7	0.171
No	18	6.5	78	12.4	112	13.9	92	11.3	
Feeding difficulty assessed (*N* = 2529)									
Yes	244	88.1	496	78.6	664	82.2	734	90.3	<0.001
No	33	11.9	135	21.4	144	17.8	79	9.7	
General child development counseling received (*N* = 2675)									
Yes	64	21.8	256	38.2	519	59.9	554	65.6	<0.001
No	229	78.2	415	61.9	347	40.1	291	34.4	
Playthings and stimulating activities in the home assessed (*N* = 2529)									
Yes	7	2.5	32	5.1	58	7.2	69	8.5	<0.001
No	270	97.5	599	94.9	750	92.8	744	91.5	
Next rendez-vous recorded (*N* = 2787)									
Yes	309	98.1	694	96.9	869	97.6	841	97.1	0.658
No	6	1.9	22	3.1	21	2.4	25	2.9	

**P*-values were calculated using a non-parametric test for trend.

completion of screening for danger signs and developmental counselling improved significantly. Possible explanations for this finding are that over time, providers became more familiar and more comfortable with assessing these components. Additionally, mentorship visits were conducted at least monthly by the hospital staff to health center clinics where the district hospital PDC team provided practice-based guidance on care protocols, referral processes, and nutrition and development counseling to health center teams. These visits have likely contributed to this improvement. Percent complete recording of adjusted age, although improved since the first 6 months of PDC, have fluctuated over time. Interval growth calculation was steadily above 70% until the last 6 months, when we saw a sharp reduction in percent complete recording. These quality gaps highlight the particular challenges of growth monitoring in preterm infants where growth standards are unique and gestational age is often not known. We found that variables requiring calculation, such as adjusted age for preterm infants and interval growth calculation, were completed less frequently than those variables requiring simple recording, such as age, weight and head circumference. These well-done components are also captured in other clinics, such as the Integrated Management of Childhood Illness, and clinicians are accustomed to recording them. Although a clinician's ability to calculate interval growth will be impacted if the weight of the previous visit was not recorded in patient charts, the fact that weight was recorded more than 95% of the time makes this less likely to be an issue. Qualitative exploration of factors leading to the reduction in recording are needed to understand these findings. Automated calculation tools, such as job aids or mHealth tools, could facilitate the completion of these assessments, provide clinical reminders, and video teaching and counseling supports, as has been successfully done in other task-shifted programs [38, 39].

More than the half of PDC children who were eligible for ASQ had one completed. The integration of developmental screening has proven challenging as nurses have to read questions to caretakers due to low literacy and it takes time to administer, which can be particularly burdensome as patient volume increases. Furthermore, the ASQ-3 was a new tool in our setting and nurses from PDCs needed time to become familiar with the process. Further efforts are needed to be able to appropriately translate the findings of a developmental screening into direct intervention in settings such as Rwanda where no locally validated tools exist [18]. Some promising tools have emerged that were designed specifically for easy assessment and intervention in low- and middle-income countries including the International Guide for Monitoring Child Development [40] and the Caregiver-Reported Early Childhood Development Index (CREDI) [41], which could be more appropriate but require additional study for feasibility in the PDC. In the meantime, a play and communication module has been introduced more recently into the protocol and provider training in order to help boost the developmental assessment and intervention skills of PDC providers.

This study has some limitations. Because we used routinely-collected data from patient charts entered into EMR, data were missing or incomplete for several variables. However, we believe the data available gives an accurate description of the clinic's patients and services. In addition, when possible, we verified discrepant data in patient charts and in the EMR. Another limitation could be the generalizability of the study findings to other settings, as the pilot for PDC was conducted in rural southern Kayonza District in Rwinkwavu District Hospital catchment area which has received support from Partners In Health/Inshuti Mu Buzima since 2005.

Conclusion

Our study demonstrates that the PDC model is a feasible design that supports early identification and intervention for medical, nutritional, and developmental complications among high-risk children in a rural African setting. Using a task-shifting model, nurses and social workers were able to follow a standardized protocol for patient visits; however as a new program there are areas for ongoing improvement in the quality of care. Future research is needed to understand the outcomes of the children benefiting from the PDC program as well as costs of PDC implementation.

Acknowledgements

We acknowledge Partners In Health/Inshuti Mu Buzima for the support of this work. This study was developed under the Partners In Health/Inshuti Mu Buzima Intermediate Operational Research Training Program, developed and facilitated by Bethany Hedt-Gauthier and Jackline Odhiambo. Ann Miller and Catherine Kirk provided direct mentorship to this paper as part of this training. Training costs were covered by the Harvard Global Health Initiative Burke Global Health Fellowship grant and by Partners In Health/Inshuti Mu Buzima. Some training facilitators and mentors are Rwanda Human Resources for Health faculty, funded with the support of the Government of Rwanda, the Global Fund to Fight AIDS, Tuberculosis and Malaria and Centers for Disease Control and Prevention. Support for some mentors was provided by the Global Health Research Core at Harvard Medical School. We also acknowledge the contributions of Stephanie Bazubagira, Jean de Dieu Uwihaye, and Emmanuel Ndayishimiye for data collection as well as Kaya Hedt for her support of data cleaning.

Funding

This manuscript was developed under the Partners In Health/Inshuti Mu Buzima Intermediate Operational Research Training Program, training costs were covered by the Harvard Global Health Initiative Burke Global Health Fellowship grant and by Partners In Health/Inshuti Mu Buzima. Some training facilitators and mentors are Rwanda Human Resources for Health faculty, funded with the support of the Government of Rwanda, the Global Fund to fight AIDS, Tuberculosis and Malaria and Centers for Disease Control and Prevention. Support for some mentors was provided by the Global Health Research Core at Harvard Medical School. Data collection costs were covered by UNICEF Rwanda.

Authors' contributions
CM & EN designed the protocol, analyzed the data, and wrote the first and subsequent drafts of the manuscript. HM & KW designed the PDC program, assisted with protocol design, analysis contextualization, and reviewed all drafts of the manuscript. AM & CK mentored the protocol design, data analysis and drafts of the paper, and reviewed all versions of the manuscript. CK also cleaned the data. ED and FN reviewed the manuscript, OB and SE work on PDC implementation directly and reviewed the manuscript. All authors read and approved the final manuscript.

Competing interests
The authors declare that they have no competing interests.

Author details
[1]Rwinkwavu District Hospital, Ministry of Health, Rwinkwavu, Rwanda. [2]Department of Pediatrics, Partners In Health/Inshuti Mu Buzima, Rwinkwavu, Rwanda. [3]Division of Global Health Equity, Brigham and Women's Hospital, Boston, USA. [4]Division of General Pediatrics, Boston Children's Hospital, Boston, USA. [5]Harvard Medical School, Department of Global Health and Social Medicine, Boston, USA. [6]Division of Clinical Services, Ministry of Health, Kigali, Rwanda. [7]P.O. Box 3432, Kigali, Rwanda.

References

1. Darmstadt GL, Shiffman J, Lawn JE. Advancing the newborn and stillbirth global agenda: priorities for the next decade. Arch Dis Child. 2015;100(Suppl 1):S13–8.
2. Lu C, Black MM, Richter L. Risk of poor development in young children in low-income and middle-income countries: an estimation and analysis at the global, regional, and country level. Lancet Glob Health. 2016;4(12):e916–e22.
3. Lawn JE, Blencowe H, Oza S, You D, Lee AC, Waiswa P, et al. Every Newborn: progress, priorities, and potential beyond survival. Lancet. 2014; 384(9938):189–205.
4. Gilmore JH, Lin W, Prastawa MW, Looney CB, Vesta YS, Knickmeyer RC, et al. Regional gray matter growth, sexual dimorphism, and cerebral asymmetry in the neonatal brain. J Neurosci. 2007;27(6):1255–60.
5. Ford ND, Stein AD. Risk factors affecting child cognitive development: a summary of nutrition, environment, and maternal child interaction indicators for Sub- Saharan Africa. J Dev Orig Health Dis. 2016;7(2):197–217.
6. Casale D, Desmond C, Richert L. The association between stunting and psychosocial development among preschool children: a study using the South African Birth to Twenty cohort data. Child Care Health Dev. 2014; 40(6):900–10.
7. Aarnoudse-Moens CS, Weisglas-Kuperus N, Van Goudoever JB, Oosterlaan J. Meta- Analysis of Neurobehavioral Outcomes in Very Preterm and/ or Very Low Birth Weight Children. Pediatrics. 2009;124(2):717–28.
8. Colella-Santos MF, Hein TA, de Souza GL, do Amaral MI, Casali RL. Newborn Hearing Screening and Early Diagnostic in the NICU. Biomed Res Int. 2014; 2014:845308. doi:10.1155/2014/845308.
9. Zerbeto AB, Cortelo FM, Filho EB C. Association between gestational age and birth weight on the language development of Brazilian children: a systematic review. J Pediatr. 2015;91(4):326–32.
10. Ballot DE, Potterton J, Chirwa T, Hilburn N, Cooper PA. Developmental outcome of very low birth weight infants in a developing country. BMC Pediatr. 2012;12:11. doi:10.1186/1471-2431-12-11.
11. Sudfeld CR, McCoy DC, Fink G, Muhihi A, Bellinger DC, Masanja H, et al. Malnutrition and Its Determinants Are Associated with Suboptimal Cognitive, Communication and Motor Development in Tanzanian Children. J Nutr. 2015;145(12):2705–14.
12. Doyle LW, Anderson PJ, Battin M, Bowen JR, Brown N, Callanan C, et al. Long term follow up of high risk children: who, why and how? BMC Pediatr. 2014;14:279. doi:10.1186/1471-2431-14-279.
13. Huang KY, Nakigudde J, Calzada E, Boivin MJ, Ogedegbe G, Brotman LM. Implementing an early childhood school- based mental health promotion intervention in low-resource Ugandan Schools: study protocol for a cluster randomized controlled trial. Trails. 2014;15(1):471. doi:10.1186/ 1745-6215-15-471.
14. Yousfazai AK, Rasheed MA, Rizvi A, Amstrong R, Bhutta ZA. Parenting Skills and Emotional Availablity: An RCT. Pediatrics. 2015;135(5):e1247–57.
15. Wallender JL, Bann CM, Biasini FJ, Goudar SS, Pasha O, Chomba E, et al. Development of children at risk for adverse outcomes participating in early intervention in developing countries: a randomized controlled trial. J Child Psychol Psychiarty. 2014;55(11):1251–9.
16. Farmer PE, Nutt CT, Wagner CM, Sekabaraga C, Nuthulaganti T, Weigel JL, et al. Reduced premature mortality in Rwanda: lessons from success. BMJ. 2013;346:f65.
17. Katz J, Lee AC, Kozuki N, Lawn JE, Cousens S, Blencowe H, et al. Mortality risk in preterm and small-for-gestational-age infants in low-income and middle-income countries: a pooled country analysis. Lancet. 2013;382(9890): 417–25.
18. Rwanda Ministry of Health. National Community Health Policy. 2015. http://www.moh.gov.rw/fileadmin/templates/policies/NATIONAL_COMMUNITY_HEALTH_POLICY.pdf. 24 Jan 2017.
19. UNICEF. Early Childhood Development and Family Services: Baseline Evaluation in 2016 Sites in Rwanda. https://www.unicef.org/evaldatabase/files/ECD_and_F_Baseline_Evaluation_Rwanda.pdf. 12 Dec 2016.
20. USAID. An Evaluation of the Kuraneza Project: Good Growth for Children in Rwanda. 2015. http://www.mcsprogram.org/wp-content/uploads/2015/08/CARE-Rwanda-FE-Brief1.pdf. Accessed 16 Nov 2016.
21. World Health Organization. Health workforce requirements for universal health coverage and the sustainable development goals. 2016. http://apps.who.int/iris/bitstream/10665/250330/1/9789241511407-eng.pdf?ua=1. Accessed 12 Jan 2016.
22. Shumbusho F, van Griensven J, Lowrance D, Turate I, Weaver MA, Price J, et al. Task shifting for scale-up of HIV Care: evaluation of nurse- centered antiretroviral treatment at rural health centers in Rwanda. PLoS Med. 2009; 6(10):e1000163.
23. National Institute of Statistics of Rwanda. Fourth Population and Housing Census, Rwanda, 2012: Final Results Main Indicators Report 2014. 16 Nov 2016.
24. Hansen A, Magge H, Labrecque M, Munyaneza RB, Nahimana E, Nyishime M, et al. The development and implementation of a newborn medicine program in a resource-limited setting. Public Health Action. 2015;5(1):17–22.
25. World Health Organization. WHO Child Growth Standards: Length/height-for-age, weight-for-age, weight-for-length, weight-for-height and body mass index-for-age: Methods and Development. Geneva: World Health Organization; 2006.
26. World Health Organization. WHO Child Growth Standards: Head Circumference-for-age, Arm Circumference-for- age, Triceps Skinfold-for-age and Subscapular Skinfold-for-age: Methods and Development. Geneva: World Health Organization; 2007.
27. Squires J, Twombly E, Bricker D, Potter L. ASQ-3 User's Guide. 2009. Baltimore: Paul H. Brookes Publishing Company. 2009.
28. Ministry of Finance and Economic Planning. The Government of Rwanda, Poverty Reduction Strategy Paper. 2002. http://www.unrwanda.org/undp/prsp2002.pdf. Accessed 25 Jan 2017.
29. Cuzick J. A Wilcoxon-type test for trend. Stat Med. 1985;4:87–90.
30. World Health Organization. Task shifting to tackle health worker shortages. 2007. http://www.who.int/healthsystems/task_shifting_booklet.pdf. Accessed 11 Nov 2016.
31. Blencowe H, Cousens S, Chou D, Oestergaard M, Say L, Moller AB, et al. Borrn To Soon: The global epidemiology of 15 million preterm births. Reprod Health. 2013;10(suppl 1):S2. doi:10.1186/1742-4755-10-S1-S2.
32. Masulani-Mwale C, Mathanga D, Silungwe D, Kauye F, Gladstone M. Parenting children with intellectual disabilities in Malawi: the impact that reaches beyond coping? Child Care. Health Dev. 2016;42(6):871–80.
33. Mugeni C, Levine AC, Munyaneza RM, Mulindahabi E, Crokrell HC, Glavis-Bloom J, et al. Nationwide implementation of integrated community case management of childhood illness in Rwanda. Glob Health Sci Pract. 2014; 2(3):328–41.
34. Britto PR, Lye SL, Proulx K, Yousfazai AK, Matthews SG, Vaivada T, et al. Nurturing care: promoting early childhood development. Lancet. 2017; 389(10064):91–102.
35. Jeong J, McCoy DC, Yousafzai AK, Salhi, C, Fink G. Paternal Stimulation and Early Child Development in Low- and Middle- Income Countries. Pediatrics. 2016;138(4):e20161357.
36. Pinto-Foltz MD, Logsdon C, Derrick A. Engaging adolescent mothers in a longitudinal mental health intervention study: challenges and lessons learned. Issues Ment Health Nurs. 2011;32(4):214 9.

8

Early onset fetal growth restriction

Andrea Dall'Asta[1,2†], Valentina Brunelli[3†], Federico Prefumo[3], Tiziana Frusca[2] and Christoph C Lees[1,4,5*]

Abstract

Fetal growth restriction (FGR) diagnosed before 32 weeks is identified by fetal smallness associated with Doppler abnormalities and is associated with significant perinatal morbidity and mortality and maternal complications. Recent studies have provided new insights into pathophysiology, management options and postnatal outcomes of FGR. In this paper we review the available evidence regarding diagnosis, management and prognosis of fetuses diagnosed with FGR before 32 weeks of gestation.

Keywords: Fetal Doppler, Fetal complications, Iatrogenic preterm delivery, Antenatal counseling, Neonatal intensive care unit

Background

Fetal growth restriction (FGR) is both a common obstetric condition and a major cause of perinatal morbidity and mortality [1, 2]. Early FGR by definition is diagnosed at or below 32 weeks and differs from late onset FGR also in terms of its clinical manifestations, association with hypertension [3], patterns of deterioration and severity of placental dysfunction [4, 5].

The perinatal outcome of FGR is dependent on the severity of growth restriction; an estimated fetal weight below the 3rd centile and/or abnormal umbilical artery Doppler are strongly associated with adverse perinatal outcome [6]. A recent study has shown how the incidence of perinatal death is highest in those with a birth weight below the 2.3rd centile, falling gradually with an increasing birth weight up to the 80th and 90th centiles, at which the lowest death rates occur [7].

FGR is a complex and multifactorial disorder affecting the fetal development that often results in multiple perinatal complications [8–10] and currently represents a major risk factors for long term poor neurological outcome. FGR is also associated with poor postnatal growth and numerous studies in both humans and animals have shown an association between low birth weight and development of cardiovascular disease including increased risk of hypertension, diabetes, dyslipidemia and coagulation in children and adults [9–16]. These observations were first made in 1989 by Barker and colleagues and confirmed in the last few decades [17, 18]. It has been postulated that cardiovascular remodelling is due to hemodynamic redistribution and adaptation to hypoxia and insufficient nutrition [17–22].

At present there is no effective treatment to reverse the course of FGR except delivery. Fetal growth restriction is probably among the obstetric entities where there is the greatest variation in clinical practice, in terms of monitoring and recommended gestational age at delivery. Prenatal recognition of FGR remains the main challenge in daily obstetric practice. Correct surveillance, antenatal management and timing of delivery can improve fetal and neonatal outcomes.

Etiology

The causes of FGR are heterogeneous and can be classified as fetal, maternal, environmental, and placental. Small fetuses can be divided into two groups: non-placenta mediated growth restriction and placenta mediated [23].

The first group includes structural and chromosomal/genetic anomalies (trisomies 13 and 18; genetic conditions such as Russel Silver Syndrome), congenital infections (rubella, cytomegalovirus, toxoplasmosis) [24] and inborn errors of metabolism. The second and much more common group includes medical conditions that can affect placental function: pre-eclampsia, chronic hypertension and gestational hypertension are complicated by FGR in 30 to 40% of cases [23]; diabetes is complicated by FGR in 10 to 20% of cases

* Correspondence: christoph.lees@imperial.nhs.uk
†Equal contributors
1Centre for Fetal Care, Queen Charlotte's and Chelsea Hospital, Imperial College Healthcare NHS Trust, Du Cane Road, London W12 0HS, United Kingdom
4Department of Surgery and Cancer, Imperial College London, London, United Kingdom
Full list of author information is available at the end of the article

irrespective of glycemic control [25]; maternal vascular disease, renal disease, thrombophilia, autoimmune disease, can lead to uteroplacental hypoperfusion thereby impairing fetal growth [26]; hypoxemia secondary to cardiac, respiratory and hematological disorders may also cause FGR.

Others maternal risk factors associated with an increased risk of a SGA neonate are maternal age ≥35 years and particulalry in women ≥40 years old [27], African American [28] or Indian/Asian ethnicity [29], nulliparity [30], social deprivation [31], body mass index (BMI) <20, BMI > 25 [32], alcohol intake [33], drug use (with cocaine use during pregnancy being the most significant) [34] and cigarette smoking [35]. Singleton pregnancies following IVF are also at increased risk for SGA [36]. Twin pregnancies have a high incidence of FGR: about 20–30% of dichorionic and 40% of monochorionic twin pregnancies will suffer from FGR [37].

Definition and diagnosis

Multiple definitions of FGR have been suggested over the decades by National and Internationl Societies and experts (Table 1) [38, 39]. Despite this, there is currently no agreed upon diagnostic criteria for FGR. The American College of Obstetricians and Gynecologists (ACOG) defines FGR as an estimated fetal weight less than the 10th centile [40]. The Royal College of Obstetricians and Gynaecologists (RCOG) uses fetal abdominal circumference (AC) or estimated fetal weight (EFW) <10th centile to diagnose a FGR fetus [41]. Other Authors have suggested a cut off of the 3rd centile to detect pregnancies at higher risk of adverse outcomes [42]. In 2002 the TRUFFLE group, which included 20 European Perinatal experts, defined fetal growth restriction as the combination of abdominal circumference <10th centile and umbilical artery Doppler pulsatility index (PI) >95th percentile [3]. Similarly, after prospectively assessing the adverse perinatal outcomes in over 1100 pregnancies where EFW at inclusion was <10th centile, the PORTO group defined FGR as a combination of fetal smallness (EFW <5th centile) and umbilical artery Doppler PI >95th percentile [6]. More recently, early FGR has been defined by a consensus committe of international fetal medicine experts with solitary parameters ither EFW <3rd centile, AC <3rd centile or absent umbilical artery end diastolic flow [43].

Table 1 FGR definition in recent literature

Institution / Author	FGR definition
Baschat et al 2007 [101]	Combination of small fetal AC with elevated UA Doppler blood flow resistance
Cochrane 2013 [65]	Failure to reach the growth potential
DIGITAT 2012 [38]	EFW or AC <10th centile for gestational age
ACOG 2013 [40]	Fetuses with EFW <10th centile for gestational age
RCOG 2013 [41]	Small–for–gestational age (SGA) refers to an infant born with a birth weight less than the 10th centile. Fetal growth restriction (FGR) is not synonymous with SGA.
SOGC 2013 [39]	Intrauterine growth restriction refers to a fetus with a EFW <10th centile on ultrasound that, because of a pathologic process, has not attained its biologically determined growth potential.
PORTO 2013 [6]	EFW < 5th percentile & umbilical artery PI >95th percentile
TRUFFLE 2013 [3]	AC < 10th percentile & umbilical artery PI >95th percentile
Gordijin et al 2016 [43]	AC <3rd centile OR EFW <3rd centile OR AREDF OR Both of the following: 1) EFW or AC < 10th centile and 2) UtA PI >95th centile OR UA PI >95th centile.

AC abdominal circumference
AREDF absent/reversed umbilical artery end diastolic flow
EFW estimated fetal weight
PI pulsatility index
UtA uterine artery
UA umbilical artery

In its latest practice bulletin the ACOG acknowledges the fact that terminology for classifying fetuses and newborns who have failed to achieve normal weight is inconsistent [40]. Indeed, the acronyms SGA and FGR are often used interchangeably. However, fetuses with a weight <10 th percentile may be constitutionally small but healthy and not necessarily growth restricted. On the other hand, an estimated weight >10th percentile does not necessarily denote normal fetal growth. Because of this, FGR shouldbe referred to fetuses with pathological smallness caused by an underlying functional problem and hence a definition including not only a biometric cut off but also Doppler indices of feto-placental function is currently agreed in most Fetal Medicine Units [3, 6, 43, 44].

FGR may also be classified by gestational age at onset as early and late, with an arbitrary cut-off conventionally set at 32 weeks: the extremes of the clinical spectrum of FGR differ not only for gestation at onset, but also for clinical manifestations, patterns of fetal deterioration, association with hypertensive disorders of the pregnancy and severity of placental dysfunction [45, 46]. Fetuses with late-onset disease do not present the same sequence of Doppler deterioration described for early-onset FGR [6]. Early-onset FGR represents 20–30% of all FGR and is associated with gestational hypertension and/or pre-eclampsia in up to 70%. On the other hand, late-onset FGR, which represents approximately 70–80% of cases of FGR, shows a weaker association with hypertensive disorders of the pregnancy, roughly 10% [6].

A prerequisite for a correct diagnosis of FGR is accurate dating of the pregnancy, most usually in the first trimester. The Hadlock formula is the most widely accepted method of estimating fetal weight using a composite sonographic measurement of fetal head, abdomen, and femur [47]. Fetal size is influenced by race, ethnicity, sex, parity, maternal size and genetic factors [48, 49]. In the 1990s, Gardosi et al. developed a method that used customized birth weights to identify the growth potential for individual fetuses: antenatal growth charts were customized for maternal characteristics including height, weight, ethnic origin and parity [50, 51]. The use of customized growth charts is purported to increase the antenatal detection of fetal growth restriction, improving the distinction between normal and abnormal growth, but whether this improves clinical outcomes still has to be demonstrated [51]. Customization is questioned by Intergrowth-21st according to which growth patterns in healthy pregnancies are not considered to be modulated by ethnic and environmental conditions [52].

Ultrasound assessment of fetal anatomy and amniotic fluid volume is complementary to the Doppler investigation of fetoplacental circulation to distinguish FGR from constitutionally small fetuses and to identify the most likely underlying etiology of the fetal smallness (e.g., aneuploidy, viral infection, genetic syndromes). The role of determining the karyotype is very controversial; it may be offered in cases where there is a dissociation between growth, amniotic fluid and Doppler.

Screening

Early screening to predict the likelihood of a FGR fetus include medical and obstetric history, uterine artery Doppler and maternal serum parameters [53]. Uteroplacental Doppler is the most powerful predictor of the clinical deterioration and the circumstances surrounding delivery [54]. The systematic review and meta-analysis conducted by Cnossen et al. in 2008 established uterine artery Doppler ultrasonography as a predictor of FGR, providing a more accurate prediction when performed in the second trimester than in the first-trimester [55]. Numerous studies have also shown that some maternal biochemical markers (e.g. pregnancy assoiciasted plasma protein-a, PAPP-A; alfa-fetoprotein, AFP; human chorionic gonadotropin, hCG; Inhibin A) are associated with placental function and fetal growth, and their levels are altered in SGA and FGR pregnancies [56]. A low level first trimester PAPP-A should be considered a major risk factor for delivering a SGA neonate; the combination of uterine artery Doppler and maternal serum markers appears promising for improving prediction of SGA fetus, although predictive values are still poor [57–59]. Use of combination testing in the second trimester appears to predict adverse outcome related to placental insufficiency more effectively than first trimester screening [60].

Role of fetal Doppler in FGR

The fetal vessels that are more commonly examined include umbilical artery, middle cerebral artery, and ductus venosus [61].

Early-and late-onset FGR epitomize two distinct clinical phenotypes of placental dysfunction and differ significantly in clinical progression. Early-onset FGR is associated with high impedance utero placental perfusion which in turn leads to elevated umbilical artery blood flow resistance once villous damage exceeds 30% [45].

The relationship between fetal size and growth and fetal Doppler indices in FGR is complex but in general Doppler deterioration is associated with absolute fetal size rather than growth velocity [62].

Late-onset FGR is more common but less severe with absent or mild placental abnormalities; umbilical artery Doppler may be normal, but fetuses may react with decreased middle cerebral artery (MCA) impedance in response to hypoxemia [63].

Umbilical artery Doppler

Umbilical artery Doppler is the only measure that provides both diagnostic and prognostic information for the management of FGR [64]. A Cochrane systematic review reported that the use of umbilical artery Doppler was associated with a reduction in perinatal deaths, inductions of labor and cesarean deliveries [65]. Also according to RCOG the use of umbilical artery Doppler in a high-risk population has been shown to reduce perinatal morbidity and mortality, and should be the primary surveillance tool in the SGA fetus [41].

Umbilical artery flow identifies different degrees of impaired placental function. Absent or reversed end diastolic flow (AEDF or REDF) indicates an important reduction of blood flow and severe fetal deterioration.

Thanks to longitudinal studies of high-risk pregnancies, we know that the the transition from AEDF to REDF may be slow and gradual in early FGR. Absent end-diastolic velocities in the umbilical artery, if not associated with severe maternal disease, can last for days and weeks before abnormal heart rate pattern or delivery [66].

Reverse end-diastolic flow velocity represents an extreme abnormality in waveform and resistance, with a perinatal mortality of 50% and significant perinatal morbidity [67]. It has also been demonstrated that FGR fetuses with absent or reverse end-diastolic flow in the umbilical artery not only have an increased fetal and neonatal mortality but also a higher incidence of long-term permanent neurologic damage when compared with FGR fetuses with positive diastolic flow in the umbilical circulation [68].

Middle cerebral artery Doppler

A condition of chronic hypoxia determines a fetal flow redistribution that manifests as vasodilatation in the brain circulation. Cerebral vasodilatation, easily detectable as a reduction in the PI of the middle cerebral artery (MCA) represents an adaptative mechanism in response to hypoxia.

Recently published data emphasize the association between abnormal MCA PI and adverse perinatal and neurological outcome [64]. MCA may be valuable for the identification of adverse outcome among late-onset FGR though its role in prediction is weak, independently of umbilical artery Doppler, which is often normal in these fetuses [69–71]. The cerebroplacental ratio (CPR) quantifies the redistribution of cardiac output by dividing the Doppler indices of the middle cerebral artery (MCA) with that of the umbilical artery. The PORTO study demonstrated the association between redistribution, either isolated or associated with umbilical artery PI >95th centile, and adverse perinatal outcome [6, 63]. More recent data have shown significantly lower MCA PI and CPR among fetuses with EFW <10th centile diagnosed gestation beyond 32 weeks who experienced adverse perinatal outcomes in terms of intrapartum distress and abnormal cord pH [72]. Of note, such abnormal Doppler patterns have been related to histological signs of placental insufficiency [73]. It is estimated that in late-onset FGR fetuses abnormal CPR is present before delivery in 20 to 25% of cases [74]. Of note, it is important to underline that MCA Doppler is currently not included in any protocol for the diagnosis and the management of early FGR fetuses as insufficient data exists in prospective studies to define its role.

Ductus venosus Doppler

Doppler examination of the ductus venosus (DV) plays an important role in the management of fetuses with early fetal FGR with the hope of improving the timing of delivery and outcome.

FGR is associated with increased ductus venosus (DV) shunting, and increasing impedance in the umbilical artery, has a graduated effect on the degree of shunting [20]. In contrast to alterations in umbilical artery and middle cerebral artery, which are early signs of adverse outcome, longitudinal studies have demonstrated that DV flow waveforms become abnormal only in advanced stages of fetal compromise [75–78].

It has been showed that the PI of the DV is related to pH at birth, with higher DV pulsatility associated with lower pH at birth [79].

In 2001 Hecher et al. described the time sequence of changes in fetal monitoring variables in fetal growth restriction; they found that ductus venosus PI and short-term variation of fetal heart rate are important indicators for the optimal timing of delivery before 32 weeks of gestation and correlate with fetal outcome at delivery [78]. Ferrazzi et al identified the temporal sequence of abnormal Doppler changes in the fetal circulation in early growth restricted fetuses. Early changes occurred in umbilical and middle cerebral arteries (AEDF and brain sparing respectively); late changes were significantly associated with perinatal death and included umbilical artery REDF and abnormalities in the DV Doppler (reverse A-wave in particular) [2]. Another study demonstrated that absent or reverse velocities in the DV during atrial contraction are associated with perinatal mortality independently of the gestational age at delivery [79]. Bilardo et al. showed that during the last 24 h before delivery DV pulsatility index for veins (PIV) and umbilical artery PI were significantly higher and STV lower in the adverse outcome group, while 2–7 days before delivery only DV PI was significantly higher. These results indicatc that DV PI measurement is a good predictor of perinatal outcome and may be useful in determining the timing of the delivery in of early FGR fetuses [80]. In about 50% of cases, abnormal DV precedes the loss of short-term variability in computerized cardiotocography (CTG) [79], and in about 90% of cases it is abnormal 48 to 72 h before the biophysical profile (BPP) [80].

Cardiac and aortic isthmus Doppler

Cardiac Doppler allows the evaluation of the functionality of the heart with the deterioration of FGR. Systolic and diastolic heart function, atrio-ventricular flows and ventricular outflows can be studied.

In 1988 a prospective longitudinal study by Rizzo et al. described the physiological patterns of blood flow velocity waveforms in normal and in SGA fetuses. In normal fetuses the ratio between the E velocity (early passive ventricular filling) and the A velocity (active ventricular filling during atrial contraction) increased progressively during pregnancy in both transmitral and transtricuspidal waveforms. In SGA fetuses, the E/A ratios did not increase during pregnancy and the values obtained were significantly lower than in normal fetuses [81]. In FGR fetuses the time to peak velocity at the level of the ascending aorta and pulmonary is also lower than in normal fetus, indicating an impairment of myocardial contractility [82].

The literature suggests a potential role for Doppler imaging of the aortic isthmus (AoI) in the clinical surveillance of fetuses with severe FGR. Retrograde flow in the AoI in growth-restricted fetuses correlates strongly with adverse perinatal outcome and neurological deficit in the infant [83, 84].

The myocardial performance index (MPI) is a more recently described parameter that may be useful in fetal monitoring. MPI, AoI PI, together with DV PIV, increase with progressive fetal deterioration. According to Cruz-Martinez et al., at the last examination before delivery the proportion of increased MPI (70.4%) was significantly higher than that of abnormal AoI PI (55.7%) and DV PIV (47.8%) [85]. A significantly higher MPI in growth restricted fetuses compared to appropriately grown fetuses was also demonstrated by Hassan et al, who additionally found a potential role of the MPI in the prediction of arterial and venous Doppler abnormalities in small for gestational age fetuses [86].

Management

Despite being one of the most relevant and most commonly studied conditions in modern obstetrics, there has not been consensus among International Guidelines regarding the optimal management of early onset FGR in terms of monitoring and recommended gestational age at delivery, which can be due to the lack of comparability among studies and the paucity of randomized controlled trials available [3, 65, 87, 88]. Nevertheless, more recent data suggest that reliable protocols of surveillance and management are emerging now [3, 88].

When managing FGR fetuses clinicians focus on EFW, gestational age and fetal Doppler. A threshold of about 500 grams is often considered the value of EFW above which a fetus is potentially surviving outside the uterus, and which must be considered especially when evaluating the options of termination of pregnancy, invasive testing and delivery of a potentially viable fetus. Furthermore, an EFW $<3^{rd}$ centile has been described as predictive of poor outcome [89].

Importantly, gestational age is the most significant determinant of both survival and intact survival [46]. A remarkable reduction in the gestational age cut off for neonatal survival has been achieved, and current neonatal practice has lead to the survival of fetuses born from 22 weeks onwards [90]. Recently published data report a better than expected prognosis for periviable small fetuses [91], however according to Visser et al. [92] active intervention by delivery of early FGR fetuses should not be recommended before 26 weeks as their outcome is comparable to that of AGA infants born at a 2-weeks earlier gestational age. Counseling plays a crucial role, however in a scenario of lacking evidence it is usually individualized on the basis of the clinical features and the option of pregnancy termination may be discussed when legally available.

Monitoring fetuses by using umbilical artery Doppler has been demonstrated to reduce the perinatal death rate [66, 69] though there are few clues as to when delivery should be undertaken. Abnormal umbilical artery PI is a feature of FGR according to the TRUFFLE group as a PI above the 95th centile together with AC $<10^{th}$ centile are the diagnostic criteria for FGR; a raised umbilical PI is suggestive of severe placental disease, which represents the most common cause for FGR [69]. However, as reported by Figueras et al. [64] the management based on umbilical artery alone cannot be effective in those cases of mild placental disease, which account for a proportion of the early onset FGR fetuses, which show reduced MCA pulsatility or cerebroplacental ratio (CPR) (or cerebro-umbilical C-U ratio). Unfortunately, there is not enough evidence to consider MCA Doppler effective in managing FGR fetuses. A recent review by DeVore et al [93] reports that an abnormal CPR is associated with adverse pre- and post-natal outcomes even in fetuses with early-onset SGA; however, it has never been demonstrated whether delivering earlier fetuses who show features of redistribution could add any benefit [64, 93, 94].

Ductus venosus (DV) Doppler is currently used in most European Specialist Perinatal Units as the reference for the management of FGR fetuses before 32 weeks. DV has been demonstrated to be the single strongest Doppler parameter to predict the short term risk of fetal death in early onset FGR [64] and there is good correlation between abnormal DV waveform and late stage acidemia. Absent or reversed A-wave have been reported to be associated with increased risk of intrauterine fetal death (40–70%) independently of the gestational age at delivery; DV PI >95th centile also confers higher risk of adverse outcome, although at lesser extent than that of reversed or absent A-wave [87]. According to Hecher et al. [76] DV is, together with computerized cardiotocography (cCTG), the parameter which last modifies before delivery, and the TRUFFLE group has demonstrated the benefits of a longer stay in utero, especially with regard to long term outcomes.

The biophysical profile has not been demonstrated to be beneficial in high risk pregnancies in terms of perinatal deaths and Apgar <7 at 5 min [33], it is not an accurate predictor of fetal acidemia [24, 34], and there is concern regarding the high false positive and false negative rate (up to 23% of instances of intrauterine fetal death in fetuses with BPP >6 and 11% in those with BPP >8) reported in early-onset very preterm FGR fetuses [46].

Conventional cardiotocography (CTG), along with the assessment of the baseline, the long term variability, accelerations and decelerations of the fetal heart rate, currently represents one of the main tools for the antenatal surveillance of the fetal wellbeing. CTG has been compared to no intervention in a Cochrane review of four randomized control trials. No improvement in perinatal mortality was shown [65, 95] and currently there is no other evidence supporting the use of conventional CTG in FGR fetuses [65, 89]. Short-term variability (STV) can be detected only using cCTG and becomes abnormal in the case of advanced fetal deterioration [77]. Current evidence suggests that cCTG is sensitive in the detection of advanced fetal deterioration providing information similar to DV reverse A-wave for the short-term prediction of fetal death.

Uterine artery Doppler may predict poor outcome in FGR but does not provide information sufficiently sophisticated to be considered effective in the management of the FGR fetuses [89, 96–98].

Which parameter is used to monitor FGR fetuses is not a more important issue than how often these fetuses should be assessed. A stage-based management protocol suggested by Figueras et al. [94], recommends fetal monitoring twice weekly up to 34 weeks if umbilical artery AEDF, every 24 to 48 h up to 30 weeks if reverse diastolic flow in the umbilical artery (REDV) or DV-PI > 95th centile, and every 12 to 24 h up to 26 weeks if spontaneous FHR decelerations, reduced STV (<3 ms) in the computerised cardiotocography, or reverse atrial flow in the DV.

There is no data as regards the decision for inpatient versus outpatient management of FGR fetuses. Most cases of isolated FGR are monitored in an outpatient setting even though the decision for inpatient monitoring can be taken on a subjective basis. Of note, 60–70% of cases of early FGR are associated with hypertensive complications of the pregnancy [3]. In such cases we believe that admission is advisable despite the lack of clinical data supporting this view.

Timing of delivery

At present there is no effective intervention for FGR except delivery, and especially for early-onset FGR the timing is crucial and requires a balance between the risks of prematurity and the possibility of stillbirth and organ damage due to inadequate tissue perfusion [64, 90], unless severe maternal complications supervene [3, 88, 99].

Currently there is no consensus on what is the most appropriate trigger for delivery as the evaluation of the fetal status by Doppler indices and CTG cannot be assessed independently from the gestational age, which is the most significant determinant of both survival and intact survival, and fetal weight [90].

Though the GRIT study showed no clear benefit in delivering immediately or delaying delivery when a fetus is thought to be compromised, evidence from the TRUFFLE study shows how important it is to delay delivery in order to reduce the risk of cerebral palsy and poor neurodevelopmental outcome [79, 99] in this case based on deterioration in both the ductus venosus and STV from computerized CTG. However, this can be safely achieved only through protocols that integrate the best available evidence and reducing clinical practice variation [64].

Baschat et al. suggested the absent or reversed umbilical artery end diastolic velocity (AREDV) as the trigger for delivery, as it seems to have an independent impact on neurodevelopment from the late second trimester onward as representative of deepening hypoxemia [54], though this strategy was not tested in a prospective study.

The GRIT study was the first RCT which aimed to assess the timing for delivering FGR fetuses and concluded that "uncertainty" of the clinician as to whether deliver or not to deliver is related to the timing of delivery, which varied on average by only 4 days. Furthermore, fetuses with severe DV abnormalities at or beyond 28 weeks should be delivered after completion of steroids as there is evidence that reversed A-wave in the DV increases the risk of intrauterine fetal death at any gestational age [99].

According to the stage-based management protocol suggested by Figueras et al. [94] delivery by Caesarean section should be recommended at or after 34 weeks in case of umbilical artery AEDV, at or after 30 weeks if umbilical artery REDF or DV-PI > 95th centile and at or after 26 weeks if spontaneous fetal heart rate (FHR) decelerations, reduced short-term variability (<3 ms) in the cCTG, or reverse atrial flow in the DV Doppler.

The TRUFFLE is the only randomized controlled study which has evaluated a standardized monitoring and delivery protocol focussed on computerized CTG and DV Doppler. The "late" DV group (absent or reversed A-wave) was associated with significant improval in the rate of survival without impairment when compared to computerized CTG, and delivery was recommended in case of umbilical artery REDF between 30 and 32 weeks, umbilical artery AEDF between 32 and 34 weeks, or umbilical artery PI >95th centile beyond 34 weeks. Safety nets for the computerised CTG were used in the TRUFFLE protocol, and may have contributed to the excellent outcomes in term of mortality and survival without impairment [3, 87].

Despite accumulating evidence suggesting that cerebral redistribution, defined by a reduction in the MCA PI below the 5th centile or a reduction in the C-U ratio below the 2.5th centile, may not be an entirely protective phenomenon, currently there is no evidence to recommend delivery before 34 weeks in fetuses who show features of cerebral redistribution [45, 64, 94].

Regarding the mode of delivery, 97% of women in TRUFFLE had Caesarean deliveries, compared with 98 and 85% in the cohorts reported by Baschat and GRIT, respectively [3, 87, 88, 100, 101]. It is of note that no studies have evaluated the optimal mode of delivery in early FGR fetuses.

Outcomes

Early growth restricted fetuses by definition carry at least one of the major risk factors for perinatal morbidity and mortality, *i.e.* low birthweight and prematurity. Early and late-onset FGR are both associated with poor short- and long-term neurodevelopmental outcome, and also with cardiovascular and metabolic complications particularly in case of birth weigth <3rd centile and gestation at delivery <26 weeks [64, 93]. Additionally, the cause of the growth restriction can impact on the short and long term prognosis, so especially for severely early growth restricted fetuses it is important to identify the cause by offering karyotyping and viral screen [32, 90]. This can allow to distinguish between fetuses who are affected by true FGR, and those who are constitutionally small (SGA) but with a guarded

Table 2 Short term survival across gestation at diagnosis[a]

Gestation at diagnosis	Survival N	Perinatal death (IUD + NND) N	Survival %	Perinatal death (IUD + NND) %
22–23 weeks	49	69	41%	59%
24–25 weeks	52	42	55%	45%
26–27 weeks	126	22	85%	15%
28–29 weeks	188	15	93%	7%
30–31 weeks	164	2	99%	1%

Source: Data has been collated and fused from TRUFFLE 2013 [3] and Lawin O'Brien et al [91]
IUD intrauterine death
NND neonatal death
[a]Terminations of pregnancy (TOP) excluded

prognosis, particularly if the birthweight is below the 3rd centile [102].

Few data exist regarding periviable growth restricted babies, a category which is commonly associated with poor outcome [92]. In 2014 Story et al [102] reviewed the outcomes of 20 FGR fetuses diagnosed <24 weeks and EFW <3rd centile reporting a 67% preterm delivery rate and a better than expected survival to neonatal discharge rate of 60%. Such surprisingly good outcomes were confirmed by recently published data from a wider UK cohort of 245 cases of periviable FGR fetuses who showed an overall 41% neonatal survival rate and a 15% rate of delivery beyond 36 weeks, concluding that at a periviable gestational age both SGA and FGR can present in similar ways, and differentiation at the earliest possible time is crucial to allow appropriate management and counseling [91].

After 26 weeks the best results in terms of short term and 2-year outcomes were reported by the TRUFFLE group [3, 87], with 8% overall mortality (3% beyond 30 weeks), 24% severe neonatal morbidity, and low rates of bronchopulmonary dysplasia and poor neurodevelopmental outcome despite including fetuses who were on average 1 week younger and 300 g lighter if compared to the other RCT (GRIT) conducted on FGR fetuses [88]. Overall 69% of the 503 included fetuses survived without severe neonatal morbidity and these results were explained as a consequence of a more detailed and standardized protocol of surveillance. Allocation to delivery on the basis of absent/reversed A-wave in the DV accounted for a non significant increase in the stillbirth rate and a significant lower rate of abnormal neurodevelopmental outcome compared to the computerized CTG group, irrespective of the gestational age at inclusion [87]. According to Baschat et al. in-early onset FGR the nutritional and vascular restriction in placental function is limited with umbilical artery AREDV, and particularly reversed end-diastolic velocity is an independent risk factor for adverse motor and cognitive development [54]. Later in life no differences were reported in the rates of severe disability and individual domain scores between the two delivery arms in the GRIT study [86, 98] and results were comparable to other preterm cohorts without FGR [54]. Recently published data concerning short term survival of severe growth restricted fetuses across gestation at diagnosis and delivery are reported in Tables 2, 3 and in Figs. 1 and 2.

Future directions

Delivery is acknowledged to be the only treatment for FGR at present and the most important studies have

Table 3 Short term survival across gestation at delivery[a,b]

Gestation at delivery	Survival N	Perinatal death (IUD + NND) N	Survival %	Perinatal death (IUD + NND) %
22–23 weeks	1	7	13%	87%
24–25 weeks	0	30	0%	100%
26–27 weeks	51	52	49%	51%
28–29 weeks	141	27	84%	16%
30–31 weeks	173	10	95%	5%
32–33 weeks	111	5	96%	4%
>34 weeks	87	4	96%	4%

Source: Data has been collated and fused from TRUFFLE 2013 [3] and Lawin O'Brien et al [91]
IUD intrauterine death
NND neonatal death
[a]Lawin-O'Brien et al [91] 4 cases missing gestation at delivery
[b]Terminations of pregnancy (TOP) excluded

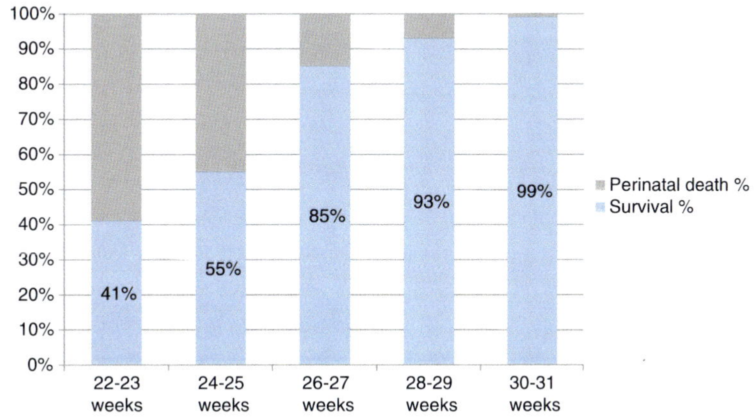

Fig. 1 Short term survival across gestation at diagnosis

focused on how to monitor and when to deliver FGR fetuses in order to optimize the perinatal outcomes.

Currently there are no evidence-based therapies for early onset FGR but over the last decades it has been suggested that other approaches, namely nitric oxide (NO), Sildenafil and maternal plasma volume expansion may play a role in prolonging pregnancies and reducing Doppler deterioration in FGR fetuses [103–106].

Early FGR is associated with hypertensive disorders of the pregnancy and preeclampsia in up to 73 and 52% of the cases respectively [3]. It is hypothesized that the syndrome of pre-eclampsia stems from a failure of placental implantation and development [107] which leads to a failure in physiologic increase of uterine perfusion during pregnancy. Nevertheless, uteroplacental insufficiency is also a widely acknowledged cause of FGR. In 2001 Parra et al [103] demonstrated that in pregnancies complicated by FGR NO production is impaired if compared to normal and hypertensive cases, whereas more recent data suggest an increased NO production in FGR fetuses [108]. It is uncertain how and why NO pathways are abnormal in FGR fetuses and, most importantly, no data have supported a significant improvement in perinatal outcomes in mothers treated with NO. On the other hand, some evidences have shown that in pregnancies complicated by hypertension and growth restriction the combined therapy consisting in plasma volume expansion with enriched physiological solution and NO donors can improve maternal hemodinamics, prolong the pregnancy and increase the birthweight [106].

Animal models of fetal growth restriction have demonstrated that the phosphodiesterase 5 inhibitor Sildenafil citrate increases birth weight and improves uteroplacental blood flow and there is also little evidence from a study done on humans that Sildenafil increases birthweight in pregnancies complicated by ealy-onset preeclampsia [109]. STRIDER is the acronim of an ongoing prospective individual participant data study which will add clinical information as to whether Sildenafil can be safely and effectively used in human pregnancies [104].

Last, but not least, studies conduced on sheep have shown that local treatment at the uteoplacental site with

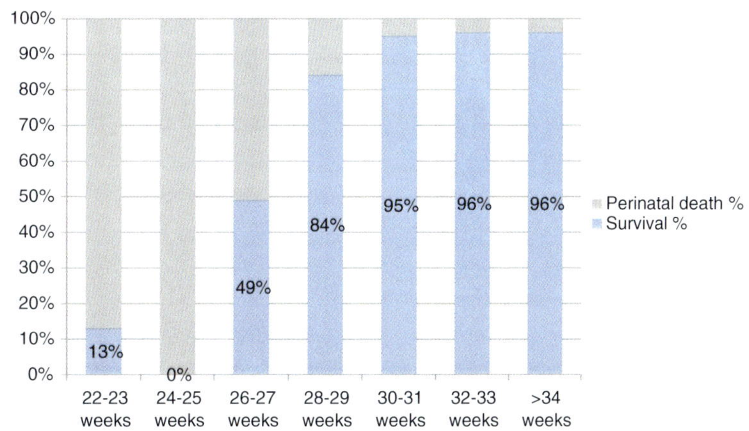

Fig. 2 Short term survival across gestation at delivery

the pro-angiogenetic factor VEGF-A improves fetal growth in growth restricted ewes [110, 111]. VEGF-A treatment was associated with a significant and long term (at least 4 weeks) increase in bloodflow and reduction in contractility of the uterine arteries in both pregnant and non pregnant animals [112]. These findings give hope that VEGF-A gene therapy can reverse the impaired uteroplacental perfusion which is associated with most cases of FGR even in humans, however further studies on both animal and human models are needed before any clinical application could be contemplated.

Conclusions

In summary, a conservative management focused on the identification of etiology in periviable growth restricted fetuses is recommended, as prognosis can vary widely despite similar ultrasound findings at diagnosis. Beyond 26 weeks the current evidence suggests that a detailed surveillance protocol integrating fetal ductus venosus Doppler and computerized CTG allows better outcomes and delivery only when one or both become abnormal.

Abbreviations

ACOG: American College of Obstetrician and Gynecologists; AEDF: Umbilical artery absent end diastolic flow; AFP: Alfa feto protein; AGA: Appropriate for gestational age; AoI: Aortic isthmus; AREDF: Umbilical absent or reverse end diastolic flow; BMI: Body mass index; BPP: Biophysical profile; CPR: Cerebro-placental ratio; CTG: Cardiotocography; C-U ratio: Cerebro-umbilical ratio; DV: Ductus venosus; EFW: Estimated fetal weight; FGR: Fetal growth restriction; FHR: Fetal heart rate; hCG: Human chorionic gonadotropin; MCA: Middle cerebral artery; MPI: Myocardial performance index; NO: Nitric oxide; PAPP-A: Pregnancy associated plasma protein-A; PI: Pulsatility index; RCOG: Royal College of Obstetricians and Gynecologists; RCT: Randomised controlled trial; REDF: Umbilical artery reverse end diastolic flow; SGA: Small for gestational age; STV: Short term variability; VEGF-A: Vascular-endotelial growth factor-A

Acknowledgements

CCL is supported by the National Institute for Health Research (NIHR) Biomedical Research Centre based at Imperial College Healthcare NHS Trust and Imperial College London.

Funding

No financial support was received for this study.

Authors' contributions

ADA and VB wrote the main text. FP and TF supervised Dr ADA and Dr VB work. CCL: comments and final review. All authors read and approved the final manuscript.

Authors' information

ADA has recently completed his Specialty Training in Obstetrics and Gynecology at the University of Parma (head Prof Tiziana Frusca) and is currently PhD Student at the same University and Clinical Fellow in Fetal Medicine at the Centre for Fetal Care, Queen Charlotte's and Chelsea Hospital (Lead Dr C Lees). His main interests have focused on prenatal diagnosis and management of fetal growth restriction.
VB has recently completed her Specialty Training in Obstetrics and Gynecology at the University of Brescia. Her main clinical interest has focused on maternal-fetal medicine.
CCL, TF and FP are Senior Consultants in Maternal-Fetal Medicine. They all have taken part in the TRUFFLE Study, which is currently the largest available randomized controlled trial on diagnosis, management and prognosis of severe early fetal growth restriction.

Competing interests

The authors declare that they have no competing interests.

Author details

[1]Centre for Fetal Care, Queen Charlotte's and Chelsea Hospital, Imperial College Healthcare NHS Trust, Du Cane Road, London W12 0HS, United Kingdom. [2]Department of Obstetrics & Gynecology, University of Parma, Parma, Italy. [3]Department of Obstetrics and Gynaecology, Maternal-Fetal Medicine Unit, University of Brescia, Brescia, Italy. [4]Department of Surgery and Cancer, Imperial College London, London, United Kingdom.
[5]Department of Development and Regeneration, KU, Leuven, Belgium.

References

1. Alberry M, Soothill P. Management of fetal growth restriction. Arch Dis Child Fetal Neonatal Ed. 2007;92:62–7.
2. Damodaram M, Story L, Kulinskaya E, Rutherford M, Kumar S. Early adverse perinatal complications in preterm growth-restrcited fetuses. Aust N Z J Obstet Gynaecol. 2011;51:204–9.
3. Lees C, Marlow N, Arabin B, Bilardo CM, Brezinka C, Derks JB, et al. Perinatal morbidity and mortality in early-onset fetal growth restriction: cohort outcomes of the trial of randomized umbilical and fetal flow in Europe (TRUFFLE). Ultrasound Obstet Gynecol. 2013;42:400–8.
4. Gardosi J, Chang A, Kalyan B, Sahota D, Symonds EM. Customised antenatal growth charts. Lancet. 1992;339:283–7.
5. Gardosi J, Giddings S, Buller S, Southam M, Williams M. Preventing stillbirths through improved antenatal recognition of pregnancies at risk due to fetal growth restriction. Public Health. 2014;128:698–702.
6. Unterscheider J, Daly S, Geary MP, Kennelly MM, McAuliffe FM, O'Donoghue K, Hunter A, Morrison JJ, Burke G, Dicker P, Tully EC, Malone FD. Optmizing the definition of intrauterine growth restriction: the multicenter prospective PORTO Study. Am J Obstet Gynecol. 2013;208(4):290. e1-290 e6.
7. Vasak B, Koenen SV, Koster MP, Hukkelhoven CW, Franx A, Hanson MA, Visser GH. Human fetal growth is constrained below optimal for perinatal survival. Ultrasound Obstet Gynecol. 2015;45:162–7.
8. Mcintire DD, Bloom SL, Casey BM, Leveno KJ. Birth weight in relation to morbildity and mortality among newborn infants. N Engl J Med. 1999; 340:1234–8.
9. Jones RA, Robertson NR. Problems of the small for dates baby. Clin Obstet Gynaecol. 1984;11:499–524.
10. Alkalay AL, Graham JM, Pomerance JJ. Evaluation of neonates born with intrauterine growth retardation: review and practice guidelines. J Perinatol. 1998;18:142–51.
11. Yanney M, Marlow N. Paediatric consequences of fetal growth restriction. Semin Fetal Neonatal Med. 2004;9:411–8.
12. Marlow N, Wolke D, Bracewell MA, Samara M, The Epicure Study Group. Neurologic and developmental disability at six years of age after extremely preterm birth. N Engl J Med. 2005;352:9–19.
13. Walker DM, Marlow N. Neurocognitive outcome following fetal growth restriction. Arch Dis Child Fetal Neonatal Ed. 2008;93:322–5.
14. Low J, Handley M, Burke S, et al. Association of intrauterine growth retardation and learning deficits at age 9 to it years. AJOG. 1992;162:1499.
15. Robertson CT, Etches PC, Kyle M. Eight years school performance and growth of preterm, small for gestational age infants: a comparative study with subjects matched for birth weight or for gestational age. J Pediatrics. 1990;116:19.
16. Tideman E, Marsal K, Ley D. Cognitive function in young adults following intrauterine growth restriction with abnormal fetal aortic blood flow. Ultrasound Obstet Gynecol. 2007;29:614–8.

17. Barker DJ, Osmond C, Golding J, Kuh D, Wadsworth ME. Growth in utero, blood pressure in childhood and adult life, and mortality from cardiovascular disease. BMJ. 1989;298:564–7.
18. Barker DJ. Fetal origins of coronary heart disease. BMJ. 1995;311:171–4.
19. Tintu A, Rouwet E, Verlohren S, Brinkmann J, Ahamd S, Crispi F, van Bilsen M, Carmeliet P, Staff AC, TJwa M, Cetin I, Gratacos E, Hernandez-Andrade E, Hofstra L, Jacobs M, Lamers WH, Morano I, Safak E, Ahmed A, le Noble F. Hypoxia induces dilated cardiomyopathy in the chick embryo: mechanism, intervention, and long-term consequences. PLoS One. 2009;4:e5155.
20. Kiserud T, Kessler J, Ebbing C, Rasmussen S. Ductus venosus shunting in growth-restricted foetuses and the effect of umbilical circulatory compromise. Ultrasound Obstet Gynecol. 2006;28:143–9.
21. Leon DA, Lithell HO, Vagero D, Koupilova I, Mohsen R, Berglund L, Lithell UB, McKeigue PM. Reduced fetal growth rate and increased risk of death from ischemic heart disease: cohort study of 15,000 Swedish men and women born 1915-29. BMJ. 1998;317:241–5.
22. Rich-Edwards JW, Stampfer MJ, Manson JE, Rosner B, Hankinson SE, Colditz GA, Willet WC, Hennekens CH. Birth weight and risk of cardiovascular disease in a cohort of women followed up since 1976. BMJ. 1997;315:369–400.
23. Villar J, Altman DG, Purwar M, Noble JA, Knight HE, Ruyan P, Cheikh Ismail L, Barros FC, Lambert A, Papageorghiou AT, Carvalho M, Jaffer YA, Bertino E, Gravett MG, Bhutta SH K, the International Fetal and Newborn Growth Consortium for the 21st century (INTERGROWTH-21ST). The objectives, design and implementation of the INTERGROWTH-21ST Project. BJOG. 2013;120 Suppl 2:9–26.
24. Sibai BM, Abdella TN, Anderson GD. Pregnancy outcome in 211 patients with mild chronic hypertension. Obstet Gynecol. 1983;61(5):571–6.
25. McCowan L, Horgan RP. Risk factors for small for gestationalage infants. Best Pract Res Clin Obstet Gynaecol. 2009;23:779–93.
26. Langer O, Levy J, Brustman L, Anyaegbunam A, Merkatz R, Divon M. Glycemic control in gestational diabetes mellitus–how tight is tight enough: small for gestational age versus large for gestational age? Am J Obstet Gynecol. 1989; 161(3):646–53.
27. Alfirevic Z, Roberts D, Martlew V. How strong is the association between maternal thrombophilia and adverse pregnancy outcome? A systematic review. Eur J Obstet Gynecol Reprod Biol. 2002;101(1):6–14.
28. Odibo AO, Nelson D, Stamilio DM, Sehdev HM, Macones GA. Advanced maternal age is an independent risk factor for intrauterine growth restriction. Am J Perinatol. 2006;23:325–8.
29. Kramer MS. Determinants of low birth weight: methodological assessment and meta–analysis. Bull World Health Organ. 1987;65:663–737.
30. Alexander GR, Wingate MS, Mor J, Boulet S. Birth outcomes of Asian–Indian–americans. Int J Gynaecol Obstet. 2007;97:215–20.
31. Shah PS. Knowledge Synthesis Group on Determinants of 45. LBW/PT Births. Parity and low birth weight and pre–termbirth: a systematic review and meta–analyses. Acta Obstet. Gynecol Scand. 2010;89:862–75.
32. Blumenshine P, Egarter S, Barclay CJ, Cubbin C, Braveman PA. Socioeconomic disparities in adverse birth outcomes: a systematic review. Am J Prev Med. 2010;39:263–72.
33. Han Z, Mulla S, Beyene J, Liao G, McDonald SD, Knowledge Synthesis Group. Maternal underweight and the risk of preterm birth and low birth weight: a systematic review and meta–analyses. Int J Epidemiol. 2011;40:65–101.
34. Jaddoe VW, Bakker R, Hofman A, Mackenbach JP, Moll HA, Steegers EA, et al. Moderate alcohol consumption during pregnancy and the risk of low birth weight and preterm birth. The generation R study. Ann Epidemiol. 2007;17:834–40.
35. Gouin K, Murphy K, Shah PS. Knowledge Synthesis Group on Determinants of LBW/PT Births. Effects of cocaine use during pregnancy on low birthweight and preterm birth: systematic review and metaanalyses. Am J Obstet Gynecol. 2011;204(340):1–12.
36. McCowan LM, Dekker GA, Chan E, Stewart A, Chappell LC, Hunter M, et al. Spontaneous preterm birth and small for gestational age infants in women who stop smoking early in pregnancy: prospective cohort study. BMJ. 2009; 338:b1081.
37. Jackson RA, Gibson KA, Croughan MS, Wu YW. Perinatal outcomes in singletons following in vitro fertilization: a meta- analysis. Obstet Gynecol. 2004;103:551–63.
38. Boers KE, Vijgen SM, Bijlenga D, van der Post JA, Bekedam DJ, Kwee A, van der Salm PC, van Pampus MG, Spaanderman ME, de Boer K, Duvekot JJ, Bremer HA, Hasaart TH, Delemarre FM, Bloemenkamp KW, van Meir CA, Willekes C, Wijnen EJ, Rijken M, le Cessie S, Roumen FJ, Thornton JG, van Lith JM, Mol BW, Scherjon SA, DIGITAT study group. Induction versus expectant monitoring for intrauterine growth restriction at term: randomised equivalence trial(DIGITAT). BMJ. 2010;341:c7087.
39. Lausman A, Kingdom J, Maternal Fetal Medicine Committee, Gagnon R, Basso M, Bos H, Crane J, Davies G, Delisle MF, Hudon L, Menticoglou S, Mundle W, Ouellet A, Pressey T, Pylypjuk C, Roggensack A, Sanderson F. Intrauterine growth restriction: screening, diagnosis and management. J Obstet Gynaecol Can. 2013;35(8):741–57.
40. American College of Obstetricians and Gynecologists. ACOG Practice bulletin no. 134: fetal growth restriction. Obstet Gynecol. 2013;121:1122–33.
41. RCOG Green Top Guidline No.31. The Investigation and Management of the Small-for-Gestational Age Fetus. January 2014.
42. Growth restriction in Oski's paediatrics. McMillan JAF, DeAngelis CD, Jones MD, editors. Principles and practice. Philadelphia: Lippincot Williams and Wilkins,2006.
43. Gordijn SJ, Beune IM, Thilaganathan B, Papageorghiou A, Baschat AA, Baker PN, Silver RM, Wynia K, Ganzevoort W. Consensus definition of fetal growth restriction: a Delphi procedure. Ultrasound Obstet Gynecol. 2016;48(3):333–9.
44. Turan S, Miller J, Baschat AA. Integrated testing and management in fetal growth restriction. Semin Perinatol. 2008;32:194–2000.
45. Baschat AA. Fetal growth restriction – from observation to intervention. J Perinat Med. 2010;38:239–46.
46. Savchev S, Figueras F, Sanz-Cortes M, Cruz-Lemini M, Triunfo S, Botet F, Gratacos E. Evaluation of an optimal gestational age cut-off for the definition of early- and late-onset fetal growth restriction. Fetal Diagn Ther. 2014;36(2):99–105.
47. Crovetto F, Crispi F, Scazzocchio E, Mercade I, Meler E, Figueras F, Gratacos E. Performance of first-trimester integrated screening for early and late small for gestational age newborns. Ultrasound Obstet Gynecol 2013 (E-pub ahead of print).
48. Hadlock FP, Harrist RB, Sharman RS, Deter RL, Park SK. Estimation of fetal weight with the use of head, body, and femur measurements-a prospective study. Am J Obstet Gynecol. 1985;151:333–7.
49. Brenner WE, Edeman DA, Hendrincks CH. A standard of fetal growth for the United States of America. Am J Obstet Gynecol. 1976;126:555–64.
50. Zhang J, Bowes Jr WA. Birth-weight-for gestational-age patterns by race, sex, and parity in the United States population. Obstet Gynecol. 1995;86:200–8.
51. Gardosi J, Mongelli M, Wilcox M, Chang A. An adjustable fetal weight standard. Ultrasound Obstet Gynecol. 1995;6:168–74.
52. Resnik R. to customize or not to customize: that is the question. Paediatr Perinat Epidemiol. 2011;25:17–9.
53. Baschat AA, Weiner CP. Umbilical artery Doppler screening for detection of the small fetus in need of antepartum surveillance. Am J Obstet Gynecol. 2000;182:154–8.
54. Baschat AA. Neurodevelopment after Fetal Growth Restriction. Fetal Diagn Ther. 2014;36:136–42.
55. Cnossen JS, Morris RK, ter Riet G, Mol BW, van der Post JA, Coomarasamy A, et al. Use of uterine artery Doppler ultrasonography to predict pre-eclampsia and intrauterine growth restriction: a systematic review and bivariate meta–analysis. CMAJ. 2008;178:701–11.
56. Maulik D, Frances Evans J, Ragolia L. Fetal growth restriction: pathogenic mechanisms. Clin Obstet Gynecol. 2006;49:219–27.
57. Pilalis A, Souka AP, Antsaklis P, Daskalakis G, Papantoniou N, Mesogitis S, et al. Screening for pre-eclampsia and fetal growth 80. restriction by uterine artery Doppler and PAPP–A at 11–14weeks gestation. Ultrasound Obstet Gynecol. 2007;29:135–40.
58. Filippi E, Staughton J, Peregrine E, Jones P, Huttly W, Peebles DM, et al. Uterine artery Doppler and adverse pregnancy outcome in women with extreme levels of fetoplacental proteins used for Down syndrome screening. Ultrasound Obstet Gynecol. 2011;37:520–7.
59. Dane B, Dane C, Kiray M, Cetin A, Koldas M, Erginbas M. Correlation between first–trimester maternal serum markers second trimester uterine artery doppler indices and pregnancy outcome. Gynecol Obstet Invest. 2010;70:126–31.
60. Costa SL, Proctor L, Dodd JM, Toal M, Okun N, Johnson JA, et al. 83. Screening for placental insufficiency in high risk pregnancies:Is earlier better? Placenta. 2008;29:1034–40.
61. Harman CR, Baschat AA. Comprehensive assessment of fetal wellbeing: which Doppler tests should be performed? Curr Opin Obstet Gynecol. 2003; 15:147–57.
62. Talmor A, Daemen A, Murdoch E, Missfelder-Lobos H, Timmerman D, Bourne T, Giussani DA, Lees C. Defining the relationship between fetal

Doppler indices, abdominal circumference and growth rate in severe fetal growth restriction using functional linear discriminant analysis. J R Soc Interface. 2013;10(88):20130376.
63. Flood K, Unterscheider J, Daly S, Geary MP, Kennelly MM, McAuliffe FM, O'Donoghue K, Hunter A, Morrison JJ, Burke G, Dicker P, Tully EC, Malone FD. The role of brain sparing in the prediction of adverse outcomes in intrauterine growth restriction: results of the multicenter PORTO study. Am J Obstet Gynecol. 2014;211:288. e1-5.
64. Figueras F, Gratacos E. Update on the Diagnosis and Classification of Fetal Growth Restriction and Proposal of a Stage-Based Management Protocol. Fetal Diagn Ther. 2014;36:86–98.
65. Alfirevic Z, Stampalija T, Gyte GM. Fetal and umbilical Doppler ultrasound in high-risk pregnancies. Cochrane Database Syst Rev. 2013;11:CD007529.
66. Arduini D, Rizzo G, Romanini C. The development of abnormal heart rate pattern after absent end diastolic velocity in umbilical artery: analysis of risk factors. Am J Obstet Gynecol. 1993;168:43.
67. Brar H, Platt L. Reverse end diastolic flow velocity on umbilical artery velocimetry in high pregnancies: an ominous finding with adverse pregnancy outcome. Am J Obstet Gynecol. 1988;159:559.
68. Valcamonico A, Danti L, Frusca T, Soregaroli M, Zucca S, Abrami F, Tiberti A. Absent end diastolic velocity in umbilical artery: risk of neonatal morbidity and brain damage. Am J Obstet Gynecol. 1994;170:796.
69. Eixarch E, et al. Neurodevelopmental outcome in 2-year-old infants who were small-for-gestational age term fetuses with cerebral blood flow redistribution. Ultrasound Obstet Gynecol. 2008;32(7):894–9.
70. Hershkovitz R, et al. Fetal cerebral blood flow redistribution in late gestation: identification of compromise in small fetuses with normal umbilical artery Doppler. Ultrasound Obstet Gynecol. 2000;15(3):209–12.
71. Cruz-Martinez R, et al. Longitudinal brain perfusion changes in near-term small-for-gestational-age fetuses as measured by spectral Doppler indices or by fractional moving blood volume. Am J Obstet Gynecol. 2010;203(1):42. e1-e6.
72. Figueras F, Savchev S, Triunfo S, Crovetto F, Gratacos E. An integrated model with classification criteria to predict small-for-gestational-age fetuses at risk of adverse perinatal outcome. Ultrasound Obstet Gynecol. 2015;45(3):279–85.
73. Parra-Saavedra M, Crovetto F, Triunfo S, Savchev S, Peguero A, Nadal A, Gratacós E, Figueras F. Association of Doppler parameters with placental signs of underperfusion in late-onset small-for-gestational-age pregnancies. Ultrasound Obstet Gynecol. 2014;44(3):330–7.
74. Ferrazzi E, Bozzo M, Rigano S, Bellotti M, Morabito A, Pardi G, Battaglia FC, Galan HL. Temporal sequence of abnormal Doppler changes in the peripheral and central circulatory systems of the severely growth-restricted fetus. Ultrasound Obstet Gynecol. 2002;19:140–6.
75. Cosmi E, et al. Doppler, cardiotocography, and biophysical profile changes in growth-restricted fetuses. Obstet Gynecol. 2005;106(6):1240–5.
76. Hecher K, Bilardo CM, Stigter RH, Ville Y, Hackelöer BJ, Kok HJ, Senat MV, Visser GHA. Monitoring of fetuses with intrauterine growth restriction: a longitudinal study. Ultrasound Obs Gyn. 2001;18:564–70.
77. Baschat AA, Gembruch U, Harmann CR. The sequence of changes in Doppler and biophysical parameters as severe fetal growth restriction worsens. Ultrasound Obstet Gynecol. 2001;18(6):571–7.
78. Francisco RPV, Miyadahira S, Zugaib M. Predicting pH at birth in absent or reversed end-diastolic velocity in the umbilical arteries. Obstet Gynecol. 2006;107:1042–8.
79. Schwarze A, et al. Qualitative venous Doppler flow waveform analysis in preterm intrauterine growth-restricted fetuses with ARED flow in the umbilical artery-correlation with short-term outcome. Ultrasound Obstet Gynecol. 2005;25(6):573–9.
80. Bilardo CM, Wolf H, Stigter RH, Ville Y, Baez E, Visser GHA, Hecher K. Relationship between monitoring parameters and perinatal outcome in severe, early intrauterine growth restriction. Ultrasound Obstet Gynecol. 2004;23:119–25.
81. Rizzo G, Arduini D, Romanini C, et al. Doppler echocardiographic assessment of atrioventricular velocity waveforms in normal and small for gestational age fetuses. Br J Obst Gynaecol. 1988;95:65.
82. Rizzo G, Arduini D, Romanini C, et al. Doppler echocardiographic evaluation of time to peak velocity in the aorta and pulmonary artery of small for gestational age fetuses. Br J Obst Gynaecol. 1990;97:603.
83. Del Río M, Martínez JM, Figueras F, Bennasar M, Olivella A, Palacio M, Coll O, Puerto B, Gratacós E. Doppler assessment of the aortic isthmus and perinatal outcome in preterm fetuses with severe intrauterine growth restriction. Ultrasound Obstet Gynecol. 2008;31(1):41–7.
84. Fouron JC, Gosseli J, Raboisson MJ, Lamoureux J, Tison CA, Fouron C, Hudon L. The relationship between an aortic isthmus blood flow velocity and the postnatal neurodevelopmental status of fetuses with placental circulatory insufficiency. AJOG. 2005;192:497–503.
85. Cruz-Martinez R, Figueras F, Benavides-Serralde A, Crispi F, Hernandez-Andrade E, Gratacos E. Sequence of changes in myocardial performance index in relation to aortic isthmus and ductus venosus Doppler in fetuses with early-onset intrauterine growth restriction. Ultrasound Obstet Gynecol. 2011;38(2):179–84.
86. Hassan WA, Brockelsby J, Alberry M, Fanelli T, Wladimiroff J, Lees CC. Cardiac function in early onset small for gestational age and growth restricted fetuses. Eur J Obstet Gynecol Reprod Biol. 2013;171(2):262–5.
87. Lees CC, Marlow N, van Wassenaer-Leemhuis A, Arabin B, Bilardo CM, Brezinka C, Calvert S, Derks JB, Diemert A, Duvekot JJ, Ferrazzi E, Frusca T, Ganzevoort W, Hecher K, Martinelli P, Ostermayer E, Papageorghiou AT, Schlembach D, Schneider KT, Thilaganathan B, Todros T, Valcamonico A, Visser GH, Wolf H, TRUFFLE study group. 2 year neurodevelopmental and intermediate perinatal outcomes in infants with very preterm fetal growth restriction (TRUFFLE): a randomised trial. Lancet. 2015;385(9983):2162–72.
88. GRIT Study Group. A randomised trial of timed delivery for the compromised preterm fetus: short term outcomes and Bayesian interpretation. BJOG. 2003; 110(1):27–32.
89. Savchev S, Figueras F, Cruz-Martinez R, Illa M, Botet F, Gratacos E. Estimated weight centile as a predictor of perinatal outcome in small-for gestational-age pregnancies with normal fetal and maternal Doppler indices. Ultrasound Obstet Gynecol. 2012;39:299–303.
90. Raju TN, Mercer BM, Burchfield DJ, Joseph Jr GF. Periviable birth: executive summary of a joint workshop by the Eunice Kennedy Shriver National Institute of Child Health and Human Development, Society for Maternal-Fetal Medicine, American Academy of Pediatrics, and American College of Obstetricians and Gynecologists. Obstet Gynecol. 2014;123(5):1083–96.
91. Lawin-O'Brien AR, Dall'Asta A, Knight C, Sankaran S, Scala C, Khalil A, Bhide A, Heggarty S, Rakow A, Pasupathy D, Papageorghiou AT, Lees CC. Short-term outcome of periviable small-for-gestational-age babies: is our counseling up to date? Ultrasound Obstet Gynecol. 2016;48(5):636–41.
92. Visser GH, Bilardo CM, Lees C. Fetal growth restriction at the limits of viability. Fetal Diagn Ther. 2014;36(2):162–5.
93. DeVore GR. The importance of the cerebroplacental ratio in the evaluation of fetal well-being in SGA and AGA fetuses. Am J Obstet Gynecol. 2015;213(1):5–15.
94. Figueras F, Gratacos E. Stage-based approach to the management of fetal growth restriction. Prenat Diagn. 2014;34:655–9.
95. Alfirevic Z, Neilson JP. Doppler ultrasonography in high-risk pregnancies: Systematic review with meta-analysis. Am J Obstet Gynecol. 1995;172(5):1379–87.
96. Grivell RM, Wong L, Bhatia V. Regimens of fetal surveillance for impaired fetal growth. Cochrane Database Syst Rev. 2012;6:CD007113.
97. Severi FM, Bocchi C, Visentin A, Falco P, Cobellis L, Florio P, Zagonari S, Pilu G. Uterine and fetal cerebral Doppler predict the outcome of third-trimester small-for-gestational age fetuses with normal umbilical artery Doppler. Ultrasound Obstet Gynecol. 2002;19:225–8.
98. Ghosh GS, Gudmundsson S. Uterine and umbilical artery Doppler are comparable in predicting perinatal outcome of growth-restricted fetuses. BJOG. 2009;116:424–30.
99. Vergani P, Roncaglia N, Andreotti C, Arreghini A, Teruzzi M, Pezzullo JC, Ghidini A. Prognostic value of uterine artery Doppler velocimetry in growth-restricted fetuses delivered near term. Am J Obstet Gynecol. 2002;187:932–6.
100. Thornton JG, Hornbuckle J, Vail A, Spiegelhalter DJ, Levene M, GRIT study group. Infant wellbeing at 2 years of age in the Growth Restriction Intervention Trial (GRIT): multicentred randomised controlled trial. Lancet. 2004;364(9433):513–20.
101. Baschat AA, Cosmi E, Bilardo CM, Wolf H, Berg C, Rigano S, Germer U, Moyano D, Turan S, Hartung J, Bhide A, Muller T, Bower S, Nicolaides KH, Thilaganathan B, Gembruch U, Ferrazzi E, Hecher K, Galan HL, Harman CR. Predictors of neonatal outcome in early-onset placental dysfunction. Obstet Gynecol. 2007;109:253–61.
102. Story L, Sankaran S, Mullins E, Tan S, Russell G, Kumar S, Kyle P. Survival of pregnancies with small for gestational age detected before 24 weeks gestation. Eur J Obstet Gynecol Reprod Biol. 2015;188:100–3.
103. Parra MC, Lees C, Mann GE, Pearson JD, Nicolaides KH. Vasoactive mediator release by fetal endothelial cells in intrauterine growth restriction and preeclampsia. Am J Obstet Gynecol. 2001;184(3):497–502.

104. Ganzevoort W, Alfirevic Z, von Dadelszen P, Kenny L, Papageorghiou A, van Wassenaer-Leemhuis A, Gluud C, Mol BW, Baker PN. STRIDER: Sildenafil Therapy In Dismal prognosis Early-onset intrauterine growth Restriction–a protocol for a systematic review with individual participant data and aggregate data meta-analysis and trial sequential analysis. Syst Rev. 2014;3:23.
105. Vasapollo B, Valensise H, Novelli GP, Altomare F, Galante A, Arduini D. Abnormal maternal cardiac function precedes the clinical manifestation of fetal growth restriction. Ultrasound Obstet Gynecol. 2004;24(1):23–9.
106. Valensise H, Vasapollo B, Novelli GP, Giorgi G, Verallo P, Galante A, Arduini D. Maternal and fetal hemodynamic effects induced by nitric oxide donors and plasma volume expansion in pregnancies with gestational hypertension complicated by intrauterine growth restriction with absent end-diastolic flow in the umbilical artery. Ultrasound Obstet Gynecol. 2008;31(1):55–64.
107. Lees C, Valensise H, Black R, Harrington K, Byiers S, Romanini C, Campbell S. The efficacy and fetal-maternal cardiovascular effects of transdermal glyceryl trinitrate in the prophylaxis of pre-eclampsia and its complications: a randomized double-blind placebo-controlled trial. Ultrasound Obstet Gynecol. 1998;12(5):334–8.
108. Pisaneschi S, Strigini FA, Sanchez AM, Begliuomini S, Casarosa E, Ripoli A, Ghirri P, Boldrini A, Fink B, Genazzani AR, Coceani F, Simoncini T. Compensatory feto-placental upregulation of the nitric oxide system during fetal growth restriction. PLoS One. 2012;7(9):e45294.
109. Samangaya RA, Mires G, Shennan A, Skillern L, Howe D, McLeod A, Baker PN. A randomised, double-blinded, placebo-controlled study of the phosphodiesterase type 5 inhibitor sildenafil for the treatment of preeclampsia. Hypertens Pregnancy. 2009;28(4):369–82.
110. Eremia SC, de Boo HA, Bloomfield FH, Oliver MH, Harding JE. Fetal and amniotic insulin-like growth factor-I supplements improve growth rate in intrauterine growth restriction fetal sheep. Endocrinology. 2007;148:2963–72.
111. David AL, Torondel B, Zachary I, Wigley V, Abi-Nader K, Mehta V, et al. Local delivery of VEGF adenovirus to the uterine artery increases vasorelaxation and uterine blood flow in the pregnant sheep. Gene Ther. 2008;15:1344–50.
112. Mehta V, Abi-Nader KN, Peebles DM, Benjamin E, Wigley V, Torondel B, Filippi E, Shaw SW, Boyd M, Martin J, Zachary I, David AL. Long-term increase in uterine blood flow is achieved by local overexpression of VEGF-A(165) in the uterine arteries of pregnant sheep. Gene Ther. 2012;19(9):925–35.

A review of selected Arboviruses during pregnancy

Penélope Saldanha Marinho[1,4*], Antonio José Cunha[2], Joffre Amim Junior[1,2] and Arnaldo Prata-Barbosa[2,3]

Abstract

Arboviruses are emerging infectious diseases with the ability to expand geographically and rapidly affect large populations. The recent epidemic caused by the Zika virus in the Americas and congenital Zika syndrome associated with maternal infection has called out attention to the importance of studying arboviruses during pregnancy.

This is a review on selected arboviruses infections during gestation, including Zika, Chikungunya, Dengue and Yellow Fever viruses. Issues such as historical overview, pathogenesis, transmission, clinical conditions, diagnosis, treatment and prevention are addressed.

Keywords: Arboviruses, Pregnancy, Dengue, Zika, Chikungunya, Yellow fever, Review

Background

Arboviruses are emerging infectious diseases which have gained importance in the last 50 years due to their ability to expand geographically and rapidly affect large populations. The spread of these diseases in the human population occurs through the introduction of the pathogen into the environment, associated with other factors such as ecological changes and human behavior. As the mosquito vectors breed in standing water, events like heavy rain with flooding and construction of dams are associated with the emergence of infections by arboviruses. In addition, urbanization, migration and international travel are also contributing factors to the transmission of these disease [1, 2].

Recently, the epidemic caused by the Zika virus in the Americas has led the World Health Organization to declare a state of international emergency, providing global visibility to the issue, which has become a public health priority.

The present study consists in a review on arboviruses during gestation, addressing infections caused by the Zika, Chikungunya, Dengue and Yellow Fever viruses.

* Correspondence: penelope@me.ufrj.br
[1]Maternidade Escola da Universidade Federal do Rio de Janeiro, Rio de Janeiro, RJ, Brazil
[4]Rua das Laranjeiras, 180 – Laranjeiras, Rio de Janeiro CEP: 22240-003, RJ, Brazil
Full list of author information is available at the end of the article

History of arboviruses

Arboviruses are thus designated since they are viruses essentially transmitted by arthropods, predominantly mosquitoes. At least 135 types of arboviruses are capable of causing human infection, with the vast majority being RNA viruses [3].

Zika

The Zika virus was initially isolated in 1947 from Rhesus monkey blood during epidemiological studies on Yellow Fever in the Zika Forest, in Uganda [4]. This virus was first isolated in humans in 1954, in Nigeria [5] and, in 1969, it was identified outside the African continent, in Malaysia, in the *Aedes aegypti* mosquito [6]. Throughout the following years, until 2007, the Zika virus was known to causes sporadic infections in both Africa and Asia.

The first recognized major outbreak occurred on Yap Island, Micronesia, in 2007 [7], followed by a major outbreak from October 2013 to March 2014 in French Polynesia [8, 9].

In 2015, the Zika virus reached the Americas, and was initially identified in Brazil, where a phylogenetic analysis indicated it was the Asian strain of the virus [10]. According to the Pan American Health Organization report of July 2017, cases of autochthonous transmission have been reported at least in 50 other countries or territories of the American continent, totaling more than 200,000 confirmed cases, with approximately 3300 cases of congenital syndrome associated with the Zika infection [11].

Chikungunya

The Chikungunya virus was reported for the first time in Tanzania in 1952. After the first epidemic, the virus became endemic in Africa. It reached Asia in 1958 and was responsible for several outbreaks in subsequent years [12].

The virus remained restricted to the African and Asian continents until 2013, when it was introduced in the Latin Caribbean and established the first human cycle in the Americas [13]. Subsequently, cases of autochthonous transmission were reported in South and Central America and in Florida, United States of America [14].

In September 2014, the first autochthonous case was confirmed in Brazil, in the northern region. After 7 days, new cases were identified in the northeastern region and, in just 1 month, the Ministry of Health of Brazil had already confirmed 682 cases of this virus infection [15].

Dengue

Although numerous epidemics with Dengue-like characteristics have been described for centuries, the Dengue virus was first isolated in 1943 in Japan (DENV1) and in 1945 in Hawaii (DENV2) [16].

The spread of its vector, the *Aedes aegypti* mosquito, created an environment conducive to the virus transmission, which reached a pandemic status after World War II [17].

In the Americas, Dengue was controlled through a campaign conducted by the Pan American Health Organization in 1947 to eliminate mosquitoes. However, in the 1970s, the region was reinfested and, since then, the incidence of the disease has increased in the Americas, as well as in other regions [18].

Yellow fever

Yellow Fever originated in Africa and was brought to the Americas in the seventeenth century as a consequence of the slave trade, and was responsible for the deaths of thousands of people in the 18th and 19th centuries. In 1900, transmission was confirmed through the *Aedes aegypti* mosquito and, in the 1930s, two live attenuated virus vaccines were developed. The combination of extensive vaccination campaigns and vector control significantly reduced the number of cases of this disease [19].

Over the years, outbreaks in Africa and South and Central America continued to occur [20]. In December 2015, an urban Yellow Fever epidemic occurred in Angola and expanded to other locations, and in 2017, an outbreak of the disease affected the Brazilian states of Minas Gerais, Espírito Santo, São Paulo and Rio de Janeiro [21].

Pathogenesis and transmission

Mechanical transmission

The Zika, Dengue and Yellow Fever viruses belong to the Flaviviridae family and Flavivirus genus, while the Chikungunya virus belongs to the Togaviridae family and Alphavirus genus. All are transmitted in the urban cycle, mainly by mosquito species *A. aegypti* and *A. alpobictus*.

Arboviruses display a transmission cycle between the mosquito and the human host, with periods of both extrinsic and intrinsic incubation. Extrinsic incubation refers to the period that elapses between the vector infection until the virus spreads to the mosquito's saliva, which then infects the new host. The intrinsic incubation period refers to the time interval between inoculation in the human host until the virus reaches the bloodstream.

The pathogenesis of arboviruses still remains unknown in several respects, but it is recognized that, upon primary inoculation, viral particles infect target cells such as fibroblasts, monocyte, dendritic cells and host endothelial cells. The viruses then replicate, reaching the regional lymph nodes, and, subsequently, the bloodstream [22].

Sexual transmission and blood transfusion

Sexual transmission of the Dengue, Chikungunya or Yellow Fever viruses has not been described. However, transmission of the Zika virus through infected semen has already been well established [23]. In addition, regarding the identification of virus RNA in semen, which may persist for more than 60 days after the onset of the symptoms [24], some studies have confirmed the disease in people who have not been in endemic areas but who have had sexual contact with infected persons.

A review of a study of sexually active women of Rio de Janeiro highlights the contribution of sexual transmission of the Zika virus. Women between the ages of 15 and 65 presented 90% more cases recorded in 100,000 women than men of the same age group. This was not repeated in groups <15 years and > 65 years [25].

Arboviruses can also be transmitted by blood transfusion or transplantation of organs or tissues from infected and asymptomatic donors at the time of donation. In the case of Yellow Fever, transmission is also possible during the viremia period after donor vaccination [26–30].

Maternal-fetal transmission

The occurrence of arboviruses during pregnancy is of additional concern, due to the possibility of vertical transmission and fetal involvement. In 2015, a significant increase in the number of newborns diagnosed with microcephaly in several regions of Brazil presenting a high incidence of Zika virus was observed. Maternal-fetal transmission of the virus was verified during all gestation stages [31–34].

Torres et al. found a vertical transmission rate for the Chikungunya virus ranging from 27.7 to 48.29%, occurring more frequently when maternal viremia coincided with the time of birth. However, the birth route showed no relation to the incidence of congenital disease [35].

Infection of pregnant women with the Dengue virus is associated with the risk of miscarriage, fetal death, prematurity and vertical transmission. Although gestation is considered a risk factor for the clinical course of the disease, no association was found between the severity of the maternal infection and neonatal disease [36, 37].

Few studies on yellow fever are available, but perinatal transmission of the disease has been described [38].

Clinical conditions

The clinical presentation of these arboviruses during pregnancy is supposed to be similar to the general population. However, there is a lack of studies specifically addressing pregnant women.

Zika

The incubation period of this disease is of 4 to 5 days. The most frequently reported symptoms are a rash, fever, arthritis or arthralgia, and conjunctivitis. Other symptoms include myalgia, headache, retro-orbital pain, edema and vomiting. It is estimated that only 20% of the people infected with the Zika virus manifest symptoms [39].

In a cohort of pregnant women in Rio de Janeiro, where exanthema was used as the inclusion criterion, in addition to macular or maculopapular exanthema in 100% of the cases, the following symptoms were also observed: pruritus (90%), arthralgia (62%), conjunctivitis (58%), fatigue and malaise (52%), myalgia (41%) and a short mild fever in less than 1/3 of women with acute infection [40]. Another study, carried out during the outbreak in Micronesia in 2007, found a similar symptom frequency, differing only in the fever incidence, which occurred in 65% of the cases [39].

Chikungunya

Since its discovery, four different genotypes of the Chikungunya virus have been identified: East-Central-South-African (ECSA), West African, Asian and Indian Ocean lineage (IOL). The incubation period is usually from 3 to 7 days (ranging from 1 to 12 days) and 80% of the cases are symptomatic [41].

Fever is typically elevated, with a sudden onset, associated with arthralgia in almost all cases. Joint pain is usually symmetrical and can be disabling, more intense in the morning, improving with moderate exercise. The joints most often involved are the ankle, wrists and fingers. About 50% of the patients present a maculopapular rash and, occasionally, vesicular-bullous lesions and ulcers. Other symptoms include headache, myalgia, conjunctivitis, nausea and vomiting [42].

Symptoms typically resolve within 7 to 10 days, but some patients may still present rheumatologic symptoms for long periods after the initial infection.

Dengue

Pregnant women are considered a risk group and are more likely to progress to more severe forms of the illness and death [43, 44].

Four serotypes of the Dengue virus exist: DENV-1, DENV-2, DENV-3 and DENV-4. Primary infection by one serotype confers immunity against reinfection by the homologous virus, but when infection by another serotype occurs, which is common in endemic areas, the risk of severe disease is increased due to a phenomenon known as antibody-dependent enhancement [45].

The incubation period varies from 4 to 10 days. About 50% of the infections are symptomatic and may present a broad clinical spectrum. The classification for dengue severity is divided into Dengue without warning signs, Dengue with warning signs, and severe Dengue. For the symptomatic patients three phases may occur:

1st phase - febrile, lasting from 2 to 7 days. The first manifestation is fever, usually high, associated with headaches, myalgia, arthralgia and retro-orbital pain. The rash, predominantly maculopapular, is present in 50% of the cases. Nausea and vomiting may be present. Most patients present improvements in their general state, but 5% progress to the critical phase.

2nd phase - critical, beginning with the defervescence of the fever, between the third and seventh day of the onset of the disease, accompanied by the appearance of one or more warning signs, including:

- Abdominal pain or tenderness;
- Persistent vomiting;
- Clinical fluid accumulation (i.e., pleural effusion or ascites);
- Mucosal bleeding;
- Lethargy or restlessness;
- Liver enlargement (≥2 cm);
- Increases in hematocrit concurrent with rapid decrease in platelet count.

3rd phase - recovery, lasting from 3 to 5 days, after which there is progressive clinical improvement of patients who have suffered the critical phase.

Severe Dengue is defined in the presence of one of the following criteria:

- Severe plasma leakage, leading to shock or fluid accumulation with respiratory distress;
- Severe bleeding;
- Severe organ involvement (AST or ALT ≥1000; impaired consciousness; failure of heart and other organs).

The process that determines the infection progression to severe forms appears to be multifactorial, involving individual immunological status and virus-related factors.

Yellow fever

Like other infectious diseases, Yellow Fever has a wide spectrum of severity, ranging from asymptomatic patients to fatal cases.

The incubation period of the disease ranges from 3 to 6 days. Most symptomatic patients present with fever, headache, chills, muscle aches, and nausea, usually lasting a week. About 10 to 25% develop hemorrhagic manifestations and hepatic and renal impairment, with mortality occurring in 20 to 50% of the symptomatic cases [46].

The disease manifests itself in three stages: infection, remission and intoxication. In milder cases, patients recover without sequelae within a few days. In severe cases, patients develop a more severe form of the disease after the remission period, lasting from 24 to 48 h, called the intoxication period, and may present coagulopathy, haemorrhagic manifestations, jaundice, urinary albuminuria and acute renal failure [19].

Fetal and neonatal outcomes

Zika

A cohort of pregnant women with suspected Zika virus infections was carried out in Rio de Janeiro, between September 2015 and May 2016. Among the 125 pregnant women with confirmed diagnoses, 46.4% presented adverse pregnancy outcomes. Acute infection occurred between 6 and 39 weeks of gestation and complications were observed in 55% of cases when the infection occurred in the first trimester, 52% when infection occurred in the second trimester and 29% when the pregnant women were infected in the last trimester. Abortion cases accounted for 25% of first trimester outcomes and 3% of second trimester outcomes, with 2 fetal deaths among 34 pregnant women with a positive third trimester examination [40].

Of the 117 neonates, 42% displayed abnormal findings in the first month of life, with almost all cases presenting central nervous system abnormalities. Microcephaly was diagnosed in 3.4% of cases and restriction of fetal growth in 9%. The neurological abnormalities, similar to other studies [47, 48], included cerebral calcification, cerebral atrophy, ventriculomegaly, hypoplasia of the cerebral structures and hemorrhage of the cerebral parenchyma [40].

The neurological findings, observed even in late infections, result from central nervous system tropism of the virus, leading to the occurrence of fetal microcephaly and Guillain-Barré syndrome in adults [49, 50].

A previous case–control study, had already established the association of the Zika virus with the occurrence of fetal and neonatal neurological abnormalities. The analysis included 32 neonates with microcephaly, considered cases, and 62 neonates without microcephaly as controls, born in eight public maternity units in the metropolitan northeastern region of Brazil. Eleven of 32 cases showed severe microcephaly and significantly higher proportions of cases compared to controls were born with low birth weight and were small for their gestational age. Of the 27 cases investigated by brain imaging, 11 presented one or more abnormalities [51].

Another study analyzed the data extracted from the epidemiologic reports published by the Secretary of Health Surveillence of the Brazilian Ministry of Health, that monitors cases of microcephaly associated with congenital infection in Brazil. Considering the confirmed cases of microcephaly and related deaths associated with Zika virus in Brazil, from November 2015 to October 2016, the estimated case fatality rate is 8.3% [52].

Chikungunya

Maternal-fetal transmission occurs mainly when there is maternal viremia at the time of delivery, with onset of neonatal symptoms 3 to 9 days after birth.

The main clinical manifestations in symptomatic newborns are fever, irritability, exanthema, lower or generalized lower limb edema, hyperalgesia, vesicular-bullous dermatosis, meningoencephalitis and hemodynamic instability [35]. Some cases may progress with neonatal encephalopathy and microcephaly.

A 2-year follow-up of a cohort of children exposed to the virus during the perinatal period showed a delay in global neurodevelopment, with low developmental rates of those exposed compared to negative controls for infections [53].

Dengue

Two possible mechanisms may be responsible for fetal and neonatal morbidity due to dengue virus infection during pregnancy: the presence of maternal hemodynamic changes, which may compromise the placenta and cause fetal hypoxia, and the direct effect of infection on the fetus.

Paixão et al. conducted a systematic review and meta-analysis of adverse fetal outcomes resulting from Dengue infection during gestation. Sixteen studies were included in the systematic review and eight were eligible for the meta-analysis, totaling 292 women exposed to the Dengue virus during gestation. The review indicated an association of Dengue in pregnancy with abortion (OR 3.51), fetal death (RR 6.7), preterm birth (OR 1.71) and low birth weight (OR 1.41) [54]. Other studies have verified similar results, especially with regard to prematurity and low birth weight [55–58].

Ribeiro et al. studied the fetal outcome of 24 pregnant women with laboratory-confirmed Dengue infections and observed an increase in the incidence of abortions (20,8%), fetal death (8.3%) and prematurity (12.5%). After birth, 29% of the newborns presented symptoms of the disease [59].

The Dengue virus is endemic in many localities and the prevalence of infection during pregnancy, with consequent fetal impairment, may vary according to the local scenario and the cumulative period of exposure to the virus [43, 60]. The analysis of the prevalence and incidence of Dengue during pregnancy in a great epidemic in the central region of Brazil indicated an incidence of 2.8%, diagnosed through the presence of maternal IgM and a prevalence of 53.9% identified by maternal IgG. When umbilical cord blood was analyzed in IgG positive pregnant women, the transfer of maternal antibodies to the fetus was observed to be 99.3% [55].

Yellow fever

Most studies regarding Yellow Fever analyzed fetal and neonatal effects after inadvertent vaccinations during pregnancy.

In 2009, a case of perinatal transmission of Yellow Fever was described during an epidemic in the state of São Paulo, Brazil. The 30-year-old woman presented with fever, headache and jaundice 3 days before vaginal delivery. The female newborn was discharged after 2 days and on the third day was readmitted with fever and cyanosis, progressing with hemorrhage, liver enzyme alterations, oliguria and death with 12 days of life. The neonate underwent antibiotic therapy and intensive support during hospitalization. Confirmation of newborn infection was obtained by RT-PCR harvested after 5 days of the onset of symptoms. The maternal infection was confirmed by IgM positive for Yellow Fever and negative for Dengue [38].

Diagnoses

Clinical presentation

Due to the similarity between these arboviruses symptoms and the possibility of rapid evolution to severe forms, it is recommended that infection by the Dengue virus be considered as the main differential diagnosis in patients who have been in endemic areas. Infections with the Zika and Chikungunya virus should also be considered, since they present the same vector and many regions are endemic for different arboviruses.

Table 1, released by the Fiocruz Agency, summarizes the characteristics and frequencies of symptoms in Dengue, Zika and Chikungunya.

Laboratory tests

Some endemic areas display multiple arboviruses which present the same symptoms, such as fever, rash, myalgia, and arthralgia. Therefore, laboratory evaluation of the Dengue, Zika and Chikungunya viruses, as well as other TORCH group diseases (Toxoplasmosis, Rubella, Cytomegalovirus and Herpes) is recommended to establish the diagnosis.

In the acute phase, which occurs within the first 7 days after the onset of the symptoms, virus RNA can be identified in the patient's serum, with RT-PCR as the test of choice for the diagnosis of Dengue, Zika and Chikungunya. In the case of Dengue infection, the NS1 antigen can also be detected in the acute phase by the ELISA test. However, this test is not widely available. A negative result, however, does not exclude the infection, and a serological test for IgM antibodies is necessary.

In the convalescence phase, the ELISA test for IgM antibodies, which are usually detectable between 2 and 12 weeks after infection, should be performed for Dengue, Zika and Chikungunya. However, due to cross-reactions, a positive serology (IgM) for Dengue or Zika only indicates a recent flavivirus infection and it is not possible to distinguish the type of virus in question. In case of positive IgM antibodies, the Plaque Reduction Neutralization Test (PRNT), which characterizes and quantifies circulating levels of anti-Dengue virus neutralizing antibody, is necessary to confirm the diagnosis. Patients who have received a Yellow Fever vaccine in the past may also present serology cross-reactivity [61, 62].

The Trioplex RT-PCR is a laboratory test designed to detect Zika, Dengue and Chikungunya virus RNA, authorized by the FDA to be used under an Emergency Use Authorization (USA) [63].

The diagnosis of a Yellow Fever infection follows the same protocol with RT-PCR, and the detection of the NS1 antigen with high sensitivity and specificity, possible during the acute phase. The identification of Yellow Fever antibodies by IgM ELISA can also be performed. Serology assays, however, present limitations due to the possibility of cross-reactivity with other flaviviruses [64].

In addition to serum, RT-PCR can also be performed on urine and saliva samples. Musso et al. analyzed saliva samples from symptomatic patients during the French Polynesia epidemic from October 2013 to March 2014, and, although there was no increase in the virus detection window, the saliva sample increased the molecular detection rate of viral RNA [65].

Treatment

There is no specific medication for infections caused by Dengue, Zika, Chikungunya or Yellow Fever viruses. The treatment consists in rest, drinking fluids to prevent dehydration and the use of analgesics, such as acetaminophen. In the presence of warning signs (section Dengue), the patients must be admitted to a hospital where they can receive intensive care. Gestation, since it is considered a risk condition for Dengue infection, should present a follow-up in the maternity hospital or health unit.

Table 1 Comparison of symptoms of symptomatic presentation[a] between Dengue, Zika and Chikungunya

Signs/Symptoms	Dengue	Zika	Chikungunya
Fever	Above 38 °C (4 to 7 days)	No fever or subfebrile ≤38 °C (1 to 2 days)	Above 38 °C (2 to 3 days)
Rash	Appears from the 4th day 30–50% of the cases	Appears on the 1st or 2nd day 90–100% of cases	Appears on the 2nd or 5th day 50% of cases
Myalgia	+++/+++	++/+++	+/+++
Arthralgia	+/+++	++/+++	+++/+++
Conjunctivitis	Rare	50–90% of cases	30%
Headache	+++	++	++
Pruritus	Slight	Moderate/Intense	Slight
Blood dyscrasia	Moderate	Absent	Slight
Neurological impairment	Rare	More frequent than Dengue and Chikungunya	Rare (predominant in neonates)

[a]Estimated symptomatic presentation in 50% of Dengue virus, 20% of Zika virus and 80% of Chikungunya virus infection

The use of aspirin or other non-steroidal anti-inflammatory drugs must be avoided. The use of these medicines may aggravate the hemorrhagic condition in case of Dengue virus infection [66].

Prevention

Vaccines

The Dengue vaccine CYD-TDV has recently been licensed but still remains largely unused. It is a tetravalent live attenuated viral vaccine, licensed for the prevention of Dengue illness caused by Dengue virus serotypes 1, 2, 3 and 4 in individuals ranging from 9 to 45 years old or 9 to 60 years old, depending on the license, living in Dengue endemic areas. The vaccination schedule consists of 3 0,5 mL injections administered at 6-month intervals, with an average efficiency of approximately 60%.

There is no recommendation concerning CYD-TDV during pregnancy and breastfeeding, due to lack of sufficient data in this population. However, the limited data collected during the clinical trials on unintentional immunization in pregnancy have yielded no evidence of harm to the fetus or pregnant women. To date, no studies evaluating the effects of inadvertent use in pregnant women are available [67].

Yellow Fever 17D vaccine is widely used for the prevention of Yellow Fever in travelers, for routine immunization in endemic areas and for emergency response during outbreaks. It is given in a volume of 0,5 ml by the subcutaneous route in a dose of no less than 1000 International Units. Approximately 90% of vaccines seroconvert by 10 days and 99% seroconvert by 30 days post immunization.

The Yellow Fever vaccine is not recommended during gestation or breastfeeding, since it is composed of a live attenuated virus, except in situations of a severe epidemic or unavoidable trip to high-risk locations [68]. However, studies analyzing Yellow Fever vaccination in pregnant women found no increased risk of adverse events in gestation and newborns, except in a study that presented insufficient statistical power [69–73]. The risk of miscarriage, malformations, fetal death and prematurity is similar to that of the general population [74]. It is noteworthy that many of these studies reported small series.

If vaccination is required during pregnancy, it is preferable to be administered during the first trimester, when the immune response appears to be more satisfactory. The vaccine may be administered during breastfeeding, which should be discontinued for 10 days during the post-vaccine viremia phase. Regarding breastfeeding, a case of vaccine-induced encephalitis in one infant was reported 8 days after the mother's primary vaccination [75].

At the time of publication of this article, no vaccines against Zika and Chikungunya were available. Future vaccine programs should consider the serological cross-reaction between the Zika virus and Dengue virus and the implications for disease pathogenesis [76].

Vector control

The preventive strategy considered most efficient is vector control, through the use of repellents and long-sleeved clothes, placement of screens in houses, sleeping in rooms with air conditioning and avoiding the accumulation of standing water, which serves as a breeding ground for the mosquito vectors. The WHO recommends the use of repellents containing DEET, IR3535, aminopropionic or icaridine [77].

Other measures during pregnancy

The CDC recommends sexual abstinence or condom use for men suspected of contracting a Zika virus infection over a period of 6 months. For those residing or returning from a region with active transmission of the virus but who do not show symptoms, such measures should be adopted for at least 8 weeks after the person's return.

Women who are interested in childbearing and pregnant women should not travel to areas with the risk of Zika. If travel is unavoidable, or with regard to pregnant couples living in Zika areas, condoms from start to finish every time sex is performed is recommended, during the entire pregnancy. Populations in endemic areas or who have been exposed should conduct early and serial ultrasounds during pregnancy [78].

Conclusions

Arboviruses are emerging infectious diseases endemic in several localities, but with unpredictable and devastating potential, as seen recently with the viral epidemics in the Americas.

Despite the recent publications on infections by the Zika virus and the repercussions of congenital infection, research in this area is still modest and many arboviruses aspects need to be clarified, especially regarding gestational infection.

Some issues that should be focused on are the improvement of diagnostic tests, including specific and sensitive molecular tests, associated to ultrasound screening; more accurate estimates of maternal, fetal and neonatal risks and the development of preventive vaccines, among other therapeutic options.

Only after the advancement of these issues will it be possible to develop effective intervention strategies aimed at the prevention or eradication of arbovirus infections and their deleterious maternal-fetal outcomes.

Acknowledgements
Not applicable.

Funding
This study received no funding.

Authors' contributions
PSM: concept, collection of data, writing the manuscript, critique and revision. AJC: mentor, concept, collection of data, writing the manuscript, critique and revision. JAJ: contributed to management, critique and revision. APB: contributed to management, critique and revision. All authors read and approved the final manuscript.

Competing interests
The authors declare that they have no competing interests.

Author details
[1]Maternidade Escola da Universidade Federal do Rio de Janeiro, Rio de Janeiro, RJ, Brazil. [2]Faculdade de Medicina da Universidade Federal do Rio de Janeiro, Rio de Janeiro, RJ, Brazil. [3]Instituto D'Or de Pesquisa e Ensino – IDOR, Rio de Janeiro, RJ, Brazil. [4]Rua das Laranjeiras, 180 – Laranjeiras, Rio de Janeiro CEP: 22240-003, RJ, Brazil.

References

1. Morse SS. Factors in the emergence of infectious diseases. Emerg Infect Dis. 1999;1(1):7–15.
2. Scrag SJ, Wiener P. Emerging infectious disease: what are the relative roles of ecology and evolution? Trends Ecol Evol. 1995;10(8):319–24.
3. Mayer SV, Robert BT, Nikos V. The emergence of arthropod-borne viral disease: a global prospective on dengue, chikungunya and zika fevers. Acta Trop. 2017;166:155–63.
4. Dick GW, Cozinha SF, Haddow AJ. Zika virus. I: isolations and serological specificity. Trans R Soc Trop Med Hyg. 1952;46(5):509–20.
5. Macnamara FN. Zika virus: a report on three cases of human infection during an epidemic of jaundice in Nigeria. Trans R Soc Trop Med Hyg. 1954;48(2):139–45.
6. Marchette NJ, Garcia R, Rudnick A. Isolation of zika virus from aedes aegypti mosquitoes in Malaysia. Am J Trop Med Hyg. 1969;18(3):411–5.
7. Duffy MR, Chen TH, Hancock WT, Powers AM, Kool JL, Lanciotti RS, et al. Zika outbreak on Yap Island, Federated States of Micronesia. N Engl J Med. 2009;360:2536–43.
8. Cao-Lormeau VM, Roche C, Teissier A, Robin E, Anne-Laure B, Henri-Pierre M, et al. Zika virus, French Polynesia, South Pacific 2013. Emerg Infect Dis. 2014;20(6):1085–6.
9. Musso D, Nilles EJ, Cao-Lormeau VM. Rapid spread of emerging zika virus in the Pacific area. Clin Microbiol Infect. 2014;20:595–6.
10. Zanluca C, Melo VCA, Mosimann ALP, Santos GIV, Santos CND. First report of autochthonous transmission of Zika virus in Brazil. Mem Inst Oswaldo Cruz. 2015;110(4):569–72.
11. PAHO/WHO. Regional Zika Epidemiological. http://www.paho.org/hq/index.php?option=com_content&view=article&id=12390&Itemid=42090&lang=en (2017). Accessed 16 July 2017.
12. Sudeep AB, Parashar D. Chikungunya: an overview. J Biosci. 2008;33:443–9.
13. Leparc-Goffart I, Nougairede A, Cassadou S, Prat C, Lamballerie X. Chikungunya in the Americas. Lancet. 2014;383(9916):514.
14. Weaver SC, Forrester NL. Chikungunya: evolutionary history and recent epidemic spread. Antivir Res. 2015;120:32–9.
15. Nunes MRT, Faria NR, Vasconcelos JM, Golding N, Kraemer MUG, Oliveira LF, et al. Emergence and potential for spread of Chikungunya virus in Brazil. BMC Med. 2015;13:102.
16. Messina JP, Brady OJ, Scott TW, Zou C, Pigott DM, Duda KA, et al. Global spread of dengue virus types: mapping the 70 year history. Trends Microbiol. 2014;22:138–46.
17. Gubler DJ. Human behaviour and cultural context in disease control. Tropical Med Int Health. 1997;2(11):A1–2.
18. Gubler DJ. The global emergence/resurgence of arboviral diseases as public health problems. Arch Med Res. 2002;33(4):330–42.
19. Gardner CL, Ryman KD. Yellow fever: a reemerging threat. Clin Lab Med. 2010;30:237–60.
20. Monath TP, Vasconcelos PF. Yellow fever. J Clin Virol. 2015;64:160–73.
21. Paules CI, Fauci AS. Yellow fever – once again on the radar screen in the Americas. N Engl J Med. 2017;376(15):1397–9.
22. Abushouk AI, Negida A, Ahmed H. An updated review of zika vírus. J Clinl Virology. 2016;84:53–8.
23. D'Ortenzio E, Matheron S, Yazdanpanah Y, Lamballerie X, Hubert B, Piorkowski G, et al. Evidence of sexual transmission of zika virus. New Engl J Med. 2016;374(22):2195–8.
24. Atkinson B, Hearn P, Afrough B, Lumley S, Carter D, Aarons EJ. Detecção do vírus Zika no sêmen. Emerg Infect Dis. 2016;22(5):940. Https://dx.doi.org/10.3201/eid2205.160107.
25. Coelho FC, Durovni B, Saraceni V, Lemos C, Codeco CT, Camargo S, et al. Higher incidence of zika in adult women than adult men in Rio de Janeiro suggests a significant contribution of sexual transmission from men to women. Int J Infect Dis. 2016;51:128–32. doi:10.1016/j.ijid.2016.08.023.
26. Busch MP, Sabino EC, Brambilla D, Lopes ME, Capuani L, Chowdhury D, et al. Duration of dengue viremia in blood donos and relationships between donor viremia, infection incidence and clinical case reports during a large epidemic. J Infec Diseases. 2016;214:49–54.
27. Sabino EC, Loureiro P, Lopes ME, Capuani L, McClure C, Chowdhury D, et al. Transfusion-transmitted dengue and associated clinical symptoms during the 2012 epidemic in Brazil. J Infec Diseases. 2016;231:694–702.
28. Motta IJ, Spencer BR, Silva CSG, Arruda MB, Dobbin JA, Gonzaga YB, et al. Evidence for transmission of Zika virus by platelet transfusion. N Engl J Med. 2016;375(11):1101–3.

29. Lanteri MC, Kleinman SH, Glynn SA, Musso D, Keith HW, Custer BS, et al. Zika virus: a new threat to the safety of the blood supply with worldwide impact and implications. Transfusion. 2016;56:1907–14.
30. Centers for Disease Control and Prevention (CDC). Transfusion-related transmission of yellow fever vaccine vírus – California, 2009. MMWR. 2010;59(2):34–7.
31. Faria NR, Azevedo RS, Kraemer MU, Souza R, Cunha MS, Hill SC, et al. Zika virus in the Americas: early epidemiological and genetic findings. Science. 2016;352(6283):345–9. doi:10.1126/science.aaf5036.
32. Martines RB, Bhatnagar J, Ramos AMO, Davi HPF, Iglezias SD'A, Kanamura CT. Pathology of congenital zika syndrome in Brazil: a case series. Lancet. 2016; 388: 898–904. Doi: https://doi.org/10.1016/S0140-6736(16)30883-2.
33. França GV, Schuler-Faccini L, Oliveira WK, Henriques CM, Carmo EH, Pedi VD. Livebirths with complete investigation. Lancet. 2016;388(10047):891–7. doi:10.1016/S0140-6736(16)30902-3.
34. Mlakar J, Korva M, Tul N, Popović M, Poljšak-Prijatelj M, Mraz J, et al. Zika virus associated with microcephaly. N Engl J Med. 2016;374:951–8. doi:10.1056/NEJMoa1600651.
35. Torres JR, Falleiros-Arlant LH, Dueñas L, Pleitez-Navarrete J, Salgado DM, Castillo JB. Congenital and perinatal complications of chikungunya fever: a Latin American experience. Int J Infect Dis. 2016;51:85–8. doi:10.1016/j.ijid.2016.09.009.
36. Ribeiro CF, Lopes VG, Brasil P, Coelho J, Muniz AG, Nogueira RM. Perinatal transmission of dengue: a report of 7 cases. J Pediat. 2013;163(5):1514–6.
37. Kariyawasam S, Senanayake H. Dengue infections during pregnancy: case series from a tertiary care hospital in Sri Lanka. J Infect Dev Ctries. 2010;4(11):767–75.
38. Bentlin MR, Almeida RA, Coelho KI, Ribeiro AF, Siciliano MM, Suzuki A, et al. Transmissão perinatal de febre amarela, Brasil, 2009. Infect Emerg Dis. 2011;17(9):1779–80. Https://dx.doi.org/10.3201/eid1709.110242
39. Duffy MR, Chen TH, Hancokc WT, Powers AM, Kool JL, Lanciotti RS, et al. Zika virus outbreak on Yap Island, Federated States of Micronesia. New Engl J Med. 2009;360:2536–43.
40. Brasil P, Pereira JP Jr, Moreira ME, Nogueira RMR, Damaceno L, Pharm LD, et al. Zika virus infection in pregnant women in Rio de Janeiro. N Engl J Med. 2016;375(24):2321–34. doi:10.1056/NEJMoa1602412.
41. Moro ML, Gagliotti C, Silvi G, Angelini R, Sambri V, Rezza G, et al. Chikungunya virus in north-eastern Italy: a seroprevalence survey. Am J Trop Med Hyg. 2010;82(3):508–11.
42. Centers for Disease Control and Prevention. Chikungunya: information for healthcare providers. https://www.cdc.gov/chikungunya/hc/clinicalevaluation.html. Acessado em 23 de março de 2017.
43. Adam I, Jumaa AM, Elbashir HM, Karsany MS. Maternal and perinatal outcomes of dengue in PortSudan, eastern. Sudan Virology J. 2010;7:153.
44. Machado CR, Machado ES, Rohloff RD, Azevedo M, Campos DP, Oliveira RB, Brasil P. Is pregnancy associated with severe dengue? A review of data from the rio de janeiro surveillance information system. PLoS Negl Trop Dis. 2013;7(5):e2217. doi:10.1371/journal.pntd.0002217.
45. Guzman MG, Alvarez M, Halstead SB. Secondary infection as a risk factor for dengue hemorrhagic fever/dengue shock syndrome: an historical perspective and role of antibody-dependent enhancement of infection. Arch Virol. 2013;158(7):1445–59.
46. Wilder-Smith A, Gubler DJ, Weaver SC, Monath TP, Heymann DL, Scott TW. Epidemic arboviral disease: priorities for research and public health. Lancet Infect Dis. 2017;17:e101–6.
47. Oliveira-Szejnfeld PS, Levine D, Melo ASO, Amorim MMR, Batista AGM, Chimelli L, et al. Congenital brain abnormalities and Zika virus: what the radiologista can expect to see prenatally and postnatally. Radiology. 2016;281(1):203–18.
48. Honein MA, Dawson AL, Petersen EE, Jones AM, Lee EH, Yazdy MM. Birth defects among fetuses and infants of US women with evidence of possible Zika virus infection during pregnancy. JAMA. 2017;317(1):59–68. doi:10.1001/jama.2016.19006.
49. Suwanmanee S, Luplertlop N. Dengue and Zika viruses: lessons learned from the similarities between these Aedes Mosquito-vectored arboviruses. J Microbiol. 2017;55(2):81–9. doi:10.1007/s12275-017-6494-4.
50. França GV, Schuler-Faccini L, Oliveira WK, Henriques CM, Carmo EH, Pedi VD, et al. Congenital zika virus syndrome in Brazil: a case series of the first 1501 livebirths with complete investigation. Lancet. 2016;388:891–7.
51. Araújo TVB, Rodrigues LC, Ximenes RAA, Miranda-Filho DB, Montarroyos UR, Melo APL, et al. Association between Zika virus infection and microcephaly in Brazil, January to may, 2016: preliminary report of a case–control study. Lancet Infect Dis. 2016;16:1356–63.
52. Cunha AJ, de Magalhães-Barbosa MC, Lima-Setta F, Medronho RA, Prata-Barbosa A. Microcephaly case fatality rate associated with Zika virus infection in Brazil: current estimates. Pediatr Infect Dis J. 2017;36(5):528–30. doi:10.1097/INF.0000000000001486.
53. Gérardin P, Sampériz S, Ramful D, Boumahni B, Bintner M, Alessandri JL, et al. Neurocognitive outcome of children exposed to perinatal mother-to-child chikungunya virus infection: the chimere cohort study on reunion Island. PLoS Negl Trop Dis. 2014;8(7):e2996. doi:10.1371/journal.pntd.0002996.
54. Paixão ES, Teixeira MG, Costa MC, Rodrigues LC. Dengue during pregnancy and adverse fetal outcomes: a systematic review and meta-analysis. Lancet Infect Dis. 2016;16:857–65.
55. Xiong X, Harville E, Paz-Soldão V, Tomashek KM, Breart L, Buekens P. Maternal dengue and pregnancy outcomes: a systematic review. Obstet GynecoSurv. 2010;65(2):107–18.
56. Alvarenga CF, Silami VG, Brasil P, Boechat MEH, Coelho J, Nogueira RMR. Dengue during pregnancy: a study of thirteen cases. American J Infect Diseases. 2009;5(4):288–93.
57. Tan PC, Soe MZ, Si Lay K, Wang SM, Sekaran SD, Omar SZ. Dengue infection and miscarriage: a prospective case control study. PLoS Negl Trop Dis. 2012;6(5):e1637. doi:10.1371/journal.pntd.0001637.
58. Friedman EE, Dallah F, Harville EW, Myers L, Buekens P, Breart G, Carles G. Symptomatic dengue infection during pregnancy and infant outcomes: a retrospective cohort study. PLoS Negl Trop Dis. 2014;8(10):e3226. doi:10.1371/journal.pntd.0003226.
59. Christiane FR, Lopes VGS, Brasil P, Pires ARC, Rohloffe R, Nogueira RMR. Dengue infection in pregnancy and its impact on the placenta. Internat J Infect Diseases. 2017;55:109–12.
60. Argolo AF, Féres VC, Silveira LA, Oliveira AC, Pereira LA, Júnior JB, Braga C, Martelli CM. Prevalence and incidence of dengue virus and antibody placental transfer during late pregnancy in central Brazil. BMC Infect Dis. 2013;13:254.
61. World Health Organization (WHO) and the Special Programme for Research and Training in Tropical Diseases (TDR). Dengue: guidelines for diagnosis, treatment, prevention and control. 9a ed. Genebra: WHO; 2009. http://apps.who.int/iris/bitstream/10665/44188/1/9789241547871_eng.pdf. Acessado em 08 de abril de 2017.
62 Centers for Disease Control and Prevention (CDC). Guidance for U.S. laboratories testing for zika virus infection. https://www.cdc.gov/zika/laboratories/lab-guidance.html. Acessado em 08 de abril de 2017.
63 Centers for Disease Control and Prevention (CDC). Dengue laboratory guidance and diagnostic testing. https://www.cdc.gov/dengue/clinicallab/laboratory.html. Acessado em 08 de abril de 2017.
64 Monath TP, Vasconcelos PFC. Yellow fever. J Clinical Virology. 2015;64:160–73.
65. Mussoa D, Rocheb C, Tu-Xuan N, Robina E, Teissierb A, Van-Mai CL. Detection of zika virus in saliva. J Clinical Virology. 2015;68:53–5.
66. Centers for Disease Control and Prevention. Symptoms and what to do if you think you have dengue. https://www.cdc.gov/dengue/symptoms/. Acessado em 08 de abril de 2017.
67. Scott, L.J. Drugs (2016) 76: 1301. doi:10.1007/s40265-016-0626-8.
68. Staples JE, Gershman M, Fischer M. Yellow fever vaccine: recommendations of the advisory committee on immunization Practise (ACIP). MMWR Reccomm Rep. 2010;59:1–279.
69. Cavalcanti DP, Salomão MA, Lopez-Camelo J, Pessoto MA. Early exposure to yellow fever vaccine during pregnancy. Tropical Med Int Health. 2007;12(7):833–7.
70. D'Acremont V, Tremblay S, Genton B. Impact of vacines given during pregnancy on the offspring of women consulting a travel clinic: a longitudinal study. J Travel Med. 2008;15:77–81.
71. Nasidi A, Monath TP, Vanderberg J. Yellow fever vaccination and pregnancy: a four year prospective study. Trans R Soc Trop Med Hyg. 1993;87:337–9.
72. Robert E, Vial T, Schaefer C, Arnon J, Reuvers M. Exposure to yellow fever vaccine in early pregnancy. Vaccine. 1999;17:283–5.
73. Nishioka SA, Nunes-Araújo FR, Pires WP, Silva FA, Costa HL. Yellow fever vaccination and pregnacy and spontaneous abortion: a case–control study. Tropical Med Int Health. 1998;3:29–33.
74. Suzano CE, Amaral E, Sato HK, Papaiordanou PM. The effects of yellow fever immunization (17DD) inadvertently used in early pregnancy during a mass campaign in Brazil. Vaccine. 2006;24:1421–6.
75. Imbert P, Moulin F, Mornand P, Mechai F, Rapp C. Should yellow fever vaccination be recommended during pregnancy or breastfeeding? Med Trop. 2010;70(4):321–4.

10

Circadian changes and sex-related differences in fetal heart rate parameters

Habiba Kapaya[3*], Fiona Broughton Pipkin[1], Barrie Hayes-Gill[2] and Pamela V. Loughna[1]

Abstract

Background: Previous researchers have studied circadian changes in the fetal heart rate (FHR) on small sample sizes and in a strictly controlled environment. This study was undertaken to investigate these changes during the late second and third trimesters, using a portable fetal electrocardiogram recording device (Monica AN24) in pregnant women in home and hospital environments with unrestricted mobility.

Methods: This was a prospective cohort study of 54 pregnant women with uncomplicated singleton pregnancies between 25 and 40 weeks gestation. FHR recordings were made up to 16 h at home or in the hospital setting in the United Kingdom. FHR data over 90 min periods were averaged and the day (7:00 am–11:00 pm) and night (11:00 pm–7:00 am) data from the same individual were compared. Data were examined for evidence of sex-related differences.

Results: During the night, there was a significant reduction in basal heart rate (bFHR) and a significant increase in short term variation (STV) and long term variation (LTV) ($P < 0.05$). Basal FHR decreased ($P < 0.002$), whereas LTV increased ($P = 0.014$) with advancing gestation. Male fetuses showed greater day: night variation than females regardless of gestation ($P = 0.014$). There was a higher bFHR in fetuses monitored during the day in hospital ($P = 0.04$).

Conclusion: This study demonstrates that there are sex-, environment and time-related differences in the FHR parameters measured. These differences may need to be considered taken when interpreting FHR data.

Keywords: Circadian, Fetal heart rate, Fetal heart rate monitoring, Electronic fetal monitoring, Fetal electrocardiogram, Fetal sex, Pregnancy

Abbreviations: ANS, Autonomic nervous system; bFHR, Basal fetal heart rate; ECG, Electrocardiogram; Fetal ECG, fECG; FHR, Fetal heart rate; GA, Gestational age; HRV, Heart rate variability; HV, High-variation; LTV, Long-term variation; ms, Millisecond; RMS, Root-mean square; RMSSD, Root mean square of successive difference; STV, Short-term variation

Background

The presence of a circadian pattern in fetal heart rate (FHR) [1, 2] and activity [3] is well documented. However, the origin of this variation is uncertain. Animal work has confirmed that in the adult information on circadian variation, which is driven by the biological clock located in the suprachiasmatic nuclei of the hypothalamus, is conveyed to the heart via the autonomic nervous system (ANS) [4]. It is less clear whether the fetal suprachiasmatic nucleus plays such a role in the generation of prenatal diurnal patterns, particularly as the fetus is influenced by the mother's rhythm from late mid-trimester [5]. Whilst circadian rhythms are affected by daylight exposure, the fetus is not directly exposed to light but still retains a clear circadian pattern.

Circadian variation in FHR in the human fetus has been reported from as early as 20–22 weeks through to the end of pregnancy [1]. The fetal suprachiasmatic nucleus can be clearly identified from 23 weeks gestation [6] and it therefore seems logical that fetal circadian patterns should be discernible from early in the mid-trimester. FHR variability increases markedly with gestational age [7], suggesting development of fetal ANS. In addition, fetal behavioural state and maturation [8] fetal rest-activity cycles [9] and general body and breathing movements can also influence FHR and its variability [10].

* Correspondence: h.kapaya@sheffield.ac.uk
[3]Department of Oncology and Metabolism, Academic Unit of Reproductive & Developmental Medicine, 4th Floor Jessop Wing, Tree Root Walk, Sheffield S102SF, UK
Full list of author information is available at the end of the article

It is unclear to what extent the fetus is influenced by the maternal rhythm. Studies from 26 weeks gestation to term have suggested that there is a direct relationship between the mother's and fetal heart rates, implying that the fetus is not autonomous in this respect [5, 2]. A twin pregnancy discordant for anencephaly did not show any correlation in heart rate patterns with maternal activity, particularly in the anencephalic twin suggesting that an intact fetal central nervous system is required for the circadian rhythm to be evident [11].

Differences in heart rate variability (HRV) with respect to sex have been reported in fetuses [12], adults [13] and both pre-pubertal children and fetuses, with boys having a higher HRV than girls [14, 15].

Previous studies on circadian patterns of FHR variables including basal fetal heart rate (bFHR), short and long term variation (STV, LTV), and high variation (HV) have been conducted in hospital under laboratory conditions with controlled maternal activity (including diet) and most have studied small numbers [1, 3, 5, 16].

The introduction of a small, portable fetal electrocardiogram (ECG) recording device capable of continuous recording for up to 16 h (Monica AN24) enabled us to examine changes in the day and night FHR patterns while the women continued their-day-today activities. This investigation was undertaken in home and hospital environments to assess if place of monitoring affected FHR patterns.

Methods

This was an observational prospective cohort study, which was approved by the local Research Ethics Committee (REC reference number: 07/Q0108/127). All eligible women over 20 weeks gestation, attending maternity assessment unit, antenatal clinic and antenatal wards at City Campus, Nottingham University Hospitals NHS Trust, Nottingham, UK were invited to participate.

Fifty-four pregnant women (28 women with gestational age (GA) ≤ 34 completed weeks and 26 with GA >34 weeks) with uncomplicated singleton pregnancies consented and participated in the study. GA varied between 25 and 40 weeks (median GA was 34 weeks). At the time of recording, none of the women used tobacco, alcohol or received any medication.

Exclusion criteria were known fetal malformation, fetal growth restriction, maternal hypertension, inability to provide informed consent, maternal smoking or alcohol dependence, in active labour, multiple pregnancies and pre-existing medical conditions such as diabetes, thyroid and cardiac disease. Inclusion criteria were a singleton pregnancy >24 weeks gestation confirmed by early ultrasound scan and maternal age at least 18 years and above. After giving informed written consent, women were recruited for a single recording, using the Monica AN24, to be made either at home ($n = 30$) or during admission to the antenatal ward ($n = 24$) starting between 13.00 and 16.00 h and lasting for up to 16 h. All women recruited for the study were given instruction on how to turn the monitor off and, if they had home monitoring, returned it to the hospital at their convenience. Women were requested to fill in a questionnaire to identify any concerns and to record their views on the comfort of the monitoring session.

Fetal electrophysiological data recorded within the monitor were downloaded via a USB connection. The methodology used for FHR signal extraction and analysis has been described in detail by others before [17]. The software programme installed in the device not only extracts the traditional FHR data obtained from conventional Doppler-based CTG monitors, it also generates beat-to-beat information on FHR providing a deeper insight into the understanding of complex development of FHR and its variation. In addition, the device also records the FHR parameters which are part of Dawes and Redman analysis [17–19].

In order to investigate changes in FHR pattern between the day and night times, three consecutive 30 min frames with FHR acquisition success rate of ≥80 % were selected randomly during the "day" (07.00–23.00) and "night" (23.00–07.00) periods for each subject.

The FHR parameters studied from the Dawes Redman analysis in this paper were:

- bFHR: basal FHR or resting level of the FHR once accelerations and decelerations have subsided,
- number of accelerations:,defined as a rise in FHR above the baseline greater than 10 bpm and lasting for more than 15 s
- STV: Short Term Variation. Computed from any minute which does not contain a deceleration or part of a deceleration and does not have a high signal loss (>10 %). For each valid minute, the STV is calculated as the average difference of adjacent 3.75 s epochs of FHR
- LTV: Long Term Variation or sometimes referred to as Mean Minute range. In any valid minute (i.e. no deceleration or large signal loss) this is the difference between the largest 3.75 s FHR and the smallest 3.75 s FHR and is expressed in milliseconds (ms)
- HV: High Variation. This is a section of the 3.75 s FHR trace where the minute range is above 32 ms for 5 out of 6 consecutive minutes.
- RMSSD: Root Mean Square of Successive Differences. This is – a measure of true beat to beat variability and is calculated from the beat to beat fetal ECG (fECG) data and not the average 3.75 s FHR (hence strictly it is not part of the traditional

FHR Dawes Redman extracted parameters). The RR interval is determined for each pair of (fECG) beats and the difference is determined between consecutive RR intervals. From each 1 min of RR interval differences a root mean square (RMS) value is calculated in milliseconds (ms).

The above FHR parameters were averaged over the three 30 min epochs and compared between the day and night of the same individual.

Statistical analysis

Kolmogorov Smirnoff analysis was first used to test for normality of the FHR data. Most FHR parameters followed a normal distribution; therefore parametric testing was used for statistical analysis. Independent sample t test was used to compare the demographics between the recordings made at home and in hospital. In order to analyse the day and night recording of the same individual, the paired sample t-Test was used for bFHR, STV, LTV and RMSSD or the Wilcoxon paired sample test for accelerations and HV. Univariate analysis of variance was considered to measure the association of FHR parameters with time and place of recording. Correlation between FHR parameters and gestational age was assessed using Pearson's rank-order correlation coefficient.

Results

Table 1 summarises the basic demographic data for the women and their fetuses monitored at home and in hospital.

One hundred eight recordings (54 day and 54 night) made over 90 min epochs were analysed from 30 women recruited at home and 24 at hospital (Table 2). A significant reduction in basal heart rate and a significant increase in STV and LTV was observed in all fetuses at night, whether monitored at home or in hospital. Although all fetuses exhibited an increased number of accelerations at night, statistically significant results were observed only for the fetuses recruited at home ($P < 0.001$ home; $P > 0.1$ hospital)).

Having demonstrated a significant day: night effect, we calculated the day: night difference for each measurement, to allow further analysis in relation to absolute difference. Regression analysis showed the change in bFHR to be strongly reciprocally-associated with GA at the time of recording (Fig. 1; $P < 0.002$); the addition of place of recording to the analysis significantly ($P < 0.01$) improved the final r to 0.554 ($P < 0.001$). The change in LTV was directly related to GA ($r = 0.331$; $P = 0.014$); there was no effect of GA at recording or place of recording on day: night change in either STV or RMSSD ($P > 0.1$, >0.3 respectively).

In our study, 30 fetuses were male and 24 female. Although bFHR was very similar in male and female fetuses (day: 139.2 ± 7.4 and 138.8 ± 12.2 bpm; night 131.2 ± 6.4 and 132.4 ± 9.4 bpm), males had significantly higher night-time STV and RMSSD than did females (12.5 ± 3.0 compared with 10.6 ± 2.7 ms, and 11.0 ± 1.5 compared with 9.7 ± 1.8 ms; $P = 0.014$, $P = 0.004$ respectively); the sex-related difference also approached significance for LTV ($P = 0.057$). There were no sex-associated differences during the daytime recordings.

Table 3 shows the day-night differences with respect to sex. This difference was significant for LTV ($P = 0.01$) and remained significant when GA at recording was included in the analysis (Fig. 2), and was independent of birth weight.

When place of recording was taken as a fixed factor in our univariate model of analysis, a significantly higher bFHR ($P = 0.04$) was observed in the day time (142.5 ± 9.3 bpm) for the recordings made in hospital compared to the home setting (136.1 ± 9.2 bpm). None of the other normally-distributed parameters showed any significant difference when place of the recording was taken into account as well as sex.

Discussion

This study has demonstrated that there is a clear circadian pattern of changes in the FHR, with a greater influence of time on bFHR and LTV with advancing gestation. Male fetuses show a greater difference than females in STV when day and night recordings are compared, regardless of gestation. The bFHR is higher in fetuses monitored in hospital than those monitored in the home.

Table 1 Basal demographic data for the women and fetuses studied at home and in hospital setting

Variables	Home setting ($n = 30$)	Hospital setting ($n = 24$)	P value
Age (y)	28.9 ± 5.6	28.1 ± 7.1	$P = 0.7$
Body mass index (kg/m^2)	26.3 ± 5.7	27.5 ± 5.8	$P = 0.5$
Gestational age at recording (completed weeks)	33.8 ± 3.9	34.2 ± 3.0	$P = 0.5$
Gestational age at delivery (days)	273 ± 17	273 ± 17	$P = 0.7$
Birth weight of the babies (kg)	3.46 ± 0.55	3.48 ± 0.53	$P = 0.9$
Birth weight of the babies (centiles)	57 [38–74][30]	47 [34–77]	$P > 0.5$

Data are shown as mean ± SD or median [interquartile]

Table 2 Basic comparison of day and night fetal heart rate (FHR) parameters in normal fetuses at home and in hospital setting

	Home ($n = 30$)			Hospital ($n = 24$)		
Parameters	Day recordings	Night recordings	*P* value	Day recordings	Night recordings	*P* value
bFHR (bpm)	136.1 ± 9.2	131.6 ± 7.4	=0.005	142.6 ± 9.3	131.9 ± 8.6	<0.0001
STV (ms)	10.9 ± 2.7	11.8 ± 2.8	0.04	10.5 ± 2.7	11.7 ± 3.1	=0.024
LTV (ms)	58.3 ± 14.1	63.3 ± 14.8	=0.009	56.3 ± 14.2	63.4 ± 16.6	=0.017
Accelerations (numbers)	10.0 [6.5–14.0]	13.0 [9.8–17.0]	<0.0001	10.2 [7.0–13.8]	13.5 [9.0–17.0]	>0.1
HV (ms)	58.5 [43.3–68.3]	58.5 [51.4–73.5]	=0.09	51.7 [37.1–66.7]	67.2 [54.1–72.8]	<0.001
RMSSD (ms)	11.0 ± 1.6	10.7 ± 1.6	>0.3	10.7	10.3	>0.5

Data are shown as mean ± SD or median [IQR]
bFHR basal fetal heart rate, *STV* short term variation, *ms* milliseconds, *LTV* long term variation, *HV* high variation, *RMSSD* root mean square of successive difference

Maternal activity, diet intake, psychological and physiological conditions can influence FHR [8, 20, 21]. The fact that information regarding these maternal factors were not collected can be considered as a limitation of this study. However, the ability to achieve good quality recordings of the FHR over prolonged periods (up to 16 h) whilst the mother continued with normal activities at home is a novel approach, permitting the assessment of the FHR under normal (uncontrolled) conditions. This is the first study to report changes seen in the FHR in relation to time of day in pregnancies where maternal mobility was not restricted.

Because we did not investigate the relationship of the FHR to that of the mother, it is not possible to comment on whether the control of the circadian pattern in the fetus is partially under fetal control or partially or totally under maternal influence. However, the fact that advancing GA has a clear influence on the size of the day: night differences in both bFHR and LTV supports the theory that there is a major fetal component. This is supported by a small study looking at nine pregnancies at term that did not demonstrate a significant relationship between maternal and fetal heart rates [21]. In addition, although this study did not collect data as regards the quality of the mothers sleep, a prospective

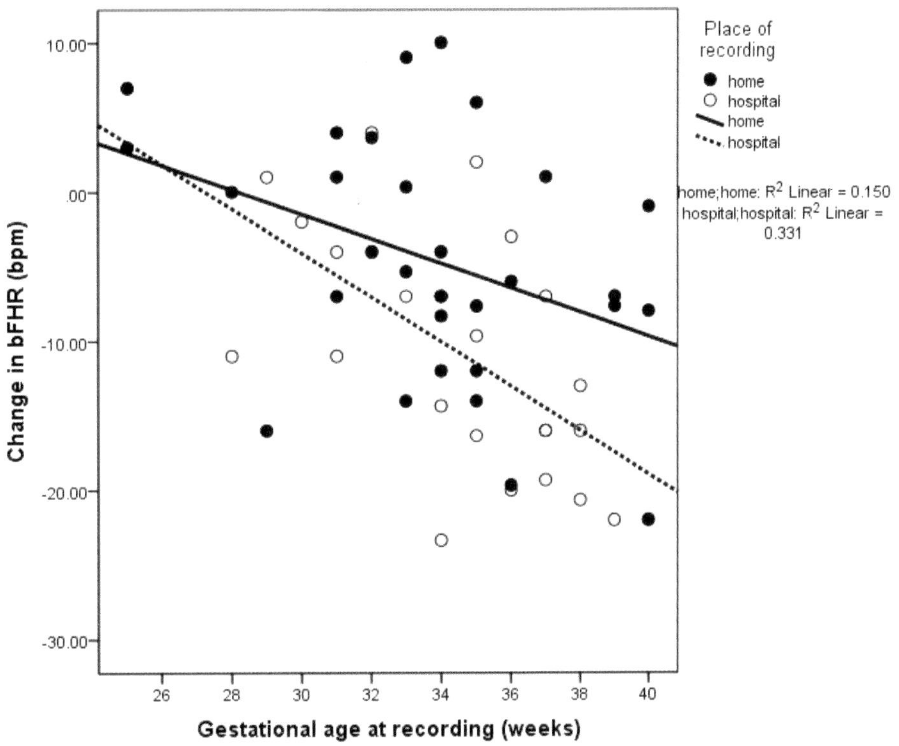

Fig. 1 Analysis of Day: Night Changes in Basal Fetal Heart Rate. The day:night change in basal fetal heart rate (bFHR) increased significantly with gestation age at the time of recording ($r = -0.409$; $P < 0.002$). The place of recording also exerted an additive significant effect (final $r = -0.554$; $P < 0.001$)

Table 3 Day: night differences in fetal heart rate (FHR) parameters with respect to sex

	Male ($n = 30$)	Female ($n = 24$)	*P* value
Change in bFHR (bpm)	−7.3 [−3.3, −14.0]	−5.7 [+1.0, −15.6]	>0.4
Change in STV (ms)	1.2 [3.1, 0.2]	0.6 [1.6, −1.1]	0.076
Change in LTV (ms)	7.7 [17.6, 5.0]	3.5 [7.5, −5.6]	0.010
Change in RMSSD (ms)	0.0 [1.3 -1.3]	−0.31 [0.4, −1.5]	>0.2

Data are shown as mean median [IQR]
The day: night change in all measures of FHR variability was greater in male than female fetuses; this difference was significant with respect to long-term variation (LTV)
bFHR basal fetal heart rate, *STV* short term variation, *LTV* long term variation, *RMSSD* root mean square of successive differences

trial on the effect of obstructive sleep apnea in pregnancy on fetal heart rate monitoring found there was no effect [22].

In order to assess day: night changes in FHR pattern, we randomly selected the best 90 min FHR data with good fetal signals from the day and night recording of the same individual. Therefore we recognise that our study suffered from selection bias. However, selection of 90 min data FHR data guaranteed the analysis of high variation episodes as in human fetus the cycle of active and quiet sleep ranges from 60–90 min [23]. Nonetheless, our results are in keeping with previous studies, all performed under strictly controlled laboratory conditions, confirming the presence of a circadian pattern in the FHR. The night time reduction in bFHR is also in keeping with previously published data [5, 24]. Not all researchers have confirmed the increase in measures of variability during the night that we have described, but some have been small studies using visual rather than computerised analysis of the heart rate recordings [25]. The increase in variability is in keeping with the known increase in fetal activity seen at night [3]. However, there are also longer rest phases seen at night [23] which could, at least in part, explain the lower bFHR.

To date, few studies have evaluated sex-related FHR differences and most of them have failed to demonstrate significant difference in the antepartum period. It has been suggested that sex does not need to be considered when assessing FHR variability [26], this was based on a small study looking at 5 min recordings of FHR whereas our data were obtained from recordings over three hours (90 min day and 90 min night). Both Fleisher et al. [27], in a longitudinal study of 14 male and 17 female fetuses studied over 15 min periods and Amorim-Costa et al. [12], in a cross-sectional retrospective study of 5172 male and 4529 female fetuses studied for an average duration of 30 min, reported significant sex-related differences in FHR parameters at various gestational ages.

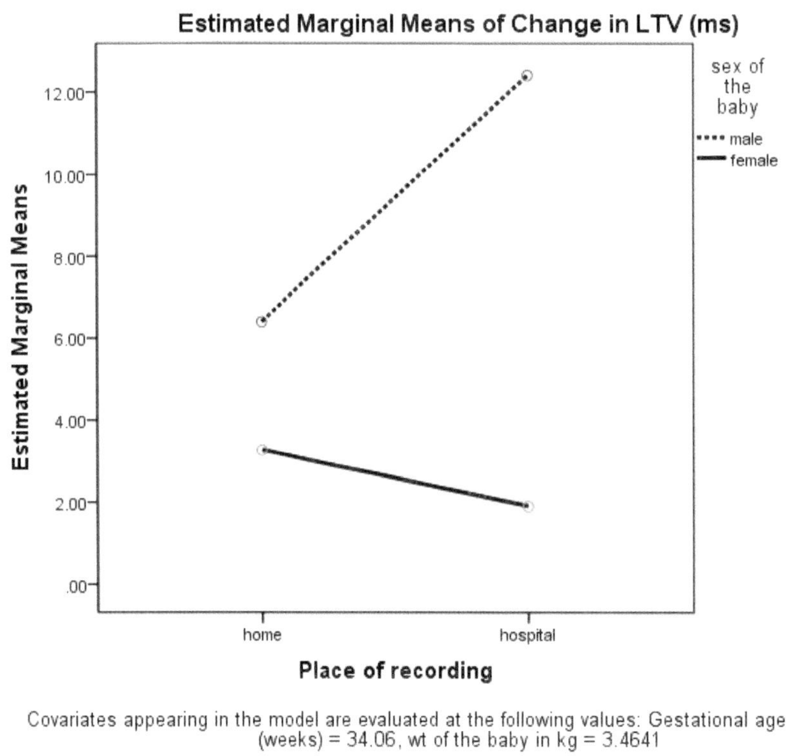

Fig. 2 Analysis of Day: Night Changes in Long Term Variation. Analysis of the day:night change in long-term variation (LTV) showed significant effects of both gestational age (GA) at recording ($P = 0.030$) and sex ($P = 0.029$); birthweight (used as a surrogate for weight at recording) did not have a significant additional effect ($P > 0.1$)

Baseline FHR was consistently found to be higher in female fetuses whereas STV and LTV tend to be lower at most stages of pregnancy. Our data confirm greater heart rate variability, expressed as several indices, in male than female fetuses. This adds to existing knowledge by showing that this increased variability in males is significant at night (when bFHR is lower and maternal conditions are at their most stable) but not during the day. Possible mechanisms for this sex-related difference seem not to have been addressed. Animal work has shown that female fetuses have significantly greater adrenomedullary mRNA expression of catecholamine-synthesizing enzymes than males [28]. The greater heart rate variability in male fetuses suggests the possibility of increased sensitivity to circulating catecholamine. Sex-related differences in catecholamine receptor density or affinity have not yet been investigated.

Conclusions

The existence of circadian rhythms has been demonstrated in most living organisms including plants and some bacteria. This study confirms that the human fetus demonstrates a clear circadian pattern in both the underlying heart rate and other variables. It is probable that there is, at least, a large fetal component to the control of this pattern. The demonstration of sex-related differences, particularly in terms of the size of the differences seen between day and night, supports this.

The changes in both fetal activity and heart rate variables with the time of day [29] have implications for the assessment of fetal well-being. Knowledge of the circadian pattern of fetal activity and heart rate will improve the interpretation of fetal monitoring.

Acknowledgements

We gratefully acknowledge Monica Healthcare, Nottingham, UK for providing the fetal ECG monitors and electrodes in kind for the study.

Funding

The authors report no funding.

Authors' contributions

All authors contributed significantly to the manuscript and approved the final version. Dr Habiba Kapaya did the analysis and drafted the report. Professor Fiona Broughton Pipkin provided guidance on the analysis and edited the report. Professor Barrie Hayes-Gill and Dr Pamela Loughna provided input, oversaw the process, edited the report and supported throughout.

Competing interests

Professor Barrie Hayes-Gill is an Executive Director and shareholder at Monica Healthcare, Ltd. Other authors have no conflicts of interest.

Author details

[1]Division of Child Health, Obstetrics and Gynaecology, School of Medicine, University of Nottingham, Nottingham NG7 2RD, UK. [2]Electrical Systems and Optics Research Division, University of Nottingham, University Park, Nottingham NG7 2RD, UK. [3]Department of Oncology and Metabolism, Academic Unit of Reproductive & Developmental Medicine, 4th Floor Jessop Wing, Tree Root Walk, Sheffield S102SF, UK.

References

1. de Vries JI, Visser GH, Mulder EJ, Prechtl HF. Diurnal and other variations in fetal movement and heart rate patterns at 20–22 weeks. Early Hum Dev. 1987;15:333–48.
2. Patrick J, Campbell K, Carmichael L, Natale R, Richardson B. Daily relationships between fetal and maternal heart rates at 38 to 40 weeks of pregnancy. Can Med Assoc J. 1981;124:1177–8.
3. Patrick J, Campbell K, Carmichael L, Natale R, Richardson B. Patterns of gross fetal body movements over 24-hour observation intervals during the last 10 weeks of pregnancy. Am J Obstet Gynecol. 1982;142:363–71.
4. Warren WS, Champney TH, Cassone VM. The suprachiasmatic nucleus controls the circadian rhythm of heart rate via the sympathetic nervous system. Physiol Behav. 1994;55:1091–9.
5. Lunshof S, Boer K, Wolf H, van Hoffen G, Bayram N, Mirmiran M. Fetal and maternal diurnal rhythms during the third trimester of normal pregnancy: Outcomes of computerized analysis of continuous twenty-four—hour fetal heart rate recordings. Am J Obstet Gynecol. 1998;178: 247–54.
6. Koutcherov Y, Mai JK, Paxinos G. Hypothalamus of the human fetus. J Chem Neuroanat. 2003;26:253–70.
7. Schneider U, Schleussner E, Fiedler A, Jaekel S, Liehr M, Haueisen J, Hoyer D. Fetal heart rate variability reveals differential dynamics in the intrauterine development of the sympathetic and parasympathetic branches of the autonomic nervous system. Physiol Meas. 2009;30:215–26.
8. Marzbanrad F, Kimura Y, Palaniswami M, Khandoker AH. Quantifying the interactions between maternal and fetal heart rates by transfer entropy. PLoS One. 2015;10:e0145672.
9. Swartjes JM, van Geijn HP, Mantel R, Schoemaker HC. Quantitated fetal heart rhythm at 20, 32 and 38 weeks of gestation and dependence on rest-activity patterns. Early Hum Dev. 1992;28:27–36.
10. Pillai M, James D. The importance of the behavioural state in biophysical assessment of the term human fetus. BJOG. 1990;97:1130–4.
11. Lunshof S, Boer K, van Hoffen G, Wolf H, Mirmiran M. The diurnal rhythm in fetal heart rate in a twin pregnancy with discordant anencephaly: comparison with three normal twin pregnancies. Early Hum Dev. 1997;48:47–57.
12. Amorim-Costa C, Cruz J, Ayres-de-Campos D, Bernardes J. Gender-specific reference charts for cardiotocographic parameters throughout normal pregnancy: a retrospective cross-sectional study of 9701 fetuses. Eur J Obstet Gynecol Reprod Biol. 2016;199:102–7.
13. Bonnemeier H, Richardt G, Potratz J, Wiegand U, Brandes A, Kluge N, Katus H. Circadian profile of cardiac autonomic nervous modulation in healthy subjects: differing effects of aging and gender on heart rate variability. J Cardiovasc Electrophysiol. 2003;14:791–9.
14. Aziz W, Schlindwein F, Wailoo M, Biala T, Rocha F. Heart rate variability analysis of normal and growth restricted children. Clin Autonomic Res. 2012; 22:91–7.
15. Bernardes J, Goncalves H, Ayres-de-Campos D, Rocha F. Sex differences in linear and complex fetal heart rate dynamics of normal and acidemic fetuses in the minutes preceding delivery. J Perinat Med. 2012;37:168–76.
16. Visser GH, Goodman JD, Levine DH, Dawes GS. Diurnal and other cyclic variations in human fetal heart rate near term. Am J Obstet Gynecol. 1982; 142:535–44.
17. Cohen W, Ommani S, Hassan S, Mirza F, Solomon M, Brown R, Schifrin B, Himsworth J, Hayes-Gill B. Accuracy and reliability of fetal heart rate monitoring using maternal abdominal surface electrodes. Acta Obstet Gynecol Scand. 2012;91:1306–13.

18 Dawes G, Meir YJ, Mandruzzato GP. Computerized evaluation of fetal heart-rate patterns. J Perinat Med. 1994;22:491–9.
19 Pardey J, Moulden M, Redman CW. A computer system for the numerical analysis of nonstress tests. Am J Obstet Gynecol. 2002;186:1095–103.
20 Esin S. Factors that increase reactivity during fetal nonstress testing. Curr Opin Obstet Gynecol. 2014;26:61–6.
21 Muro M, Shono H, DShono M, Ito Y, Uchiyama A, Iwasaka T. Analysis of the influence of diurnal variation in maternal movements on fetal heart rate pattern. Psych Clin Neurosci. 2002;56:247–8.
22 Olivarez SA, Maheshwari B, McCarthy M, Zacharias N, van den Veyver I, Casturi L, Sangi-Haghpeykar H, Aagaard-Tillery K. Prospective trial on obstructive sleep apnea in pregnancy and fetal heart rate monitoring. Am J Obstet Gynecol. 2010;202:552.e551–557.
23 Muro M, Shono H, Kohara M, Ito Y, Uchiyama A, Sugimori H. Diurnal variations in resting-active cycles in full-term fetal heart rate changes. Early Hum Dev. 1996;44:51–8.
24 de Vries JIP, Visser GHA, Mulder EJH, Prechtl HFR. Diurnal and other variations in fetal movement and heart rate patterns at 20–22 weeks. Early Hum Dev. 1987;15:333–348.
25 Morokuma S, Horimoto N, Nakano H. Diurnal changes in the power spectral characteristics of eye movements and heart rate variability in the human fetus at term. Early Hum Dev. 2001;64:27–36.
26 Lange S, van Leeuwen P, Geue D, Hatzmann W, Gronemeyer D. Influence of gestational age, heart rate, gender and time of day on fetal heart rate variability. Med Biol Eng Comput. 2005;43:481–6.
27 Fleisher L, Dipietro J, Johnson T, Pincus S. Complementary and non-coincident increases in heart rate variability and irregularity during fetal development. Clin Sci (Lond). 1997;92:345–9.
28 Bibeau K, Battista M-C, Houde V, Brochu M. Fetal adrenal gland alterations in a rat model of adverse intrauterine environment. Am J Physiol. 2010;298: R899–911.
29 Ozkaya E, Baser E, Cinar M, Korkmaz V, Kucukozkan T. Does diurnal rhythm have an impact on fetal biophysical profile? J Mat Fet Neonat Med. 2012;25: 335–8.
30 Patrick J, Campbell K, Carmichael L, Probert C. Influence of maternal heart rate and gross fetal body movements on the daily pattern of fetal heart rate near term. Am J Obstet Gynecol. 1982;144:533–8.

11

Urogenital fistula reviewed: a marker of severe maternal morbidity and an indicator of the quality of maternal healthcare delivery

Margo S. Harrison[1*], Hillary Mabeya[2], Robert L. Goldenberg[1] and Elizabeth M. McClure[3]

Abstract

Background: While obstetric fistula has been recognized as a major maternal morbidity since the 1980s, it has become an indicator of access to and quality of women' s health care.

Findings: Obstetric fistula still exists in low-income countries (LIC) because health care systems fail to provide adequate family planning, skilled birth attendance, basic and emergency obstetric care, and affordable treatment of fistula, while concurrently lacking social networks to serve as safety nets for affected girls and women [WHO, 2007].

Conclusion: This review explores the most recent published experience with respect to the definition of fistula, its diagnosis, treatment, and management, and further steps for prevention of fistula on a global scale.

Keywords: Urogenital fistula, Obstetric fistula, Maternal morbidity, Low and middle income countries

Introduction

An urogenital fistula is defined as an abnormal communication between the bladder, ureter, urethra, vagina, and/or rectum with resulting incontinence of urine and/or stool. It may occur as a sequela of childbirth or as a result of surgical injury, malignancy, infection, trauma, or endometriosis. The term obstetric fistula refers to fistulae resulting from the 'obstructed labor injury complex,' which describes the injury that occurs when the presenting fetal part becomes impacted against the bony pelvis during labor causing hypoperfusion of the soft tissues in between, resulting in ischemia, necrosis, and an abnormal communication between two pelvic organs [2]. Not all obstetric fistulae result from obstructed labor. A recent review of almost 6,000 cases of urogenital fistula suggested that just over thirteen percent of fistulae were iatrogenic, 80 % of which followed surgery for obstetric complications including cesarean section (57 %), repair of ruptured uterus (20 %), and hysterectomy for ruptured uterus or obstetric indications (3 %), with the remainder occurring during gynecologic surgery unrelated to pregnancy [3]. Of note, urogenital fistulae are often referred to by the organs they involve; for example, a vesicovaginal fistula involves the bladder and vagina, rectovaginal the rectum and vaginal, ureterovaginal the ureter and vagina, and vesicouterine the bladder and uterus. Urogenital fistulas are quiet varied and can include any and/or all of the genitourinary system, but those involved are often reflected by how the fistula is named.

Epidemiology, incidence, and prevalence

With the recognition of urogenital fistula as a public health indicator related to both the availability and quality of women's healthcare services, there has been much interest in determining its incidence and prevalence around the world. Fistula patients are a literal embodiment of healthcare system failure to provide appropriate maternal healthcare and delivery services, and as such, fistula occurrence can be used as a measure to determine the quality of the healthcare system in a given area. Commonly quoted numbers suggest that there are 3.5 million women currently living with urogenital fistula and that 50,000 to 100,000 women develop fistula annually [4, 5]. A recent meta-analysis estimated a pooled prevalence of 0.29 fistulae per 1000 reproductive age women in all regions with a rate of 1.6/1000 in sub-Saharan Africa and 1.2/1000 in south Asia [6]. The pooled incidence was 0.09 fistulae per 1000 recently pregnant women [6]. Prior to this

* Correspondence: msh2154@cumc.columbia.edu
[1]Department of Obstetrics/Gynecology, Columbia University, New York, NY, USA
Full list of author information is available at the end of the article

publication, the previously accepted numbers regarding incidence came from the 2000 Global Burden of Disease report that suggested the incidence was 0.08 % of all births and 2.15 % of births complicated by neglected obstructed labor [7].

Current methods for assessing the prevalence of urogenital fistula include self-reporting and general communication with surgeons, studies by advocacy groups, and reviews of hospital services; they mostly use community or facility sampling or a combination of both [8]. Because of the relative rarity of fistula, the desire of affected women to hide their condition, and the poor quality of data collection methods in areas where women are affected, obtaining quality data is very difficult [8]. A recent review published on determining the worldwide incidence and prevalence of urogenital fistula suggests that data need to be collected through routine surveillance and monitoring systems that are currently integrated into established health systems and national programs [8]. An example given is the Demographic and Health Surveys that many countries conduct, which include home births; questions should be added to the survey regarding urogenital fistula to garner better data [8]. Additionally, follow-up data collection on women seeking care is also important to track the met need for surgical care and to observe how targeted prevention or treatment interventions are affecting outcomes related to urogenital fistula [8]. The aforementioned review also suggests that fistula care be part of the full continuum of maternal health services provided in maternity wards, and that providers should be trained to assess for urogenital fistula at postpartum visits [8].

The global public health community has recognized the necessity of good data collection regarding urogenital fistula not only in terms of incidence and prevalence, but also in terms of availability of centers for fistula care and providers capable of providing high quality treatment. As such, the WHO developed the Global Fistula Map in an attempt to show not only where women are affected around the world, but also where providers are available [9]. The map was unable to be reproduced for this review, but can be accessed online at http://www.globalfistulamap.org/. Information on how the data was collected is explained on the website and the actual data itself can be downloaded for review.

Risk factors and causes

Obstetric fistula is associated with age < twenty years, first pregnancy, labor greater than 24 h, delivery at home, height < 150 cm (<59 in.), low levels of maternal education, poor contraceptive utilization, low rates of antenatal care utilization, and having a male fetus [10–12]. A given woman's risk for obstetric fistula formation is also determined by her overall health, socioeconomic status, and her access to and utilization of health care services [11]. While the immediate cause of obstetric fistula is the lack of safe labor and delivery services, root causes include poor health care infrastructure such as transportation and communication, as well as cultural norms that devalue women, including lack of female autonomy, economic and social independence, and education [11].

Socioeconomic and psychosocial implications

Urogenital fistula follows acute physical trauma, but it causes continued physical and psychosocial trauma through exclusion from social networks, divorce, impoverishment, and major depression [12]. Role loss, isolation, and economic deprivation were the most common consequences for women with fistula, and the majority of these women were abandoned by husbands, shunned by family, and struggled severely with hygiene associated with incontinence and wound care, as well as frequent infections [13]. The women suffer from post-traumatic stress disorder, social isolation, feeling like the object of stigma, low quality of life, and general mental health dysfunction, including suicidal ideation [14–16].

Diagnosis, treatment and management

Timing and symptomatology

Women with urogenital fistula classically present with continuous urinary incontinence, as compared to incontinence with a valsalva maneuver, or stress urinary incontinence, which is common after normal labor and delivery [17, 18]. While timing of presentation after delivery can be affected by socioeconomic as much as clinical factors, it can also be determined by the type of fistula from which a woman suffers. For example, fistula from cesarean delivery may present seven to ten days post-operatively due to formation of a fistulous tract over time, while obstetric fistula due to obstructed labor can usually be noted immediately after delivery [1, 19, 20]. Fistulas that involve the uterus can involve irregular bleeding patterns and loss of blood in urine [19, 21]. Additionally, if the ureter is transected, the presentation will likely occur immediately post-operatively as an intra-abdominal urinoma when the patient begins to experience the pain, pressure, and symptoms produced by the mass effect of extravasated urine, but may not present as a fistula until the anomalous tract has formed with the vagina or another body cavity [19].

Diagnosis

Diagnosis involves a full medical and social history, including details about the incident pregnancy, the labor course, the delivery, and the fetal outcome. Review of systems should be performed with attention to urinary and fecal symptoms, as well as general mobility and musculoskeletal function [1]. The physical examination begins with collecting vital signs and performing a neurologic and gait evaluation [1]. Visual inspection should always be the first step in the genital exam with evaluation for perineal dermatitis, ulceration, infection, and scarring from prior episiotomy, circumcision, or fistula repair [1]. The examiner should then proceed to abdominal and bimanual examination noting the severity and nature of vaginal and rectal scarring; location, size, and number of fistulae; and involvement of crucial structures such as the urethral sphincter, anal sphincter, and urethra itself [1]. Further diagnostic testing may be necessary, such as a vaginal speculum exam for improved exposure, or a dye test [22]. Dye tests generally involve back-filling the bladder and temporarily occluding the urethra for evaluation of dye leakage. If the fistula cannot be immediately located, some authors recommend vaginal packing, with the location of dye leakage on the pack used to help narrow down the fistula position [17]. Additionally, oral pyridium or intravenous indigo carmine can be administered to assess ureteral involvement [17, 19]. Hemoglobin determination and testing for sexually transmitted infections are also recommended, as the former is important for pre-operative planning, and the latter because sexually transmitted infections can be the cause of a fistula (and their treatment may allow for spontaneous fistula closure), and they can also cause friability of the tissue which will complicate fistula closure. Additionally, patients who are HIV positive may require treatment and rehabilitation prior to surgery to improve their surgical outcomes.

Treatment

The primary goal of fistula treatment is continence. Obtaining continence generally requires surgery, but may be achieved by conservative treatment with catheters or stents, or require a more aggressive diversionary procedure [1, 23].

Conservative management

Women with a small simple fistula discovered shortly after delivery, or those presenting to a facility with obstructed labor, may be treated conservatively with insertion of a Foley catheter for somewhere between two and six weeks, twice daily sitz baths, high volume oral intake of fluids, and treatment of any obvious concurrent infections [1]. Currently available data are of poor quality and no clear recommendations can be made as to whether initial conservative management with a Foley catheter is appropriate or effective [24]. However, since 1942, papers have been published suggesting use of a Foley catheter as a method of assisting spontaneous closure of vesicovaginal fistulae less than one centimeter in size [24]. Similarly, ureteral stents placed for one to two months may result in spontaneous resolution of fistulas involving the ureter in greater than half of cases [17, 23]. Ureteral stents are usually placed, in this context, by way of cystoscopy, which may not be available in LIC.

Surgical management

For most patients, surgery is the only option. The overriding principle of fistula repair is that the first attempt offers the best chance of successful closure [1]. The basic principles of surgical repair are: 1) achieving adequate exposure, 2) mobilizing the fistula from surrounding scar tissue, so that 3) a tension-free closure can be performed that is water-tight [1, 4].

Timing of surgery

While the traditional teaching is that patients undergo surgery three months after diagnosis to allow time for the fistulae to become less inflamed, more recent data suggest that fistulae be repaired immediately if diagnosed within 72 h of delivery, or even within the three month window, as repair within this timeframe prevents a significant amount of the negative social, economic, and physical sequelae associated with incontinence [17, 19, 23, 25]. Some patients, however, may present years after fistula formation. For these patients, if there is no residual edema, erythema, or persistent granulation tissue, and no need for treatment of infections, anemia, or malnutrition, surgery can be pursued without additional delay [19]. Iatrogenic fistulae should undergo surgical repair with diagnosis, unless the fistula is the result of retained suture. In that case, waiting until the suture is resorbed is in order [3, 19].

Pre-operative care

The WHO advises pre-operative management include anesthesia evaluation, skin preparation, hair clipping, high oral fluid intake, bowel preparation, and nothing by mouth from midnight of the night before surgery [1]. Issues such as nutritional supplementation and pre-operative estrogen usage, as well as transfusion or supplementation for anemia and empiric treatment with anti-malarials, antibiotics, or antiparasitics are topics for further research.

Surgical methods

The WHO guidelines recommend a vaginal approach to urogenital fistula repair. The optimal surgical position is high lithotomy, and the optimal anesthetic technique is regional [1]. Vaginal repair is associated with less blood loss, results in shorter operative time, leads to decreased use of analgesics, and overall accounts for shorter hospital length of stays [19]. Various antibiotic regimens, which include single-dose gentamicin, appear to be equally effective at decreasing post-operative urinary tract infections and improving leakage and incontinence profiles on discharge from the hospital [19, 26]. Commonly performed initial surgical steps include episiotomy for exposure, placement of retractors that assist with visualization, Foley catheterization to divert urine from the operative field, protection of the ureters with stents, and placement of a probe into the fistula to delineate its course and establish its boundaries [17].

Closure methods include the Latzko technique (partial colpocleisis without excision of the fistula tract), layered closure (excision of the fistulous tract), and use of flaps, which may be biologic (such as the Martius flap—a labial fat pad), but also include more recent experimentation with synthetic materials [17, 19, 23]. Studies have shown the Latzko technique to be quite effective with success rates quoted as 93 to 100 %, and placement of the Martius flap to have 70 – 100 % success rates, with the caveat that the latter method is used in the setting of more complicated fistulae with greater fibrosis and necrosis, or lack of tissue available for closure [19]. There is also a role for more invasive procedures that necessitate an abdominal approach for patients with reduced bladder capacity or pliability, involvement of the ureter, trigone, ureteral orifice, or cervix, and inability to access the fistula by way of the vagina, or for patients who have not achieved continence after multiple repairs or those whose fistula is too large, or the remaining tissue is too scarce, that anatomic closure is not possible [17, 27].

Minimally invasive surgery

Although minimally invasive surgery (MIS) such as laparoscopy and robotics is more accessible in high-income countries (HIC), a group in India is utilizing MIS to repair urogenital fistulae resulting from obstetric complications [28]. This group reportedly closed vesicovaginal fistulae with a single layer continuous laparoscopic suture with interposition of an omental flap; urethral catheters were left in situ for a month post-operatively [28]. As the capacity for MIS in LIC builds, it will be interesting to see how this experience contributes to the surgical literature.

Post-operative care

The WHO guidelines recommend regularly scheduled vital signs, pad checks and catheter monitoring for genitourinary bleeding, intravenous fluids, strict tracking of intake and output of fluids, and regularly scheduled analgesia for pain control, which will allow earlier patient mobility [1]. Patients are encouraged to continue to maintain very high fluid consumption in the early days following surgery, and the catheter is advised to be left in situ for a minimum of 10 – 14 days, with removal of any necessary vaginal packing after 24 – 72 h [1, 19, 26]. There are no recommendations regarding post-operative antibiotic use, but some research suggests that if used, antibiotics should cover all vaginal flora [17].

Outcomes

No straightforward framework exists for analyzing the determinants of successful fistula treatment and outcomes. This also applies to fistula classification—no generally accepted method exists: there are currently 25 proposed systems in practice, none of which were developed based on empiric evidence or with prognosis in mind [29]. Standardization of terminology regarding urogenital fistula will not only allow development of an evidence-based prognostic classification system, but will also facilitate research, guideline development, and the analysis of clinical outcomes to determine the safety, efficacy, and quality of preventative, diagnostic, and treatment interventions [24, 30]. Even the definitions of 'success' and 'failure' of fistula treatment are poorly defined; many studies define success as physical closure of the fistula while others define success as continence immediately after surgery and then at a later point in time. These assessments are made by back-filling the bladder with dye and evaluating leakage and continence after catheter removal; the time point at which this exam is performed is usually at surgery to confirm fistula closure, and then two weeks post-operatively.

Despite the lack of uniform definitions of type of fistula and measures of success, if success is defined as physical closure of the fistula, then the literature reports a 55 % to 95 % closure rate with an average success rare of about 85 % [30]. If success is defined as urinary continence then outcomes range from about a 40 % to 90 % success rate with an average success rate of about 70 % [30]. According the WHO guidelines, when establishing a fistula treatment program, it is expected that the closure rate for fistula should be 85 % and the continence rate should be 90 % after a patient's first fistula repair surgery [1]. Clinical factors that can affect surgical outcome and success rates include degree of urethral involvement (some damage versus circumferential involvement); size, location, and number of fistulae; amount of scar tissue and remaining healthy tissue, including bladder capacity; and whether or not the patient has previously undergone repair [30].

Psychosocial

Beyond documenting the distress experienced by fistula patients, researchers are implementing interventions to improve the mental health of this population. A Tanzanian trial of a six-session treatment plan based on psychological theory (cognitive behavioral therapy) was integrated into the clinical flow of a fistula ward (two sessions pre-operatively, four sessions post-operatively) and conducted by a non-specialist mental health provider, to improve mental health outcomes for fistula survivors [31]. The ratings from participants were very positive. While that study worked with patients individually, other studies have looked at group therapy and also achieved measureable success

[32]. The data suggests that mental health interventions are very important for fistula patients and can be executed concurrently with surgical treatment during the time when patients are preparing for and recovering from surgery [31].

Physiotherapy

The WHO practice guidelines recommend including physiotherapy as part of the treatment program (deep breathing, hip stretches, lower extremity range of motion stretches, and core strengthening exercises) as well as post-operative workouts that include sitting, standing, walking, and balancing, with graduated strength training, and a detailed program of special movement, positioning, and passive stretches for patients affected by contractures and nerve injuries [1]. A study of pre- and post-operative health education and physiotherapy of urogenital fistula patients reported that those who underwent physiotherapy were almost three times more likely to recover with less post-operative stress incontinence, and in a follow-up study conducted by the same group a year later, the results were maintained and quality of life had significantly improved [33, 34].

Socioeconomic practices & reintegration

The guiding principles for reintegration programs are that patients should be taught self-sustaining skills, which may require literacy training or workshops in making clothes or crafts. These skills become especially important for women who are single and no longer have the ability to bear children or function as homemaker, and who otherwise have no one to support them. They should be offered counseling services and should be helped to reintegrate into their social support network, which includes their communities and families, but might also involve enrollment in a women's or fistula survivors support group [1]. Currently utilized interventions include training in income generating skills, literacy training, and microcredit programs, as well as post-operative financial support in the form of clothing, supplies, food, water, and actual stipends [35]. While data in the area of economic repercussions of fistula are lacking, recent research from Tanzania reported that fistula patient's hopes and concerns about the future are primarily related to their ability to work, in addition to social acceptance and future fertility [13, 36, 37].

Post-fistula

Some data exist on long-term follow-up of fistula patients after repair. A Nigerian study evaluated 150 women six months after repair to assess quality of life, physical health, mental health, social health, and environment (available income, ability to perform activities of daily living, and level of participation in leisure activities), comparing those indicators before and after surgery; the results were significantly improved on all measures except 'environment' [38]. A study of Ethiopian women reported that, the majority felt a dramatic sensation of relief and happiness following repair, yet some continued to experience mental anguish, stigma, and physical problems regardless of the outcome of the procedure. All women suffered intense fear of developing another fistula, most commonly from sex or childbirth. Despite this, the majority of women had sex or planned to, while a smaller cohort avoided intercourse and childbearing, thus subjecting them to isolation, marital conflict, and/or economic vulnerability [39].

A study of fertility in 32 women with fistula from Malawi showed that about half of pregnancies conceived with an active fistula, and 70 % of those conceived post-repair, ended in spontaneous abortion or perinatal death [40]. Findings suggest that pregnancies conceived post-repair may result in poor outcomes years out from surgery; whether these results are related to fistula or occur from coincident damage to the pelvis or some other etiology is not clear. Data on contraception use in women with fistula or post fistula repair is scarce. However, a study of almost 200 women in Nigeria, showed that almost all knew about contraception, but less than half actually utilized it, suggesting that contraceptive uptake after fistula repair was poor for fear of adverse effects (41 % of participants), desire for fertility (30 %), religious prohibition (22 %), cultural beliefs (25 %), and partner disapproval (36 %) [41]. No studies were found on interventions providing contraceptive counseling to urogenital fistula patients.

Findings

Prevention & awareness

Whether the fistula results from poor labor and delivery care or poor surgical technique, both are avoidable, and the key is prevention. Improved access to high-quality emergency obstetrical care including cesarean section is essential, but so is improved access to family planning services [25]. Over the longer term, attention should be devoted to developing programs that combat the root causes of fistula formation including improved education, economic opportunity, and gender equality for women [25]. While many of the factors leading to fistula formation may be out of the control of the individual woman, the decision to seek care for a dysfunctional labor falls to the patient and birth attendant. Seeking timely care for prolonged labor is a critical component of obstetrical fistula prevention programs in resource-limited settings [25]. To achieve the goal of overcoming this initial delay to care, patients must value the services provided by health institutions and understand the consequences of not seeking care in a time-sensitive fashion. To accomplish this, the care women anticipate receiving must be effective and of high quality, and be socially, physically, and economically accessible. Overcoming these barriers requires utilization of prenatal care and education of men and the greater community regarding dysfunctional labor and the risk of fistula [25].

A recent review article examined current evidence supporting fistula prevention strategies in sub-Saharan Africa [42]. The authors advise promoting a minimum of post-primary education for girls; providing sexual education that includes information about fistula; educating communities about cultural, social, and physiological factors that influence and contribute to fistula; delaying early marriage and childbirth; eradicating malnutrition; and defining time limits for labor at home without progress [42]. The health system based strategies that have shown success in prevention of fistula include scaling up access to, availability of, and provision of emergency obstetric care; provision of affordable, safe, and timely interventions for women in need of care; reducing the distance to access care; and providing affordable transportation to health facilities [42]. Clearly, additional training or re-training of surgical providers is also crucial, since iatrogenic fistulae due to poor surgical technique are also preventable.

In terms of actual interventions to prevent fistula that have been published, there exist a few. One author applied a fistula index he developed, which is the multiplication of a given patient's height in centimeters by her intertuberous distance (the distance between the ischial tuberosities of her pelvis), which was measured by the number of knuckles on the surgeon's hand that he could fit between the pelvic bones [43]. He applied his index in a case-controlled study of 39 fistula patients and 54 controls with normal vaginal deliveries [43]. His results were significantly different between the groups, which was not the case when height alone was compared, suggesting that such a measure of clinical pelvimetry could be useful in identifying women at risk for fistula development [43]. Another study conducted in Niger employed a community-mobilization program to reduce maternal and neonatal mortality and reduce urogenital fistula formation [44]. The intervention utilized village volunteers to identify and evacuate women with protracted labor, provide education, and collect data on pregnancies, births, and deaths [44]. Over three years the intervention significantly reduced maternal and perinatal mortality and reduced the occurrence of fistula from seven cases in the first six months of the study to zero cases in the next 24 months [44]. These interventions suggest that some combination of prenatal risk assessment and education with access to emergency obstetrical care can reduce and potentially prevent urogenital fistula from obstetric causes.

Training & facility capacity

Even though efforts have been underway to address the problem of urogenital fistula on a global scale for at least 30 years, it was not until 2003 that the United Nations established the Campaign to End Fistula, and it was not until almost ten years later that attention was paid to issues such as the availability of providers and facilities to address the issue. Thus, WHO developed the Global Fistula Map to assess how many providers provided fistula repair services and to provide an illustration of available services for women with fistula [43]. The Map demonstrates that currently, despite increased international attention to the issue, the number of women with fistula is increasing because the number of repairs is less than the number of new cases [22]. It is estimated that up to 80 % of women living with fistula do not receive appropriate care [22, 45]. Given the lack of providers, the International Federation of Gynecology and Obstetrics, published a competency-based fistula-training manual in 2011 [22]. The manual, available on their website at no cost, is meant to promote standardization of surgical training for fistula repair and increased the number of appropriately trained providers able to provide high quality surgical repair [22, 46].

The next question on the topic of training and capacity building is how much money will programs cost, and what results can be expected from the investment. On the issue of what gains can be expected from preventing fistula, a recent paper was published on the surgically avertable burden of obstetric conditions in low and middle-income regions (LMIC) [47]. This manuscript examines five conditions (maternal hemorrhage, obstructed labor, obstetric fistula, abortion, and neonatal encephalopathy) and uses demographic and epidemiological data from the 2010 Global Burden of Disease study to estimate avertable disability adjusted life years (DALYs)—or years of healthy life lost caused by the burden of a disease [47]. The analysis suggests that 37 % of DALYs are avertable by the provision of universal, quality obstetric surgery in LMIC. The study suggests that obstructed labor and obstetric fistula have the highest rates of avertable burden and that sub-Saharan Africa and South Asia carry the largest proportion of this burden [47]. According to these authors, 1,121,346 DALYs (100 % of associated DALYs) and 996,555 DALYs (89 % of associated DALYs) would be averted if quality obstetric surgical services were available to prevent fistula formation [47]. As for cost estimates, it has been suggested that the investment required to scale up provision of comprehensive universal obstetric care through from the prenatal through postnatal period in the 75 LMIC most in need of such care would require 39 billion dollars [48]. For comparison, as of 2012 UNAIDS estimates that 122.5 billion dollars had been invested in the global HIV/AIDS response [49].

Ethical considerations

Fistula patients deserve high quality care when they present for fistula treatment. As such, a bill of rights for the fistula patient has been developed, as has a code of ethics for the fistula surgeon [50–52]. The bill of rights states that fistula patients should be treated with compassion, dignity, and respect; they should have a right to privacy and to full information and education regarding their condition; they should have the right to direct their own care—including refusal of treatment; and they have the right to receive high quality care, and to be fed, clothed, and sheltered during that process [51]. The code of ethics of the fistula surgeon holds the provider to the standard of providing the highest quality care to the fistula patient and holding her welfare above all else; treating her with dignity, respect, compassion, honesty, and keeping her care confidential; taking responsibility for her total care including appropriate pre-operative and follow-up care; to not experiment on her or provide care in which the surgeon is not trained; to be committed to evidence-based care and to be willing to alter methods based on best-practice guidelines; to not take advantage or allow others to take advantage of the fistula patient (physically, emotionally, economically, sexually); to exercise good stewardship over the financial resources entrusted to them for the care of the fistula patients; to work as part of a fistula care team and obey the laws of the country in which they practice; and to be an advocate on behalf of fistula patients to help remove barriers that hinder access to emergency obstetrical care [50].

Future research

More research would improve clinical care as well as the full spectrum of supportive care services that accompany fistula treatment, such as psychosocial and economic support, in addition to guiding the training and health system capacity building expected by the global community. That being said, specialists in the field formulated recommendations regarding the clinical topics they feel would most benefit from rigorous controlled trials, which include: the "efficacy/safety of short-term catheterization; efficacy of surgical and nonsurgical therapies for urinary incontinence; technical measures during fistula repair to reduce the incidence of post-surgery incontinence; identification of predictive factors for 'incurable fistula'; usefulness of urodynamic studies in the management of urinary incontinence; incidence and significance of multi-drug resistant bacteria in the fistula population; primary management of small, new fistulae by catheter drainage; and antibiotic prophylaxis in fistula repair" [53].

Conclusion

This review has addressed the multifaceted nature of urogenital fistula and that it may be a natural sequela of obstructed labor or iatrogenic. Fistula formation is primarily rooted in poor access to quality labor and delivery care. It deeply affects and disorganizes women's lives, plaguing the poorest and most marginalized populations, and clinical management of urogenital fistula is in dire need of an evidence-base, despite published guidelines. In conclusion, successful treatment of a fistula patient not only means closure of her fistula, but incorporation into a comprehensive treatment program aimed at achieving continence, mental health, physical rehabilitation, and socioeconomic training and support. Urogenital fistula resulting from childbirth is an historical footnote in HIC, and the provision of high-quality comprehensive emergency obstetrical care in LIC would render it extinct on a global scale. With a manageable price tag of 39 billion dollars, a massive burden of death and disability would be lifted from the human race, resulting in the survival of healthy women and children who bring near limitless potential for their own and the common good.

Competing interests
The authors declare that they have no competing interests

Authors' contributions
MSH and RLG conceived of the review. MSH wrote the review and RLG, HM, EMM edited the review for content and readability. All authors read and approved the final manuscript.

Acknowledgments
The authors wish to thank all those involved in the field of urogenital fistula diagnosis, treatment, management, and activism.

Author details
[1]Department of Obstetrics/Gynecology, Columbia University, New York, NY, USA. [2]Moi University School of Medicine, Eldoret, Kenya. [3]RTI International, Durham, NC, USA.

References

1. Lewis G, de Bernis L. Obstetric fistula: guiding principles for clinical management and programme development. Publication of the World Health Organization, 2006.
2. Arrowsmith S, Hamlin C, Wall LL. Obstructed labor injury complex: obstetric fistula formation and the multifaceted morbidity of maternal birth trauma in the developing world. Obstet Gynecol Surv. 1996;51(9):568–74.
3. Raassen TJIP, Ngongo CJ, Mahendeka MM. Iatrogenic genitourinary fistula: an 18-year retrospective review of 805 injuries. Int J Urol. 2014;25:1699–706.
4. Wall LL. Obstetric vesicovaginal fistula as an international public-health problem. Lancet. 2006;368:1201–9.
5. World Health Organization. "Ten Facts on obstetric fistula." Internet: http://www.who.int/features/factfiles/obstetric_fistula/en/, 2014.
6. Adler AJ, Ronsmans C, Calvert C, Filippi V. Estimating the prevalence of obstetric fistula: a systematic review and meta-analysis. BMC Pregnancy Childbirth. 2013;13(246):1–14.
7. Dolea C, AbouZhar C. Global burden of obstructed labour in the year 2000. World Health Organ. 2003; 1–17. http://www.who.int/healthinfo/statistics/bod_obstructedlabour.pdf
8. Tunçalp O, Tripathi V, Landry E, Stantonc CK, Ahmed S. Measuring the incidence and prevalence of obstetric fistula: approaches, needs and recommendations. Bull World Health Organ. 2015;93(1):60–2.
9. Campaign to End Fistula. Campaign to End Fistula. 4 8, 2015. http://www.endfistula.org/ (accessed 4 8, 2015).
10. Tebeu PM, Fomulu JN, Khaddaj S, de Bernis L, Delvaux T, Rochat CH. Risk factors for obstetric fistula: a clinical review. Int Urogynecol J. 2012;23(4):387–94.

11. Wall LL. Preventing Obstetric Fistulas in Low-Resource Countries: Insights From a Haddon Matrix. Obstet Gynecol Surv. 2012;67(2):111–21.
12. Roka ZG, Akech M, Wanzala P, Omolo J, Gitta S, Waiswa P. Factors associated with obstetric fistulae occurrence among patients attending selected hospitals in Kenya, 2010: a case control study. BMC Pregnancy Childbirth. 2013;13(56):1–7.
13. Roush KM. Social Implications of Obstetric Fistula: An Integrative Review. J Midwifery Womens Health. 2009;54(2):e21–33.
14. Weston K, Mutiso S, Mwangi J, Qureshi Z, Beard J, Venkat P. Depression among women with obstetric fistula in Kenya. Int J Gynaecol Obstet. 2011;115:31–3.
15. Alio AP, Merrell L, Roxburgh K, Clayton HB, Marty JP, Bomboka L, et al. The psychosocial impact of vesico-vaginal fistula in Niger. Arch Gynecol Obstet. 2011;284:371–8.
16. Wilson SM, Sikkema KJ, Watt MH, Masenga GG. Psychological Symptoms Among Obstetric Fistula Patients Compared to Gynecology Outpatients in Tanzania. Int J Behav Med; 2015: 1–9.
17. Mellano E, Tarnay CM. Management of genitourinary fistula. Curr Opin Obstet Gynecol. 2014;26:415–23.
18. Rortveit G, Kjersti A, Hannestad Y, Hunskaar S. Urinary Incontinence after Vaginal Delivery or Cesarean Section. N Engl J Med. 2003;348:900–7.
19. Wong MJ, Wong K, Rezvan A, Tate A, Bhatia NN, Yazdany T. Urogenital Fistula. Female Pelvic Med Reconstr Surg. 2012;18(2):71–8.
20. Wall LL. Birth Trauma and the Pelvic Floor: Lessons from the Developing World. J Womens Health. 1999;8(2):149–55.
21. Rajamaheswari N, Chhikara AB. Vesicouterine fistulae: our experience of 17 cases and literature review. Int Urogynecol J. 2013;24:275–9.
22. Hampton BS, Kay A, Pilzek A. Urinary Fistula and Incontinence. Semin Reprod Med. 2015;3(1):47–52.
23. Waaldijk K. The immediate management of fresh obstetric fistulas. Am J Obstet Gynecol. 2004;191:795–9.
24. Bazi T. Spontaneous closure of vesicovaginal fistulas after bladder drainage alone: review of the evidence. Int Urogynecol J Pelvic Floor Dysfunct. 2007;18:329–33.
25. Wall LL. Overcoming phase 1 delays: the critical component of obstetric fistula prevention programs in resource-poor countries. BMC Pregnancy Childbirth. 2012;12(68):1–13.
26. Nardos R, Browning A, Member B. Duration of bladder catheterization after surgery for obstetric fistula. Int J Gynaecol Obstet. 2008;103(208):30–2.
27. Frajzyngier V, Ruminjo J, Asiimwe F, Barry TH, Bello A, Danladi D, et al. Factors influencing choice of surgical route of repair of genitourinary fistula, and the influence of route of repair on surgical outcomes: findings from a prospective cohort study. Br J Obstet Gynaecol. 2012;11:1344–1353.
28. Singh V, Sinha RJ, Mehrotra S, Gupta DK, Gupta S. Transperitoneal Transvesical Laparoscopic Repair of Vesicovaginal Fistulae: Experience of a Tertiary Care Centre in Northern India. Current Urology. 2013;7:75–82.
29. Frajzyngier V, Li G, Larson E, Ruminjo J, Barone MA. Development and comparison of prognostic scoring systems for surgical closure of genitourinary fistula. Am J Obstet Gynecol. 2013;208(2):1–19.
30. Arrowsmith SD, Barone MA, Rominjo J. Outcomes in obstetric fistula care: a literature review. Curr Opin Obstet Gynecol. 2013;25:399–403.
31. Watt MH, Wilson SM, Sikkema KJ, Velloza J, Mosha MV, Masenga GG, et al. Development of an intervention to improve mental health for obstetric fistula patients in Tanzania. Eval Program Plann. 2015;50:1–9.
32. Ojengbede OA, Baba Y, Morhason-Bello IO, Armah M, Dimiti A, Buwa D, et al. Group Psychological Therapy in Obstetric Fistula Care: A Complementary Recipe for the Accompanying Mental Ill Health Morbidities? Afr J Reprod Health. 2014;18(1):156–60.
33. Castille YJ, Avocetien C, Zaongo D, Colas JM, Peabody JO, Rochat CH. Impact of a program of physiotherapy and health education on the outcome of obstetric fistula surgery. Int J Gynaecol Obstet. 2014;124:77–80.
34. Castille YJ, Avocetien C, Zaongo D, Colas JM, Peabody JO, Rochat CH. One-year follow-up of women who participated in a physiotherapy and health education program before and after obstetric fistula surgery. Int J Gynaecol Obstet. 2015;128:264–6.
35. Lombard L, Jorre J, Geddes R, El Ayadi AM, Grant L. Rehabilitation experiences after obstetric fistula repair: systematic review of qualitative studies. Trop Med Int Health. 2015;20(5):554–68.
36. Mselle LT, Evjen-Olsen B, Moland KM, Polit C, Mvungi A, Kohi TW. "Hoping for a Normal Life Again": Reintegration after Fistula Repair in Rural Tanzania. J Obstet Gynaecol Can. 2012;34(10):927–38.
37. Pope R, Bangser M, Ruquejo JH. Restoring dignity: Social reintegration after obstetric fistula repair in Ukerewe, Tanzania. Glob Public Health. 2011;6(8):859–73.
38. Umoiyoho AJ, Inyang-Etoh EC, Abah GM, Abasiattai AM, Akaiso OE. Quality of life following successful repair of vesicovaginal fistula in Nigeria. Rural Remote Health. 2011;11:1–7.
39. Donnelly K, Oliveras E, Tilahun Y, Belachew M, Asnake M. Quality of life of Ethiopian women after fistula repair: implications on rehabilitation and social reintegration policy and programming. Cult Health Sex. 2015;17(2):150–64.
40. Wilson AL, Chipeta E, Kalilani-Phiri L, Taulo F, Tsui AO. Fertility and pregnancy outcomes among women with obstetric fistula in rural Malawi. Int J Gynaecol Obstet. 2011;113:196–8.
41. Lawani L, Iyoke CA, Ezeonu PO. Contraceptive practice after surgical repair of obstetric fistula in southeast Nigeria. Int J Gynaecol Obstet . 2015;1–7.
42. Banke-Thomas AO, Wilton-Waddell OE, Kouraogo SF, Mueller JE. Current Evidence Supporting Obstetric Fistula Prevention Strategies in Sub Saharan Africa: A Systematic Review of the Literature. Afr J Reprod Health. 2014;18(3):118–27.
43. Browning A, Lewis A, Whiteside S. Predicting women at risk for developing obstetric fistula: a fistula index? An observational study comparison of two cohorts. Br J Obstet Gynaecol. 2014;121:604–9.
44. Seim AR, Alassoum Z, Bronzan RN, Mainassara AA, Jacobsen JL, Gali YA. Pilot community-mobilization program reduces maternal and perinatal mortality and prevents obsetric fistula in Niger. Int J Gynaecol Obstet. 2014;127:269–74.
45. EngenderHealth. Obstetric Fistula Needs Assessment Report: Findings from Nine African Countries. Needs Assessment, New York: UNFPA & EngenderHealth; 2003.
46. FIGO. Global competency-based fistula surgery training manual. Training Manual, London: FIGO; 2011.
47. Higashi H, Barendregt JJ, Kassebaum NJ, Weiser TG, Bickler SW, Vos T. Surgically avertable burden of obstetric conditions in low- and middle-income regions: a modelled analysis. Br J Obstet Gynaecol. 2015;122:228–37.
48. Johns B, Sigurbjörnsdóttir K, Fogstad H, Zupan J, Mathai M, Edejer TTT. Estimated global resources needed to attain universal coverage of maternal and newborn health services. Int J Gynaecol Obstet. 2007;85:256–63.
49. UNAIDS. Fact sheet HIV/AIDS. Accessed 7/2/15. http://www.unaids.org/en/resources/campaigns/globalreport2013/factsheet
50. Wall LL, Wilkinson J, Arrowsmith SD, Ojengbede O, Mabeya H. A Code of Ethics for the fistula surgeon. Int J Gynaecol Obstet. 2008;101:84–7.
51. Wall LL. A bill of rights for patients with obstetric fistula. Int J Gynaecol Obstet. 2014;127:301–4.
52. Wall LL. Ethical Concerns Regarding Operations by Volunteer Surgeons on Vulnerable Patient Groups: The Case of Women with Obstetric Fistulas. HEC Forum. 2011;23:115–27.
53. Arrowsmith SD, Ruminjo J, Landry EG. Current practices in treatment of female genital fistula: a cross sectional study. BMC Pregnancy Childbirth. 2010;10(73):1–11.

12

Nasal high flow treatment in preterm infants

Calum T. Roberts[1,2*] and Kate A. Hodgson[1]

Abstract

Nasal High Flow (HF) is a mode of 'non-invasive' respiratory support for preterm infants, with several potential modes of action, including generation of distending airway pressure, washout of the nasopharyngeal dead space, reduction of work of breathing, and heating and humidification of inspired gas. HF has several potential advantages over continuous positive airway pressure (CPAP), the most commonly applied form of non-invasive support, such as reduced nasal trauma, ease of use, and infant comfort, which has led to its rapid adoption into neonatal care. In recent years, HF has become a well-established and commonly applied treatment in neonatal care.

Recent trials comparing HF and CPAP as primary support have had differing results. Meta-analyses suggest that primary HF results in an increased risk of treatment failure, but that 'rescue' CPAP use in those infants with HF failure results in no greater risk of mechanical ventilation. Even in studies with higher rates of HF failure, the majority of infants were successfully treated with HF, and rates of important neonatal morbidities did not differ between treatment groups. Importantly, these studies have included only infants born at ≥28 weeks' gestational age (GA). The decision whether to apply primary HF will depend on the value placed on its advantages over CPAP by clinicians, the approach to surfactant treatment, and the severity of respiratory disease in the relevant population of preterm infants.

Post-extubation HF use results in similar rates of treatment failure, mechanical ventilation, and adverse events compared to CPAP. Post-extubation HF appears most suited to infants ≥28 weeks; there are few published data for infants below this gestation, and available evidence suggests that these infants are at high risk of HF failure, although rates of intubation and other morbidities are similar to those seen with CPAP. There is no evidence that using HF to 'wean' off CPAP allows for respiratory support to be ceased more quickly, but given its advantages it would appear to be a suitable alternative in infants who require ongoing non-invasive support. Safety data from randomised trials are reassuring, although more evidence in extremely preterm infants (<28 weeks' GA) is required.

Keywords: Nasal high flow, Continuous positive airway pressure, Non-invasive ventilation, Infant, premature

Background

Respiratory distress syndrome (RDS) and sequelae such as bronchopulmonary dysplasia (BPD) are substantial contributors to adverse outcomes in preterm infants. The use of 'non-invasive' respiratory support (without an endotracheal tube) is one strategy clinicians have adopted to improve management of these conditions. For several decades, nasal continuous positive airway pressure (CPAP) has been the principal mode of non-invasive respiratory support for preterm infants. CPAP is effective as post-extubation support, [1] and as primary respiratory support (the first respiratory support applied after initial stabilisation). CPAP is a feasible and effective alternative to routine intubation and ventilation after birth, even for those infants born at <28 weeks' gestational age (GA) [2–5]. The use of CPAP as primary respiratory support may also improve long-term outcomes such as death or BPD, [6] and is recommended in current consensus guidelines for preterm infants with RDS [7].

While effective, CPAP does have some disadvantages: it requires the use of bulky interfaces, must be managed by highly skilled nursing staff to be effective, and has been associated with adverse outcomes, such as nasal trauma [8] and pneumothorax [3]. There is

* Correspondence: calum.roberts@thewomens.org.au
[1]Newborn Research Centre, The Royal Women's Hospital, Locked Bag 300, Flemington Road, Parkville 3052, Melbourne, VIC, Australia
[2]Department of Obstetrics and Gynaecology, The University of Melbourne, Melbourne, Australia

also significant heterogeneity of CPAP devices and interfaces, which may influence efficacy in research and clinical settings [9].

Interest in nasal High Flow (HF), an alternative mode of non-invasive respiratory support, has grown dramatically in recent years. HF treatment refers to the delivery of heated, humidified, blended air and oxygen, via small loose-fitting nasal cannulae (Fig. 1), at >1 Litre per minute (L/min) [10]. Initially HF was applied clinically without good quality evidence of efficacy and safety. However, the publication of several recent large randomised clinical trials has allowed clinicians to make more informed decisions about which infants can appropriately receive HF treatment [11–14].

Mechanisms of action

Several mechanisms of action for HF have been proposed, which can be summarised as follows: generation of distending pressure; 'washout' of the nasopharyngeal dead space; provision of gas flow sufficient to reduce inspiratory resistance and work of breathing; and provision of adequate gas conditioning [15].

Distending pressure

CPAP systems generate a continuous distending pressure, which is set and usually measured. In comparison, HF devices use a set gas flow, but do not target, or measure, the applied pressure. Early clinical studies of HF in neonates focused on measuring the distending pressure resulting from HF therapy, both as a proposed mechanism of action, and due to concern that application of an uncontrolled, potentially high pressure may lead to pulmonary over-distension. Studies have identified three key factors that result in increased distending pressure during HF treatment: increasing gas flow, increased ratio of the diameter of the cannulae to that of the nares, and lower infant weight [16–18]. Appropriate sizing of the cannulae, such that there is a gas 'leak' around them in the nares, is an important aspect of applying HF safely. Studies in which the prongs are sized according to these recommendations have found that within the flow range currently applied in neonates (up to 8 L/min), upper airway pressures are similar to those routinely used with CPAP [19–21].

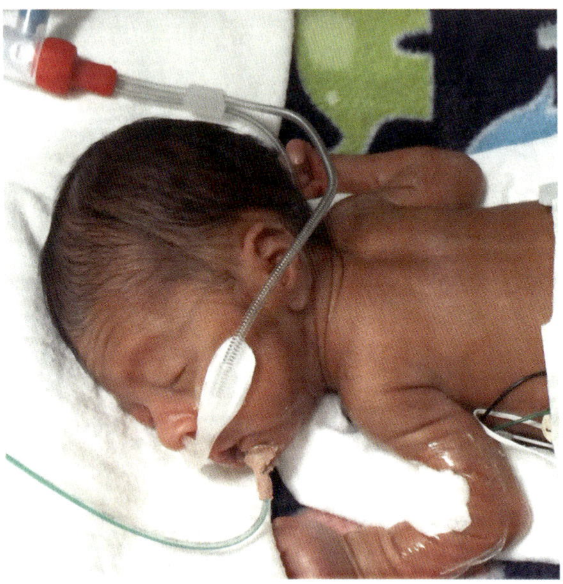

Fig. 1 A preterm infant receiving High Flow support

Dead space washout

The anatomical dead space is the volume of gas between external nares and terminal bronchioles, which usually has gas concentrations similar to the alveoli (i.e. higher carbon dioxide and lower oxygen concentrations than atmospheric air) [22]. In theory, the 'wash out' of the nasopharyngeal gas space by HF may reduce anatomical dead space and improve gas exchange, although data supporting this concept come mostly from lab and animal studies [15, 23]. A recent benchtop study, using a neonatal model with simulated spontaneous breathing, found that with the mouth closed, carbon dioxide washout times were significantly shorter with HF than with CPAP, although the two modes did not differ with the mouth open. The authors noted that this effect might be particularly important in more preterm infants, who have a high dead space-to-tidal volume ratio [24]. There are no in vivo data specifically supporting this mechanism of action from studies of neonatal patients.

Work of breathing

The nasopharynx has a relatively large surface area with resulting resistance to gas flow, which might be minimised by the use of HF to provide a gas flow at or above the peak inspiratory flow of the patient [15]. Physiological studies, using measures such as respiratory inductance plethysmography and diaphragmatic electrical activity, have generally supported the concept that work of breathing can be reduced by HF treatment. Results of comparisons with CPAP however have been conflicting, with some studies finding HF to be of similar efficacy, [25–27] and others finding CPAP more effective [28, 29].

Gas conditioning

Delivery of unconditioned gases can have a number of adverse effects on respiratory function, including impaired mucociliary function and thickening of secretions, damage to the airway mucosa, [30–32] and a reduction in pulmonary compliance and functional residual capacity [33]. Furthermore, heating and humidification of environmental gas by the upper airway mucosa is associated with both caloric and evaporative heat loss, [34] and can result in hypothermia, factors that are all specifically important to preterm infants [35–37]. Therefore, appropriate gas conditioning has been postulated as a potential benefit resulting from HF treatment [15]. Lab studies have found HF devices to produce absolute humidity levels similar to, or slightly below, those achieved by CPAP devices [38, 39]. Whether these differences are clinically significant is unclear.

Advantages of high flow

The perception that HF has several advantages over CPAP, and is a 'less invasive' mode of therapy, was a major contributory factor in the growth of its use in neonatal units. In surveys conducted in Australia and the UK, cited benefits included reduced nasal trauma, increased infant comfort, easier access for parental feeding and skin-to-skin care, and ease of set-up and use for staff [40–42]. Over time, evidence has accumulated to support the veracity of many of these perceived benefits.

The majority of HF randomised controlled trials (RCTs) have shown a reduction in nasal trauma with HF in comparison with CPAP, [11, 12, 14, 43, 44] although two showed no difference in trauma rates [45, 46]. The Cochrane Review included pooled analyses of several of these studies: as post-extubation treatment HF was associated with a significant reduction in nasal trauma versus CPAP (RR 0.64, 95% confidence interval [CI] 0.51, 0.79), but as primary respiratory support the difference was not significant (RR 0.62, 95% CI 0.34, 1.15) [10].

Of two studies to assess patient comfort using validated scales, one showed no difference in pain score between HF and CPAP, [47] whereas a second found HF infants to have significantly lower pain scores and salivary cortisol levels [48].

Another perceived advantage is that HF better enables oral feeding, specifically for infants attempting to breastfeed. However, neither individual RCTs, nor pooled analysis, have demonstrated any advantage in feeding outcomes with HF support [14, 46, 49, 50]. Non-randomised studies suggest that oral feeds can be introduced in infants receiving HF [51, 52].

Studies in both the lab and clinical setting indicate that noise levels produced by HF are generally greater than, or similar to, those produced by CPAP [53, 54].

Studies that have more systematically assessed the response of parents and nursing staff have borne out initial reports that they find HF preferable to CPAP. Klingenberg et al. [47] reported that parents scored HF significantly higher in three domains: their child's satisfaction, contact and interaction, and parental ability to take part in infant care. A single-centre survey of neonatal nurses revealed that they preferred HF to CPAP for infants of 28 weeks' GA and above, believing it to be easier to set up and use, less likely to cause nasal trauma, more comfortable, and preferred by parents [55].

HF might also present the advantage of reduced cost, although there are currently few data to support this. A 2016 systematic review and economic evaluation performed by the National Institute for Health Research (UK), based on the results of four post-extubation RCTs, concluded that there was insufficient evidence to indicate whether HF treatment is cost-effective [56].

Primary respiratory support

Prior to 2016, there was little published evidence from RCTs assessing the role of HF as primary respiratory support. Available data came from small studies, each including approximately 70 infants, [43, 46] and a subgroup of a larger trial that principally assessed post-extubation support. [14] Meta-analyses published in 2015 and 2016, including infants from these 4 studies, found no differences in treatment failure, intubation, or other important outcomes, and concluded that further adequately powered studies were required [10, 57]. The latter half of 2016 saw the publication of two larger studies, of differing methodology, designed to better evaluate primary HF.

A single-centre Italian study by Lavizzari et al. [49] randomised 316 preterm infants, of mean GA 33 weeks and birth weight 1.9 kg, to primary treatment with either HF, or CPAP/biphasic positive airway pressure (BiPAP). The primary outcome was treatment failure within 72 h, defined as the need for mechanical ventilation. The study allowed infants to receive intubation, surfactant treatment, and extubation (INSURE treatment), without regarding them as having treatment failure. The authors found similar rates of treatment failure (10.8% with HF and 9.5% with CPAP/BiPAP), with resultant risk difference (RD) 1.3% (one-sided 95% CI -6.0, 8.6), and concluded that HF was non-inferior to CPAP/BiPAP, relative to their specified non-inferiority margin of 10 percentage points. Despite the relatively low treatment failure rates, surfactant administration was common, occurring in >40% of infants in both treatment groups. Other outcomes did not differ significantly between treatment groups.

The authors acknowledged that their centre had relatively limited HF experience, and that treatment allocation could not be blinded. Other limitations included that the age at randomisation was not reported, and it was unclear if patients received respiratory support before randomisation took place. Furthermore, the trial was not prospectively registered in a clinical trials registry, and preliminary data from this trial had previously been published part way through recruitment, [58] so the authors were unblinded to the study outcomes, creating a risk of bias.

The HIPSTER trial, [13] led by our research group, included 564 infants of mean 32 weeks' GA and 1.7 kg; infants had not received surfactant treatment and were median 1.4 h of age at randomisation. The study was designed to assess non-inferiority of HF, with a margin of 10%, but was stopped early on the advice of the independent safety monitoring committee due to a highly significant difference in the primary outcome: treatment failure within 72 h, defined by objective oxygenation, blood gas, apnoea and intubation criteria. Infants received surfactant treatment only after meeting treatment failure criteria.

Treatment failure occurred significantly more frequently in the HF infants (25.5% vs. 13.3%; RD 12.3%, 95% CI 5.8 to 18.7), but infants with HF failure could receive 'rescue' CPAP prior to intubation, and the resulting intubation rates were similar in the two treatment groups (15.5% vs. 11.5%; RD 3.9%, 95% CI -1.7 to 9.6). Again, blinding of the two treatments was not possible, and just over half of infants received a brief period of CPAP (median 1.5 h) prior to randomisation, which could have influenced outcomes.

Recently, another RCT comparing HF and CPAP as primary support in a single Korean unit was published [59]. This study included 85 of 87 randomised infants, mean 33 weeks' GA and 2.0 kg, in a per-protocol analysis. Objective treatment failure criteria (respiratory acidosis, apnoea or hypoxia) were defined. Infants in both groups were permitted to receive nCPAP or bilevel CPAP at clinician discretion, prior to mechanical ventilation. Reported rates of treatment failure were 38.1% with HF compared to 20.9% with CPAP (RD 17.2%, 95% CI -1.9 to 36.2).

The higher rate of treatment failure seen in HF infants may be a reflection of the more consistent and slightly higher distending pressure produced by CPAP [16, 21]. This is likely to be beneficial in infants with acute RDS, and may explain the difference in risk of treatment failure seen with HF in HIPSTER, and the findings of the Lavizzari and post-extubation studies, in which many infants had received surfactant prior to determination of the primary outcome.

There are now >900 additional infants randomised in trials of primary HF support since the Cochrane Review was published in early 2016. An updated pooled analysis of key outcomes from published RCTs comparing HF and CPAP is shown in Fig. 2. Ultimately, whether clinicians choose to apply HF as primary support for preterm infants will depend on several factors. Those who place a high value on HF's advantages (e.g. in units with high rates of nasal trauma associated with CPAP) may choose to use HF frequently, with the option of 'rescue' CPAP in those infants with HF failure. Those who have low rates of nasal trauma, or deal with populations with more severe RDS (e.g. those with low rates of antenatal steroid exposure) may prefer to use primary CPAP. Strategies to prospectively identify the infants most likely to be successfully treated with HF may facilitate wider use in this clinical setting. These studies have all included infants of 28 weeks' GA or higher, and primary HF use in infants of lower gestations is not recommended based on current evidence.

Post-extubation support

Early RCTs of post-extubation HF published between 2006 and 2010 (whether comparing HF and CPAP, or different HF devices) included relatively small study samples (≤40 infants), and low gas flows in comparison to current practice [44, 60, 61]. In 2013, the publication of three larger RCTs significantly added to the evidence base for HF use. The first included 132 very preterm infants (<32 weeks' GA), who were randomised to either HF or CPAP at extubation [11]. Rates of extubation failure did not differ significantly (22% in the HF group and 34% in the CPAP group), nor did rates of reintubation (17% versus 24% respectively).

A similar study compared HF and CPAP using a non-inferiority design, designating a RD for treatment failure of 20 percentage points as the margin of non-inferiority for HF treatment [12]. This trial included 303 very preterm infants, and treatment failure (defined by prespecified criteria) occurred in 34.2% of HF infants and 25.8% of CPAP infants; the RD for treatment failure with HF was 8.4% (95% CI -1.9, 18.7), thereby meeting the defined non-inferiority margin. This study also included 'rescue' CPAP treatment for those infants with HF failure, with the result that approximately half of these infants avoided reintubation within 7 days: 17.8%, versus 25.2% of CPAP infants. In those infants <26 weeks' GA, the risk of HF failure was particularly high (81%) compared with 61% for CPAP. Although the 63 infants <26 weeks' GA represent a small sample, given the high rate of HF failure and 20 percentage point increase compared with CPAP, the authors advised caution with HF use in this group.

The third RCT included infants between 28 and 42 weeks' GA at birth. [14] Of the 432 infants included, 291 were randomised to HF or CPAP at extubation, and the primary outcome of reintubation within 72 h did not differ significantly between groups: 11.6% and 6.5% respectively.

A Cochrane Review, [10] updated in 2016, identified 6 published studies including 934 infants, who were randomised to either HF or CPAP as post-extubation support. Meta-analysis demonstrated that infants treated with HF were at no additional risk of treatment failure (typical risk ratio [RR] 1.21, 95% CI 0.95 to 1.55),

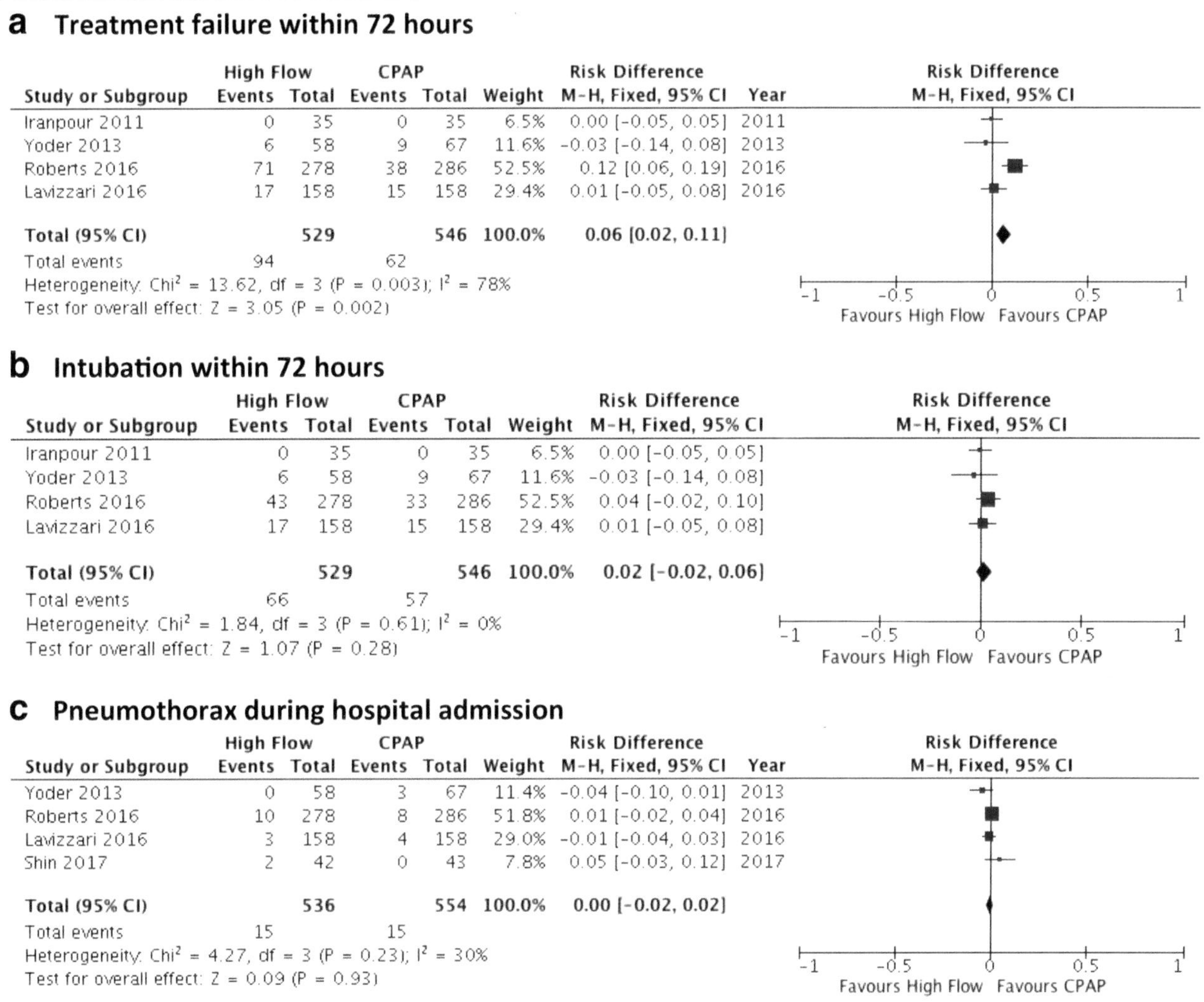

Fig. 2 Pooled analyses of published randomised trials comparing High Flow and CPAP as primary support for preterm infants, for the outcomes: **a**. Treatment failure within 72 h; **b**. Intubation within 72 h; **c**. Pneumothorax during hospital admission

reintubation (RR 0.91, 95% CI 0.68 to 1.20), or other adverse outcomes including death or BPD. The Cochrane Review authors noted that RCTs thus far have included relatively few extremely preterm infants (<28 weeks' GA). Within the subgroup of infants from 28 to 32 weeks' GA, HF resulted in a RR (95% CI) of 0.80 (0.44, 1.44) for treatment failure, and 0.51 (0.27, 0.97) for intubation in comparison to CPAP, suggesting that post-extubation HF (with the availability of rescue CPAP) may be a particularly appropriate strategy in this group of infants.

Three studies published since the Cochrane Review have included similar populations and methods to those previously published, and results were consistent with the previous Cochrane conclusions. Two studies showed similar rates of treatment failure and intubation with HF and CPAP, [62, 63] and the third small study found a higher rate of intubation in HF infants, although outcomes were reported for only half of the 108 infants randomised [64].

The available data seem to support the use of HF as an alternative to CPAP as post-extubation support for infants ≥28 weeks' GA, but it is advised that 'rescue' CPAP, which prevented intubation of infants with HF failure in several studies, is available. Routine use of post-extubation HF in infants <28 weeks' GA should be approached with caution.

Weaning from CPAP

HF may also be used as a 'weaning' mode, to transition infants off CPAP support. Randomised trials assessing this approach have included far fewer infants than those assessing primary and post-extubation support, and have produced conflicting outcomes. One study found HF use to be associated with a significant increase in duration of oxygen therapy, and of respiratory support, in comparison to weaning directly from CPAP, [65] another found HF infants to have a significantly shorter duration of oxygen treatment and of hospital stay, [66] and other studies reported similar outcomes with either approach [67, 68]. There is no convincing evidence that use of HF in this manner is beneficial in weaning infants from CPAP, although given its advantages, it may be viewed as an alternative to CPAP in those infants who continue to require non-invasive support.

Safety and later outcomes of high flow

The first major safety concern associated with HF therapy was an outbreak of infection with the Gram-negative species *Ralstonia,* resulting from contaminated humidifier cartridges in the Vapotherm 2000i device in 2005 [69]. Following the introduction of stricter infection control guidance by the manufacturer, there have been no further infection concerns since.

A further area of concern for clinicians, in keeping with the potential to generate high airway pressures discussed above, was the risk of over-distension and pulmonary air leak. Case reports of infants with complications including pneumothorax, pneumomediastinum, subcutaneous scalp emphysema, pneumocephalus and pneumo-orbitis gave some weight to these concerns [70–72]. Fortunately, available data from randomised trials have been reassuring, with no evidence of an increased pneumothorax risk with HF. The Cochrane Review in fact found a small reduction in the rate of pneumothorax (typical RD −0.02, 95% CI −0.03 to −0.00) in a pooled analysis of 896 infants from post-extubation studies. [10] Recent primary support trials have also reported similar rates of pneumothorax with HF and CPAP; a pooled analysis of these results is shown in Fig. 2 [13, 14, 49, 59].

Several RCTs have reported no increase in duration of support with HF, [11, 12, 49, 59] and in those that have, the difference has usually been small (1–2 days). [13, 14, 46] There is no evidence from RCTs to suggest that HF treatment is associated with an increased risk of BPD or death, either as individual or combined outcomes. Nor have these studies shown an increase in duration of hospitalisation, or other important clinical outcomes [10–14, 43, 49, 59].

Recent publications based on non-randomised data have raised concerns about the effect of HF use on respiratory outcomes, [73, 74] in particular prolonged respiratory support and BPD. However, limitations such as differing demographics in infants treated with HF, inconsistencies in the definition of BPD, and changes in practice during the study period, mean that these data do not allow firm conclusions to be drawn. HF is commonly applied after mechanical ventilation and/or CPAP, [75, 76] and it is conceivable that the infants receiving HF in these studies were those with the most significant lung disease, who required the most prolonged respiratory support. However, there are relatively few extremely preterm infants included in RCTs, and further research in this population is required. Exposure to prolonged respiratory support may be influenced in part by the approach to weaning HF applied by clinicians, and care should be taken to avoid unnecessarily prolonging support when weaning or cessation of treatment may be possible.

Use in neonatal units

HF devices were incorporated into neonatal care before good quality RCT data were available to guide their use. The Vermont Oxford Network reported that HF use in infants born between 501 and 1500 g increased from 45% to 58% between 2006 and 2009 [77]. Surveys conducted between 2009 and 2011 showed HF to be in use in the majority of UK and Australasian NICUs, with the majority using gas flows of ≤8 L/min [40, 42, 78]. Concerningly in one UK survey, half of units stated that they selected the cannulae size that best fit the nostrils, rather than allowing a gas 'leak' around the prongs, which is an important safety mechanism. Many units also had no written HF guideline or policy in place [42]. Common reasons for HF use in Australian and UK units were as an alternative to CPAP, to wean from CPAP, and as post-extubation support [40].

Data reported from the 56 neonatal units in The Australian and New Zealand Neonatal Network (ANZNN) show that HF use increased from 8% of NICU registrants in 2009, to 27% in 2014. [79] HF use was most common in infants born at <28 weeks' GA. Amongst all very preterm infants from 2009 to 2012, HF was commenced at a median 17 days of age, and the majority of infants had received CPAP (90%), endotracheal ventilation (71%), or both (64%) prior to HF, with primary HF use being rare (2% of infants) [75].

More recent publications indicate further growth in HF use in the UK, [76] use in the majority of Japanese NICUs, [80] and the introduction of HF use during neonatal inter-hospital transport [81].

Future research directions

There remain several areas of HF practice in which further evidence is needed. Given the concerns raised about prolonged exposure to respiratory support, studies assessing the best approach to weaning and ceasing HF should be conducted. Extremely preterm infants, who are those at greatest risk of BPD, should be further studied, to ensure that HF use is not associated with important adverse outcomes.

Studies thus far have evaluated HF at the gas flows suggested by device manufacturers, which are currently a maximum of 8 L/min in the neonatal population.

Given that evidence suggests adverse events (particularly pneumothorax) at these flows are rare, there is the possibility to study the use of higher gas flows, which may produce a greater distending pressure, potentially beneficial in conditions such as RDS. Some clinicians continue to report an anecdotal preference for one HF device over another and, with the exception of a single underpowered study, [61] there has been little research in this area. HF may be of value as a method of stabilisation in the delivery room, as reported in a small observational study of infants <30 weeks' GA at birth, [82] but this has yet to be assessed in a randomised trial.

The available RCT evidence for neonatal HF use relates exclusively to NICUs, but HF use in non-tertiary neonatal units is commonly reported, and increasing. A multi-centre RCT comparing HF and CPAP in Australian non-tertiary neonatal units is currently underway (ACTRN12614001203640).

Conclusions

High Flow is now well established as an important part of neonatal respiratory care, and has a number of potential benefits for preterm infants. While it appears that HF can be applied successfully as primary support for many infants >28 weeks' GA, it is less effective than CPAP in preventing treatment failure, and factors such as severity of RDS in the treated population, and approach to surfactant should be considered. The evidence suggests that post-extubation HF is suitable for infants >28 weeks' GA. The availability of rescue CPAP is an important part of the treatment pathway in both primary and post-extubation use, ensuring infants treated with HF are not at increased risk of intubation. Research into the optimal approach to weaning HF, and its use in extremely preterm infants, is required to ensure it is applied in such a way that produces maximal benefit for infants and their families, whilst avoiding unintended adverse effects.

Acknowledgements

CR acknowledges the support of The University of Melbourne Henry and Rachael Ackman Travelling Scholarship.

Funding

The authors have no sources of funding to declare.

Authors contributions

CR prepared the first draft of the manuscript, which was reviewed and revised by KH. Both authors read and approved the final manuscript.

Competing interests

The authors declare that they have no competing interests.

References

1. Davis PG, Henderson-Smart DJ. Nasal Continuous Positive Airways Pressure Immediately After Extubation For Preventing Morbidity In Preterm Infants. Cochrane Database Syst Rev 2003, Issue 2. Art. No.:Cd000143. doi:10.1002/14651858.CD000143.
2. Dunn MS, Kaempf J, De Klerk A, et al. Randomized trial comparing 3 approaches to the initial respiratory management of preterm neonates. Pediatrics. 2011;128:E1069–76.
3. Morley CJ, Davis PG, Doyle LW, et al. Nasal CPAP or intubation at birth for very preterm infants. N Engl J Med. 2008;358:700–8.
4. Support Study Group of the Eunice Kennedy Shriver NICHD Neonatal Research Network, Finer NN, Carlo WA, et al. Early CPAP versus surfactant in extremely preterm infants. N Engl J Med. 2010;362:1970–9.
5. Sandri F, Plavka R, Ancora G, et al. Prophylactic or early selective surfactant combined with NCPAP in very preterm infants. Pediatrics. 2010;125:E1402–9.
6. Schmolzer GM, Kumar M, Pichler G, Aziz K, O'Reilly M, Cheung PY. Non-invasive versus invasive respiratory support in preterm infants at birth: systematic review and meta-analysis. BMJ. 2013;347:F5980.
7. Sweet DG, Carnielli V, Greisen G, et al. European consensus guidelines on the management of neonatal respiratory distress syndrome in preterm infants–2013 update. Neonatology. 2013;103:353–68.
8. Fischer C, Bertelle V, Hohlfeld J, Forcada-Guex M, Stadelmann-Diaw C, Tolsa JF. Nasal trauma due to continuous positive airway pressure in neonates. Arch Dis Child Fetal Neonatal Ed. 2010;95:F447–51.
9. De Paoli AG, Davis PG, Faber B, Morley CJ. Devices And Pressure Sources For Administration Of Nasal Continuous Positive Airway Pressure (Ncpap) In Preterm Neonates. Cochrane Database Syst Rev 2008, Issue 1. Art. No.: Cd002977. doi:10.1002/14651858.CD002977.pub2.
10. Wilkinson D, Andersen C, O'Donnell CP, De Paoli AG, Manley BJ. High flow nasal cannula for respiratory support in preterm infants. Cochrane Database Syst Rev. 2016, Issue 2. Art. No.: CD006405.doi: 10.1002/14651858.CD006405.pub3.
11. Collins CL, Holberton JR, Barfield C, Davis PG. A randomized controlled trial to compare heated humidified high-flow nasal cannulae with nasal continuous positive airway pressure postextubation in premature infants. J Pediatr 2013; 162:949-954 E1.
12. Manley BJ, Owen LS, Doyle LW, et al. High-flow nasal cannulae in very preterm infants after extubation. N Engl J Med. 2013;369:1425–33.
13. Roberts CT, Owen LS, Manley BJ, et al. Nasal high-flow therapy for primary respiratory support in preterm infants. N Engl J Med. 2016;375:1142–51.
14. Yoder BA, Stoddard RA, Li M, King J, Dirnberger DR, Abbasi S. Heated, humidified high-flow nasal cannula versus nasal CPAP for respiratory support in neonates. Pediatrics. 2013;131:E1482–90.
15. Dysart K, Miller TL, Wolfson MR, Shaffer TH. Research in high flow therapy: mechanisms of action. Respir Med. 2009;103:1400–5.
16. Kubicka ZJ, Limauro J, Darnall RA. Heated, humidified high-flow nasal cannula therapy: yet another way to deliver continuous positive airway pressure? Pediatrics. 2008;121:82–8.
17. Spence KL, Murphy D, Kilian C, McGonigle R, Kilani RA. High-flow nasal cannula as a device to provide continuous positive airway pressure in infants. J Perinatol. 2007;27:772–5.
18. Wilkinson DJ, Andersen CC, Smith K, Holberton J. Pharyngeal pressure with high-flow nasal cannulae in premature infants. J Perinatol. 2008;28:42–7.
19. Collins CL, Holberton JR, Konig K. Comparison of the pharyngeal pressure provided by two heated, humidified high-flow nasal cannulae devices in premature infants. J Paediatr Child Health. 2013;49:554–6.
20. Hasan RA, Habib RH. Effects of flow rate and airleak at the nares and mouth opening on positive distending pressure delivery using commercially available high-flow nasal cannula systems: a lung model study. Pediatr Crit Care Med. 2011;12:E29–33.
21. Lampland AL, Plumm B, Meyers PA, Worwa CT, Mammel MC. Observational study of humidified high-flow nasal cannula compared with nasal continuous positive airway pressure. J Pediatr. 2009;154:177–82.
22. Van Hove SC, Storey J, Adams C, et al. An experimental and numerical investigation of CO_2 distribution in the upper airways during nasal high flow therapy. Ann Biomed Eng. 2016;44:3007–19.
23. Frizzola M, Miller TL, Rodriguez ME, et al. High-flow nasal cannula: impact on oxygenation and ventilation in an acute lung injury model. Pediatr Pulmonol. 2011;46:67–74.
24. Sivieri Em, Foglia Ee, Abbasi S. Carbon Dioxide Washout During High Flow Nasal Cannula Versus Nasal Cpap Support: An In Vitro Study. Pediatr Pulmonol. 2017;52:792–98.
25. Lavizzari A, Veneroni C, Colnaghi M, et al. Respiratory mechanics during NCPAP and HHHFNC at equal distending pressures. Arch Dis Child Fetal Neonatal Ed. 2014;99:F315–20.

26. Saslow JG, Aghai ZH, Nakhla TA, et al. Work of breathing using high-flow nasal cannula in preterm infants. J Perinatol. 2006;26:476–80.
27. Shetty S, Hickey A, Rafferty GF, Peacock JL, Greenough A. Work of breathing during CPAP and heated humidified high-flow nasal cannula. Arch Dis Child Fetal Neonatal Ed. 2016;101:F404–7.
28. de Jongh BE, Locke R, Mackley A, et al. Work of breathing indices in infants with respiratory insufficiency receiving high-flow nasal cannula and nasal continuous positive airway pressure. J Perinatol. 2014;34:27–32.
29. Nasef N, El-Gouhary E, Schurr P, et al. High-flow nasal cannulae are associated with increased diaphragm activation compared with nasal continuous positive airway pressure in preterm infants. Acta Paediatr. 2015;104:E337–43.
30. Hirsch JA, Tokayer JL, Robinson MJ, Sackner MA. Effects of dry air and subsequent humidification on tracheal mucous velocity in dogs. J Appl Physiol. 1975;39:242–6.
31. Konrad F, Schiener R, Marx T, Georgieff M. Ultrastructure and mucociliary transport of bronchial respiratory epithelium in intubated patients. Intensive Care Med. 1995;21:482–9.
32. Sleigh MA, Blake JR, Liron N. The propulsion of mucus by cilia. Am Rev Respir Dis. 1988;137:726–41.
33. Noguchi H, Takumi Y, Aochi O. A study of humidification in tracheostomized dogs. Br J Anaesth. 1973;45:844–8.
34. Sottiaux TM. Consequences of under- and over-humidification. Respir Care Clin N Am. 2006;12:233–52.
35. Bickler PE, Sessler DI. Efficiency of airway heat and moisture exchangers in anesthetized humans. Anesth Analg. 1990;71:415–8.
36. Bissonnette B, Sessler DI. Passive or active inspired gas humidification increases thermal steady-state temperatures in anesthetized infants. Anesth Analg. 1989;69:783–7.
37. Stone DR, Downs JB, Paul WL, Perkins HM. Adult body temperature and heated humidification of anesthetic gases during general anesthesia. Anesth Analg. 1981;60:736–41.
38. Chang GY, Cox CA, Shaffer TH. Nasal Cannula, CPAP, and high-flow nasal cannula: effect of flow on temperature, humidity, pressure, and resistance. Biomed Instrum Technol. 2011;45:69–74.
39. Roberts CT, Kortekaas R, Dawson JA, Manley BJ, Owen LS, Davis PG. The effects of non-invasive respiratory support on oropharyngeal temperature and humidity: a neonatal manikin study. Arch Dis Child Fetal Neonatal Ed. 2016;101:F248–52.
40. Hough JL, Shearman AD, Jardine LA, Davies MW. Humidified high flow nasal cannulae: current practice in Australasian nurseries, a survey. J Paediatr Child Health. 2012;48:106–13.
41. Manley BJ, Owen L, Doyle LW, Davis PG. High-flow nasal cannulae and nasal continuous positive airway pressure use in non-tertiary special care nurseries in Australia and New Zealand. J Paediatr Child Health. 2012;48:16–21.
42. Ojha S, Gridley E, Dorling J. Use of heated humidified high-flow nasal cannula oxygen in neonates: a UK wide survey. Acta Paediatr. 2013;102:249–53.
43. Iranpour R, Sadeghnia A, Hesaraki M. High-flow nasal cannula versus nasal continuous positive airway pressure in the management of respiratory distress syndrome. J Isfahan Med School. 2011;29:761–71.
44. Woodhead DD, Lambert DK, Clark JM, Christensen RD. Comparing two methods of delivering high-flow gas therapy by nasal cannula following endotracheal extubation: a prospective, randomized, masked, crossover trial. J Perinatol. 2006;26:481–5.
45. Collaborative Group For The Multicenter Study On Heated Humidified High-Flow Nasal Cannula V. Efficacy and safety of heated humidified high-flow nasal cannula for prevention of extubation failure in neonates. Zhonghua Er Ke Za Zhi. 2014;52:271–6.
46. Kugelman A, Riskin A, Said W, Shoris I, Mor F, Bader D. A randomized pilot study comparing heated humidified high-flow nasal cannulae with NIPPV for RDS. Pediatr Pulmonol. 2015;50:576–83.
47. Klingenberg C, Pettersen M, Hansen EA, et al. Patient comfort during treatment with heated humidified high flow nasal cannulae versus nasal continuous positive airway pressure: a randomised cross-over trial. Arch Dis Child Fetal Neonatal Ed. 2014;99:F134–7.
48. Osman M, Elsharkawy A, Abdel-Hady H. Assessment of pain during application of nasal-continuous positive airway pressure and heated, humidified high-flow nasal cannulae in preterm infants. J Perinatol. 2015;35:263–7.
49. Lavizzari A, Colnaghi M, Ciuffini F, Et Al. Heated, Humidified High-Flow Nasal Cannula Vs Nasal Continuous Positive Airway Pressure For Respiratory Distress Syndrome Of Prematurity: A Randomized Clinical Noninferiority Trial. Jama Pediatr. 2016. Published online August 8, 2016. doi:10.1001/jamapediatrics.2016.1243.
50. Hegde D, Mondkar J, Panchal H, Manerkar S, Jasani B, Kabra N. Heated humidified high flow nasal cannula versus nasal continuous positive airway pressure as primary mode of respiratory support for respiratory distress in preterm infants. Indian Pediatr. 2016;53:129–33.
51. Leder SB, Siner JM, Bizzarro MJ, McGinley BM, Lefton-Greif MA. Oral alimentation in neonatal and adult populations requiring high-flow oxygen via nasal cannula. Dysphagia. 2016;31:154–9.
52. Shetty S, Hunt K, Douthwaite A, Athanasiou M, Hickey A, Greenough A. High-flow nasal cannula oxygen and nasal continuous positive airway pressure and full oral feeding in infants with bronchopulmonary dysplasia. Arch Dis Child Fetal Neonatal Ed. 2016;101:F408–11.
53. Konig K, Stock EL, Jarvis M. Noise levels of neonatal high-flow nasal cannula devices–an in-vitro study. Neonatology. 2013;103:264–7.
54. Roberts CT, Dawson JA, Alquoka E, et al. Are high flow nasal cannulae noisier than bubble CPAP for preterm infants? Arch Dis Child Fetal Neonatal Ed. 2014;99:F291–5.
55. Roberts CT, Manley BJ, Dawson JA, Davis PG. Nursing perceptions of high-flow nasal cannulae treatment for very preterm infants. J Paediatr Child Health. 2014;50:806–10.
56. Fleeman N, Mahon J, Bates V, et al. The clinical effectiveness and cost-effectiveness of heated humidified high-flow nasal cannula compared with usual care for preterm infants: systematic review and economic evaluation. Health Technol Assess. 2016;20:1–68.
57. Kotecha SJ, Adappa R, Gupta N, Watkins WJ, Kotecha S, Chakraborty M. Safety and Efficacy of High-Flow Nasal Cannula Therapy in Preterm Infants: A Meta-analysis. Pediatrics. 2015;136:542–53.
58. Ciuffini F, Pietrasanta C, Lavizzari A, et al. Comparison between two different modes of non-invasive ventilatory support in preterm newborn infants with respiratory distress syndrome mild to moderate: preliminary data. Pediatr Med Chir. 2014;36(4):88.
59. Shin J, Park K, Lee E, Choi BM. Humidified high flow nasal cannula versus nasal continuous positive airway pressure as an initial respiratory support in preterm infants with respiratory distress: a randomized, controlled non-inferiority trial. J Korean Med Sci. 2017;32:650–5.
60. Campbell DM, Shah PS, Shah V, Kelly EN. Nasal continuous positive airway pressure from high flow cannula versus Infant Flow for Preterm infants. J Perinatol. 2006;26:546–9.
61. Miller SM, Dowd SA. High-flow nasal cannula and extubation success in the premature infant: a comparison of two modalities. J Perinatol. 2010;30:805–8.
62. Kang WQ, Xu BL, Liu DP, et al. Efficacy of heated humidified high-flow nasal cannula in preterm infants aged less than 32 weeks after ventilator weaning. Zhongguo Dang Dai Er Ke Za Zhi. 2016;18:488–91.
63. Soonsawad S, Swatesutipun B, Limrungsikul A, Nuntnarumit P. Heated Humidified High-Flow Nasal Cannula for Prevention of Extubation Failure in Preterm Infants. Indian J Pediatr. 2017;84:262–6.
64. Kadivar M, Mosayebi Z, Razi N, Nariman S, Sangsari R. High flow nasal cannulae versus nasal continuous positive airway pressure in neonates with respiratory distress syndrome managed with Insure method: a randomized clinical trial. Iranian Journal Of Medical Sciences. 2016;41:494–500.
65. Abdel-Hady H, Shouman B, Aly H. Early weaning from CPAP to high flow nasal cannula in preterm infants is associated with prolonged oxygen requirement: a randomized controlled trial. Early Hum Dev. 2011;87:205–8.
66. Badiee Z, Eshghi A, Mohammadizadeh M. High flow nasal cannula as a method for rapid weaning from nasal continuous positive airway pressure. Int J Prev Med. 2015;6:33.
67. Soonsawad S, Tongsawang N, Nuntnarumit P. Heated humidified high-flow nasal cannula for weaning from continuous positive airway pressure in preterm infants: a randomized controlled trial. Neonatology. 2016;110:204–9.
68. Tang J, Reid S, Lutz T, Malcolm G, Oliver S, Osborn DA. Randomised controlled trial of weaning strategies for preterm infants on nasal continuous positive airway pressure. BMC Pediatr. 2015;15:147.
69. Jhung MA, Sunenshine RH, Noble-Wang J, et al. A national outbreak of Ralstonia mannitolilytica associated with use of a contaminated oxygen-delivery device among pediatric patients. Pediatrics. 2007;119:1061–8.
70. Iglesias-Deus A, Perez-Munuzuri A, Lopez-Suarez O, Crespo P, Couce ML. Tension pneumocephalus induced by high-flow nasal cannula ventilation in a neonate. Arch Dis Child Fetal Neonatal Ed. 2017;102:F173–F5.

71. Hegde S, Prodhan P. Serious air leak syndrome complicating high-flow nasal cannula therapy: a report of 3 cases. Pediatrics. 2013;131:E939–44.
72. Jasin LR, Kern S, Thompson S, Walter C, Rone JM, Yohannan MD. Subcutaneous scalp emphysema, pneumo-orbitis and pneumocephalus in a neonate on high humidity high flow nasal cannula. J Perinatol. 2008;28:779–81.
73. Hoffman SB, Terrell N, Driscoll CH, Davis NL. Impact of High-Flow Nasal Cannula Use on Neonatal Respiratory Support Patterns and Length of Stay. Respir Care. 2016;61:1299–304.
74. Taha DK, Kornhauser M, Greenspan JS, Dysart KC, Aghai ZH. High Flow Nasal Cannula Use Is Associated with Increased Morbidity and Length of Hospitalization in Extremely Low Birth Weight Infants. J Pediatr. 2016; 173:50–5 e1.
75. Roberts CT, Owen LS, Manley BJ, Davis PG, Australian, New Zealand Neonatal N. High-flow support in very preterm infants in Australia and New Zealand. Arch Dis Child Fetal Neonatal Ed. 2016;101:F401–3.
76. Shetty S, Sundaresan A, Hunt K, Desai P, Greenough A. Changes in the use of humidified high flow nasal cannula oxygen. Arch Dis Child Fetal Neonatal Ed. 2016;101:F371–2.
77. Soll RF, Edwards EM, Badger GJ, et al. Obstetric and neonatal care practices for infants 501 to 1500 g from 2000 to 2009. Pediatrics. 2013;132:222–8.
78. Nath P, Ponnusamy V, Willis K, Bissett L, Clarke P. Current practices of high and low flow oxygen therapy and humidification in UK neonatal units. Pediatr Int. 2010;52:893–4.
79. Chow SSW. Report of the Australian and New Zealand Neonatal Network 2014. Sydney: ANZNN; 2016.
80. Motojima Y, Ito M, Oka S, Uchiyama A, Tamura M, Namba F. Use of high-flow nasal cannula in neonates: nationwide survey in Japan. Pediatr Int. 2016;58:308–10.
81. Boyle MA, Dhar A, Broster S. Introducing high-flow nasal cannula to the neonatal transport environment. Acta Paediatr. 2017;106:1363.
82. Reynolds P, Leontiadi S, Lawson T, Otunla T, Ejiwumi O, Holland N. Stabilisation of premature infants in the delivery room with nasal high flow. Arch Dis Child Fetal Neonatal Ed. 2016;101:F284–7.

13

Logistic regression analysis on the determinants of stillbirth in Ethiopia

Kidanemariam Alem Berhie[1*] and Habtamu Gebremariam Gebresilassie[2]

Abstract

Background: Stillbirth is often defined as fetal death after 24 weeks of gestation, but a fetus greater than any combination of 16, 20, 22, 24, or 28 weeks gestational age and 350 g, 400 g, 500 g, or 1000 g birth weight may be considered stillborn depending on local law. Once the fetus has died, the mother may or may not have contractions and undergo childbirth or in some cases, a Caesarean section. Most stillbirths occur in full-term pregnancies.

Methods: This study has intended to model determinants of experiencing stillbirth among women in child bearing age group of Ethiopia using the Ethiopian demographic and health Survey data (EDHS, 2011). First, the bivariate chi-square test of association was fitted to the data and significant variables were considered for further investigation binary logistic regression models were fitted.

Results: This study revealed that the rate of experiencing stillbirth among women of child bearing age was about 25.5 per 1000 deliveries in Ethiopia. From binary logistic regression, region of residence, maternal age, place of residence, education level, parity, antenatal care utilization, place of delivery, body mass index (BMI) and anemia level were found to be significantly associated with experiencing stillbirth.

Conclusions: Researchers should use multilevel models than traditional regression methods when their data structure is hierarchical as like in Ethiopian Demographic and Health Survey data.

Keywords: Stillbirth, Antenatal care visit, Logistic regression, Ethiopia

Background

Stillbirth is often defined as fetal death after 24 weeks of gestation [1], but a fetus greater than any combination of 16, 20, 22, 24, or 28 weeks gestational age and 350 g, 400 g, 500 g, or 1000 g birth weight may be considered stillborn depending on local law [2]. Once the fetus has died, the mother may or may not have contractions and undergo childbirth or in some cases, a Caesarean section. Most stillbirths occur in full-term pregnancies. The cause is often unknown.

The 2011 Lancet Stillbirths Series reviewed the global status of stillbirths and presented the case for a triple return on investment in stillbirth prevention that also prevents newborn and maternal deaths. That Series received widespread media attention and an unprecedented response [3]. However, despite progress this new Series shows that more must be done to integrate stillbirth prevention within global and national agendas for high quality health care for women, adolescents, and babies. This message resonates with other Lancet Series, notably on maternal health, early child development, and Every Newborn.

Most of the world's 2.6 million stillbirths each year occur in low-income and middle-income countries (98 %), with three quarters in sub-Saharan Africa and south Asia. About 60 % occur in rural areas and more than half in conflict and emergency zones, affecting the families most underserved by health-care systems. Stillbirths are often not registered systematically in many low-income countries. This leads to underestimation of stillbirths in these countries, in which 98 % of all stillbirths occur. Reliable registrations exist only in countries with minor number of deaths. India, Pakistan, Nigeria, China, Bangladesh, Democratic Republic of the Congo, Ethiopia, Indonesia, Tanzania and Afghanistan are ten countries that account for two-thirds of all third

* Correspondence: kidanemariam2012@gmail.com
[1]Department of Statistics, College of Natural and Computational Sciences, University of Gondar, Gondar, Ethiopia
Full list of author information is available at the end of the article

trimester stillbirths. Ethiopia is ranked number seven out of these ten [4].

If all causes of stillbirth are taken together, the new estimates would place stillbirths fifth on the list of causes of deaths (COD) worldwide, two-thirds of stillbirths happen in rural areas, where skilled birth attendants, in particular midwives and physicians, are not always available for essential care during childbirth and for obstetric emergencies, including caesarean sections [5].

Over 98 % of the perinatal deaths occur in low and middle-income countries (LMIC), with more than 70 % occurring in community settings, often the home, far from vital registration/formal health systems [6–8], under-reporting of stillbirths is a huge problem, and reliable data about rates and causes are difficult to obtain. Hospital stillbirth data are often subject to substantial bias and the ability to generalize from these data is unknown. Nevertheless, of the stillbirths occur worldwide yearly, the vast majority in developing countries, with rates in many developing countries ten-fold higher than elsewhere. Prolonged and obstructed labor, preeclampsia and various infections, all without adequate treatment, account for the majority of stillbirths [9].

In Ethiopia, the world health statistics 2013 revealed a stillbirth rate of 26/1000 deliveries which is third highest in the east African countries next to Djibouti and Somalia (with stillbirth rates of 34 & 30 per 1000 births, respectively) [10] and seventh among the ten countries that account for two-thirds of all third trimester stillbirths in the world [11], a study reported that the prevalence of stillbirth is 19/1000 births [12]. A study done at Tikur Anbessa Hospital has shown a stillbirth rate of 53.3/1000 births and contributed to 77.2 % of gross perinatal mortality [13]. The Ethiopian Demographic and Health Survey (DHS) 2005 data indicated that the still birth rate is 1.8 % [14]. The Addis Ababa city administration health bureau 2005/06 annual activity report revealed that the rate of stillbirth is 2.5 % [15]. A study done, recently, on prenatal outcomes in Addis Ababa in 2010, also indicates that the rate of stillbirth is 3.1 % [16].

Most of the mothers and grandmothers associated the causes of stillbirth and neonatal death with malevolent spirits. As one Oromiya grandmother observed, "Families lose their new born because of an evil spirit". (Wukabi is a type of malevolent spirit that, when offended, will attack the beholder or his/her family) [17].

Goal by 2020 [18]; For countries with a current stillbirth rate of more than 5 per 1000 births, the goal by 2020 is to reduce their stillbirth rates by at least 50 % from the 2008 rates. For countries with a current stillbirth rate of less than 5 per 1000 births, the goal by 2020 is to eliminate all preventable stillbirths and close equity gaps [19].

Therefore, this study attempts to investigate the major socio-economic, demographic, medical, behavioral and environmental factors of stillbirth in Ethiopia so that the SDG and goal by 2020 for stillbirth will be met.

Objective of the study

General objective

The general objective of this study is to assess the determinants of stillbirth in Ethiopia using Ethiopian Demographic and Health Survey 2011 data.

Specific objectives

➢ To assess socio-economic, demographic, and medical factors associated with stillbirth.

➢ To identify factors that may explain the variation of rate of stillbirth

Data and methodology

Source of data

This study has used the 2011 Ethiopia Demographic and Health Survey (2011, EDHS) [20]. The 2011 EDHS was conducted under the aegis of the ministry of health and was implemented by the Central Statistical Agency and partner organizations from September 2010 through June 2011 with a nationally representative sample of nearly 18,500 households. All women age 15–49 and all men age 15–59 in these households were eligible for individual interview.

The sample for the 2011 EDHS was designed to provide population and health indicators at the national and regional levels. The sample design allowed for specific indicators, such as stillbirth experience, to be calculated for each of Ethiopia's eleven geographic/administrative regions: nine regional states (Tigray, Afar, Amhara, Oromiya, Somali, Benishangul-Gumuz, SNNPR, Gambela and Harari) and two city administrations (Addis Ababa and Dire-Dawa). The sampling frame used for the 2011 EDHS was the Population and Housing Census conducted by the Central Statistical Agency (CSA) in 2007 (2007 PHC). The 2011 EDHS sample was selected using a stratified, two-stage cluster design, and EAs were the sampling units for the first stage sampling. The 2011 EDHS sample included 624 EAs, 187 in urban areas and 437 in rural areas.

Households comprised the second stage of sampling. A complete listing of households was carried out in each of the 624 selected EAs from September 2010 through January 2011. Maps were drawn for each of the clusters and all private households were listed. The listing excluded institutional living arrangements (e.g., army barracks, hospitals, police camps, and boarding schools). A representative sample of 17,817 households was selected for the 2011 EDHS survey. Because the sample is not self-weighting at the national level, all data in this report have been weighted unless otherwise specified. Sixteen thousand five hundred fifteen women aged 15–49 are interviewed, 12,560 women after adjusting for the missing data have been taken for the analysis.

Variables of the study

Variables considered in this study were selected based on literatures which have been conducted at the global level. Potential determinant factors expected to be correlated with stillbirth among mothers of child bearing age are included as variables of the study. Variables considered in this study are categorized into dependent and explanatory or predictor variables.

Dependent variable

The 2011 EDHS asked women to report any pregnancy loss that occurred in the five years preceding the survey. For each pregnancy that did not end in a live birth, the duration of the pregnancy was recorded. Pregnancy losses occurring after seven completed months of gestation are defined as stillbirths. The response variable of this study is the occurrence of stillbirth among mothers of child bearing age.

The response variable for the ith mother (15–49) is represented by a random variable Y_i with two possible values coded as 1 and 0. So, the response variable of the ith mother Y_i was measured as a dichotomous variable with possible values $Y_i = 1$, if i^{th} mother had experienced stillbirth and $Y_i = 0$ otherwise.

Methods

In this study binary logistic regressions were employed to identify determinant risk factors of stillbirth and to determine the prevalence of stillbirth in Ethiopia. The response variable of the study is experiencing stillbirth prior to the survey. We analyzed using single level binary logistic regressions by assuming the occurrence of stillbirth is independent among mothers of child bearing age.

Results

Descriptive statistics

We analyzed data from women of child bearing age from the Ethiopian Demographic and Health Survey 2011 sample. The initial population consisted of 16,515 women of child bearing age. Out of this 12,560 (76 %) of women with complete information were selected and studied in the analysis. From the sampled women, the proportion of experiencing stillbirth was about 2.55 % (25.5 per 1000) in Ethiopia.

The analysis is carried out in two parts. In the first part, we present the bivariate analysis with its chi-square test of association and then selecting the significant variables, we analyze the data using ordinary logistic regression, for both the analyses we used SPSS 20 software.

Result of bivariate analysis

The sample distribution of region of residence, maternal age, place of residence, Education level, wealth index, Parity (Total children ever born), Antenatal care utilization, Place of Delivery (home or health center), Mode of Delivery (normal or by caesarean section), Body mass index (BMI), marital status, whether they had any STI or not, whether they smoke cigarettes or not, Anemia level (Anemic or not), whether they have job or not and frequency of consuming alcoholic drink are presented in Table 1.

Among the factors, region of residence, maternal age, place of residence, education level, parity, antenatal care utilization, place of delivery, mode of delivery, body mass index (BMI), and anemia level were found to have a significant association with experiencing stillbirth at 1 % level of significance (p-values less than 0.01), while having job was significant at the 5 % level of significance (p-values less than 0.05).

Experiencing stillbirth has varied from one region to the other. The result in Table 1 shows that region of residence is significantly associated with experiencing stillbirth ($p < 0.001$). Somali region had the highest (5.26 %) percentage of experiencing stillbirth followed by Tigray region (3.73 %). Gambela and Addis Ababa had the lowest percentages (1.49 %, 1.54 %) respectively, for experiencing stillbirth in Ethiopia.

Of the 12,560 women with complete information, 50.7 % were 15–24 years old, 33.3 % were 25–34 years old and the rest (16.1 %) were 35 or above. Maternal age was significantly associated with experiencing stillbirth and it was found that mothers with higher age were found to be with higher probability to experience stillbirth. Place of residence was also significantly associated with experiencing stillbirth and of the 71.1 % rural area resident women 4.62 % had experienced stillbirth and only 2.37 % urban area residents had experienced stillbirth.

Education level is also associated with experiencing stillbirth. 47.4 % of the women were with no educational achievement and, of this, those who had experienced stillbirth were 3.53 % as compared to that of those who completed their primary education (1.68) and to that of those who completed secondary or higher education level (1.64). 41.2 % of the women were nulliparous, having no child, with 1.01 % proportion of experiencing stillbirth as compared to 3.63 % proportion of experiencing stillbirth among multiparas.

Table 1 Distribution of factors analyzed with experiencing stillbirth among women of child bearing age in Ethiopia (EDHS, 2011)

Variables	Levels	N	N%	Experienced Stillbirth %		d.f	Chi-square	*p*-value
				No	Yes			
Region	Addis Ababa	1167	9.3	98.46	1.54	10	53.262	< .001
	Tigray	1368	10.9	96.27	3.73			
	Affar	1034	8.2	98.26	1.74			
	Amhara	1554	12.4	98.13	1.87			
	Oromiya	1705	13.6	96.48	3.52			
	Somali	703	5.6	94./4	5.26			
	Benishangul-Gumuz	975	7.8	97.23	2.77			
	SNNP	1640	13.1	97.62	2.38			
	Gambela	872	6.9	98.51	1.49			
	Harari	742	5.9	98.38	1.62			
	Dire Dawa	800	6.4	98.00	2.00			
Maternal age	15–24	6363	50.7	98.88	1.12	2	144.68	< .001
	25–34	4179	33.3	96.84	3.16			
	35+	2018	16.1	94.20	5.80			
Place of residence	Rural	8924	71.1	95.38	4.62	1	8.407	.004
	Urban	3636	28.9	97.63	2.37			
Education Level	No education	5955	47.4	96.47	3.53	2	43.691	< .001
	Primary	4835	38.5	98.32	1.68			
	Secondary & Higher	1770	14.1	98.36	1.64			
Wealth Index	Poor	4924	39.2	97.42	2.58	2	1.439	.487
	Middle	1784	14.2	97.09	2.91			
	Rich	5852	46.6	97.59	2.41			
Parity (Total children ever born)	Nulliparous	5169	41.2	98.99	1.01	1	84.097	< .001
	Multiparas	7391	58.8	96.37	3.63			
Antenatal care utilization	No antenatal visits	4101	32.7	93.34	6.66	2	97.417	< .001
	Visited at least once	3290	26.2	96.41	3.59			
	Never given birth	5169	41.2	98.99	1.01			
Place of Delivery	HOME	6166	49.1	92.40	7.60	2	138.53	< .001
	Health center	1225	9.8	96.24	3.76			
	Never given birth	5169	41.2	98.99	1.01			
Mode of Delivery	Normal	7169	57.1	94.42	5.58	2	85.725	< .001
	Caesarean section	222	1.8	96.05	3.95			
	Never given birth	5169	41.2	98.99	1.01			
Body mass index (BMI)	Thin	3541	28.2	95.83	4.17	2	134.32	< .001
	Normal	8248	65.7	97.37	2.63			
	Overweight/Obese	771	6.1	93.63	6.37			
Marital status	Never Married	4017	32.0	97.13	2.87	2	4.067	.131
	Married/Living with partner	7640	60.8	96.32	3.68			
	Divorced/separated/Widowed	903	7.2	96.46	3.54			
Had any STI	No	12498	99.5	97.46	2.54	1	0.115	.471
	Yes	62	.5	96.77	3.23			
Smokes cigarettes	No	12513	99.6	97.44	2.56	1	1.233	.297
	Yes	47	.4	100.0	0.00			

Table 1 Distribution of factors analyzed with experiencing stillbirth among women of child bearing age in Ethiopia (EDHS, 2011) *(Continued)*

Anemia level	Not anemic	10010	79.7	97.65	2.35	1	11.953	< .001
	Anemic	2550	20.3	94.67	5.33			
Has job	No	12340	98.2	97.51	2.49	1	6.190	.013
	Yes	220	1.8	96.09	3.91			
Alcoholic drink	Never	8454	67.3	97.60	2.40	3	3.669	.299
	Sometimes	2945	23.4	97.32	2.68			
	Usually	683	5.4	96.93	3.07			
	Always	478	3.8	96.44	3.56			

Table 1 displayed also that among the women of child bearing age 26.2 % has made their antenatal care visit at least once during their pregnancy times and 3.59 % of these had experienced stillbirth, which is less than that of those (32.7 %) who made no antenatal care visit during their pregnancies which was 6.66 %. 41.2 % of the women had no child and among the women who delivered a child, 49.1 % had delivered at home in which 7.6 % were stillbirth, only 9.8 % had delivered at any health center in which 3.76 % were stillbirth, 57.1 % had delivered normally in which 5.58 % were stillbirth and 1.8 % of the women delivered with caesarean section in which 3.95 % of those delivered with caesarean section had given to stillbirth.

Body mass index was found to be another significantly associated with experiencing stillbirth. The result indicates that 28.2 % of the women were thin (body mass index (BMI) < 18.5), 65.7 % were normal (weight) (BMI 18.5–24.9) and 6.1 % were overweight or obese (BMI ≥ 25). The proportion of experiencing stillbirth among women who are thin, normal and overweight were 4.17 %, 2.63 % and 6.37 % respectively. 79.7 % of the women were not anemic and with less proportion of experiencing stillbirth than those (20.3 %) with anemia whose proportion is 5.33 %. 98.2 % of the women were having no job while 1.8 % had any job. The proportion of experiencing stillbirth among those who had no job was 2.49 % which is less than that of those who had any job (3.91 %).

Results of binary logistic regression analysis

Multiple logistic regression models were fitted using the categorical predictor variables which were found to be significant in the bivariate analysis using enter selection (Likelihood ratio) method. The results are presented in Table 5. The result shows that nine of the predictor variables were significantly associated with experiencing stillbirth.

Assessment of goodness of fit of the model

For categorical data, after we fit the logistic model, it is necessary to see the appropriateness, adequacy and usefulness of the fitted model. To overcome this we have several techniques. The most commonly used techniques are Pearson's Chi-square, the likelihood ratio tests (LRT) and Hosmer and Lemeshow Goodness of fit test.

The result presented in Table 2 showed a likelihood ratio test statistic $G^2 = 277.041$ which is distributed as chi-square with 11° of freedom. The tabulated value was $X^2_{0.05}(11) = 19.675$. Since $G^2 > X^2_{0.05}(11)$, we reject the null hypothesis and conclude that at least one of the predictors was significantly related with experiencing stillbirth among mothers of child bearing age.

Based on the results in Table 3, the null hypothesis that there is no difference between the model with only a constant and the model with independent variables was rejected.

The Hosmer-Lemeshow goodness-of-fit test is found to be not significant (x^2 = 7.424, d.f = 8, p-value = 0.72). Thus, we do not have an evidence to reject the null hypothesis that the model fitted the data well.

The Nagelkerke R-square was 8.0 % indicating that explanatory variables were useful in predicting experiencing stillbirth. But, it doesn't give the meaning of variance explained as in linear regressions (33).

Validation of predicted probabilities

The degree to which predicted probabilities agree with actual outcomes is expressed as a classification table. Classification table documents the validity of predicted probabilities. According to the classification presented in Table 4, prediction for women who had not experienced

Table 2 Overall model evaluation using likelihood ratio test (EDHS, 2011)

	-2 Log likelihood	Likelihood ratio (G^2)	d.f	$X^2_\alpha(16)$
Null model	3043.857	277.041	11	19.675
Full model	2766.816			

Table 3 Omnibus tests of model coefficients (EDHS, 2011)

	Chi-square	d.f	Sig.
Step	213.727	23	0.000
Block	213.727	23	0.000
Model	213.727	23	0.000

stillbirth was more accurate than that for those who had experienced stillbirth. This observation is supported by the magnitude of sensitivity (81.6 %) compared to that of specificity (100.0 %). Sensitivity measures the proportion of correctly classified events (i.e., those women who had experienced stillbirth), whereas specificity measures the proportion of correctly classified nonevents (those women who had not experienced stillbirth). The overall correct prediction was 99.5 %, an improvement over the chance level.

Interpretation of logistic regression coefficients

A multiple logistic model was fitted to the data to test the research hypothesis regarding the relationship between the likelihood that experiencing stillbirth of woman is related with the predictor variables. Result displayed in Table 5 revealed that region of residence, maternal age, place of residence, education level, parity, antenatal care utilization, place of delivery, body mass index (BMI) and anemia level were found to be significantly associated with experiencing stillbirth.

Experiencing stillbirth was significantly associated with geographical regions. The odds of experiencing stillbirth in Tigray, Amhara, Oromiya, SNNP, Gambela, Harari, and Dire-Dawa were not significantly different from that of experiencing stillbirth in Addis Ababa. Experiencing stillbirth in Benishangul-Gumuz was 2.451 times more likely than that in Addis Ababa city. Women who live in Afar and Somali were more likely to experience stillbirth than women who live in Addis Ababa (Table 5).

According to the model, the log of the odds of a woman to experience stillbirth was positively related to maternal age group 25–34 (p = 0.000) and 35+ (p = 0.000) when compared with age group 15–24. Indicating that the older the woman the more likely to experience stillbirth. The odds of a woman in age group (25–34) of experiencing stillbirth were 3.49 times the odds of woman with age group 15–24 and the odds of a woman in age group (35+) of experiencing stillbirth were 6.80 times that of a woman with age group 15–24. This further indicates that women of older ages are vulnerable to experiencing stillbirth.

Table 4 Classification table of model with predictor variables (EDHS, 2011)

Observed		Predicted		
		Experienced stillbirth		Percentage correct
		No	Yes	
Experienced stillbirth	No	12240	0	100.0
	Yes	59	261	81.6
Overall Percentage				99.5

Table 5 has also revealed that place of residence was significantly associated with experiencing stillbirth. The likelihood of experiencing stillbirth for those women residing in urban area is 0.620 times that of those women residing in rural area. Educational level was also found to be significantly associated with experiencing stillbirth. Though women having only primary education have no significant difference in experiencing stillbirth with those having no educational attainment, women with secondary and higher education were less likely (OR = 0.178) to experience stillbirth than those with no educational attainment.

Table 5 is trying to tell us that the multipara women, those having at least one child, were 3.215 times more likely vulnerable to experience stillbirth than the nulliparous women, those having no children. Women who have made antenatal care visit for at least once during their pregnancy times were less likely (OR = 0.482) to experience stillbirth than those who haven't visited antenatal care. Women who delivered their babies at any health center were 75.8 % (0.242-1, OR = 0.242) less likely to experience stillbirth than those who preferred to deliver at home.

Experiencing stillbirth is significantly associated with the body mass index (BMI) of women. The normal weight women were found to be less likely (OR = 0.482) to experience stillbirth than those women who were thin (BMI < 18.5). Although not significant, those women who were overweight/obese (BMI ≥ 25) were more likely (1.518) to experience stillbirth than those women who were thin. Thus, normal weight women were found to be less likely to experience stillbirth than abnormal weight women. Women who were anemic are 2.499 times likely to experience stillbirth than those who were not anemic.

Discussions

This study has intended to model determinants of experiencing stillbirth among women in child bearing age group of Ethiopia using the Ethiopian demographic and health Survey data. Accordingly, different models are fitted to the data to identify potential determinants of experiencing stillbirth among women in reproductive age group. First, the bivariate chi-square test of association was fitted to the data and significant variables were considered for further investigation in binary logistic regression model.

This study revealed that the rate of experiencing stillbirth among women of child bearing age was about 25.5 per 1000 deliveries in Ethiopia consistent with the world

Table 5 Logistic regression results of experiencing stillbirth among women, in Ethiopia

	B	S.E.	Wald	Df	Sig.	Exp(B)	95 % CI for Exp(B)	
							Lower	Upper
AGE (15–24 ref.cat)			49.686	2	.000			
25–34	1.250	.183	46.463	1	.000	3.49	2.438	4.996
35+	1.917	.333	33.140	1	.000	6.8	3.541	13.062
REGION (Addis Ababa ref.cat)			41.254	10	.000			
Tigray	-.035	.359	.009	1	.922	0.966	0.478	1.952
Affar	.851	.304	7.822	1	.005	2.342	1.291	4.250
Amhara	-.089	.357	.063	1	.803	0.915	0.454	1.842
Oromiya	.103	.328	.099	1	.754	1.108	0.583	2.108
Somali	.782	.300	6.794	1	.009	2.185	1.214	3.935
Benishangul-Gumuz	.897	.314	8.167	1	.004	2.451	1.325	4.538
SNNP	.478	.332	2.074	1	.150	1.613	0.841	3.092
Gambela	.358	.317	1.276	1	.259	1.431	0.768	2.663
Harari	-.109	.387	.079	1	.779	0.897	0.420	1.915
Dire Dawa	-.063	.389	.026	1	.871	0.939	0.438	2.013
ResidPlace (Rural ref.cat)								
Urban	-.478	.176	7.370	1	.007	0.62	0.439	0.875
EucationLevel (No Educ.ref.cat)			8.254	2	.016			
Primary	-.291	.252	1.342	1	.247	0.748	0.456	1.225
Secondary & Higher	-1.728	.239	7.230	1	.007	0.178	0.111	0.284
PARITY (Nulliparous ref.cat)								
Multipara	1.168	.362	10.385	1	.001	3.215	1.582	6.537
ANC (No ANC visit ref.cat)			5.953	1	.015			
Visited atleast once	-.729	.299	5.953	1	.015	0.482	0.268	0.867
DeliveryPlace (Home ref.cat)			.201	1	.654			
Health center	-1.417	.435	10.611	1	.001	0.242	0.103	0.569
Delivery Mode (Normal ref.cat)			1.894	1	.169			
Caesarean section	-.498	.362	1.894	1	.169	0.608	0.299	1.236
BMI (Thin ref.cat)			7.757	2	.021			
Normal	-.729	.152	4.796	1	.029	0.482	0.358	0.650
Overweight/Obese	.417	.230	1.815	1	.178	1.518	0.967	2.382
ANEMIA (Not anemic ref.cat)								
Anemic	.916	.436	4.414	1	.036	2.499	1.063	5.874
OCCUPATION (No ref.cat)								
Yes	-.492	.319	2.379	1	.123	0.611	0.327	1.143
Constant	-1.522	.532	8.188	1	.004	0.218	0.077	0.619

ref.cat reference category, *SNNP* South Nations Nationalities and Peoples

health statistics 2013 report which revealed a stillbirth rate of 26/1000 deliveries and was also almost consistent with a large review of data for 190 countries which estimated a stillbirth rate of 32/1000 deliveries in South Asia and Sub-Saharan Africa [4].

Among the factors, mode of delivery and occupation were found to have a significant association with experiencing stillbirth only in the bivariate analysis. And factors like education level, parity, body mass index (BMI) and anemia level were significantly associated with experiencing stillbirth also in binary logistic regression which is consistent with most of the studies in the literature [21–23].

The rate of experiencing stillbirth in Tigray, Amhara, Oromiya, SNNP, Gambela, Harari and Dire Dawa were not significantly differing from that in Addis Ababa. This might be because of most of these regions are similarly developed as Addis Ababa. Women who live in Afar, Somali and Benishangul-Gumuz regions were significantly more likely to experience stillbirth than those women living in Addis Ababa which might be because of they were disadvantaged regions in the past reigns.

This study revealed that experiencing stillbirth among women was significantly associated with the age group they are found in. Women in higher age group, especially those above 35 years, are more likely to experience stillbirth than those at lower age group. This finding was consistent with a study done using available data from 6 study sites of The Newborn Cross-Sectional Study (NCSS), component of INTERGROWTH-21st, maternal age >40 (OR: 2.52) [22]. Silver et al. [21] has reviewed researches done on five clinical sites in America stated that the stillbirth rate is increased two-fold for women 35–39 years of age, and 3- to 4-fold for women aged forty or older. While some age-associated risk is due to higher rates of maternal complications, in uncomplicated pregnancies there may be a 50% increased risk associated only with maternal age $\geq$ 35. For older women, stillbirth risk rises more rapidly as gestational age increases beyond 37 weeks. A prospective study done in Nigeria also revealed that 35 years and above pregnancy was important factor contributing to high stillbirth rate [24]. And almost all researchers in the literature agree in that advanced maternal age is contributing factor to high stillbirth rate.

Women's place of residence was found to be significantly associated with experiencing stillbirth. Those women residing in rural areas were found to be more likely to experience stillbirth than those in urban areas which might be for the reason that in rural areas there is lack of a skilled attendant at delivery, lack of education, lack of full information and so on. This finding was in line with the finding of review of causes, risk factors and prevention strategies of stillbirth in developing countries [25].

Experiencing stillbirth was also significantly associated with utilization of antenatal care (ANC). Visiting antenatal care for at least once is found to decrease the probability of experiencing stillbirth. This finding has an agreement with a cross-sectional retrospective analysis of stillbirth among women delivering in University of Maiduguri teaching hospital (UMTH), east Nigeria in which lack of antenatal care visit (OR: 1.91) had increased the rate of experiencing stillbirth [26]. A research finding also revealed that lack of antenatal care had positive association with stillbirth [24]. In the binary logistic analysis done in Hawassa University Hospital, southern Ethiopia, both the crude and adjusted analysis showed that the stillbirth rate was highest among mothers who had no Antenatal Care follow up [27].

Delivering at health center rather than delivering at home brought about less probability to experience stillbirth. This finding was consistent with a prospective study entitled 'Causes of stillbirth in a community survey in Gombe State', Nigeria [24]. This happens because when mothers deliver at home, they might not find skilled attendant and in difficult case there is no other choice like caesarean section in health centers.

Conclusions

The purpose of this study has been to assess socio-economic, demographic, and medical factors associated with stillbirth in Ethiopia. The descriptive result showed that 25.5 per 1000 deliveries were stillbirth.

In this study single level logistic regression were used. In the single level logistic regression model, region of residence, maternal age, place of residence, education level, parity, antenatal care utilization, place of delivery, body mass index (BMI) and anemia level were found to be significantly associated with experiencing stillbirth. Women of older ages are vulnerable to experiencing stillbirth. Chi-square test of association was done to see if there is association between experiencing stillbirth and region of residence and since it revealed that region of residence was associated with experiencing stillbirth.

Recommendations

Based on the findings of this study we forward the following recommendations to whom it my concern:

- ✓ First and for most all mothers should take care of their health condition when they become pregnant, during pregnancy and when approaching to labour. This can be made by utilizing antenatal care in health centers.
- ✓ Mothers should prefer and people who are around them should advise them to give birth at health centers than delivering at home.
- ✓ Those older age women, above 35 years, should be more careful for difficulties that come with age, like hypertension and should visit antenatal care during pregnancy.
- ✓ The government should facilitate infrastructures to teach and inform women, especially those residing in rural areas about the silent killer stillbirth that it is not because of an evil spirit called "Wukabi".
- ✓ Further studies should be conducted to identify other correlates of stillbirth that are not included and confirm the variables which are insignificant in this study because of many reasons and since regional variation are found significant spatial models can be applied to investigate spatial variations of experiencing stillbirth.

Limitations of the study

Some of the limitations of the study are:-

- Since this study is based on secondary data from EDHS, 2011, we can study only the variables which are included in the questionnaire.
- Due to the presence of high missing values in 2011 EDHS data; some variables are not included in the study

Abbreviations
ANC: Antenatal care; BMI: Body mass index; CSA: Central statistical agency of Ethiopia; DHS: Demographic and health survey; EDHS: Ethiopian demographic and health survey; IUGR: Intrauterine growth restriction; LMIC: Low and middle-income countries; LRT: Likelihood ratio rest; MDGs: Millennium development goals; MLEs: Maximum likelihood estimates; NCSS: The newborn cross- sectional study; PHC: Population and housing census; PMNCH: Partnership for maternal, newborn & child health; SNNPR: South Nation Nationalities and People Regional state; WHO: World Health Organization

Acknowledgements
Not applicable.

Funding
Not applicable.

Authors' contributions
HG made contributions on conceptualized the research problem, designed the study, performed statistical analysis, interpretation of data and revised & drafting the manuscript. KA was involved in, re- vision of the research design, data analysis and revision of the manuscript for publication. Both authors read and approved the final manuscript.

Competing interests
The author(s) declare that there is no conflict (competing) of interests' regarding the publication of this manuscript.

Declaration
I, declare that the thesis is my original work, has not been presented for Degrees in any other University and all sources of materials used for the thesis have been duly acknowledged.

Author details
[1]Department of Statistics, College of Natural and Computational Sciences, University of Gondar, Gondar, Ethiopia. [2]Department of Statistics, College of Natural and Computational Sciences, Dilla University, Dilla, Ethiopia.

References
1. Robinson GE. "Pregnancy loss". Best practice & research. Clin Obstet Gynaecol. 2014;28(1):169–78. doi:10.1016/j.bpobgyn.2013.08.012.
2. Nguyen RH, Wilcox AJ. Terms in reproductive and perinatal epidemiology: Perinatal terms. J Epidemiol Community Health. 2005;59(12):1019–21. doi:10.1136/jech.2004.023465. PMC 1732966. There is probably no health outcome with a greater number of conflicting, authoritative, legally mandated definitions. The basic WHO definition of fetal death is the intrauterine death of any conceptus at any time during pregnancy. However, for practical purposes, legal definitions usually require recorded fetal deaths to attain some gestational age (16, 20, 22, 24, or 28 weeks) or birth weight (350, 400, 500, or 1000 g). In the US states, there are eight different definitions by combinations of gestational age and weight, and at least as many in Europe.
3. Frøen JF, Friberg IK, Lawn JE, The Lancet Ending Preventable Stillbirths Series study group, et al. Stillbirths: progress and unfinished business. Lancet 2016; published online 18 Jan. doi:10.1016/S0140-6736(15)00818-1.
4. Lawn JE, Blencowe H, Waiswa P, The Lancet Ending Preventable Stillbirths Series study group with The Lancet Stillbirth Epidemiology investigator group, et al. Stillbirths: rates, risk factors, and acceleration towards 2030. Lancet 2016; published online 18 Jan. doi:10.1016/S0140-6736(15)00837-5.
5. The Lancet release 2011, available at:- http://www.who.int/pmnch/media/press_materials/fs/201106_stillbirths/en/.
6. Baqui AH, Darmstadt GL, Williams EK. Rates, timing and causes of neonatal deaths in rural India: implications for neonatal health programs. Bull World Health Organ. 2006;84:706–13.
7. Engmann CMR, Kinoshita R, Ditekemena J, Moore J, Goldenberg R. Stillbirth and Early Neonatal Mortality in Rural Central Africa. Int J Gynecol Obstet. 2009. in press.
8. Ngoc NT, Merialdi M, Abdel-Aleem H. Causes of stillbirths and early neonatal deaths: data from 7993 pregnancies in six developing countries. Bull World Health Organ. 2006;84:699–705.
9. McClure EM, Phiri M, Goldenberg RL. Stillbirth in developing countries: a review of the literature. Int J Gynaecol Obstet. 2006;94(2):82–90.
10. Cousens S, Blencowe H, Stanton C. National, regional, and worldwide estimates of stillbirth rates in 2009 with trends since 1995: a systematic analysis. Lancet. 2011;377(9774):1319–30. Income-group aggregates are based on the 2010 World Bank list of economies.
11. Lawn JE, Blencowe H, Pattinson R, Cousens S, Kumar R, Ibiebele I, Gardosi J, Stanton C. Stillbirths: Where? When? Why? How to make data count? Lancet. 2011;377:1448–63.
12. Berhane Y, Hogberg U. Prolonged labor in rural Ethiopia: a community base study. Afr J Reprod Health. 1999;3(2):33–9.
13. Bisetegn D. Determinants of still Birth at Tikur Anbessa hospital: a retrospective comparative study, a thesis submitted to AAU Medical Faculty department of obstetrics and gynecology. 2001.
14. Demographic and health survey preliminary report, Ethiopia, Central statistics Agency- Addis Ababa, Ethiopia and ORC Marco, Calverton, Maryland USA. 2005.
15. Addis Ababa Health Bureau. Family health team annual report for 2006. Addis Ababa, Ethiopia. 2006.
16. Berhanu Assefa T, Fikre E, Lukman Y. Birth to pregnancy interval and its effect on perinatal outcomes in Addis Ababa, Ethiopia. Ethiopian J Reprod Health. 2010;4(1):37–51.
17. Mitike Molla S, Robel Y, Abebe Gebremariam G, Sibley LM. A Qualitative Study of Attitudes and Values Surrounding Stillbirth and Neonatal Mortality among Grandmothers, Mothers, and Unmarried Girls in Rural Amhara and Oromiya Regions, Ethiopia: Unheard Souls in the Backyard. J Midwifery Womens Health. 2014;59:S110–7.
18. Goldenberg RL, McClure EM, Bhutta ZA. The Lancet's Stillbirths Series steering committee. Stillbirths: the vision for 2020. Lancet. 2011. published online April 14. doi:10.1016/S0140-6736(10)62235-0.
19. Stanton C, Lawn J, Rahman H, Wilczynska-Ketende K, Hill K. Stillbirth rates: delivering estimates in 190 countries. Lancet. 2006;367(9521):1487–94.
20. Central Statistical Agency [Ethiopia] and ICF International. Ethiopia Demographic and Health Survey 2011. Addis Ababa, Ethiopia and Calverton, Maryland, USA: Central Statistical Agency and ICF International; 2012.
21. Silver RM, Varner MW, Reddy U, Goldenberg R, Pinar H, Conway D, Bukowski R, Carpenter M, Hogue C, Willinger M, Dudley D, Saade G, Stoll B. Work-up of stillbirth: a review of the evidence. Am J Obstet Gynecol. 2007;196(5):433–44.
22. Finkton Jr DW. The epidemiology of stillbirth: The INTERGROWTH-21st Newborn Cross-Sectional Study. America: MSc Research, University of Oxford; 2013.
23. Reddy UM, Laughon SK, Sun L, Troendle J, Willinger M, Zhang J. Pre-pregnancy risk factors for antepartum stillbirth in United States. Obstet Gynecol. 2010;116(5):1119–26.
24. Alkali YS, Jalo I, AU E –N, Bode-Thomas F. Causes of stillbirth in a community survey in Gombe State. Niger J Paed. 2014;41(2):125–8.
25. McClure EM, Robert L. Goldenberg, stillbirth in developing countries: a review of causes, risk factors and prevention strategies. J Matern Fetal Neonatal Med. 2009;22(3):183–90.

14

A cross-sectional study of determinants of birth weight of neonates in the Greater Accra region of Ghana

Margaret Atuahene[1*], David Mensah[2] and Martin Adjuik[3]

Abstract

Background: Birth weight is a major determinant of infant morbidity and mortality. Fetal undernourishment means an increased risk of dying during a baby's early months and years. Birth weight has emerged as the leading indicator of infant health and welfare and the central focus of infant health policy. The issues have not been comprehensively evaluated in part due to lack of or limited empirical data. To this end, this study is aimed to evaluate the effects of maternal determinants on the birth weights of neonates in two major hospitals.

Results: Low birth weight neonates were significantly ($p < 0.001$) associated with low gestation at birth (34.8 ± 3.8) while mothers of low birth weight neonates had significantly ($p = 0.034$) lower body mass index (27.3 ± 5.4) than their normal birth weight counterparts (29.0 ± 6.3). Gestation at birth ($p < 0.001$), diastolic blood pressure ($p = 0.008$) was the only significant determinant of birth weight.

Conclusion: An increase in gestation at birth by 1 week results in over twice more likelihood of a normal birth weight while a rise in diastolic blood pressure is less likely to give rise to a normal birth weight neonate.

Keywords: Birth weight, Anthropometric measurements, Neonates, Low birth weight, Normal birth weight

Background

Low birth weight (infants born weighing less than 2500 g) is a very important phenomenon with respect to birth outcomes in the developing world [1]. Birth weight is a major determinant of infant morbidity and mortality [2, 3]. Existing literature has established the associations between LBW and infant mortality [4]. This is a major reason that attention to determinants of LBW has to be given much priority in public health.

Many studies have been conducted all over the world and a wide range of risk factors for LBW recorded over the years [5]. These range from maternal demographic and maternal anthropometric to maternal nutrition. Among the demographic risk factors are young maternal age [6], low education [7] and primiparity [8].

A major determinant of birth outcomes is the nutritional status of mothers during pregnancy [9]. Other indicators that have shown associations with birth outcomes happen to be maternal pre pregnancy body mass index and weight gain during pregnancy, among others [10]. Determinants of birth outcomes, of which maternal anthropometric measurements are a major part, have been demonstrated to differ between developed and developing countries [11–13].

Studies have demonstrated a linear relationship between maternal weight gain and birth weight. Thus a weight gain is popularly associated with normal birth weight whereas a maternal weight loss is associated with low birth weight, among others [14]. Some studies have been conducted into the relationship between maternal anthropometric measurements, other maternal factors and birth weight [11, 14–17].

In the light of the afore-stated, this cross-sectional study was designed to evaluate the associations, if any, between the effect of maternal anthropometric measurements, other maternal factors of expectant women and birth weight of neonates, and to also assess the effect of these same factors on the birth weight of the neonates.

* Correspondence: magat2006@yahoo.com
[1]School of Public Health, University of Ghana, Legon, Accra, Ghana
Full list of author information is available at the end of the article

Methods

Selection of area, hospitals and subjects

Korle-Bu Teaching Hospital is a flagship urban teaching hospital that serves Accra and other nearby towns and villages. It is the largest hospital in the country with obstetric care at all levels. It registers approximately 10,000 pregnancies annually. It receives referrals from polyclinics and other maternity centers within Accra and surrounding towns and villages and indeed throughout the country.

Ridge Hospital serves as a regional medical centre. Catchment area extends to Winneba, Kasoa, Nsawam, including neighbourhood polyclinics in Accra. There is an open door policy, no cases are turned away.

Women with singleton pregnancies comprised the study population. Nine-hundred and sixty-six singleton pregnant women were randomly sampled in two health facilities (Ridge Hospital, the Greater Accra Regional Hospital, and Korle-Bu Teaching Hospital, a referral facility) in the Greater Accra Region with singleton pregnancies above 28 weeks at delivery and at attendance of antenatal clinics were studied. Systematic Random Sampling, specifically, was employed in this regard. Knowing, on average, the number of women within our inclusion criteria who visited each facility per day, on a daily basis, we picked a random start and thereafter, we picked successive participants, based on the sampling interval till they were all been sampled for the day. Mothers with twin or multiple births, as well as those seriously sick or had physical incapacitation, were excluded from the study.

Ethical clearance: Ethical review was granted by the Ethical Review Committee of the Ghana Health Services. Participants provided written informed consent to share data and participation was completely voluntary.

Questionnaire

Information about the maternal, demographic and anthropometric measurements were recorded on fully structured questionnaire. The questionnaire was first pretested, in a facility different from the two study-facilities, to ascertain the validity of questions enshrined in it and its potential to capture required information for the study adequately well. Questions were finally modified to reflect language simplicity, clarity and ease in comprehension.

Anthropometric measurements

Weight Weight was taken with the Seca scale. The scale was calibrated each time it was moved. A participant stood still in the middle of the scale's platform without touching anything and with the body weight equally distributed on both feet. The weight was read to the nearest 100 g (0.1 kg) and recorded immediately (two measurements taken in immediate succession should agree to within 0.1 kg).

Height Each participant was bare footed with heels together, arms to the sides, legs straight, shoulders relaxed. Heels, buttocks, scapulae (shoulder blades), and back of the head were against the vertical board of the stadiometer. The measurement was read to the nearest 0.1 cm and the eye level with the headboard to avoid errors. Since there is no data on pre-pregnancy weight, first registration weight was used. For maternal height measurement reference, 145 cm was used as cut-off for short stature, which is considered a risk criteria for birth weight.

Neonate information Neonatal measurements were obtained within 72 h of delivery. Birth weight was obtained using a calibrated electronic scale. Length was measured using a standardized plastic length board. The newborns were weighed on a paediatric Seca scale that was accurate to within 10 g by research nurses. Adjustments were made to zero for any cushion, a towel or diaper that was in place. The weight of the cushion was subtracted from the newborn's weight. Infants were weighed nude or with minimum clothing. The average of two weighing was recorded in the infant's record to the nearest 10 g (0.01 kg). Weight at delivery was used to determine birth weight >90th percentile. Weight at the anthropometric assessment was used to determine total and percent body fat . Sex of the neonate was also established.

Blood pressure After at least 10 min rest, after a woman walked in, blood pressure was measured on two occasions with a mercury sphygmomanometer with an interval of 5 min between measurements with a pressure monitor. Two readings were taken–the "systolic" pressure was recorded as the heart beats, and the second "diastolic" reading was taken during the "rest" between beats. The mean of the last two measurements was used. If BP was above 140/90 on at least two occasions within a week, a diagnosis of elevated blood pressure was made. This was followed by a referral to a competent professional for further evaluation.

Hemoglobin testing A separate consent statement was read to the eligible participants. This statement explained the purpose of the test and requested permission for the test to be carried out. It required just a small sample of easily obtained blood. Before the blood was taken, the finger was wiped with an alcohol prep swab and allowed to air-dry. Then the palm side of the end of a finger was pricked with a sterile, non-reusable, self-retractable lancet and a drop of blood collected. It measured the concentration of hemoglobin in the blood. The results were recorded in the maternal health book, and the book was returned to each mother as per hospital policy. For each participant whose hemoglobin level was lower than the cut-off point of 11 g/dl a referral was made for further evaluation. It is normal for hemoglobin levels to go down somewhat in the second half of pregnancy, when the amount of blood in the body is expanding dramatically. Follow-up hemoglobin (Hb) tests were given in late second trimester or early third trimester for monitoring. Consent was given for blood work.

Data management and statistical analyses

The questionnaire was reviewed for completeness and consistency before data was entered. To ensure that sample selection procedures were complied with, the author worked closely with the field supervisors and interviewers throughout the data collection period. Effective management of fieldwork was emphasized. Participants were screened based on inclusion criteria and sampling procedures were adhered to. The study questionnaire was pretested to provide face validity in wording and interpretation.

The general characteristics of the study population were examined using mean and standard deviation for continuous variables and frequencies for categorical variables. Cross tabulations were used to establish the relationship between two or more categorical variables. Bivariate analysis was performed by cross tabulation to determine the predictors associated with birth weight which was coded as 1 = normal, 0 = low. Wald statistics was used to test the significance of individual coefficients in the model.

P-values obtained through both chi-square analysis and binary logistic regression analysis was employed to assess any associations between BW and maternal demographic and anthropometric variables. These predictor variables in the bivariate model included sex of baby, blood pressure status, meal intake frequency, hemoglobin concentration, gestational age at the time of birth urine protein levels, age of the respondent, employment status, marital status and antenatal care visits. The basis for building the multivariate model was using the Enter approach, in SPSS. Gestational age, in weeks, was calculated from the first day of the last menstrual period (LMP), as ultrasound and sonogram systems were not available. Significance level was defined as $p < 0.05$. The strength of these associations was established using odds ratio and their 95 % Confidence Intervals (CI). Statistical analysis was performed using SPSS software version 20.0 (IBM Corporation, 2011) [18].

Results and discussion

Socio-demographic characteristics of respondents

Almost all of the respondents were on health insurance (99.1 %). Over half of the respondents (56.3 %) earned less than GH¢100.00 per month while only 2.5 % earned GH¢1000.00 or more, Table 1. Their occupations were grouped into 'Professional', referring to Teachers, Engineers, Medical Doctors, etc., followed by 'Middle Level Officers', referring to respondents engaged in white-collar jobs (whether private or public) such as secretaries, managers, etc. The rest were 'Trades', referring to artisans such as hair-dressers, seamstresses, caterers, etc., and finally traders, also referring to traders in the local markets or business women operating mini-markets or super markets, etc. It turned out that less than half of the respondents (34.5 %) were traders, 5.5 % were professionals, while 4.6 % were middle level officers. Almost 40 % of them were unemployed. The modal parity was 1 and the median was

Table 1 Socio-demographic characteristics of respondents

Variables and levels	N (%)
Health insurance status	
Yes	957 (99.1)
No	9 (0.9)
Average monthly income (in GHC)	
<100	378 (56.3)
100–499.9	211 (31.4)
500–999.9	66 (9.8)
≥1000	17 (2.5)
Occupation	
Professional	53 (5.5)
Middle level officer	44 (4.6)
Trades	245 (25.5)
Trader	331 (34.5)
Unemployed	287 (39.9)
Parity	
0–1	422 (43.7)
2–3	436 (45.1)
≥4	108 (11.2)
Marital status	
Single	141 (14.6)
Married	825 (85.4)
Education	
Primary	93 (9.6)
Secondary	526 (54.5)
Tertiary	347 (35.9)
Age (years)	
<20	48 (5.0)
20–29	471 (48.8)
30–39	416 (43.1)
≥40	31 (3.2)

Exchange rate:1US$ = 3GHC

2. Parity was however re-grouped into 0–1, 2–3 and ≥4. About 44 % were expecting up to their second child while a little over 11 % were expecting at least their fourth child. A great majority of them were married (85.4 %) while a little over half of them had completed either Junior Secondary or Senior Secondary school. About 9.6 % had either never been to school or had completed primary school, and 35.9 % had completed tertiary education. The ages of the respondents were pre-grouped from 'Under 20 years','20–29 years' all the way to'40 years and above'. The modal age group was 20–29 year (48.8 %) closely followed by 30–39 years (43.1 %) whereas the least was 40 years and above (3.2 %), Table 1.

Anthropometric measurements, gestation and hemoglobin levels of women at birth

Table 2 contains the frequencies of gestation at birth, systolic and diastolic blood pressure, hemoglobin at birth, and BMI at birth. There is a significant positive correlation between systolic blood pressure and baby's weight at birth ($r = 0.216$, $p = 0.001$), diastolic blood pressure and baby's weight at birth ($r = 0.214$, $p = 0.001$), and parity and baby's weight at birth ($r = 0.140$, $p = 0.021$) and between mother's age and baby's weight at birth (0.108, $p = 0.05$). The mean gestation at birth was almost 39 weeks, the mean BMI of mother at birth was 28.8 kg/m^2, and the mean systolic blood pressure at birth was 114.5 mmHg while that of the diastolic blood pressure at birth was 70.3 mmHg. The hemoglobin at birth was 11.3. The anthropometric measurements were re-grouped in Table 2. Majority (over 60 %) of the mothers were in the 35–39.9 gestation at birth group while a similar proportion (over 60 %) of the mothers were in the 90–119.9 mmHg group. Majority of the mothers (over 80 %) had their diastolic blood pressure in the 60–89.9 mmHg group. The most represented hemoglobin at birth (25.6 %) fell in the 11–11.9 group. The most common BMI at birth (58.0 %) fell in the 20–29.9 kg/m^2 group.

Table 2 Anthropometric measurements, gestation and hemoglobin levels of women at birth

Parameters and levels	N (%)
Gestation at birth (weeks)	
Less than 30	28 (2.9)
30–34.9	139 (14.4)
35–39.9	589 (61.1)
40 and above	208 (21.6)
Systolic blood pressure at birth (mm Hg)	
Less than 90	8 (0.8)
90–119.9	590 (61.2)
120–149.9	312 (32.4)
150 and above	54 (5.6)
Diastolic blood pressure at birth (mm Hg)	
Less than 60	74 (7.7)
60–89.9	783 (81.2)
90–119.9	97 (10.1)
120 and above	10 (1.0)
Hemoglobin at birth (g/dl)	
Less than 9	67 (7.0)
9–9.9	134 (13.9)
10–10.9	233 (24.2)
11–11.9	246 (25.6)
12–12.9	184 (19.1)
13 and above	98 (10.2)
BMI at birth (kg/m^2)	
Less than 20.0	42 (4.5)
20.0–29.9	538 (58.0)
30.0–39.9	312 (33.6)
40 and above	36 (3.9)

Whereas majority of the low birth weights were recorded among the female neonates, (60.3 %), the opposite was the case for the recorded normal birth weights (55.2 % of male neonates), Table 3. On birth weight and hemoglobin levels of mothers, whereas majority of both low birth weights and normal birth weights were non-anemic, the proportion of the anemic among the low birth weights (33.8 %) was almost twice that recorded among the normal birth weights (19.6 %). It is also interesting to quickly point out that whereas majority (64.5 %) of the low birth weights were premature births, the opposite was the case among the normal birth weights (71.8 %).

In Table 4, there is confirmation to the finding in Table 3 that the low birth weights recorded a significantly ($p < 0.001$) lower gestation (34.8 ± 3.8 weeks) than the normal birth weights (37.3 ± 3.3). It is also the case, per the underlying data, that mothers of normal weight neonates (29.0 ± 6.3) have a significantly ($p = 0.034$) higher BMI than their low birth weight counterparts (27.3 ± 5.4). However, the systolic blood pressure of mothers of normal birth weight neonates (113.3 ± 17.0) are significantly lower ($p < 0.001$) than that of the mothers of low birth weight neonates (122.2 ± 30.0). A similar picture can be seen with the case of diastolic blood pressure (69.8 ± 13.2 for normal birth weight and 75.6 ± 20.7 for low birth weight with a significance of $p = 0.001$). However, mothers' hemoglobin levels had no significant association with birth weights of neonates, Table 4.

One of the areas of interest in this study was how the mean birth weights of the neonates were affected by the various levels of the socio-demographic and anthropometric parameters of mothers, Table 5. As the BMI of the mother generally rises, the birth weight of her

Table 3 Prevalence of low birth weight and normal birth weight

		Weight of baby	
		Low birth weight (Less than 2.5)	Normal birth weight (2.5 and above)
		N (%)	N (%)
Sex of baby	Male	29 (39.7)	481 (55.2)
	Female	44 (60.3)	390 (44.8)
HB status of mother	Anaemic	24 (33.8)	168 (19.6)
	Non-anaemic	47 (66.2)	690 (80.4)
Gestation status	Pre-mature	40 (64.5)	213 (28.2)
	Normal	22 (35.5)	542 (71.8)

neonate also rises, however this association is not statistically significant at 95 % confidence level, Table 5. This same trend show in the remaining parameters investigated such as Age of mother, Educational level of mother, Mother's occupation, Mother's monthly income, Gestation at birth, Systolic and Diastolic blood pressures and Mother's haemoglobin level at birth were seen to have no significant association with the birth weight of the neonates.

For the binary logistic regression, the Nagelkerke R Square (=0.236) shows that about 23.6 % of the variation in the outcome variable (Birth Weight) is explained by this logistic model. In the Wald statistics (this determines the relative importance of the predictor variables in predicting the response, thus the higher the more important and vice versa) column of Table 6, Gestation-at-birth (Wald = 9.4) happens to be the most important predictor of a mother's likelihood of having normal birth weight. This is followed by Diastolic-blood-pressure-at-birth (Wald = 7.08), and mother's-weight-at-birth (Wald = 7.07). However the remaining variables were not significant in predicting a mother's likelihood of having normal birth weight baby.

Diastolic-blood-pressure-at-birth (0.008) was the only significant factor that predicted baby's weight at birth. The Exp (B) and 95 % C.I. columns of Table 6 give us the odds ratios and their corresponding 95 % confidence interval estimates respectively. An increase in a mother's diastolic blood pressure at birth has a 4.7 % (95 % CI 2.2 to 7.9 %) decrease in the odds of having a normal birth weight baby.

Table 4 Association between birth weight of neonates and anthropometric characteristics of mothers

Parameters	LBW	NBW	*t*-test
Gestation at birth (weeks)	34.8 ± 3.8	37.3 ± 3.3	<0.001
BMI at birth (kg/m^2)	27.3 ± 5.4	29.0 ± 6.3	0.034
SBP (mm Hg)	122.2 ± 30.0	113.3 ± 17.0	<0.001
DBP (mm Hg)	75.6 ± 20.7	69.8 ± 13.2	0.001
HB (g/dl)	11.6 ± 8.4	11.2 ± 3.4	0.39

The overall accuracy of this model to predict subjects having normal birth weight (with a predicted probability of 0.5 or greater) is 93.7 % (Table 6). The sensitivity is given as 497/498 = 99.8 % and the specificity is 6/39 = 15.4 %. The model has a positive predictive value (PPV) = 497/530 = 93.8 % and negative predictive value (NPV) = 6/7 = 85.7 %.

Discussion

The bulk of incidents of low birth weight are found in developing countries, the major cause of which is preterm birth (<37 weeks) [15]. One key finding in this study is the fact that the mothers of neonates with low birth weight had significantly lower BMI and gestation at birth than their normal birth weight counterparts. This is seen in the association between birth weight and anthropometric characteristics of mothers in this article. We could not however demonstrate, with the study data, that maternal characteristics such as age, education, occupation, monthly income and haemoglobin at birth are significant determinants of birth weight of neonates. This is unlike studies that have demonstrated that poor families are more likely to have LBW neonates than well to do ones [19]. In their study titled "Maternal anthropometric measurements and other factors: relation with birth weight of neonates", Tabrizi and Saraswathi [20] considered family income, among others, as a predictive factor of birth weight of neonates [21].

Meanwhile, several studies across the world have shown that, education affects neonatal birth weight [6, 19, 21], though it has been established in literature that the causes of LBW in neonates differ between developing and developed societies [15, 22–25]. It is also reported in de AlencarBritto et al. that age, BMI and family income were significantly associated with LBW in neonates [26]. However in this study, they were not.

There was no significant association between gestation at birth and birth weight of neonates, mother's BMI and birth weight of neonates, systolic blood pressure and birth weight of neonates, as well as diastolic blood pressure and birth weight of neonates. Though the gestation at birth, mothers' height and weight at birth were lower for LBW neonates than their NBW counterparts, that difference was not statistically significant. Whereas the systolic and diastolic blood pressures and were higher for mothers of LBW neonates than their NBW counterparts, only the diastolic blood pressure showed a statistically significant difference. These findings in the current study run through several studies over the world [20, 27, 28]. However, in developing countries, gestation at birth is a determinant of birth weight [29].

There was a significant positive association between the BMI of mothers, on one side, and the weights of

Table 5 Association between socio-demographic and anthropometric characteristics of mothers and birth weights of neonates

Parameter	Level	Number	Mean weight of baby (kg)	F (p)
Age of mother (years)	<20	46	3.001	0.975 (p>0.05) (NS)
	20–29	464	3.257	
	30–39	406	3.303	
	≥40	30	3.445	
Education of mother	Primary	89	3.185	0.225 (p>0.05) (NS)
	Secondary	517	3.283	
	Tertiary	340	3.273	
Occupation	Professional	53	3.323	0.088 (p>0.05) (NS)
	Middle level officer	43	3.303	
	Trades	241	3.246	
	Trader	320	3.272	
	Unemployed	289	3.279	
Monthly income (GHc)	<100	369	3.261	0.119 (p>0.05) (NS)
	100–500	206	3.261	
	500–1000	64	3.35	
	>1000	17	3.276	
Gestation at birth (weeks)	Less than 30	28	3.013	1.359 (p>0.05) (NS)
	30–34.9	137	3.12	
	35–39.9	576	3.289	
	40 and above	204	3.356	
Systolic blood pressure (mm Hg)	Less than 90	8	2.838	1.505 (p>0.05) (NS)
	90–119.9	579	3.25	
	120–149.9	304	3.363	
	150 and above	54	3.034	
Diastolic blood pressure (mm Hg)	Less than 60	73	3.124	0.383 (p>0.05) (NS)
	60–89.9	769	3.279	
	90–119.9	93	3.322	
	120 and above	10	3.23	
Haemoglobin at birth (g/dl)	Less than 9	66	3.013	0.606 (p>0.05) (NS)
	9–9.9	130	3.322	
	10–10.9	230	3.283	
	11–11.9	243	3.295	
	12–12.9	178	3.264	
	13 and above	96	3.295	
Body mass index (kg/m^2)	Less than 20.0	41	3.227	0.726 (p>0.05) (NS)
	20.0–29.9	529	3.226	
	30.0–39.9	306	3.349	
	40.0 and above	34	3.409	

Exchange rate:1$ = 3GHC
* $p < 0.05$; *NS* Not significant

their neonates. Thus mothers of normal birth weight neonates were also significantly taller and heavier than their low birth weight counterparts [29]. This is similar to the findings of Momen et al. [17] in their study titled *Anthropometric assessment of nutritional status of Bangladeshi pregnant women and weight of their newborns*, conducted in Bangladesh. In their study they found a positive association between the weight of mothers and that of their neonates. Similarly, these findings in the current study also run through the studies of Hassan et

Table 6 Results of binary logit - determinants of birth weight

	B	S.E.	Wald	Sig.	Exp(B)	95 % C.I. for Exp(B)	
						Lower	Upper
Age (years)	−0.046	0.276	0.028	0.868	0.955	0.557	1.64
Education	−0.3	0.172	3.048	0.081	0.741	0.529	1.037
Occupation	−0.466	0.247	3.57	0.059	0.628	0.387	1.018
Monthly income (GHc)	.013	.274	.002	0.961	1.013	.592	1.733
Haemoglobin at birth (g/dl)	.286	.446	.411	0.521	1.331	.555	3.189
Mothers BMI (kg/m^2)	.050	.030	2.688	0.101	1.051	.990	1.115
SBP at birth (mm/Hg)	−.010	.012	.780	0.377	.990	.967	1.013
DBP at birth (mm/Hg)	−.048	.018	7.069	0.008	.953	.921	.988
Gestation at birth (weeks)	−.708	.382	3.426	0.064	.493	.233	1.043

al., titled *relationship between maternal characteristics and neonatal birth size in Egypt,* in which correlation tests between maternal and neonatal anthropometric measurements revealed that for both sexes combined maternal weight had a significant positive correlation with neonatal weight [27]. The relationship between the BMIs of mothers and the birth weights of their neonates was not statistically significant in this study as a Bangladeshi study revealed that a combination of the initial weight and height of the mother was not a good determinant of neonatal birth weight [27]. The same study showed that maternal weight was the best determinant of neonatal birth weight whereas in this current study, gestation at birth proved to be the best determinant of neonatal birth weight. However, other studies have also shown that not only are BMI, weight and height predictors of birth weight of neonates but that the most important predictor of birth weight is weight at first visit, followed by BMI and then Height, in descending order [29]. On the other hand, this study found that Gestation-at-birth was the most important determinant of birth weight of neonates, followed by Diastolic Blood Pressure and mother's weight-at-birth for the study area.

Mothers' hemoglobin levels had no association with birth weights of their neonates in this current study. Other studies have however shown the contrary [30–32].

Strengths and limitations

In several other studies, factors such as birth order, antenatal care and mother's health status were found to also be significant predictors of birth weight of neonates [22, 23–35]. However, in this study we did not consider those factors together with birth order in the prediction of the birth weight of neonates. These could be a limitation with our study. Furthermore, given that the Korle-Bu teaching hospital is generally a referral hospital, and the fact that it contributed a larger portion of respondents, may suggest that factors discovered as being associated with birth weight may have been over-represented in this study. Another limitation could be the inability of this study to capture the quality of education, as well as the subjective nature in which the education and monthly income variables were captured. These limitations notwithstanding, the results of this current study are considered representative given the sampling technique. The strengths of this current study are a large sample size, collection of birth data from the cohorts of mothers studied by well-trained research staff and the fact that birth data of the neonates were obtained from reliable standard instruments, rather than recall.

Conclusions

It is evident from this study that among mothers' characteristics, Diastolic Blood Pressure was the only important determinant of birth weight of neonates. Mothers' Systolic Blood Pressure, Haemoglobin at birth and mother's height were not significant per the binary logistics regression. However among the socio-demographic characteristics of mothers, Age of mother, level of education, occupation and monthly income were not significant in determining the birth-weight of neonates'.

Mothers of neonates with low birth weight were found to have significantly higher systolic and diastolic blood pressures, lower weight and shorter in terms of height as well as lower gestation at birth than their normal birth-weight counterparts. There was no significant difference between the haemoglobin level of mothers of normal birth weight and their low birth weight counterparts.

Ethical clearance Ethical review was granted by the Ethical Review Committee of the Ghana Health Services. Informed written consent was requested from study participants. The participation by any person in the study was voluntary. A separate consent was obtained for blood work including hemoglobin. They were informed that upon completion of the work the results would be shared with them and the community. This will help inform interventions on maternal child health services.

Abbreviations

ANC: Antenatal care; IUGR: Intra uterine growth retardation; LBW: Low birth weight; LMP: Last menstrual period; MCH: Maternal child health; MOH: Ministry of health; NBW: Normal birth weight; UN: United Nations; UNICEF: United Nations Children Education Fund; WH: World Health Organization; KBTH: Korle-Bu Teaching Hospital.

Competing interest

The authors declare that they have no competing interests.

Authors' contributions

MA conceived the study, worked on the research proposal and led the field work. DM and MA2 performedstatistical analyses and contributed to the interpretation of data.MA, DM and MA2 worked on the first portionand final writing of the manuscript. All authors were involved in the revision of manuscript and haveapproved it for publication.

Acknowledgements

We thank the study participants for voluntarily offering to take part in the study. We are grateful to all research assistants and medical staff who at the various stages contributed to the study.

Author details

[1]School of Public Health, University of Ghana, Legon, Accra, Ghana. [2]National Malaria Control Programme, Accra, Ghana. [3]INDEPTH Network Secretariat, Accra, Ghana.

References

1. UNICEF. Progress for Children: A Report Card on Nutrition. Other Nutrition Indicators, Low Birthweight. New York: UNICEF; 2006.
2. Godfrey KM, Barker DJ. Fetal nutrition and adult disease. Am J Clin Nutr. 2000;71:1344S–52S.
3. Boucher BJ. Determinants of size at birth. QJM. 2002;95:331–3.
4. Joseph KS, Kramer MS. Recent trends in infant mortality rates and proportions of low-birth-weight live births in Canada. CMAJ. 1997;157:535–41.
5. Fraser AM, Brockert JE, Ward RH. Association of young maternal age with adverse reproductive outcomes. N Engl J Med. 1995;332:1113–7.
6. Lee KS, Ferguson RM, Corpuz M, Gartner LM. Maternal age and incidence of low birth weight at term: a population study. Am J Obstet Gynecol. 1988;158:84–9.
7. Karim E, Mascie-Taylor CG. The association between birthweight, sociodemographic variables and maternal anthropometry in an urban sample from Dhaka, Bangladesh. Ann Hum Biol. 1997;24:387–401.
8. Abrams B, Newman V. Small-for-gestational-age birth: maternal predictors and comparison with risk factors of spontaneous preterm delivery in the same cohort. Am J Obstet Gynecol. 1991;164:785–90.
9. Osrin D, de L Costello AM. Maternal nutrition and fetal growth: practical issues in international health. Semin Neonatol. 2000;5:209–19.
10. Neggers Y, Goldenberg RL, Cliver SP, Hoffman HJ, Cutter GR. The relationship between maternal and neonatal anthropometric measurements in term newborns. Obstet Gynecol. 1995;85:192–6.
11. Mavalankar DV, Trivedi CC, Gray RH. Maternal weight, height and risk of poor pregnancy outcome in Ahmedabad, India. Indian Pediatr. 1994;31:1205–12.
12. Elshibly EM, Schmalisch G. Correlation between anthropometric measures and birthweight of infants: value in measuring actual birthweight. Am J Perinatol. 2008;25:135–9.
13. Nahar S, Mascie-Taylor CG, Begum HA. Maternal anthropometry as a predictor of birth weight. Public Health Nutr. 2007;10(9):965–70.
14. Mathews F, Youngman L, Neil A. Maternal circulating nutrient concentrations in pregnancy: implications for birth and placental weights of term infants. Am J Clin Nutr. 2004;79:103–10.
15. Imdad A, Bhutta ZA. Nutritional management of the low birth weight/ preterm infant in community settings: a perspective from the developing world. J Pediatr. 2013;162(3 Suppl):S107–14. doi:10.1016/j.jpeds.2012.11.060. PubMed: 23445841.
16. Elshibly EM, Schmalisch G. The effect of maternal anthropometric characteristics and social factors on gestational age and birth weight in Sudanese newborn infants. BMC Public Health. 2008;8:244. doi:10.1186/ 1471-2458-8-244.
17. Momen A, Yusuf HKM, Alam R. Anthropometric assessment of nutritional status of Bangladeshi pregnant women and weight of their newborns. Bangladesh Journal of Anatomy. 2011;9(2):101–5.
18. IBM Corp. IBM SPSS Statistics for Windows, Version 20.0. Armonk, NY: IBM Corp; 2011.
19. Raum E, Arabin B, Schlaud M, Walter U, Schwartz FW. The impact of maternal education on intrauterine growth: a comparison of former West and East Germany. Int J Epidemiol. 2001;30:81–7.
20. Tabrizi FM, Saraswathi G. Maternal anthropometric measurements and other factors: relation with birth weight of Neonates. Nutr Res Pract. 2012;6(2):132–7. pISSN 1976–1457 eISSN 2005–6168.
21. Thame M, Wilks RJ, McFarlane-Anderson N, Bennett FI, Forrester TE. Relationship between maternal nutritional status and infant's weight and body proportions at birth. Eur J Clin Nutr. 1997;51:134–8.
22. Celik Y, Younis MZ. Effects of antenatal care services on birthweight: importance of model specification and empirical procedure used in estimating the marginal productivity of health inputs. J Med Syst. 2007;31:197–204.
23. Walker SP, Wachs TD, Gardner JM, Lozoff B, Wasserman GA, et al. Child development: risk factors for adverse outcomes in developing countries. Lancet. 2007;369:145–57. doi:10.1016/S0140-6736(07)60076-2. PubMed: 17223478.
24. Walton E. Residential segregation and birth weight among racial and ethnic minorities in the United States. J Health Soc Behav. 2009;50:427–42. doi:10.1177/002214650905000404. PubMed: 20099449.
25. Dibben C, Sigala M, Macfarlane A. Area deprivation, individual factors and low birth weight in England: is there evidence of an "area effect"? J Epidemiol Community Health. 2006;60:1053–9. doi:10.1136/jech.2005.042853. PubMed: 17108301.
26. de AlencarBritto RP, Florêncio TML, Silva AAB, Sesso R, Cavalcante JC, Sawaya AL. Influence of Maternal Height and Weight on Low Birth Weight: A Cross-Sectional Study in Poor Communities of Northeastern Brazil. PLoS ONE. 2013;8(11):e80159. www.plosone.org, November 2013.
27. Hassan NE, Shalaan AH, El-Masry SA. Relationship between maternal characteristics and neonatal birth size in Egypt. EMHJ. 2011;17(4):281–9.
28. Backstrand JR. Maternal anthropometry as a risk predictor of pregnancy outcome: the nutrition CRSP in Mexico. 1995.
29. Jananthan R, Wijesinghe DGNG, Sivananthawerl T. Maternal Anthropometry as a Predictor of Birth Weight. Trop Agric Res Ser. 2009;21(1):89–98.
30. Malhotra M, Sharma JB, Batra S, Sharma S, Murthy NS, Arora R. Maternal and perinatal outcome in varying degrees of anemia. Int J Gynaecol Obstet. 2002;79:93–100.
31. Steer P, Alam MA, Wadsworth J, Welch A. Relation between maternal haemoglobin concentration and birth weight in different ethnic groups. BMJ. 1995;310:489–91.
32. Yazdani M, Tadbiri M, Shakeri S. Maternal hemoglobin level, prematurity, and low birth weight. Int J Gynaecol Obstet. 2004;85:163–4.
33. Maruoka K, Yagi M, Akazawa K, Kinukawa N, Ueda K, Nose Y. Risk factors for low birthweight in Japanese infants. Acta Paediatr. 1998;87:304–9.
34. Peters TJ, Golding J, Butler NR, Fryer JG, Lawrence CJ, Chamberlain GV. Plus ca change: predictors of birthweight in two national studies. Br J Obstet Gynaecol. 1983;90:1040–5.
35. Finlay JE, Ozaltin E, Canning D. The association of maternal age with infant mortality child anthropometric failure, diarrhoea and anaemia for first births: evidence from 55 low- and middle-income countries. BMJ Open. 2014;1:e000226.

15

A review of delivery room resuscitation in very low birth weight infants in a middle income country

Daynia E. Ballot*, Faustine Agaba, Peter A. Cooper, Victor A. Davies, Tanusha Ramdin, Lea Chirwa, David Rakotsoane and Lethile Madzudzo

Abstract

Background: Advanced levels of delivery room resuscitation in very low birth weight infants are reported to be associated with death and complications of prematurity. In resource limited settings, the need for delivery room resuscitation is often used as a reason to limit care in these infants.

Methods: This was a review of delivery room resuscitation in very low birth weight infants born in a tertiary hospital in South Africa between 01 January 2013 and 30 June 2016. Outcomes included death and serious complications of prematurity. Advanced delivery room resuscitation was defined as the need for intubation, chest compressions or the administration of adrenaline.

Results: A total of 1511 very low birth weight infants were included in the study. The majority (1332/1511 (88.2%) required oxygen in the delivery room. Face mask ventilation was needed in 45.2% (683/1511). Advanced delivery room resuscitation was only required in 10.6% (160/1511). More than half the infants who required advanced delivery room resuscitation died (89/160; 55.6%). Advanced delivery room resuscitation was required in significantly more infants <1000 grams at birth than those infants >1000 grams (83/539 (15.4%) vs 77/972 (7.9%) $p < 0.001$). Advanced delivery room resuscitation was significantly associated with a 5 minute Apgar score < 6 (OR 13.8 (95%CI 8.6–22.0), supplemental oxygen at day 28 (OR 2.2 (95% CI 1.4–3.9), metabolic acidosis (OR 2.3 (95% CI 1.1–4.8) and death (OR 1.9 95% CI 1.1–3.3). Other serious complications of prematurity were not associated with advanced delivery room resuscitation. Mortality was increased in infants with a low admission temperature (35.1 °C (SD 0.92) vs 36.1 °C (SD 1.4) ($p < 0.001$).

Conclusion: There was a high mortality rate associated with advanced delivery room resuscitation; however complications of prematurity were not increased in survivors..The need for advanced delivery room resuscitation alone should not be used as a predictor of poor outcome in very low birth weight infants. Survivors of advanced delivery room resuscitation should be afforded ventilatory support if required. Special care must be taken to avoid hypothermia in very low birth weight infants requiring resuscitation at birth.

Keywords: Neonate, Resuscitation, Mortality, Delivery room

* Correspondence: daynia.ballot@wits.ac.za
Department of Paediatrics and Child Health, University of the Witwatersrand, Private Bag X 39, Johannesburg 2000, South Africa

Background

Perinatal asphyxia is an important cause of morbidity and mortality, especially in low and middle income countries. In a review in South Africa in 2007, one third of neonatal deaths were due to asphyxia – hypoxia [1]. In term infants, perinatal asphyxia may result in neonatal encephalopathy, with possible long term neurological sequelae such as tetraplegic cerebral palsy [2]. In a review from the United States, 94% of neonates with an Apgar score of zero at 10 minutes either died or had severe handicap [3]. Therapeutic hypothermia has been shown to reduce rates of both mortality and long term handicap in term infants with moderate to severe hypoxic ischaemic encephalopathy [4].

Hypoxic ischaemic brain injury in preterm infants is less well defined than in their term counterparts; the extent and type of brain damage depends on brain immaturity, cellular vulnerability and the timing and intensity of the asphyxial insult [5]. Advanced delivery room resuscitation (ADRR), defined as chest compressions, intubation or the administration of adrenaline, is significantly more likely in infants of low birth weight and gestational age [6–10]. There is a significantly increased risk of death with ADRR in VLBWI [7–11]. Serious complications of prematurity, including severe intraventricular haemorrhage (IVH), retinopathy of prematurity (ROP), respiratory distress syndrome (RDS), pneumothorax, late onset sepsis (LOS), pulmonary haemorrhage, bronchopulmonary dysplasia (BPD) and use of postnatal steroids, are more common in VLBWI who had ADRR [6–9].

South Africa is a middle income country with limited health funding and resources. There are insufficient neonatal ventilator facilities to provide mechanical ventilation to all those VLBWI who require it. In order to address this problem, mechanical ventilation was rationed to those VLBWI above 1000 grams at birth, based on the premise that extremely low birth weight infants (ELBWI) with a birth weight below 1000 grams have a poor outcome. More recently, however, there has been a move away from using a birth weight cut off alone for mechanical ventilation in VLBWI [12]. Although many VLBWI are now successfully treated with surfactant replacement therapy (SRT) and nasal continuous positive airway pressure (NCPAP) [13], the issue of limited resources for ventilatory support of VLBWI in the South African context remains an important health challenge. The need for ADRR has been suggested as a possible criterion for selecting VLBWI for ventilatory support.

Resuscitation at birth has been reported to be associated with mortality in VLBWI in South Africa [14]. There is, however, limited information on survival and complications of prematurity at different levels of delivery room resuscitation (DRR) in VLBWI in sub-Saharan Africa. The aim of this study is to review DRR in VLBWI, in a tertiary referral centre in South Africa. Primary study objectives were to determine the outcome of DRR and ADRR in VLBWI and to establish whether the need for ADRR should be used as a reason to limit care to VLBWI in resource limited settings. A secondary study objective was to evaluate the association of low admission temperature in VLBWI with the need for ADRR as well as death.

Methods

This study was conducted in the neonatal unit in a tertiary referral centre, between 01 January 2013 and 30 June 2016. All inborn VLBWI were included in the study. Infants with no record of resuscitation and those with lethal congenital abnormalities were excluded.

Delivery room resuscitation was classified as none, oxygen only, positive pressure ventilation, endotracheal intubation, chest compressions and administration of adrenaline. "Oxygen only" referred to blow –by oxygen. If the infant did not respond to supplemental oxygen alone, oxygen would then be provided using positive pressure ventilation with a T piece resuscitator. An air oxygen blender was not available in the delivery room during the time of the study. A baby could have had all levels of intervention and was analysed accordingly. All VLBWI were wrapped in plastic wrap and resuscitated under a radiant warmer. The delivery room temperature was set at 25 °C.

Study site

The study site was a tertiary referral centre for both high risk obstetric and neonatal cases. The neonatal unit comprised two areas – a neonatal intensive care unit (NICU) where mechanical ventilation was provided and a premature nursery where VLBWI were treated with surfactant and NCPAP. There were 32081 live births during the study period and the overall Caesarean section (C section) rate was 48.1%. Uncomplicated preterm labour alone was not an indication for C section. Elective C section referred planned delivery by C section e.g. for previous C section and malposition. Spinal anesthesia was routinely used during the study period. Primary indication for C section was recorded.

Preterm deliveries were attended by an intern who was supervised by a registrar. An intern was a newly qualified doctor doing compulsory training in the paediatric unit, as part of a general practical training. A registrar was a doctor specializing in paediatrics. All registrars were completing a 4 year rotation in paediatrics and all had at least 18 months of paediatric experience prior to commencing the registrar rotation. Both registrars and interns were trained in neonatal resuscitation. The intern would initiate neonatal resuscitation and call the registrar for assistance as required. Resuscitation was initiated in all VLBWI irrespective of birth weight, unless there was a known diagnosis of intrauterine fetal death. Resuscitation could be discontinued after 10 minutes of asystole, in consultation with a senior member of staff.

All VLBWI were admitted to a transitional delivery ward nursery for initial evaluation and stabilization; VLBWI were then transferred to the premature nursery or NICU as required. The duration of stay in the transitional nursery could last several hours before a bed in NICU or the premature nursery became available. Deaths that occurred in this transitional nursery or labour room were classified as delivery room deaths. Deaths that occurred within 12 hours of life included VLBWI who died in the delivery room, premature nursery or NICU. Due to limited resources (both staff and equipment), during the study period, surfactant and NCPAP were only provided to VLBWI weighing >750 grams at birth; mechanical ventilation was only provided to VLBWI > 900 grams at birth. A second dose of surfactant could be given if respiratory distress worsened in VLBWI <900 grams. There was no NCPAP or surfactant replacement therapy (SRT) available in the delivery room for resuscitation during the study period. The initial therapy for all VLBWI with respiratory distress syndrome (RDS) was SRT and NCPAP. The axillary temperature of all VLBWI was recorded on admission to the transitional nursery.

Neonatal resuscitation training

All staff was trained in neonatal resuscitation according to the South African Neonatal Resuscitation Algorithm (SANRA) approved by the South African Resuscitation Council (www. resus.co.za) and the South African Paediatric Association. The SANRA is a single standardised protocol used for training all birth attendants – both nursing and medical. The SANRA states that intubation can be done at any point with a skilled operator, but most birth attendants in South Africa are midwives or junior doctors who are not skilled in endotracheal intubation. This protocol therefore emphasizes the need for proper face mask ventilation and de-emphasizes the need for intubation. Chest compressions were initiated prior to intubation and routine intubation for VLBWI was not recommended.

Database

This was a secondary analysis of an existing neonatal database, managed using Research Electronic Data Capture (REDCAP) software [15], hosted by the University of the Witwatersrand. Information was collected for each VLBWI upon hospital discharge and entered into the database, which is kept for the purpose of clinical audit. Data was verified against the hospital records after entry into the database. Data analysed for the purpose of the study included maternal information, delivery room details, VLBWI demographics, clinical characteristics and outcome.

Data analysis

Data was analysed using IBM SPSS version 23. Continuous data was described using mean and standard deviation or median and range, as appropriate, according to the distribution of the data. Categorical variables were described using frequencies and percentages. Outcomes of interest were in hospital mortality or significant complications of prematurity including necrotising enterocolitis (NEC), ROP, IVH, supplemental oxygen at 28 days of life, postnatal steroids, RDS, SRT, NCPAP, mechanical ventilation, patent ductus arteriosus (PDA), neonatal sepsis, cystic periventricular leukomalacia (PVL). Diagnosis of PDA was confirmed on echocardiography by a cardiologist; NEC was defined as modified Bell stage 2 or 3 [16] and IVH as grade 3 or 4 according to the grading of Papile [17]. Sepsis was defined as culture proven sepsis (including coagulase negative staphylococcus) - early onset sepsis (EOS) occurred before 3 days of life, while LOS occurred after 3 days. In-hospital mortality included all deaths from any cause during the hospital stay (not only deaths from perinatal asphyxia). Metabolic acidosis referred to a base excess above-16 mmol/l at any time – not only in the perinatal period. In hospital mortality was compared between different levels of DRR. The level of resuscitation and mortality was compared between ELBWI and those infants > 1000 grams birth weight. Advanced delivery room resuscitation was defined as the need for endotracheal intubation, chest compressions or administration of adrenaline. Outcomes were compared between those VLBWI who were given ADRR and those who had no ADRR. Continuous variables were compared using unpaired t tests or Mann Whitney U as appropriate. Categorical variables were compared using Chi squared tests. A p value <0.05 was considered to be statistically significant. In all analysis, only valid cases were reported (i.e. missing data was not included). Variables which were found to have a statistically significant association with ADRR on univariate analysis were entered into a multivariate logistic regression model.

Results

Total sample

There were 2994 VLBWI admitted over the study period. There were 31 infants with congenital abnormalities, 11 infants had no recorded resuscitation, 1430 infants were born elsewhere and 11 infants had no recorded birth weight. The final sample therefore comprised 1511 VLBWI. The mean birthweight of VLBWI was1091.8 (SD260) grams and gestational age was 28.8 (SD 2.6) weeks. There were 539/1511 (35.7%) ELBWI. The majority of the VLBWI was female (822/1507; 54.5%) and most were black (1457/1511; 96.4%). Other neonatal characteristics are shown in Table 1. Caesarean section (CS) was the most common mode of delivery (961/1505; 63.9%). The mean maternal age was 28.7 years (SD 6.1). Other maternal characteristics are shown in Table 2.

Outcomes of delivery room resuscitation

Very few VLBWI did not require any DRR (179/1511; 11.8%) and 10.6% (160/1511) received ADRR. The number of VLBWI in each level of DRR is shown in Table 3. Significantly more ELBWI required DRR than bigger infants (83/539 (15.4%) vs 77/972 (7.9%) $p < 0.001$).

Outcomes of advanced delivery room resuscitation

The mean birth weight of VLBWI who received ADRR was significantly lower than that of those who did not require ADRR (992.0 grams (SD 255.4) vs 1105.1 grams (SD 256.3) $p < 0.001$). Similarly, the gestational age of VLBWI who required ADRR was significantly less than those who did not (27.9 weeks (SD 2.7) vs 29.0 weeks (SD 2.7) $p < 0.001$). Other maternal and neonatal characteristics that were significantly associated with ADRR are shown in Table 4.

All other maternal and neonatal characteristics were not significantly associated with ADRR. In particular, admission temperature, NEC, ROP, PDA, IVH, cystic PVL, LOS, pneumothorax, pulmonary haemorrhage and the need for NCPAP or mechanical ventilation were not significantly associated with ADRR. The indication for C section was recorded in 649/961 (67.5%) of VLBWI delivered by C section. There was no significant association between the indication for C section and the need for ADRR (see Table 5). Multivariable regression showed that ADRR remained significantly associated with a 5 minute Apgar score below 6, supplemental oxygen at 28 days of life, metabolic acidosis and death (See Table 6).

Table 1 Characteristics of VBLW infants

Characteristic	n/N	Percent
Five minute Apgar <6	221/1490	14.8
Early onset sepsis (<3 days)	62/1423	4.4
Grade 3 or 4 intraventricular haemorrhage	49/774	6.3
Hyperglycaemia	277/1436	19.3
Hypoglycaemia	158/1436	11.0
Metabolic acidosis	93/1436	6.5
Pneumothorax	6/1418	0.4
Respiratory distress syndrome	1260/1430	88.1
Surfactant therapy at any time	1064/1511	70.4
Pulmonary haemorrhage	22/1436	1.5
Nasal CPAP	986/1390	70.9
Mechanical ventilation	231/1359	17.0
Patent ductus arteriosus	125/1419	8.8
Retinopathy of prematurity stage 3 or 4	14/411	3.4
Oxygen on day 28	340/1294	26.3
Steroids for chronic lung disease	195/1299	15.0
Necrotising enterocolitis grade 2 or 3	100/1423	7.0
Late onset sepsis (>3 days)	396/1424	27.8
Cystic Periventricular leukomalacia	10/1019	1.0

Table 2 Maternal characteristics

Characteristic	n/N	Percent
Primiparous	448/1448	30.9
Multiple gestation	286/1495	19.1
Mode delivery -%		
Normal vaginal delivery	495/1505	32.9
Vaginal breech	49/1505	3.3
Emergency C Section	891/1505	59.2
Elective C Section	70/1505	4.7
Attended antenatal care	1229/1485	82.8
Antenatal steroids received	749/1425	52.6
Antenatal magnesium sulphate	82/1401	5.4
Chorioamnionitis	49/1444	3.4
Maternal hypertension	435/1446	30.1
Maternal HIV	431/1468	29.4
Maternal syphilis	28/1416	2.0
Teenage mother	34/1483	2.3
Attempted termination of pregnancy	17/1449	1.2

Mortality

Overall in- hospital mortality was 29.1% (439/1511); 78/439 (17.8%) of the deaths occurred in the delivery room. There were 87 of the 439 deaths (19.8%) that occurred within 12 hours of admission; the majority of these occurred within the delivery room (65/87; 74.7%). Significantly more ELBWI died compared to those with a birth weight > 1000 grams (322/546; 59.0% vs 127/983; 12.9%) ($p < 0.001$). There was no difference in mortality by gender – 210/685 (30.6%) males died compared to 229/822 (27.8%) females ($p = 0.255$). – The admission temperature of VLBWI who died was significantly lower than those who survived – 35.1 °C (SD 0.92) vs 36.1 °C (SD 1.4). ($p < 0.001$)

Mortality rates by level of resuscitation are shown in Fig. 1. Mortality was significantly associated with advancing levels of DRR (intubation, chest compressions or adrenaline administration) ($p < 0.001$). More than half the VLBWI who required ADRR died (89/160; 55.6%).

Those VLBWI who required ADRR and died within the first 12 hours of admission were compared to those who survived for more than 12 hours. In this group, death within the first 12 hours was significantly associated with

Table 3 Level of resuscitation in infants <1000 grams at birth vs those > 1000 grams at birth

Level of resuscitation	Total *N* = 1511 n (%)	<1000 grams birth weight *N* = 539 n (%)	>1000 grams birth weight *N* = 972 n (%)	*P* value
Oxygen	1332 (88.2)	507 (94.1)	825 (84.9)	<0.001
Face mask ventilation	683 (45.2)	308 (57.2)	375 (38.6)	<0.001
Intubation	25 (1.7)	11 (2.0)	14 (1.5)	0.381
Adrenaline	22 (1.5)	11 (2.0)	11 (1.1)	0.158
Chest compressions	152 (10.1)	80 (14.8)	72 (7.4)	<0.001

lower admission temperature (34.9 °C SD 1.9 vs 36.0 °C SD 1.9; $p < 0{,}001$), lighter birth weight (865 grams SD 248 vs 1035 grams SD 243; $p < 0.001$) and lower gestational age (26.5 weeks SD 2.7 vs 28.4 weeks SD 2.6; $p < 0.001$).

Discussion

This review from a tertiary hospital in South Africa shows that almost all VLBWI required some degree of resuscitation in the DR, however only 10.6% needed ADRR. These findings are similar to a report by Cho et al. [8] who found that only 5.9% of VLBWI required chest compressions or drugs. In the current study, both decreasing birth weight and gestational age were significantly associated with the need for ADRR, which is in keeping with other reports [6–10].

Mortality was significantly associated with the need for ADRR in the present study. More than half the VLBWI who needed ADRR died, most of these deaths occurred in ELBWI. Increasing mortality with advancing levels of resuscitation has been reported by other researchers [7–10]. In the current study, most neonatal resuscitation was initiated by junior house staff, senior staff was only called to assist prolonged or difficult resuscitation.Ideally experienced senior staff, including registrars and fellows, should attend all high risk deliveries, including those of VLBWI. It may not be feasible to provide this service in circumstances of limited resources, so adequate training of available staff in neonatal resuscitation should be emphasised.

Although mode of delivery, antenatal care and antenatal steroids were significantly associated with the need for ADRR on univariate analysis, the adjusted odds ratios for these variables were not significant. Similarly, perinatal risk factors, determined by the indication for C-section, were not significantly associated with the need for ADRR. The only labour room characteristic significantly associated with

Table 4 Maternal and neonatal characteristics significantly associated with the need for advanced delivery room resuscitation in very low birth weight infants

Characteristic	ADRR n/N (%)	No ADRR n/N (%)	*P* value
Antenatal care	120/157 (76.4)	1109/1328 (83.5)	0.026
Antenatal steroids	57/150 (38.0)	692/1275 (54.3)	<0.001
Mode of delivery:			
-Normal vertex delivery	54/159 (34.0)	441/1346 (32.8)	0.008
-Vaginal breech	11/159 (6.9)	38/1346 (2.8)	
-Emergency CS	92/159 (57.9)	799/1346 (59.4)	
-Elective CS	2/159 (1.3)	68/1346 (5.1)	
Five minute Apgar score <6	99/157 (63.1)	122/1333 (9.2)	<0.001
Bacterial sepsis in the first 3 days of life	10/126 (8.9)	52/1297 (4.0)	0.039
Oxygen on day 28	43/107 (40.2)	297/1187 (25.0)	0.001
Hyperglycaemia	34/128 (26.6)	243/1308 (18.6)	0.029
Hypernatraemia	21/128 (16.4)	137/1308 (10.5)	0.041
Metabolic acidosis	20/128 (15.6)	73/1308 (5.6)	<0.001
Respiratory distress syndrome	121/127 (95.3)	1139/1303 (87.4)	0.009
Surfactant therapy	127/160 (79.4)	937/1351 (69.4)	0.009
Died	89/160 (55.6%)	350/1351 (25.9)	<0.001
Died in delivery room	32/160 (20.0)	46/1351 (3.4)	<0.001
Died within 12 hours of admission	41/160 (25.6)	46/1344 (3.4)	<0.001

Table 5 The need for advanced delivery room resuscitation and indication for C section

Indication	No ADRR (582) n (%)	ADRR (67) n (%)	*p* value
Absent end diastolic placental blood flow	7 (1.2)	0 (0)	*p* = 0.243
Antepartum haemorrhage	49 (8.4)	12 (17.9)	
Cord prolapse	2 (0.3)	1 (1.5)	
Decreased liquor	4 (0.7)	0 (0)	
Fetal distress	62 (10.7)	4 (6.0)	
Malpresentation	7 (1.2)	0 (0)	
Miscellaneous	4 (0.7)	1 (1.5)	
Proteinuric hypertension	377 (64.8)	44 (65.0)	
Poor obstetric history	19 (3.3)	1 (1.5)	
Prolonged rupture of membranes	14 (2.4)	1 (1.5)	

the need for ADRR in the current study was a 5 minute Apgar score below six. Iliodromiti et al. [18] confirmed the usefulness of the Apgar score in modern day practice - both in term and preterm neonates.

Several complications of prematurity were significantly associated with ADRR on univariate analysis, but adjusted odds ratios showed that only metabolic acidosis and the need for supplemental oxygen at 28 days of life remained significant. A review of VLBWI who were entered into the Caffeine and Apnoea of Prematurity (CAP) trial showed that BPD was significantly associated with ADRR [6].

Admission hypothermia significantly increases the chance of death in very preterm infants [19, 20]. In the present study, admission temperature was significantly lower in the VLBWI who died. Of particular note, VLBWI infants who required ADRR and died within the first 12 hours of life were significantly smaller, more preterm and had a lower admission temperature. This highlights the importance of preventing hypothermia in the smallest VLBWI. Although polythene wrap, radiant warmers and a warm delivery room are routine practice in the study centre, more care needs to be taken to ensure extreme preterm infants do not become hypothermic. Other measures to prevent neonatal hypothermia should be implemented, such as use of caps, avoiding cold air for resuscitation, reducing

Table 6 Adjusted odds ratios for significant associations with advanced delivery room resuscitation

Characteristic	Odds Ratio	95% CI	*P* Value
Five minute Apgar score <6	13.8	8.6–22.0	<0.001
Supplemental oxygen at day 28	2.2	1.4–3.9	0.001
Metabolic acidosis	2.3	1.1–4.8	0.035
Died	1.9	1.1–3.3	0.027

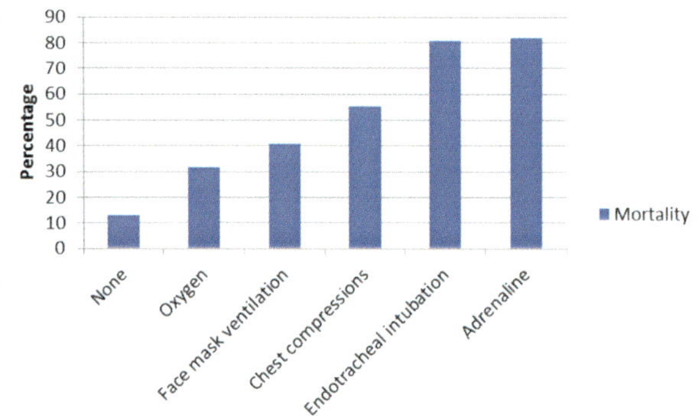

Fig. 1 Mortality by level of delivery room resuscitation

maternal hypothermia and ensuring normothermia during transfer between wards [19].

In the present study, no major complications of prematurity, including ROP, NEC, IVH, cystic PVL, sepsis, pneumothorax, pulmonary haemorrhage or the need for ventilatory support were significantly associated with ADRR. This is in contrast to many other reports which have reported an increase in complications of prematurity in VLBWI who had ADRR [6–8]. This finding may be related to the high mortality rate associated with ADRR in the present study – more than half the VLBWI needing ADRR died. Another possible reason relates to the definition of ADRR in the present study which included the need for intubation. Very few VLBWI (1.7%) were actually intubated, in strong contrast to a report from Korea where 77.7% of VLBWI were intubated at birth [8]. In addition, in the present study far more VLBWI received chest compressions than were intubated. This reflects the neonatal resuscitation training according to the South African Neonatal Resuscitation Algorithm (SANRA) (http://www.resus.co.za). Most birth attendants are midwives, so the training emphasises effective face mask ventilation, rather than intubation. In the SANRA, health workers who are not skilled in intubation are taught to intubate after chest compressions. Those VBLWI with RDS at birth would not be routinely intubated as NCPAP was the first line ventilatory support in the unit at the time of the study.

Complications of prematurity were not increased in survivors of VLBWI who required ADRR. This suggests that survivors of ADRR should be provided with ventilatory support if required– the need for ADRR alone is not sufficient reason to ration care. Some other researchers have reported that the outcome of VLBWI following ADRR is not that bad. In a study from the Vermont Oxford Network in the late 1990s Finer et al. reported that most VLBWI undergoing ADRR survive and half did not have severe IVH [7]. De Mauro et al. reported on the cohort of VLBWI enrolled in the CAP trial and found that ADRR was not associated with worse neurodevelopmental outcome at 18 months [6]. Other factors apart from the need for ADRR should be considered when making decisions to withhold or withdraw care in these VLBWI.

There was a high mortality rate in VLBWI requiring ADRR in a tertiary centre with neonatal facilities. Although there is no available information, it is very probable that the mortality rate of VLBWI is even higher in non-tertiary centres where DRR may be sub-optimal. This emphasises the need for VLBWI to be delivered in a properly equipped tertiary centre, where possible. In addition, available staff in non-tertiary centres should be properly trained and equipped to carry out neonatal resuscitation.

Limitations of the study

The retrospective nature of the study meant that some data was missing and could not be evaluated. More detailed information regarding the resuscitation e.g. dose of adrenaline, duration of chest compressions, number of attempts at intubation could not be evaluated. There was no record of the timing of cord clamping, so the effect of delayed cord clamping could not be determined. The benefit or otherwise of the seniority and experience of the attending staff members conducting the resuscitation could not be assessed. The number of VLBWI who had cranial sonars done was low due to resource constraints, so the incidence of IVH and PVL may be under estimated. Rates of death and complications are a poor proxy for the quality of resuscitation. A prospective study should be done to appraise the quality and effectiveness of DRR in VLBWI.

Conclusion

The present study showed that mortality increased with advancing levels of delivery room resuscitation in VLBWI. Extremely preterm, small VLBWI were most likely to die after ADRR. Major complications of prematurity were not increased in those VLBWI who survived ADRR. All VLBWI who survive ADRR should be provided with ventilatory support if required; the results of the present study suggest that the need for ADRR alone is not sufficient reason to limit care in these infants in the study setting. The low complication rate, however, may be related to high mortality in this group of infants – improved survival may result in an increase in complications of prematurity. There must be careful monitoring of the outcome of VLBWI who are provided with ventilatory support.

Abbreviations

ADRR: Advanced delivery room resuscitation; BPD: Bronchopulmonary dysplasia; CAP: Caffeine and apnoea of prematurity; CMJAH: Charlotte Maxeke Johannesburg Academic Hospital; CS: Caesarean section; DRR: Delivery room resuscitation; ELBWI: Extremely low birthweight infants; EOS: Early onset sepsis; IVH: Intraventricular haemorrhage; LOS: Late onset sepsis; NCPAP: Nasal continuous positive airways pressure; NEC: Necrotising enterocolitis; NICU: Neonatal intensive care unit; PDA: Patent ductus arteriosus; PVL: Periventricular leukomalacia; RDS: Respiratory distress syndrome; REDCAP: Research electronic data capture; ROP: Retinopathy of prematurity; SRT: Surfactant replacement therapy; VLBWI: Very low birthweight infants

Acknowledgements

The authors gratefully acknowledge the assistance of Ms Patricia Hanrahan, Mr Lebogang Rapola and Mr Milton Reineke in data capture and management.

Funding

There is no source of funding to declare.

Author's contributions

DEB conceptualized the study, collected and analysed the data, wrote and submitted the manuscript. FA assisted in study concept, obtained ethics approval, assisted with data collection and analysis and reviewed the various drafts of the manuscript. PAC and VAD assisted with the study concept and planning reviewed and corrected the various drafts of the manuscript, including the final draft. TR, LC, DR and LM assisted with data collection and analysis, reviewed various drafts and final submission of the manuscript. All authors read and approved the final manuscript.

Competing interests

The authors declare that they have no competing interests.

References

1. Velaphi S, Pattinson R. Avoidable factors and causes of neonatal deaths from perinatal asphyxia-hypoxia in South Africa: national perinatal survey. Ann Trop Paediatr. 2007;27(2):99–106.
2. Rennie JM, Hagmann CF, Robertson NJ. Outcome after intrapartum hypoxic ischaemia at term. Semin Fetal Neonatal Med. 2007;12(5):398–407.
3. Harrington DJ, Redman CW, Moulden M, Greenwood CE. The long-term outcome in surviving infants with Apgar zero at 10 minutes: a systematic review of the literature and hospital-based cohort. Am J Obstet Gynecol. 2007;196(5):463. e461-465.
4. Schulzke SM, Rao S, Patole SK. A systematic review of cooling for neuroprotection in neonates with hypoxic ischemic encephalopathy - are we there yet? BMC Pediatr. 2007;7:30.
5. Gopagondanahalli KR, Li J, Fahey MC, Hunt RW, Jenkin G, Miller SL, Atul M. Preterem hypoxic ischaemic encephalopathy. Frontiers in Pediatrics. 2016;4:10.
6. DeMauro SB, Roberts RS, Davis P, Alvaro R, Bairam A, Schmidt B. Impact of delivery room resuscitation on outcomes up to 18 months in very low birth weight infants. J Pediatr. 2011;159(4):546–50. e541.
7. Finer NN, Horbar JD, Carpenter JH. Cardiopulmonary resuscitation in the very low birth weight infant: the Vermont Oxford Network experience. Pediatrics. 1999;104(3 Pt 1):428–34.
8. Cho SJ, Shin J, Namgung R. Initial resuscitation at delivery and short term neonatal outcomes in very-low-birth-weight infants. J Korean Med Sci. 2015;30 Suppl 1:S45–51.
9. Handley SC, Sun Y, Wyckoff MH, Lee HC. Outcomes of extremely preterm infants after delivery room cardiopulmonary resuscitation in a population-based cohort. J Perinatol. 2015;35(5):379–83.
10. Frontanes A, Garcia-Fragoso L, Garcia I, Rivera J, Valcarcel M. Outcome of very-low-birth-weight infants who received epinephrine in the delivery room. Resuscitation. 2011;82(4):427–30.
11. Shah PS. Extensive cardiopulmonary resuscitation for VLBW and ELBW infants: a systematic review and meta-analyses. J Perinatol. 2009;29(10):655–61.
12. Velaphi SC, Mokhachane M, Mphahlele RM, Beckh-Arnold E, Kuwanda ML, Cooper PA. Survival of very-low-birth-weight infants according to birth weight and gestational age in a public hospital. S Afr Med J. 2005;95(7):504–9.
13. Jardine C, Ballot DE. The use of nasal CPAP at Charlotte Maxeke Johannesburg Academic Hospital. S Afr J Child Health. 2015;9(1):4.
14. Ballot DE, Chirwa T, Ramdin T, Chirwa L, Mare I, Davies VA, Cooper PA. Comparison of morbidity and mortality of very low birth weight infants in a Central Hospital in Johannesburg between 2006/2007 and 2013. BMC Pediatr. 2015;15:20.
15. Harris PA, Taylor R, Thielke R, Payne J, Gonzalez N, Conde JG. Research electronic data capture (REDCap)—A metadata-driven methodology and workflow process for providing translational research informatics support. J Biomed Inform. 2009;42(2):377–81.

16

Neuroprotective potential of erythropoietin in neonates; design of a randomized trial

Sandra E. Juul[1*], Dennis E. Mayock[1], Bryan A. Comstock[2] and Patrick J. Heagerty[2]

Abstract

Background: In 2013, nearly four million babies were born in the U.S., among whom 447,875 were born preterm. Approximately 30,000 of these infants were born before 28 weeks of gestation. These infants, termed Extremely Low Gestational Age Neonates (ELGANs), experience high morbidity and mortality despite modern therapies: approximately 20 % of ELGANs admitted to an NICU die before discharge, 20 % of survivors have severe, and 20 % moderate neurodevelopmental impairment (NDI). New approaches are needed to improve neonatal outcomes. Recombinant erythropoietin (Epo) is a promising neuroprotective agent that is widely available, affordable, and has been used safely in neonates to stimulate erythropoiesis. There are extensive preclinical data to support its use as a neuroprotective intervention: Epo promotes normal brain maturation by increasing neurogenesis, angiogenesis, and by protecting oligodendrocytes. Epo also decreases acute brain injury following hypoxia ischemia by decreasing inflammation, oxidative and excitotoxic injury, resulting in decreased apoptosis. Despite the availability of both preclinical and safety data there has not been a definitive clinical evaluation of the benefit of Epo, and a large phase III trial is necessary to provide evidence to support potential changes in practice guidelines.

Findings: We first review the preclinical data motivating further clinical trials, and then describe in detail the design of the PENUT study (Preterm Epo Neuroprotection). PENUT is a phase III study evaluating the effect of neonatal Epo treatment on the combined outcome of death or severe NDI among ELGANS. 940 subjects will be randomized to determine: 1) whether Epo decreases the combined outcome of death or NDI at 22–26 months corrected age; 2) the safety of high dose Epo administration to ELGANs; 3) whether Epo treatment decreases serial measures of circulating inflammatory mediators, and improves biomarkers of brain injury; and 4) whether Epo treatment improves brain structure at 36 weeks postmenstrual age as measured by MRI.

Conclusions: Epo neuroprotection is an exciting new approach to preterm neuroprotection, and if efficacious, will provide a much-needed therapy for this group of vulnerable infants.

Keywords: Prematurity, Neuroprotection, ELGANS, Biomarkers

Introduction

Extremely Low Gestational Age Neonates (ELGANs) are at high risk of death or neurodevelopmental impairment (NDI). Data from 9575 ELGANs born between 2003 and 2007 and admitted to Neonatal Research Network intensive care units showed that death or NDI occurred in 91, 80, 66 and 56 % of those born at 24, 25, 26 and 27 weeks gestation, respectively [1]. These sobering statistics do not include infants that died before admission to a NICU, or those who died within 12 h of admission. Major neurologic morbidities, which include cerebral palsy (CP), deafness, blindness, and cognitive disabilities, are present in up to 50 % of surviving extremely preterm infants at school age [2–7]. In addition to the traditional measures of impairment, long-term follow-up studies are now also increasingly identifying behavioral dysfunctions such as attention deficit disorder and autism spectrum disorder [8–11]. Sequelae of extreme prematurity are a tremendous burden to the individuals, their families, and to our health care system, accounting for nearly half of the health care dollars spent on newborn care [12]. Clearly, a neuroprotective intervention that improves outcomes for ELGANs would be profoundly beneficial to the individual, the family and to society [13].

* Correspondence: sjuul@uw.edu
[1]Department of Pediatrics, Division of Neonatology, University of Washington, 1959 Pacific Ave NE, Box 356320, Seattle, WA 98195-6320, USA
Full list of author information is available at the end of the article

Findings

A phase III study to test the safety and efficacy of high dose Epo is indicated, based on current preliminarypre-clinical and clinical data.

The PENUT (Preterm Epo Neuroprotection) Trial is a randomized, placebo controlled, double blind study ofEpo neuroprotection in an ELGAN population.

Review

Vulnerabilities of the preterm brain

ELGANs are born at a time when the fetal brain is rapidly increasing in size, shape and complexity [14, 15]. Brain development is vulnerable to interruption by hypoxia-ischemia, oxidant stress, inflammation, and excitotoxicity, as evidenced by structural, biochemical, and cell-specific injury [16, 17]. Oligodendrocytes, which emerge and mature between 24 and 32 weeks of development, are particularly susceptible to injury, resulting in the white matter injury (WMI) characteristic of preterm infants [18]. Although the transition from fetal to early postnatal life is the period of greatest vulnerability [19], ELGANs remain at risk for brain injury throughout the period of oligodendrocyte development.

Perinatal inflammation (chorioamnionitis, necrotizing enterocolitis, or sepsis) is associated with increased risk of NDI [2, 20, 21]. Microglial activation [22] and increased cytokine expression, particularly TNF-α, interleukin (IL)-6, and IL-8, have been associated with brain injury in preterm infants [23, 24] and in animal models of neonatal brain injury [25].

Epo neuroprotection

Epo has anti-inflammatory, anti-excitotoxic, anti-oxidant, and anti-apoptotic effects on neurons and oligodendrocytes, and promotes neurogenesis and angiogenesis, which are essential for repair of injury and normal neurodevelopment [26–30]. Epo effects are dose-dependent, and multiple doses are more effective than single doses [31–33]. Epo reduces neuronal loss and learning impairment following brain injury [34]. Even when initiated as late as 48–72 h after injury, there is evidence of improved behavioral outcomes, enhanced neurogenesis, increased axonal sprouting, and reduced white matter injury [35, 36]. Epo has demonstrated anti-inflammatory effects, which may contribute to neuroprotection in the scenario of preterm birth and increased inflammatory activity [37–43]. Epo also stimulates growth factors required for normal brain growth such as brain-derived neurotrophic factor (BDNF) and glial cell derived neurotrophic factor (GDNF) [27, 44].

Epo decreases WMI in adult and neonatal animal models of brain injury [35, 45–50]. Preliminary work in preterm infants suggests this holds true for developing human brain [51]. This protective effect may be mediated by the effect of Epo on oligodendrocytes: Epo promotes the proliferation, maturation and differentiation these cells [52], and protects them from injury induced by interferon-γ, LPS, and hypoxic-ischemia [35, 53, 54].

In addition to cell specific effects in brain, Epo increases iron utilization as erythropoiesis is increased. Iron is highly reactive and normally sequestered by transport proteins. Unbound iron produces free radicals and subsequent oxidative injury. Preterm infants have measurable free iron, which increases after transfusions of red blood cells or during metabolic instability such as sepsis [55, 56]. Epo may contribute to neuroprotection by decreasing free iron.

Epo dosing

In rodent, ovine and nonhuman primate models of neonatal brain injury, repeated Epo doses of 1000–5000 U/kg/dose result in sustained neuroprotection, improving both short and long-term structure and function [31, 32, 49, 57–59]. Higher doses are needed for neuroprotection than for erythropoiesis, due to the low percentage of circulating Epo that crosses the blood brain barrier [60]. In acute models of brain injury, including a late dose (7 days post injury) significantly improves outcomes [32, 61]. Preclinical data suggest that Epo neuroprotection has a U-shaped dosing curve, with too little or too much Epo resulting in diminished efficacy [31, 62]. To estimate how neuroprotective Epo doses in rat pups relate to human pharmacokinetics, plasma Epo concentrations were measured in extremely low birth weight infants (<1000 g birth weight) after 500, 1000, and 2500 U/kg/dose [63]. Nonlinear kinetics were noted, consistent with previous studies in neonates [64]. In these infants, intravenous administration of 500 and 1000 U/kg resulted in similar peak concentrations but faster clearance than were achieved in rat pups after 5000 U/kg (Fig. 1). Doses of 1000 U/kg Epo resulted in area under the curve (AUC) measurements most similar to the most protective dose in rats [31]. The 500 U/kg dose fell short (one third to one quarter the protective AUC), while 2500 U/kg was close to three times the optimal dose in rats. Minimum steady-state concentrations (mean = 576 mU/ml) were produced using the 1000 U/kg/dose. Thus, we estimate that multiple doses of 1000 U/kg would be safe and achieve neuroprotective circulating concentrations in human neonates.

Translational trials of neonatal Epo neuroprotection for preterm infants are in progress

Enrollment in a randomized, double masked phase II trial of Epo neuroprotection for preterm infants has been completed (NCT00413946). 443 infants (gestational age 26 0/7-31 6/7 weeks) were randomized to Epo (3000 U/kg, $N =$ 229) or saline ($N = 214$) at 3, 12–18, and 36–42 h after birth. This dose and dosing regimen was found to be safe [65], and those treated with Epo showed improved white matter integrity [51, 66]. Long term follow up is ongoing.

Two additional preliminary reports of preterm infants treated prospectively show benefit: 1) Preterm infants 500 to 1250 g treated with either Epo (400 U/kg 3x/

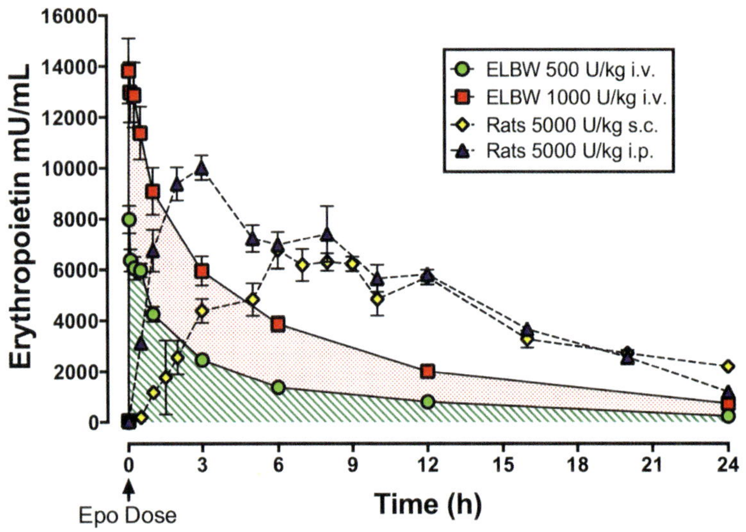

Fig. 1 Epo pharmacokinetics in neonatal rats compared to extremely low birth weight infants (ELBW). Epo concentration in mU/mL is shown on the Y axis, and time in hours on the X axis. Serum concentration in neonatal rats is shown following subcutaneous injection (s.c.) or intraperitoneal injection (i.p.) of 5000 U/kg/dose of Epo. This is compared to dosing in human ELBW infants with 500 U/kg/dose or 1000 U/kg/dose by intravenous injection (i.v.). The area under the curve (AUC) of 1000 U/kg/dose most closely approximates the neuroprotective concentrations noted in rats treated with 5000 U/kg/dose

week, $N = 29$) or Darbepoetin (10 U/kg/dose once a week, $N = 27$) from birth to 35 weeks postmenstrual age (PMA) had an average cumulative cognitive score 8 to 10 points higher than placebo/controls with Epo-treated infants earning scores of 97.9 ± 14, and Darbepoetin-treated infants scoring 96.2 ± 7.3 compared to 88 ± 14 for controls ($N = 24$). Epo recipients also performed statistically better than controls on object permanence testing [67]. The combined scores for NDI or death were significantly better in both Epo and Darbepoetin treated groups, with combined scores of 15.5 % compared to 48.2 % in the control group. 2) Follow-up of ELBW infants that received 500 to 2500 U/kg Epo x 3 doses in a phase I/II trial [63] showed that Epo treatment correlated with improvement of cognitive ($R = .22$, $p < 0.05$) and motor ($R = .15$, $p < 0.05$) scores [68].

Risks of intervention

In adults, complications of prolonged Epo treatment include polycythemia, seizures, hypertension, stroke, myocardial infarction, congestive heart failure, tumor progression, and shortened time to death. None of these adverse effects have been reported in Epo-treated neonates in over 3000 patients enrolled in randomized controlled trials [69]. Epo trials in neonates for the purposes of testing its erythropoietic effect have shown it to be a safe drug for use in this population. There is robust data from preclinical animal work showing that Epo, when used at optimal doses (1000–5000 U/kg), shows short and long term improvement in brain injury that approximates 50–80 %, and no safety issues have been discovered. Even the risk of retinopathy of prematurity (ROP) has not been substantiated in randomized controlled trials [70, 71]. Safety data for high dose Epo (3000 U/kg x 3 doses) have recently been published [65]. However, as yet unknown rare complications may occur, so safety data must still be collected as studies of Epo neuroprotection are done.

The **PENUT** (**P**reterm **E**po **Neu**roprot**e**ction) **Trial** is a randomized, placebo controlled, double blind study of Epo neuroprotection in an ELGAN population. Figure 2 provides an overview of the study. 940 patients will be enrolled at 19 sites across the United States in order to evaluate 752 infants at 22–26 months corrected age. Enrollment and initial treatment with study drug will occur by 24 h after birth. Subjects will be randomized to either Epo treatment or placebo, and treatment will continue until 32-6/7 weeks PMA. Short term, intermediate and long-term safety measures will be determined by comparing Epo-treated and control infants. Mechanisms of Epo neuroprotection and potential biomarkers of outcome will be sought by measuring sequential inflammatory cytokines and markers of brain injury. In a subset of subjects, a brain MRI will be done at 36 weeks PMA to determine whether Epo treatment preserves brain growth and decreases injury. After discharge from the hospital, phone contact will be made at 4 to 6 month intervals. Data will be collected on interval medical history and functional status. In- person follow-up will occur at two years corrected age (22–26 months), at which time standardized neurodevelopmental assessments will be made. The primary outcome is death or severe

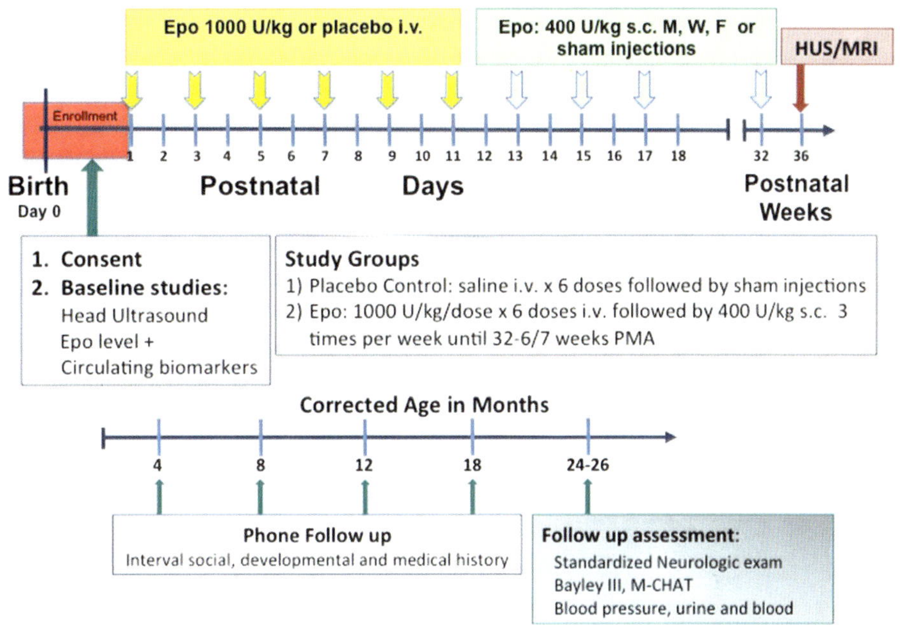

Fig. 2 PENUT Trial Overview. Significant events each subject will undergo when participating in the PENUT trial

NDI at 22–26 months corrected age, with a secondary outcome of death, severe or moderate NDI. This study of high dose Epo for the purposes of neuroprotection of preterm infants is registered with the FDA (IND # 12656) and ClinicalTrials.gov (NCT01378273).

Eligibility and enrollment

Patients will be eligible if they are NICU inpatients between 24–0/7 and 27–6/7 weeks of gestation and less than 24 h of age with arterial or venous access. Parental consent may be obtained prenatally or postnatally, as dictated by each recruitment site's IRB. Patients will be excluded if there are known major life-threatening anomalies, known or suspected chromosomal anomalies, severe hematologic crises such as disseminated intravascular coagulopathy, twin-twin transfusion such that 1 twin is not eligible due to polycythemia or hydrops, polycythemia (hematocrit > 65 %), hydrops fetalis, or known congenital infection such as toxoplasmosis, CMV, rubella or syphilis.

Randomization

We will use block randomization within site using variable blocks of size 4 to 10 subjects. Using block randomization ensures that equal numbers of subjects are randomized to the intervention and control arm and that the two groups are balanced at period enrollment intervals. For multiple births (twins, triplets, etc.), all infants will be randomized to the same treatment group (e.g. effective randomization of the mother). Randomization sequences will be provided to the research pharmacy at each site. Randomization will be stratified on site, gestational age category (24–25 weeks, 26–27 weeks), and on multiple gestation (number of babies carried to birth: singleton, twins, triplets, or more).

Epo dose justification

The Epo dose, and duration of therapy chosen for this study is based upon available preclinical and clinical data for Epo neuroprotection. Although doses as high as 3000 U/kg/dose are being tested in preterm infants without apparent adverse effects [65], we chose 1000 U/kg/dose based on our phase I/II data [63]. We will treat with high dose during the first weeks of life when physiologic vulnerability is highest, followed by maintenance Epo through 32 weeks postmenstrual age (the period of oligodendrocyte vulnerability).

Iron supplementation

Maintaining iron sufficiency in a growing preterm infant is important for normal brain growth. Because of this, iron guidelines were established for the PENUT trial. When enteral feedings are started, a standard iron containing formula is used if breast milk is unavailable. Once infants (all subjects) reach an enteral intake of 60 mL/kg/d and are at least one week old, they are started on enteral iron at a dose of 3 mg/kg/d total. Enteral iron is increased to 6 mg/kg/d when infants achieve an enteral intake of 100 to 120 mL/kg/d [72]. Serum ferritin or ZnPP/H ratios are checked at 14 and 42 days, and iron adjusted accordingly. If subjects are not able to tolerate enteral feedings and oral iron supplements, they will be given maintenance iron parenterally (3 mg/kg/week, adjusted based on iron indices).

Study procedures

Five 0.5 mL blood samples will be drawn from each enrolled subject on the following schedule: prior to the first study drug dose, 30 min after the 4th study drug dose (peak), 30 min prior to the 5th study drug dose (trough), on day 14 ± 1 day, and at the 22–26 month in-person visit (Fig. 3). These samples will be used to determine circulating Epo concentrations, cytokine measurements, and biomarkers of brain injury. The following inflammatory markers and growth factors will be assayed: BDNF, Interferon-gamma (IFN-γ), IL-1β, IL-6, IL-8, IL-10, tumor necrosis factor-α (TNF-α), transforming growth factor (TGF)-β, matrix metalloproteinase (MMP)-2 and MMP-9, macrophage inflammatory protein-1α (MIP-1α), MIP-1β, monocyte chemotactic protein-1 (MCP-1) and tissue inhibitor of metalloproteinase (TIMP)-1 [50, 73–75]. Markers of neurotoxicity and brain injury will include: S100B, glial fibrillary acidic protein (GFAP), neuron specific enolase (NSE), Tau, Activin A, and Ubiquitin C-terminal hydrolase-L1 (UCH-L1) [76–78].

Brain magnetic resonance imaging (MRI) will be obtained on 110 subjects from each study arm at 36 weeks PMA (220 total). All scans will be done on 3 T scanners using an optimized, standardized protocol. MRI's will be evaluated centrally, and analysis will include both quantitative [79, 80] and qualitative evaluations [81].

Outcomes

The primary outcome variable is the composite outcome of death or neurodevelopmental impairment at 22–26 months. All personnel involved in the neurodevelopmental assessments will undergo standardized training, and will be blind to study treatment. Assessment at 22–26 months corrected age will include: Bayley III Scales of Infant and Toddler Development, a standardized neurological examination, Gross Motor Function Classification System (GMFCS) assessment, the Child Behavior Checklist, and the Modified Checklist for Autism in Toddlers (M-CHAT-R). Neurodevelopmental impairment (NDI) is defined as the presence of any one of the following: CP, Bayley III cognitive or motor scale < 70. There is a known inflation of scores from the Bayley II to III [82–84] and we will therefore also consider a threshold of <85 for secondary analysis. Cerebral palsy will be categorized based on features present on standardized neurologic exam, and classified as mild, moderate, or severe, with hemiplegia or diplegia. Two stepped outcomes will be used: the primary outcome is very stringent, and uses a cut off of two standard deviations below the mean for cognitive or motor scales (<70). The secondary outcome uses a cut off of one standard deviation below the mean for these criteria (<85), which will still have a significant impact on the child, family, and healthcare system. The 2-year assessment will provide a window into early language development and early gross- and fine-motor development. We plan to submit further grant applications for long-term follow-up at 5 years of age, which correlates better with ultimate function [85].

Power and sample size for primary outcome

In order to determine the necessary sample size for efficacy evaluation, we formulated assumptions for the primary outcome rate in the treated and untreated groups. The primary outcome measure is the rate of death or severe NDI. Using data from two sources, we computed the expected rates of death or NDI for the neonates that we will enroll. The Vermont Oxford Network 2008 Follow-up Report [86] evaluated the disability status of infants born in 2008 only, and the combined 2004–2008 cohorts. Follow-up status was determined at age 18–24 months and information regarding death and NDI is provided for subgroups of children based on their gestational age. Therefore, we used these data to forecast expected trial results for our eligible subjects (24–27 weeks gestational age). In order to estimate the overall rate observed among treated neonates we have assumed that there will be no effect of treatment on death, but

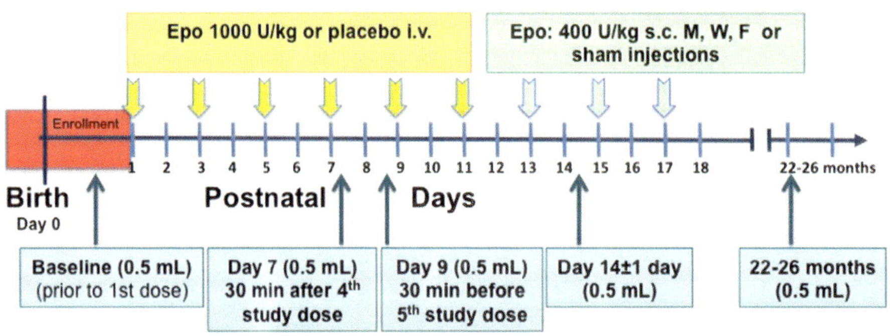

Fig. 3 PENUT Trial Blood Draws. The timing of all PENUT related blood draws is shown schematically

that Epo will lead to a decrease in the rate of NDI. If we assume a multiplicative reduction in the NDI rate of 0.45 then we expect a treated NDI rate of 12 % and an overall rate of death + NDI of 30.4 % as compared to the control rate of 40.4 %. Therefore, in order to obtain a target sample size we assumed: an overall control rate of 40 %, and an overall treated rate of 30 % corresponding to an overall treatment rate ratio of 0.75. Using the control and treated rates of 40 % and 30 % respectively leads to a sample size of 376 evaluated subjects per arm or a total evaluated sample size of 752 subjects in order to have 80 % power. We inflated the sample size by 20 % to account for correlation among multiple births (clustering) and potential loss to follow-up to arrive at a total enrollment target of 940 subjects.

Statistical analysis

A modified intent-to-treat (ITT) approach will be used [87], with all randomized infants who receive the first dose of study treatment included in the analysis. All pre-specified hypotheses will be tested using a two-sided type I error of 0.05 with no formal adjustment for multiple comparisons unless otherwise specified (such as with safety outcomes). Secondary analyses that focus on separate hypotheses will not require correction for multiple comparisons, but those analyses that use multivariate measures such as multiple brain image parameters would be corrected for multiple comparisons using standard methods.

Given that we anticipate enrollment of multiple births we require that all analyses properly account for the within-sibship correlation of outcomes. We will use Generalized Estimating Equations (GEE), which is a versatile regression approach for the analysis of discrete and continuous outcomes [88]. Use of "robust" standard errors will provide valid statistical inference and fully account for the clustering of data.

Data and safety monitoring

A data safety monitoring board (DSMB) created by National Institute of Neurological Disorders and Stroke (NINDS) will review the accruing data to ensure that the study is adequately enrolling and to ensure that there are no serious safety concerns. The research coordinators at each site monitor each subject daily for the presence of any complications. Serious adverse events are brought to the attention of an independent Medical Monitor, the DSMB, and IRB in writing. A potential risk that is unique to preterm infants is the risk of ROP [89]. In the published studies of preterm neonates receiving potentially neuroprotective doses of Epo, no difference has been noted between treatment and control groups [63, 90–92]. The DSMB will conduct formal interim safety monitoring analysis at approximately 25, 50, and 75 % and 100 % of target enrollment of $n = 940$ using O'Brien-Fleming [93] boundaries for death (net alpha = 0.05) and 10 serious adverse events (Bonferroni corrected alpha = 0.005).

Discussion

Ample preclinical, and growing phase I and II data support the neuroprotective effects of Epo as an approach to improving the neurologic outcomes of ELGANS. In designing the PENUT Trial, we considered the issue of what constitutes a clinically significant effect size. Characteristics of trials that lead to changes in clinical practice include: the estimated magnitude of benefit; the number of subjects studied; and the risk of the therapy. Ibrahim et al. performed a 13-item web-based questionnaire asking 226 neonatologists what would convince them to adopt a new therapy in infants <28 weeks of gestation. The survey assumed no adverse results of treatment. The survey results suggest that a reduction of Bayley scores < 80 by 25 % of subjects would change behavior in 40 % of clinicians, while the same change in 50 % of subjects would persuade two thirds of neonatologists to adopt the intervention. A sample size of 200 per arm resulted in one third of neonatologists changing their behavior, while a sample size of 400 per arm resulted in two thirds changing behavior. The PENUT study is powered to detect a 45 % reduction in NDI, with a large enough sample size to be judged of sufficient quality to change practice for 64 % of clinicians surveyed [personal communication]. Epo neuroprotection is an exciting new approach to preterm neuroprotection, and if efficacious, will provide a much-needed therapy for this group of vulnerable infants.

Conclusion

Current neuroprotective strategies include prenatal steroids, magnesium sulfate, delayed cord clamping, postnatal caffeine, breast milk, and avoiding postnatal growth retardation. Despite these measures, outcomes of extreme prematurity have not improved significantly over the last decades, with survivors remaining at significant risk of neurodevelopmental impairment. Erythropoietin has great potential to improve these outcomes. There is ample preclinical data showing beneficial effects of Epo on brain injury. Clinical trials to determine whether these preclinical findings translate to clinical improvement are ongoing.

Competing interests

The authors declare that they have no competing interests.

Authors' contributions

All authors have made significant and substantial contributions to this review and to the conception, design and acquisition of data for the PENUT Trial. SJ wrote the first draft of this manuscript, and is the principal investigator of the PENUT Trial. DM contributed to the design and execution of the PENUT Trial and provided editing of the review. BC and PH provided all of the statistical design of the PENUT trial and developed a portal for the acquisition of data for the PENUT trial. They also edited this review. All authors read and approved the final manuscript.

Acknowledgements

We thank Stephanie Hauge MS, for her considerable contributions to organization and smooth running of the PENUT trial, to Todd Richards PhD, Colin Studholme PhD, Dennis Shaw MD, and Christopher Traudt MD for their development of the imaging aspects of this study, and to Michael O'Shea MD, Karl Kuban MD and Jean Lowe MD for their input into the follow up aspects of the study.

Funding

S Juul: NINDS U01NS077953, NICHD R01HD073128, NICHD R21NS093154-01, NIDDK R01DK103608

D Mayock: NINDS U01NS077953, Thrasher Research Fund 30002250-14-01 AM01, NHLBI U01-HL-094338

B Comstock: NINDS U01NS077955, AHRQ R01HS22972, NIAMS UH3AT0007766, NHGRI U01HG006507

P Heagerty: NINDS U01NS077955, NHLBI R01HL072966, NCI P01CA053996, PCORI R-D2C-1310-07253, NIDDK R01DK103608, NIMH UH2MH106338, AHRQ R01HS22972, NHGRI U01HG006507, NIAMS UH3AT0007766, NCATS UL1TR000423

Author details

[1]Department of Pediatrics, Division of Neonatology, University of Washington, 1959 Pacific Ave NE, Box 356320, Seattle, WA 98195-6320, USA. [2]Department of Biostatistics, University of Washington, 4333 Brooklyn Avenue NE, Box 359461, Seattle, WA 98195-9461, USA.

References

1. Stoll BJ, Hansen NI, Bell EF, Shankaran S, Laptook AR, Walsh MC, et al. Neonatal outcomes of extremely preterm infants from the NICHD Neonatal Research Network. Pediatrics. 2010;126(3):443–56. doi:10.1542/peds.2009-2959.
2. Hintz SR, Kendrick DE, Stoll BJ, Vohr BR, Fanaroff AA, Donovan EF, et al. Neurodevelopmental and growth outcomes of extremely low birth weight infants after necrotizing enterocolitis. Pediatrics. 2005;115(3):696–703. doi:10.1542/peds.2004-0569.
3. Beauchamp MH, Thompson DK, Howard K, Doyle LW, Egan GF, Inder TE, et al. Preterm infant hippocampal volumes correlate with later working memory deficits. Brain. 2008;131(Pt 11):2986–94. doi:10.1093/brain/awn227.
4. Edgin JO, Inder TE, Anderson PJ, Hood KM, Clark CA, Woodward LJ. Executive functioning in preschool children born very preterm: relationship with early white matter pathology. J Int Neuropsychol Soc. 2008;14(1):90–101.
5. Gargus RA, Vohr BR, Tyson JE, High P, Higgins RD, Wrage LA, et al. Unimpaired outcomes for extremely low birth weight infants at 18 to 22 months. Pediatrics. 2009;124(1):112–21. doi:10.1542/peds.2008-2742.
6. Ancel PY, Goffinet F, Group E-W, Kuhn P, Langer B, Matis J, et al. Survival and Morbidity of Preterm Children Born at 22 Through 34 Weeks' Gestation in France in 2011: Results of the EPIPAGE-2 Cohort Study. JAMA Pediatr. 2015;169(3):230–8. doi:10.1001/jamapediatrics.2014.3351.
7. Ancel PY, Livinec F, Larroque B, Marret S, Arnaud C, Pierrat V, et al. Cerebral palsy among very preterm children in relation to gestational age and neonatal ultrasound abnormalities: the EPIPAGE cohort study. Pediatrics. 2006;117(3):828–35. doi:10.1542/peds.2005-0091.
8. Johnson S, Hollis C, Kochhar P, Hennessy E, Wolke D, Marlow N. Autism spectrum disorders in extremely preterm children. J Pediatr. 2010;156(4):525–31. doi:10.1016/j.jpeds.2009.10.041.
9. Buchmayer S, Johansson S, Johansson A, Hultman CM, Sparen P, Cnattingius S. Can association between preterm birth and autism be explained by maternal or neonatal morbidity? Pediatrics. 2009;124(5):e817–25. doi:10.1542/peds.2008-3582.
10. Kuban KC, O'Shea TM, Allred EN, Tager-Flusberg H, Goldstein DJ, Leviton A. Positive screening on the Modified Checklist for Autism in Toddlers (M-CHAT) in extremely low gestational age newborns. J Pediatr. 2009;154(4):535–40. doi:10.1016/j.jpeds.2008.10.011.
11. Scott MN, Taylor HG, Fristad MA, Klein N, Espy KA, Minich N, et al. Behavior Disorders in Extremely Preterm/Extremely Low Birth Weight Children in Kindergarten. J Dev Behav Pediatr. 2012. doi:10.1097/DBP.0b013e3182475287.
12. Petrou S, Abangma G, Johnson S, Wolke D, Marlow N. Costs and health utilities associated with extremely preterm birth: evidence from the EPICure study. Value Health. 2009;12(8):1124–34. doi:10.1111/j.1524-4733.2009.00580.x.
13. Petrou S, Johnson S, Wolke D, Marlow N. The association between neurodevelopmental disability and economic outcomes during mid-childhood. Child: care, health and development. 2012. doi:10.1111/j.1365-2214.2012.01368.x.
14. Lodygensky GA, Vasung L, Sizonenko SV, Huppi PS. Neuroimaging of cortical development and brain connectivity in human newborns and animal models. J Anat. 2010;217(4):418–28. doi:10.1111/j.1469-7580.2010.01280.x.
15. Huppi PS. Growth and development of the brain and impact on cognitive outcomes. Nestle Nutr Workshop Ser Pediatr Program. 2010;65:137–49. doi:10.1159/000281156. discussion 49–51.
16. Volpe JJ. Brain injury in premature infants: a complex amalgam of destructive and developmental disturbances. Lancet Neurol. 2009;8(1):110–24. doi:10.1016/S1474-4422(08)70294-1.
17. Volpe JJ. Systemic inflammation, oligodendroglial maturation, and the encephalopathy of prematurity. Ann Neurol. 2011;70(4):525–9. doi:10.1002/ana.22533.
18. Back SA, Riddle A, McClure MM. Maturation-dependent vulnerability of perinatal white matter in premature birth. Stroke. 2007;38(2 Suppl):724–30.
19. Volpe JJ. Neurology of the Newborn. 4th ed. Philadelphia, Pennsylvania: W.B. Saunders; 2001. p. 435-437.
20. Martin CR, Dammann O, Allred EN, Patel S, O'Shea TM, Kuban KC, et al. Neurodevelopment of extremely preterm infants who had necrotizing enterocolitis with or without late bacteremia. J Pediatr. 2010;157(5):751–6. doi:10.1016/j.jpeds.2010.05.042. e1.
21. Leviton A, Fichorova R, Yamamoto Y, Allred EN, Dammann O, Hecht J, et al. Inflammation-related proteins in the blood of extremely low gestational age newborns. The contribution of inflammation to the appearance of developmental regulation. Cytokine. 2011;53(1):66–73. doi:10.1016/j.cyto.2010.09.003.
22. Ivacko JA, Sun R, Silverstein FS. Hypoxic-ischemic brain injury induces an acute microglial reaction in perinatal rats. Pediatr Res. 1996;39(1):39–47.
23. Foster-Barber A, Dickens B, Ferriero DM. Human perinatal asphyxia: correlation of neonatal cytokines with MRI and outcome. Dev Neurosci. 2001;23(3):213–8.
24. Bartha AI, Foster-Barber A, Miller SP, Vigneron DB, Glidden DV, Barkovich AJ, et al. Neonatal encephalopathy: association of cytokines with MR spectroscopy and outcome. Pediatr Res. 2004;56(6):960–6.
25. Juul S, Felderhoff-Mueser U. Epo and other hematopoietic factors. Semin Fetal Neonatal Med. 2007;12(4):250–8. doi:10.1016/j.siny.2007.01.015.
26. Kumral A, Gonenc S, Acikgoz O, Sonmez A, Genc K, Yilmaz O, et al. Erythropoietin increases glutathione peroxidase enzyme activity and decreases lipid peroxidation levels in hypoxic-ischemic brain injury in neonatal rats. Biol Neonate. 2005;87(1):15–8.
27. Wang L, Zhang Z, Wang Y, Zhang R, Chopp M. Treatment of stroke with erythropoietin enhances neurogenesis and angiogenesis and improves neurological function in rats. Stroke. 2004;35(7):1732–7.
28. Iwai M, Cao G, Yin W, Stetler RA, Liu J, Chen J. Erythropoietin promotes neuronal replacement through revascularization and neurogenesis after neonatal hypoxia/ischemia in rats. Stroke. 2007;38:2795–803.
29. Shingo T, Sorokan ST, Shimazaki T, Weiss S. Erythropoietin regulates the in vitro and in vivo production of neuronal progenitors by mammalian forebrain neural stem cells. J Neurosci. 2001;21(24):9733–43.
30. Osredkar D, Sall JW, Bickler PE, Ferriero DM. Erythropoietin promotes hippocampal neurogenesis in in vitro models of neonatal stroke. Neurobiol Dis. 2010;38(2):259–65. doi:10.1016/j.nbd.2010.01.015.
31. Kellert BA, McPherson RJ, Juul SE. A comparison of high-dose recombinant erythropoietin treatment regimens in brain-injured neonatal rats. Pediatr Res. 2007;61(4):451–5. doi:10.1203/pdr.0b013e3180332cec.
32. Gonzalez FF, Abel R, Almli CR, Mu D, Wendland M, Ferriero DM. Erythropoietin sustains cognitive function and brain volume after neonatal stroke. Dev Neurosci. 2009;31(5):403–11. doi:10.1159/000232558.
33. Gonzalez FF, McQuillen P, Mu D, Chang Y, Wendland M, Vexler Z, et al. Erythropoietin enhances long-term neuroprotection and neurogenesis in neonatal stroke. Dev Neurosci. 2007;29:321–30.
34. Demers EJ, McPherson RJ, Juul SE. Erythropoietin protects dopaminergic neurons and improves neurobehavioral outcomes in juvenile rats after neonatal hypoxia-ischemia. Pediatr Res. 2005;58(2):297–301. doi:10.1203/01.PDR.0000169971.64558.5A.
35. Iwai M, Stetler RA, Xing J, Hu X, Gao Y, Zhang W, et al. Enhanced oligodendrogenesis and recovery of neurological function by erythropoietin after neonatal hypoxic/ischemic brain injury. Stroke. 2010;41(5):1032–7. doi:10.1161/STROKEAHA.109.570325.

36. Reitmeir R, Kilic E, Kilic U, Bacigaluppi M, ElAli A, Salani G, et al. Post-acute delivery of erythropoietin induces stroke recovery by promoting perilesional tissue remodelling and contralesional pyramidal tract plasticity. Brain. 2011;134(Pt 1):84–99. doi:10.1093/brain/awq344.
37. Gorio A, Gokmen N, Erbayraktar S, Yilmaz O, Madaschi L, Cichetti C, et al. Recombinant human erythropoietin counteracts secondary injury and markedly enhances neurological recovery from experimental spinal cord trauma. PNAS. 2002;99(14):9450–5. doi:10.1073/pnas.142287899.
38. Villa P, Bigini P, Mennini T, Agnello D, Laragione T, Cagnotto A, et al. Erythropoietin selectively attenuates cytokine production and inflammation in cerebral ischemia by targeting neuronal apoptosis. J Exp Med. 2003;198(6):971–5. doi:10.1084/jem.20021067.
39. Sun Y, Calvert JW, Zhang JH. Neonatal hypoxia/ischemia is associated with decreased inflammatory mediators after erythropoietin administration. Stroke. 2005;36(8):1672–8.
40. Siren AL, Fratelli M, Brines M, Goemans C, Casagrande S, Lewczuk P, et al. Erythropoietin prevents neuronal apoptosis after cerebral ischemia and metabolic stress. PNAS. 2001;98(7):4044–9.
41. Bian XX, Yuan XS, Qi CP. Effect of recombinant human erythropoietin on serum S100B protein and interleukin-6 levels after traumatic brain injury in the rat. Neurol Med Chir (Tokyo). 2010;50(5):361–6.
42. Juul SE, Beyer RP, Bammler TK, McPherson RJ, Wilkerson J, Farin FM. Microarray analysis of high-dose recombinant erythropoietin treatment of unilateral brain injury in neonatal mouse hippocampus. Pediatr Res. 2009;65(5):485–92. doi:10.1203/PDR.0b013e31819d90c8.
43. Yatsiv I, Grigoriadis N, Simeonidou C, Stahel PF, Schmidt OI, Alexandrovitch AG, et al. Erythropoietin is neuroprotective, improves functional recovery, and reduces neuronal apoptosis and inflammation in a rodent model of experimental closed head injury. FASEB J. 2005;19(12):1701–3.
44. Dzietko M, Felderhoff-Mueser U, Sifringer M, Krutz B, Bittigau P, Thor F, et al. Erythropoietin protects the developing brain against N-methyl-D-aspartate receptor antagonist neurotoxicity. Neurobiol Dis. 2004;15(2):177–87. doi:10.1016/j.nbd.2003.10.006.
45. Vitellaro-Zuccarello L, Mazzetti S, Madaschi L, Bosisio P, Fontana E, Gorio A, et al. Chronic erythropoietin-mediated effects on the expression of astrocyte markers in a rat model of contusive spinal cord injury. Neuroscience. 2008;151(2):452–66.
46. Li L, Jiang Q, Ding G, Zhang L, Zhang ZG, Li Q, et al. MRI identification of white matter reorganization enhanced by erythropoietin treatment in a rat model of focal ischemia. Stroke. 2009;40(3):936–41. doi:10.1161/STROKEAHA.108.527713.
47. Zhang L, Chopp M, Zhang RL, Wang L, Zhang J, Wang Y, et al. Erythropoietin amplifies stroke-induced oligodendrogenesis in the rat. PLoS ONE. 2010;5(6), e11016. doi:10.1371/journal.pone.0011016.
48. Yamada M, Burke C, Colditz P, Johnson DW, Gobe GC. Erythropoietin protects against apoptosis and increases expression of non-neuronal cell markers in the hypoxia-injured developing brain. J Pathol. 2011. doi:10.1002/path.2862.
49. Rees S, Hale N, De Matteo R, Cardamone L, Tolcos M, Loeliger M, et al. Erythropoietin is neuroprotective in a preterm ovine model of endotoxin-induced brain injury. J Neuropathol Exp Neurol. 2010;69(3):306–19. doi:10.1097/NEN.0b013e3181d27138.
50. Savino C, Pedotti R, Baggi F, Ubiali F, Gallo B, Nava S, et al. Delayed administration of erythropoietin and its non-erythropoietic derivatives ameliorates chronic murine autoimmune encephalomyelitis. J Neuroimmunol. 2006;172(1–2):27–37. doi:10.1016/j.jneuroim.2005.10.016.
51. Leuchter RH, Gui L, Poncet A, Hagmann C, Lodygensky GA, Martin E, et al. Association between early administration of high-dose erythropoietin in preterm infants and brain MRI abnormality at term-equivalent age. JAMA. 2014;312(8):817–24. doi:10.1001/jama.2014.9645.
52. Sugawa M, Sakurai Y, Ishikawa-Ieda Y, Suzuki H, Asou H. Effects of erythropoietin on glial cell development; oligodendrocyte maturation and astrocyte proliferation. Neurosci Res. 2002;44(4):391–403.
53. Genc K, Genc S, Baskin H, Semin I. Erythropoietin decreases cytotoxicity and nitric oxide formation induced by inflammatory stimuli in rat oligodendrocytes. Physiol Res. 2006;55(1):33–8.
54. Mizuno K, Hida H, Masuda T, Nishino H, Togari H. Pretreatment with low doses of erythropoietin ameliorates brain damage in periventricular leukomalacia by targeting late oligodendrocyte progenitors: a rat model. Neonatology. 2008;94(4):255–66. doi:10.1159/000151644.
55. Buonocore G, Perrone S, Longini M, Paffetti P, Vezzosi P, Gatti MG, et al. Non protein bound iron as early predictive marker of neonatal brain damage. Brain. 2003;126(Pt 5):1224–30.
56. Ozment CP, Turi JL. Iron overload following red blood cell transfusion and its impact on disease severity. Biochim Biophys Acta. 2009;1790(7):694–701. doi:10.1016/j.bbagen.2008.09.010.
57. Loeliger MM, Mackintosh A, De Matteo R, Harding R, Rees SM. Erythropoietin protects the developing retina in an ovine model of endotoxin-induced retinal injury. Invest Ophthalmol Vis Sci. 2011;52(5):2656–61. doi:10.1167/iovs.10-6455.
58. van der Kooij MA, Groenendaal F, Kavelaars A, Heijnen CJ, van Bel F. Neuroprotective properties and mechanisms of erythropoietin in in vitro and in vivo experimental models for hypoxia/ischemia. Brain Res Rev. 2008;59(1):22–33.
59. Traudt CM, McPherson RJ, Bauer LA, Richards TL, Burbacher TM, McAdams RM, et al. Concurrent erythropoietin and hypothermia treatment improve outcomes in a term nonhuman primate model of perinatal asphyxia. Dev Neurosci. 2013;35(6):491–503. doi:10.1159/000355460.
60. Juul SE, McPherson RJ, Farrell FX, Jolliffe L, Ness DJ, Gleason CA. Erytropoietin concentrations in cerebrospinal fluid of nonhuman primates and fetal sheep following high-dose recombinant erythropoietin. Biol Neonate. 2004;85(2):138–44.
61. Gonzalez FF, Larpthaveesarp A, McQuillen P, Derugin N, Wendland M, Spadafora R, et al. Erythropoietin increases neurogenesis and oligodendrogliosis of subventricular zone precursor cells after neonatal stroke. Stroke. 2013;44(3):753–8. doi:10.1161/STROKEAHA.111.000104.
62. Weber A, Dzietko M, Berns M, Felderhoff-Mueser U, Heinemann U, Maier RF, et al. Neuronal damage after moderate hypoxia and erythropoietin. Neurobiol Dis. 2005;20(2):594–600.
63. Juul SE, McPherson RJ, Bauer LA, Ledbetter KJ, Gleason CA, Mayock DE. A phase I/II trial of high-dose erythropoietin in extremely low birth weight infants: pharmacokinetics and safety. Pediatrics. 2008;122(2):383–91.
64. Widness JA, Veng-Pedersen P, Peters C, Pereira LM, Schmidt RL, Lowe LS. Erythropoietin pharmacokinetics in premature infants: developmental, nonlinearity, and treatment effects. J Appl Physiol. 1996;80(1):140–8.
65. Fauchere JC, Koller BM, Tschopp A, Dame C, Ruegger C, Bucher HU, et al. Safety of Early High-Dose Recombinant Erythropoietin for Neuroprotection in Very Preterm Infants. J Pediatr. 2015;167(1):52–7. doi:10.1016/j.jpeds.2015.02.052. e3.
66. O'Gorman RL, Bucher HU, Held U, Koller BM, Huppi PS, Hagmann CF, et al. Tract-based spatial statistics to assess the neuroprotective effect of early erythropoietin on white matter development in preterm infants. Brain. 2015;138(Pt 2):388–97. doi:10.1093/brain/awu363.
67. Ohls RK, Kamath-Rayne BD, Christensen RD, Wiedmeier SE, Rosenberg A, Fuller J, et al. Cognitive Outcomes of Preterm Infants Randomized to Darbepoetin, Erythropoietin, or Placebo. Pediatrics. 2014. doi:10.1542/peds.2013-4307.
68. McAdams RM, McPherson RJ, Mayock DE, Juul SE. Outcomes of extremely low birth weight infants given early high-dose erythropoietin. J Perinatol. 2013;33(3):226–30. doi:10.1038/jp.2012.78.
69. Juul S. Erythropoietin in anemia of prematurity. J Matern Fetal Neona. 2012;25 Suppl 5:80–4. doi:10.3109/14767058.2012.716987.
70. Ohlsson A, Aher SM. Early erythropoietin for preventing red blood cell transfusion in preterm and/or low birth weight infants. Cochrane Database Syst Rev. 2014;4, CD004863. doi:10.1002/14651858.CD004863.pub4.
71. Ohls RK, Christensen RD, Widness JA, Juul SE. Erythropoiesis Stimulating Agents Demonstrate Safety and Show Promise as Neuroprotective Agents in Neonates. J Pediatr. 2015. doi:10.1016/j.jpeds.2015.03.054.
72. Franz AR, Mihatsch WA, Sander S, Kron M, Pohlandt F. Prospective randomized trial of early versus late enteral iron supplementation in infants with a birth weight of less than 1301 grams. Pediatrics. 2000;106(4):700–6.
73. Bednarek N, Svedin P, Garnotel R, Favrais G, Loron G, Schwendiman L, et al. Increased MMP-9 and TIMP-1 in mouse neonatal brain and plasma and in human neonatal plasma after hypoxia-ischemia: a potential marker of neonatal encephalopathy. Pediatr Res. 2012;71(1):63–70. doi:10.1038/pr.2011.3.
74. O'Shea TM, Allred EN, Kuban KC, Dammann O, Paneth N, Fichorova R, et al. Elevated concentrations of inflammation-related proteins in postnatal blood predict severe developmental delay at 2 years of age in extremely preterm infants. The Journal of Pediatrics. 2012;160(3):395–401. doi:10.1016/j.jpeds.2011.08.069. e4.
75. Chen G, Shi JX, Hang CH, Xie W, Liu J, Liu X. Inhibitory effect on cerebral inflammatory agents that accompany traumatic brain injury in a rat model:

a potential neuroprotective mechanism of recombinant human erythropoietin (rhEPO). Neurosci Lett. 2007;425(3):177–82.

76. Douglas-Escobar M, Yang C, Bennett J, Shuster J, Theriaque D, Leibovici A, et al. A pilot study of novel biomarkers in neonates with hypoxic-ischemic encephalopathy. Pediatric Research. 2010;68(6):531–6. doi:10.1203/PDR.0b013e3181f85a03.
77. Ehrenreich H, Kastner A, Weissenborn K, Streeter J, Sperling S, Wang KK, et al. Circulating damage marker profiles support a neuroprotective effect of erythropoietin in ischemic stroke patients. Mol Med. 2011;17(11–12):1306–10. doi:10.2119/molmed.2011.00259.
78. Ennen CS, Huisman TA, Savage WJ, Northington FJ, Jennings JM, Everett AD, et al. Glial fibrillary acidic protein as a biomarker for neonatal hypoxic-ischemic encephalopathy treated with whole-body cooling. Am J Obstet Gynecol. 2011;205(3):251 e1–7. doi:10.1016/j.ajog.2011.06.025.
79. Habas PA, Corbett-Detig JM, Kim K, Rousseau F, Glenn OA, Barkovich AJ et al., editors. Global and regional patterns of tissue volume growth in the normal fetal brain from in utero MRI. 16th Annual Meeting of the Organization for Human Brain Mapping; 2010; Barcelona, Spain.
80. Rodriguez-Carranza CE, Mukherjee P, Vigneron D, Barkovich J, Studholme C. A framework for in vivo quantification of regional brain folding in premature neonates. Neuroimage. 2008;41(2):462–78. doi:10.1016/j.neuroimage.2008.01.008.
81. Kidokoro H, Neil JJ, Inder TE. New MR imaging assessment tool to define brain abnormalities in very preterm infants at term. AJNR Am J Neuroradiol. 2013;34(11):2208–14. doi:10.3174/ajnr.A3521.
82. Moore T, Johnson S, Haider S, Hennessy E, Marlow N. The Bayley-III cognitive and language scales: how do scores relate to the Bayley II? Arch Dis Child. 2011;96 Suppl 1:A1–100. doi:10.1136/adc.2011.212563.85.
83. Msall ME. Measuring outcomes after extreme prematurity with the Bayley-III Scales of infant and toddler development: a cautionary tale from Australia. Arch Pediatr Adolesc Med. 2010;164(4):391–3. doi:10.1001/archpediatrics.2010.25.
84. Anderson PJ, De Luca CR, Hutchinson E, Roberts G, Doyle LW. Underestimation of developmental delay by the new Bayley-III Scale. Arch Pediatr Adolesc Med. 2010;164(4):352–6. doi:10.1001/archpediatrics.2010.20.
85. Johnson S, Wolke D, Hennessy E, Marlow N. Educational outcomes in extremely preterm children: neuropsychological correlates and predictors of attainment. Dev Neuropsychol. 2011;36(1):74–95. doi:10.1080/87565641.2011.540541.
86. Vermont Oxford Network ELBW Follow-up Report Birth Year 2008 All Centers [database on the Internet] Sept 2011. Accessed.
87. Fisher L, Dixon DO, Herson J, Frankowski RK, Hearron MS, Peace KE, et al. Intention to treat in clinical trials. In: Peace KE, editor. Statistical Issues in Drug Research and Development. New York: Marcel Dekker; 1991. p. 331–50.
88. Diggle PJ, Heagerty PJ, Liang KY, Zeger SL. Analysis of Longitudinal Data. Second Edition ed. Oxford University Press; 2002.
89. Ohlsson A, Aher SM. Early erythropoietin for preventing red blood cell transfusion in preterm and/or low birth weight infants. Cochrane Database Syst Rev. 2006;3, CD004863.
90. Fauchere JC, Dame C, Vonthein R, Koller B, Arri S, Wolf M, et al. An approach to using recombinant erythropoietin for neuroprotection in very preterm infants. Pediatrics. 2008;122(2):375–82. doi:10.1542/peds.2007-2591.
91. Bierer R, Peceny MC, Hartenberger CH, Ohls RK. Erythropoietin concentrations and neurodevelopmental outcome in preterm infants. Pediatrics. 2006;118(3):e635–40.
92. Neubauer AP, Voss W, Wachtendorf M, Jungmann T. Erythropoietin improves neurodevelopmental outcome of extremely preterm infants. Ann Neurol. 2010;67(5):657–66. doi:10.1002/ana.21977.
93. O'Brien PC, Fleming TR. A multiple testing procedure for clinical trials. Biometrics. 1979;35(3):549–56.

17

Docosahexaenoic acid and the preterm infant

Stephanie L. Smith[1*] and Christopher A. Rouse[1,2]

Abstract

Docosahexaenoic acid (DHA) is a long chain poly-unsaturated fatty acid (LCPUFA) that has a role in the cognitive and visual development, as well as in the immune function of newborns. Premature infants are typically deficient in DHA for several reasons, to include fetal accretion of DHA that typically occurs during the third trimester. These premature infants are reliant on enteral sources of DHA, most commonly through breast milk. The DHA content in breast milk varies in direct correlation with maternal DHA intake and mothers consuming a Western diet typically have lower levels of DHA in their breast milk. Maternal DHA supplementation and direct supplementation of DHA to the infant has been tried successfully but there are still conflicting results on the optimal dosage and method of delivery of DHA to the infant. This has led to inconsistent results in trials evaluating the effects of DHA supplementation to the preterm infant in terms of cognitive and immunological outcomes. While short-term benefits have been seen in several studies, long-term benefits are not consistent. Future studies continue to be needed to optimize DHA intake in our premature infants.

Keywords: Docosahexaenoic acid, Preterm infants, DHA supplementation, Breast milk, Inflammation, Neurodevelopment

Background

Docosahexaenoic acid (DHA) is a long chain poly-unsaturated fatty acid (LCPUFA) that has a role in the cognitive and visual development, as well as in the immune function of newborns [1]. DHA is derived from α-linolenic acid (ALA), an essential omega-3 fatty acid, through the enzyme **Δ6-desaturase** [1]. ALA, along with its omega-6 counterpart linoleic acid (LA), are essential fatty acids that must be obtained from the diet as the human body is unable to synthesize them. CLA is the most common essential fatty acid consumed in the Western diet and can be found in vegetable oils, nuts and seeds. ALA is commonly found in flaxseed, walnuts and soy while DHA is found in fatty fishes such as salmon and tuna. While there is no consensus on the recommended DHA intake for pregnant or lactating women, several organizations, including the March of Dimes, American Academy of Pediatrics, and the Food and Agriculture Organization of the United Nations agree that pregnant and lactating women should have a minimal intake of 200–300 mg of DHA per day [2]. However, it is uncommon for women eating a Western diet to consume the recommended amount of DHA. A study published in 2017 by Nordgren et al. focused on evaluating the omega-3 fatty acid intake in pregnant women as well as women of childbearing age in the United States [3]. The authors found that DHA intake in both pregnant and non-pregnant women was well below the recommended minimal intake of 200–300 mg/day [3]. On average, a pregnant women's DHA intake in the United States was only 66 mg/day and only 9.0% of women took DHA supplements during pregnancy [3]. Lower levels of DHA intake were correlated with lower economic status and education [3]. In addition, DHA crosses the placenta with the highest fetal accretion rates of LA, AA and DHA occur in the last 5 weeks of pregnancy [4]. Fetuses born to women who consume a typical Western diet have a DHA accretion rate of approximately 42–67 mg/day in the last trimester, though this rate may not be ideal based on the low DHA intake and high LA intake of the Western diet [4, 5].

Following delivery, infants rely on enteral sources to meet their DHA requirement, whether through breast milk or formula. The DHA content of breast milk is correlated to maternal intake of DHA. To add to this, obesity is becoming more prevalent in the United States

* Correspondence: Stephanie.l.smith230.mil@mail.mil
[1]Uniformed Services University of Health Sciences, 4301 Jones Bridge, Bethesda, MD 20814, USA
Full list of author information is available at the end of the article

and has an effect on the omega-3 fatty acids in breast milk [6]. Breast milk analyzed from obese mothers with BMI >30 kg/m^2, was significantly lower in long-chain n-3 FA and had a higher n-6:n-3 ratio. These findings were also seen in the plasma of breastfed neonates of obese mothers [6]. The n-3 concentration, which includes the concentration of DHA, in the breast milk of obese mothers could be improved by enrolling the mothers into a clinic for weight control and dietary support [6]. Vegetarian and vegan diets are also becoming more prevalent in today's society and it is also crucial to consider these diets' effects on DHA. Sanders reviewed published studies on the DHA status in vegetarians and vegans and found a lower DHA status in vegetarians and vegans compared to omnivores [7]. The concentration of DHA in breast milk is important because of DHA's contribution to brain and visual development as well as its affect on the immune system, which is vital for the premature infant. The objective of this paper is to review DHA and the premature infant looking specifically at: 1) DHA supplementation and its effect on breast milk; 2) DHA and the premature infant; 3) DHA and its effect on the neurodevelopment in the premature infant; and 4) DHA and its effect on the immune response in the premature infant.

DHA and Breast milk

Following delivery, infants become reliant on an enteral source of DHA, commonly through maternal breast milk. DHA content in breast milk is affected by several factors including maternal nutrition, gestational age at delivery, genetics, and the stage of lactation. The DHA content in breast milk varies in direct correlation with maternal DHA intake. The worldwide mean DHA concentration of breast milk is 0.32 ± 0.22% (mean ± standard error) [8]. Mothers who have the highest DHA concentration in their breast milk typically live in coastal areas such as the Canadian Artic, Japan and the Dominican Republic, as these areas have high seafood intake [8]. These locales have DHA concentrations ranging from 0.6%–1.4% [8]. Jackson and Harris examined evidence toward obtaining a goal for DHA concentration in breast milk and suggested that 0.3% is a reasonable initial target as it provides some improvement over the typical Western diet DHA breast milk level of 0.2% [9]. Other studies have shown that it is possible to raise the DHA concentration in breast milk by maternal supplementation [10, 11]. Dunstan et al. demonstrated that women who were supplemented with fish oil starting in pregnancy had a significantly higher DHA level in their breast milk over the first 6 postpartum weeks compared to controls [11]. Another study randomized lactating mothers to receiving a placebo, 200 mg of DHA daily, or 400 mg of DHA daily and compared DHA concentrations in breast milk [10]. The authors found that not only was the DHA content of breast milk higher in the high dose DHA group but that after 6 weeks of maternal supplementation the infants in the high maternal dose DHA group also had the lowest n-6:n-3 ratio in their plasma [10]. This study concluded that maternal supplementation with DHA can help increase DHA concentration in breast milk and thus increase the amount of DHA that infants receive. Gestational age and stage of lactation has also been shown to have an effect on DHA content of breast milk. Breast milk from mothers who delivered preterm had a significantly higher initial DHA content compared to mothers who delivered at term [12]. DHA has also been shown to significantly decrease in breast milk over the first month of lactation in both term and preterm human milk samples [12]. While DHA decreases in breast milk over the first month of lactation, total fat, LA and ALA tend to increase [13]. Lastly, genetics can also contribute to the DHA content of breast milk. Fatty acid desaturase (FADS)1 and FADS2 code the enzymes Δ5-desaturase and Δ6-desaturase that are involved in the synthesis of ARA, EPA and DHA [14]. There is an association between maternal FADS genotype and the DHA content in breast milk with certain genotypes leading to a lower proportion of DHA in breast milk regardless of increased omega-3 intake [14, 15].

Donor breast milk is a significant component of nutrition for the premature infant and has been shown to have low amounts of DHA due to maternal diet as well as donor milk frequently coming from a later stage of lactation [16–19]. There is a large variance in DHA content in donor breast milk obtained through various donor milk banks across the United States [16]. DHA levels were found to vary from 0.07% to 0.2% in various studied United States milk banks [16]. A recent cross-sectional sample of five donor breast milk banks (Ohio, Michigan, Texas, Colorado, and California) found that the average DHA concentration in donor milk was 7.1 mg/100 ml which would provide preterm infants a DHA intake much lower than the fetal accretion rate of 42–67 mg/day in the third trimester [17, 20, 21]. Another study by Valentine et al. evaluating DHA concentration in donor breast milk in Ohio also found a low donor milk DHA concentration of ~0.1% [18]. In a subsequent study, Valentine et al. demonstrated that supplementing breast milk donors with 1 g of DHA daily increased the absolute milk concentration of DHA in donor breast milk to 4 times as high as the control group after 4 days of supplementation [19]. Based on an estimated intake of 150 ml/kg/day of donor milk in the preterm infant, the donor breast milk obtained from mothers receiving this DHA supplementation regimen would meet the expected intrauterine accretion levels for the preterm infant [19]. More recently, liquid human milk fortifier added to breast milk has been shown to increase the DHA content of breast milk [22]. Fortifier, with a DHA concentration of ~0.15%, can increase the level of DHA in the breast milk to 0.29%. This is considerably closer to the world wide mean DHA level of 0.32%, though still falls short of the intrauterine accretion rate. Per Lapillonne et al., milk containing a DHA concentration of ~0.8% given at 150 ml/kg/day provides 45 mg/kg/day of DHA which is very similar to the intrauterine accretion rate [13].

Breast and donor milk obtained from mothers eating a Western diet typically have low concentrations of DHA that is below the worldwide mean of 0.32%. By giving DHA supplements to mothers, it is possible to raise the DHA concentration of breast milk. Alternatively, for donor breast milk, where the milk is obtained from a later stage of lactation, using liquid human milk fortifier that contains DHA also raises DHA concentration level closer to the worldwide mean. This could potentially be vital for premature infants who typically are deficient in DHA.

DHA and preterm infants

While DHA is important to the term infant, it is particularly critical to the premature infant who is delivered early in or prior to the third trimester. Overall, fetal DHA accretion is estimated to be 10 g, with the majority being acquired in the third trimester. [23]. The placenta aids with DHA accretion by allowing for preferential transfer of DHA over other fatty acids including LA and ALA [23]. As previously stated, the intrauterine accretion rate of DHA during the third trimester is approximately 42–67 mg/day or ~43 mg/kg/day [4, 5, 24]. This increase in DHA accretion in the third trimester coincides with brain and retina maturation [25]. DHA intake during pregnancy is not only important to ensure the fetus obtains adequate levels, but a systematic review by Kar et al. also showed that omega-3 fatty acids decrease the risk of delivery prior to 34 weeks by 58% [26]. Per Shireman et al., in a post-hoc analysis of their KUDOS study that showed a daily DHA intake of 600 mg led to decrease length of hospitalization for the infant; thus having mothers take daily DHA could lead to cost savings for the health care system [27].

Premature infants are typically deficient in DHA for several reasons including missing the in utero accumulation of DHA in the third trimester, their inability to convert precursor fatty acids to DHA in large amounts, and deficient postnatal DHA intake [16]. Infants delivered at the lowest gestational ages are at the highest risk for DHA deficiencies [28]. De Rooy et al. published a study that evaluated the levels of DHA in extremely premature infants receiving standard care [29]. This longitudinal study evaluated omega-6 and omega-3 intake from all sources in infants <28 weeks. The authors showed that the total amount of DHA that infants received at the end of 6 weeks represented only 36.6% of DHA that they would have received in utero [29]. Extremely low birth weight infants who are exposed to IV lipids for a prolonged time also have a significant decline in their DHA levels [30]. This decline in DHA was seen when evaluating RBC DHA levels and was more significant in ELBW infants who received intravenous lipids for greater than 28 days [30]. This is not surprising as Intralipid, the lipid emulsion commonly used in the United States, is virtually barren of DHA and was originally created for adults who have a greater capability of converting DHA from its precursor [31]. As breast milk typically does not have the quantity of DHA needed to make up for the deficiency in DHA in preterm infants, researchers have studied other ways to increase DHA levels in infants.

Collins et al. examined the effects of providing infants delivered at <33 weeks different doses of DHA [32]. Infants were randomized to receive 40 mg/kg/day, 80 mg/kg/day or 120 mg/kg/day of DHA orally for 28 days with the primary outcome being erythrocyte phospholipid DHA levels [32]. The authors found that supplementing infants with 120 mg/kg/day of DHA prevented the drop in DHA typically seen in premature infants at this age [32]. The benefit of this oral emulsion was that it allowed infants to receive a larger amount of DHA early on than what they would receive from breast milk, even from breast milk obtained from mothers taking supplementation. While this study discontinued supplements at 28 days, a study performed by Baack et al. randomized preterm infants to receive a DHA supplement or from the first week of life until term or discharge [33]. Infants in the DHA supplement group received 50 mg/day of DHA to match in utero DHA accretion rates. While DHA supplementation did significantly increase DHA levels in infants, the DHA levels at discharge in supplemented preterm infants remained significantly lower than term infant values [33]. Another recent study looking at delivering DHA via the buccal method found that this method did not alter DHA levels after 8 weeks of supplementation [34].

While term infants can achieve adequate DHA levels in breast milk through maternal supplementation, preterm infants struggle to overcome their DHA deficit. While directly supplementing preterm infants, as shown by both Collins et al. and Baack et al., does successfully increase their DHA level, the optimal amount of supplementation still needs to be determined [32, 33].

DHA and cognitive/visual outcomes in preterm infants

DHA is one of the most abundant LCPUFAs in the brain and has an important role in brain development including roles in neurotransmission and neurogenesis [35–37]. It is also found in high levels in the visual system, especially in rod photoreceptors and M retinal ganglion cells [38]. From reviews of previous studies, the most consistent benefit from DHA supplementation was seen in earlier premature infants with lower birthweights, typically <1500 g, as these infants missed the majority of the third trimester with the highest fetal accretion rates of DHA. Therefore, a focus of DHA research has been to explore its role on cognitive and visual outcomes in the premature infant.

Previous studies have examined the association between DHA levels in the premature infant and cognitive outcomes. Tam et al. observed a cohort of 60 preterm infants between 24 and 32 weeks gestational age and noted an association between higher early red blood cell DHA levels and a decrease in both the incidence and severity of intraventricular hemorrhage (IVH) [39]. The authors showed that a 1% increase in early postnatal DHA was associated with a 4.3 fold decrease in the odds of intraventricular hemorrhage [39]. At 30–36 months corrected age (mean age of 33 months corrected), neurodevelopment outcome was able to be assessed in 45 of the 60 enrolled infants using the Bayley Scales of Infant Development, 3rd edition (BSID-3). The study showed an association with higher early DHA levels and improved developmental outcome at 30–36 months old that was not fully explained by the decreased risk of IVH [39]. Sabel et al. performed a longitudinal study on the development of premature infants at 3, 6, 10 and 18 months corrected age using the Bayley's Scales of Infant Development, Second Edition (BSID-II) [40]. They found that in the initial 6 months, developmental scores were positively associated with breast milk DHA concentration [40]. Development was positively associated with DHA and negatively associated with n-6 fatty acids up to 18 months of age [40]. While these studies looked at the association between infant DHA level and cognitive outcome, there have been several studies evaluating the effects of DHA supplementation in premature infants on cognitive outcomes.

The DHA for the Improvement of Neurodevelopmental Outcome in preterm infants (DINO) trial was an Australian trial that randomized premature infants delivered at <33 weeks gestation to a high-DHA or standard-DHA diet until they reach 40 weeks corrected age [41]. Mothers of infants in the high-DHA group took 6 capsules daily, containing DHA-rich tuna oil and the mothers of infants in the standard-DHA diet received placebo soy capsules. When analyzing the breast milk of the two groups, the high-DHA group had milk with a mean DHA concentration of 0.85% versus 0.25% in the standard DHA group. At 18 months the Mental Development Index (MDI) of the BSID-II was performed. Overall, there was no statistically significant difference between the high DHA and the standard DHA group. Although the MDI in infants with birth weights <1250 g was higher, it did not reach statistical significance when adjusted for gestational age, sex, maternal education and birth order. When comparing only the girls in the high-DHA and standard-DHA groups, there was a statistically significant improvement in MDI scores in the high-DHA group [41]. The proportion of infants with severe developmental delay was also significantly less in the high-DHA group. Subsequently, the participants in this study were followed up at 7 years of age to assess their general intellectual ability using the Full Scale IQ of the Wechsler Abbreviated Scale of Intelligence (WASI) [42]. The researchers found no significant difference between the two groups in Full Scale, Verbal or Performance IQ [42].

While the DINO study supplemented mothers to achieve higher DHA levels in the breast milk, a randomized controlled trial by Henriksen et al. enrolled very low birth weight infants born at one of three hospitals in Norway and randomized them to receive a DHA/AA supplement or placebo for approximately 9 weeks after birth [43]. This supplement was directly added to their milk. The intervention group received supplemented human milk with a DHA concentration of 0.86% of total fatty acids, which is considered a high dose compared to the 0.3% level typical in preterm formula. At the corrected age of 6 months, the Ages and Stages Questionnaire was administered and the intervention group scored significantly higher on the problem solving section of the Ages and Stages Questionnaire compared to the control group [43]. There was also a trend toward an overall higher score in the intervention group that did not reach statistical significance (221 vs 215 points, *p*-value not given) [43]. In a study published by Almaas et al., the subjects were then followed up at 8 years of age, although no significant difference in cognitive functions was found between the two groups [44].

While the above studies demonstrated some early benefit with DHA supplementation, this benefit was not seen once the children reached school-age. A Cochrane review, updated in 2017, assessed whether giving premature infants formula milk supplemented with LCPUFA improved development, both cognitively and visually. The median concentration of DHA in formula in the included studies was 0.33% with a range of 0.15% to 1%. Based on their analysis, the authors concluded that premature infants did not obtain a benefit from receiving formula milk supplemented with LCPUFAs. Importantly, however, the review stated that outcomes should be evaluated based on a yet to be determined optimal dose [45].

Studies have also evaluated the effects of DHA on the development of visual function in the premature infant.

The DIAMOND (DHA Intake and measurement of neural development) study, though done in term infants is an important study which evaluated how DHA supplementation of infant formula, administered in one of four concentrations (0%, 0.32%, 0.64%, or 0.96%), effected visual acuity in term infants at 12 months of age [46]. This study found that infants who received any of the formula supplemented with DHA had significantly better visual evoked potential (VEP) visual acuity at 12 months of age. There was no significant difference in VEP visual acuity between DHA concentrations, however, and the authors concluded that additional DHA above 0.32% had no additional benefit [46]. In another study, performed by Smithers et al., visual responses were assessed in premature infants at two months corrected age. The infants had been randomized into either a high-DHA group receiving 1% DHA or the standard-DHA group receiving 0.3%DHA. This study found that infants in the high-DHA group had significantly better visual acuity at 4 months corrected age compared to infants in the standard-DHA group [47]. Molloy et al. evaluated the effects of high-DHA versus standard-DHA on visual function at school age on a subgroup of children from the DINO trial described previously [48]. They assessed the participants' visual function using the Freiburg Visual Acuity Test at 7 years old. The authors found that infants who received the human milk supplemented with high-DHA had no significant long-term benefit in their visual processing compared to infants who received standard-DHA [48].

Premature infants are deficit in DHA at birth and while short-term developmental benefits have been seen with DHA supplementation, no effects on long-term development have been shown. Because studies vary in the dosage, delivery, and length of DHA supplementation, it remains difficult to come to a decisive conclusion on DHA and cognitive outcomes. Until an optimal method for supplementing DHA to a preterm infant is found, it will continue to be a challenge to determine the true effect DHA supplementation has on the cognitive development of a premature infant.

DHA and inflammation

Premature infants are at risk for inflammatory diseases such as bronchopulmonary dysplasia (BPD) and necrotizing enterocolitis (NEC), risks which may be mitigated by DHA's anti-inflammatory properties. Atopic sensitization is also known to occur early in life and it is thought that omega-3 may help prevent this. As mentioned previously, without supplementation, DHA levels in preterm infants drop following birth [31]. Martin et al. showed an association between DHA levels in the first four weeks of life and the development of chronic lung disease (CLD) in premature infants. Lower DHA levels in these infants were significantly associated with the development of CLD. This study showed that a 1% decrease in the total fatty acid mass of DHA in the blood gave a 2.5 fold increase in the odds of developing CLD [31]. Similarly for late-onset sepsis, the authors found an association between decreased DHA concentration and an increased risk for developing late-onset sepsis. Lower AA and higher LA levels were also significantly associated with the development of late-onset sepsis in this cohort of premature infants. The authors did not find an association between mean DHA levels and IVH, NEC or ROP [31]. In addition to DHA levels, the authors also found that increased ratios of LA:DHA, AA:DHA, and n-6: n-3 were associated with CLD. A similar study was completed in Tunisia evaluating plasma DHA levels where improved control of the n-6:n-3 ratio may help prevent certain neonatal morbidities, such as RDS, sepsis and IVH in the premature infant [49]. Because infants who are born extremely premature often require TPN, a study in Greece examined the effects of various lipid emulsions on certain cytokine levels known to be proinflammatory: tumor necrosis factor (TNF)-α, interleukin (IL)-6, and IL-8. Infants who received a lipid emulsion which contained omega-3's had significantly lower IL-6 and IL-8 levels compared to infants receiving a typical soybean oil-based lipid emulsion [50]. Prior studies have shown an association with these cytokines and BPD in premature infants and subsequent studies have evaluated the effects of DHA on BPD in premature infants [51–53]. Another study showed that maternal fish oil supplementation of 1.5 g/day of n-3 long-chain PUFA can continue to have an effect on a child's immune system up to at least two years after the supplement was given [54].

In a follow-up to the DINO trial that initially evaluated cognitive outcomes with DHA supplementation in premature infants, the authors evaluated the long-term respiratory and allergy outcomes in these infants. The infants were evaluated at 18 months for history of BPD as well as parental reports of atopic conditions such as hay fever, asthma, eczema or food allergies [52]. Of the 657 infants originally enrolled in the study 614 infants completed the 18-month follow-up, though the allergy data was incomplete, as some families did not complete these questionnaires. The authors found a statistically significant reduction in parental reported hay fever at either 12 months or 18 months in the high –DHA group compared to the standard DHA group, but no reported reductions in food allergies, eczema or asthma. The risk of developing BPD was not significantly different between the two groups but there was a significant reduction of oxygen requirement at 36 weeks in both male infants and infants with birth weights <1250 g. Of note, these findings should be interpreted with caution as the study was not powered to detect these differences [52].

Based on these previous studies suggesting that DHA may reduce the risk of BPD, the N-3 Fatty Acids for Improvement in Respiratory Outcomes (N3RO) study was developed [55]. This was a large randomized, blinded controlled trial conducted in Australia, New Zealand and Singapore that was designed to assess the effect of DHA given to premature infants delivered prior to 29 weeks on the incidence of BPD [55]. This study randomized 1273 infants to receiving either 60 mg/kg/day DHA enteral emulsion or to receive no additional DHA. There was no statistically significant difference in the development of BPD between the groups and though not significant, the DHA group actually had a higher percentage of infants who developed physiological BPD (49.1% vs 43.9%, p-value 0.07) [55]. The authors concluded that supplementing premature infants with DHA enterally did not reduce the incidence of BPD and actually may have increased the risk [55].

Conclusion

DHA is an important LCPUFA that has roles in several physiological processes including brain and visual development as well as the inflammatory process. Mothers in the United States typically consume a Western diet that is low in omega-3 fatty acids which can also lead to breast milk that has a low concentration of DHA. Premature infants, especially those born before 30 weeks, have been shown to have a deficit in DHA shortly after delivery for several reasons including foregoing third trimester DHA accretion, receiving enteral breast milk or donor milk feeds that are typically low in DHA, and having an increased risk of requiring prolonged TPN. Despite numerous studies evaluating the effects of DHA on development in the premature infant, there are still conflicting results on whether DHA actually improves the cognitive outcomes in premature infants. While short-term benefits have been seen in several studies, long-term benefits are not consistent. Future studies continue to be needed to assess the optimal DHA dosage, method of delivery (maternal supplementation, direct supplementation, IV lipid emulsions, etc.), and length of supplementation to optimize DHA intake in very premature infants.

Abbreviations

ALA: α-linolenic acid; BPD: Bronchopulmonary dysplasia; BSID: Bayley Scales of Infant Development; CLD: Chronic lung disease; DHA: Doxosahexaenoic acid; FADS: Fatty acid desaturase; IVH: Intraventricular hemorrhage; LA: Linoleic acid; LCPUFA: Long-chain polyunsaturated fatty acids; MDI: Mental Development Index; NEC: Necrotizing enterocolitis; ROP: Retinopathy of prematurity; TNF: Tumor necrosis factor; VEP: Visual evoked potential; WASI: Wechsler Abbreviated Scale of Intelligence

Acknowledgements

Not applicable

Funding

No funding obtained for this article.

Disclaimer

The views expressed in this article are those of the authors and do not reflect the official policy or position of the United States Air Force, United States Army, United States Navy, Department of Defense, or the U.S. Government.

Authors' contributions

SS helped to draft the manuscript. CR helped to draft the manuscript. Both authors read and approved the final manuscript.

Competing interests

The authors declare that they have no competing interests.

Author details

[1]Uniformed Services University of Health Sciences, 4301 Jones Bridge, Bethesda, MD 20814, USA. [2]Walter Reed National Military Medical Center, 8901 Rockville Pike, Bethesda, MD 20814, USA.

References

1. Carlson SJ, Fallon EM, Kalish BT, Gura KM, Puder M. The role of the ω-3 fatty acid DHA in the human life cycle. JPEN J Parenter Enteral Nutr. 2013;37(1): 15–22.
2. Global Recommendations for EPA and DHA Intake (Rev 16 April 2014). http://www.goedomega3.com/index.php/files/download/304. Accessed 10 June 2017.
3. Nordgren TM, Lyden E, Anderson-Berry A, Hanson C. Omega-3 Fatty Acid Intake of Pregnant Women and Women of Childbearing Age in the United States: Potential for Deficiency? Nutrients. 2017; doi: 10.3390/nu9030197.
4. Kuipers RS, Luxwolda MF, Offringa PJ, Boersma ER, Dijck-Brouwer DA, Muskiet FA. Fetal intrauterine whole body linoleic, arachidonic and docosahexaenoic acid contents and accretion rates. Prostaglandins Leukot Essent Fat Acids. 2012;86(1–2):13–20.
5. Innis SM. Essential fatty acid transfer and fetal development. Placenta. 2005; 26(Suppl A):S70–5.
6. Storck Lindholm E, Strandvik B, Altman D, Möller A, Palme KC. Different fatty acid pattern in breast milk of obese compared to normal-weight mothers. Prostaglandins Leukot Essent Fat Acids. 2013;88(3):211–7.
7. Sanders TA. DHA status of vegetarians. Prostaglandins Leukot Essent Fat Acids. 2009;81(2–3):137–41.
8. Brenna JT, Varamini B, Jensen RG, Diersen-Schade DA, Boettcher JA, Arterburn LM. Docosahexaenoic and arachidonic acid concentrations in human breast milk worldwide. Am J Clin Nutr. 2007;85(6):1457–64.
9. Jackson KH, Harris WS. Should there be a target level of docosahexaenoic acid in breast milk? Curr Opin Clin Nutr Metab Care. 2016;19(2):92–6.
10. Sherry CL, Oliver JS, Marriage BJ. Docosahexaenoic acid supplementation in lactating women increases breast milk and plasma docosahexaenoic acid concentrations and alters infant omega 6:3 fatty acid ratio. Prostaglandins Leukot Essent Fat Acids. 2015;95:63–9.
11. Dunstan JA, Mitoulas LR, Dixon G, Doherty DA, Hartmann PE, Simmer K, Prescott SL. The effects of fish oil supplementation in pregnancy on breast milk fatty acid composition over the course of lactation: a randomized controlled trial. Pediatr Res. 2007;62(6):689–94.
12. Kovács A, Funke S, Marosvölgyi T, Burus I, Decsi T. Fatty acids in early human milk after preterm and full-term delivery. J Pediatr Gastroenterol Nutr. 2005;41(4):454–9.

13. Lapillonne A, Groh-Wargo S, Gonzalez CH, Uauy R. Lipid needs of preterm infants: updated recommendations. J Pediatr. 2013;162(Supple 3):S37–47.
14. Xie L, Innis SM. Genetic variants of the FADS1 FADS2 gene cluster are associated with altered (n-6) and (n-3) essential fatty acids in plasma and erythrocyte phospholipids in women during pregnancy and in breast milk during lactation. J Nutr. 2008;138(11):2222–8.
15. Moltó-Puigmartí C, Plat J, Mensink RP, Müller A, Jansen E, Zeegers MP, Thijs C. FADS1 FADS2 gene variants modify the association between fish intake and the docosahexaenoic acid proportions in human milk. Am J Clin Nutr. 2010;91(5):1368–76.
16. Baack ML, Norris AW, Yao J, Colaizy T. Long-chain polyunsaturated fatty acid levels in US donor human milk: meeting the needs of premature infants? J Perinatol. 2012;32(8):598–603.
17. Valentine CJ, Morrow G, Reisinger A, Dingess KA, Morrow AL, Rogers LK. Lactational Stage of Pasteurized Human Donor Milk Contributes to Nutrient Limitations for Infants. Nutrients. 2017; doi: 10.3390/nu9030302.
18. Valentine CJ, Morrow G, Fernandez S, Gulati P, Bartholomew D, Long D, Welty SE, Morrow AL, Rogers LK. Docosahexaenoic Acid and Amino Acid Contents in Pasteurized Donor Milk are Low for Preterm Infants. J Pediatr. 2010;157(6):906–10.
19. Valentine CJ, Morrow G, Pennell M, Morrow AL, Hodge A, Haban-Bartz A, Collins K, Rogers LK. Randomized controlled trial of docosahexaenoic acid supplementation in midwestern U.S. humanmilk donors. Breastfeed Med. 2013;8(1):86–91.
20. Haggarty P. Fatty Acid Supply to the Human Fetus. Annu Rev Nutr. 2010;30: 237–55.
21. Haggarty P. Placental Regulation of Fatty Acid Delivery and its Effect on Fetal Growth–A Review. Placenta. 2002; doi:10.1053/plac.2002.0791.
22. Berseth CL, Harris CL, Wampler JL, Hoffman DR, Diersen-Schade DA. Liquid human milk fortifier significantly improves docosahexaenoic and arachidonic acid status in preterm infants. Prostaglandins Leukot Essent Fat Acids. 2014;91(3):97–103.
23. Haggarty P. Effect of placental function on fatty acid requirements during pregnancy. Eur J Clin Nutr. 2004;58(12):1559–70.
24. Lapillonne A, Jensen CL. Reevaluation of the DHA requirement for the premature infant. Prostaglandins Leukot Essent Fat Acids. 2009;81(2–3):143–50.
25. Rogers LK, Valentine CJ, Keim SA. DHA supplementation: current implications in pregnancy and childhood. Pharmacol Res. 2013;70(1):13–9.
26. Kar S, Wong M, Rogozinska E, Thangaratinam S. Effects of omega-3 fatty acids in prevention of early preterm delivery: a systematic review and meta-analysis of randomized studies. Eur J Gynecol Reprod Biol. 2016;198:40–6.
27. Shireman TI, Kerling EH, Gajewski BJ, Colombo J, Carlson SE. Docosahexaenoic acid supplementation (DHA) and the return on investment for pregnancy outcomes. Prostaglandins Leukot Essent Fat Acids. 2016;111:8–10.
28. Baack ML, Puumala SE, Messier SE, Pritchett DK, Harris WS. What is the relationship between gestational age and docosahexaenoic acid (DHA) and arachidonic acid (ARA) levels? Prostaglandins Leukot Essent Fat Acids. 2015; 100:5–11.
29. De Rooy L, Hamdallah H, Dyall SC. Extremely preterm infants receiving standard care receive very low levels of arachidonic and docosahexaenoic acids. Clin Nutr. 2016; https://doi.org/10.1016/j.clnu.2016.09.033.
30. Robinson DT, Carlson SE, Murthy K, Frost B, Li S, Caplan M. Docosahexaenoic and arachidonic acid levels in extremely low birth weight infants with prolongedexposure to intravenous lipids. J Pediatr. 2013;162(1): 56–61.
31. Martin CR, Dasilva DA, Cluette-Brown JE, Dimonda C, Hamill A, Bhutta AQ, Coronel E, Wilschanski M, Stephens AJ, Driscoll DF, Bistrian BR, Ware JH, Zaman MM, Freedman SD. Decreased postnatal docosahexaenoic and arachidonic acid blood levels in premature infants are associated with neonatal morbidities. J Pediatr. 2011;159(5):743–9.
32. Collins CT, Sullivan TR, McPhee AJ, Stark MJ, Makrides M, Gibson RA. A dose response randomised controlled trial of docosahexaenoic acid (DHA) in preterm infants. Prostaglandins Leukot Essent Fat Acids. 2015;99:1–6.
33. Baack ML, Puumala SE, Messier SE, Pritchett DK, Harris WS. Daily Enteral DHA Supplementation Alleviates Deficiency in Premature Infants. Lipids. 2016; 51(4):423–33.
34. Robinson DT, Caplan M, Carlson SE, Yoder R, Murthy K, Frost B. Early docosahexaenoic and arachidonic acid supplementation in extremely-low-birth-weight infants. Pediatr Res. 2016;80(4):505–10.
35. Harris WS, Baack ML. Beyond building better brains: bridging the docosahexaenoic acid (DHA) gap of prematurity. J Perinatol. 2015;35(1):1–7.
36. Innis SM. Dietary (n-3) fatty acids and brain development. J Nutr. 2007; 137(4):855–9.
37. Janssen CI, Kiliaan AJ. Long-chain polyunsaturated fatty acids (LCPUFA) from genesis to senescence: the influence of LCPUFA on neural development, aging, and neurodegeneration. Prog Lipid Res. 2014;53:1–17.
38. Molloy C, Doyle LW, Makrides M, Anderson PJ. Docosahexaenoic acid and visual functioning in preterm infants: a review. Neuropsychol Rev. 2012; 22(4):425–37.
39. Tam EW, Chau V, Barkovich AJ, Ferriero DM, Miller SP, Rogers EE, Grunau RE, Synnes AR, Xu D, Foong J, Brant R, Innis SM. Early postnatal docosahexaenoic acid levels and improved preterm brain development. Pediatr Res. 2016;79(5):723–30.
40. Sabel KG, Strandvik B, Petzold M, Lundqvist-Persson C. Motor, mental and behavioral developments in infancy are associated with fatty acid pattern in breast milk and plasma of premature infants. Prostaglandins Leukot Essent Fat Acids. 2012;86(4–5):183–8.
41. Makrides M, Gibson RA, McPhee AJ, Collins CT, Davis PG, Doyle LW, Simmer K, Colditz PB, Morris S, Smithers LG, Willson K, Ryan P. Neurodevelopmental outcomes of preterm infants fed high-dose docosahexaenoic acid: a randomized controlled trial. JAMA. 2009;301(2):175–82.
42. Collins CT, Gibson RA, Anderson PJ, McPhee AJ, Sullivan TR, Gould JF, Ryan P, Doyle LW, Davis PG, McMichael JE, French NP, Colditz PB, Simmer K, Morris SA, Makrides M. Neurodevelopmental outcomes at 7 years' corrected age in preterm infants who were fed high-dose docosahexaenoic acid to term equivalent: a follow-up of a randomised controlled trial. BMJ Open. 2015; doi: 10.1136/bmjopen-2014-007314.
43. Henriksen C, Haugholt K, Lindgren M, Aurvåg AK, Rønnestad A, Grønn M, Solberg R, Moen A, Nakstad B, Berge RK, Smith L, Iversen PO, Drevon CA. Improved cognitive development among preterm infants attributable to early supplementation of human milk with docosahexaenoic acid and arachidonic acid. Pediatrics. 2008;121(6):1137–45.
44. Almaas AN, Tamnes CK, Nakstad B, Henriksen C, Walhovd KB, Fjell AM, Due-Tønnessen P, Drevon CA, Iversen PO. Long-chain polyunsaturated fatty acids and cognition in VLBW infants at 8 years: an RCT. Pediatrics. 2015;135(6):972–80.
45. Moon K, Rao SC, Schulzke SM, Patole SK, Simmer K. Longchain polyunsaturated fatty acid supplementation in preterm infants. In: Cochrane Neonatal Group Cochrane Database of Systematic Reviews; 2017, Issue 2. Art. No.: CD000375. doi: 10.1003/14651858.CD000375.pub5.
46. Birch EE, Carlson SE, Hoffman DR, Fitzgerald-Gustafson KM, Fu VL, Drover JR, Castañeda YS, Minns L, Wheaton DK, Mundy D, Marunycz J, Diersen-Schade DA. The DIAMOND (DHA Intake And Measurement Of Neural Development) Study: a double-masked, randomized controlled clinical trial of the maturation of infant visual acuity as a function of the dietary level of docosahexaenoic acid. Am J Clin Nutr. 2010;91(4):848–59.
47. Smithers LG, Gibson RA, McPhee A, Makrides M. Higher dose of docosahexaenoic acid in the neonate improves visual acuity of preterm infants: results of a randomized controlled trial. Am J Clin Nutr. 2008;88:1049–56.
48. Molloy CS, Stokes S, Makrides M, Collins CT, Anderson PJ, Doyle LW. Long-term effect of high-dose supplementation with DHA on visual function at school age in children born at < 33 wk gestational age: results from a follow-up of a randomized controlled trial. Am J Clin Nutr. 2016;103:268–75.
49. Fares S, Sethom M, Kacem S, Khouaja-Mokrani C, Feki M, Kaabachi N. Plasma arachidonic and docosahexaenoic acids in Tunisian very low birth weight infants: status and association with selected neonatal morbidities. J Health Popul Nutr. 2015; doi: 10.1186/s41043-015-0011-3.
50. Skouroliakou M, Konstantinou D, Agakidis C, Kaliora A, Kalogeropoulos N, Massara P, Antoniadi M, Panagiotakos D, Karagiozoglou-Lampoudi T. Parenteral MCT/ω-3 Polyunsaturated Fatty Acid-Enriched Intravenous Fat Emulsion Is Associated With Cytokine and Fatty Acid Profiles Consistent With Attenuated Inflammatory Response in Preterm Neonates: A Randomized. Double Blind Clin Trial Nutr Clin Pract. 2016;31(2):235–44.
51. De Dooy JJ, Mahieu LM, Van Bever HP. The role of inflammation in the development of chronic lung disease in neonates. Eur J Pediatr. 2001;160(8): 457–63.
52. Manley BJ, Makrides M, Collins CT, McPhee AJ, Gibson RA, Ryan P, Sullivan TR, Davis PG, DINO Steering Committee. High-dose docosahexaenoic acid supplementation of preterm infants: respiratory and allergy outcomes. Pediatrics. 2011;128(1):e71–7.
53. Collins CT, Gibson RA, Makrides M, McPhee AJ, Sullivan TR, Davis PG, Thio M, Simmer K, Rajadurai VS, N3RO Investigative Team. The N3RO trial: a randomised controlled trial of docosahexaenoic acid to

18

Prevalence and correlates of unintended pregnancy in Ghana: Analysis of 2014 Ghana Demographic and Health Survey

Edward Kwabena Ameyaw

Abstract

Background: Unintended pregnancies increase levels of stress, adoption of risky behaviours and impact on women's general quality of life. In Ghana, in spite of the paucity of literature on unintended pregnancies, the phenomenon is high especially among women in the early years of their reproductive health. This study therefore sought to investigate the prevalence and correlates of unintended pregnancies in Ghana.

Methods: This study made use of data from the 2014 Ghana Demographic and Health Survey. Descriptive statistics were conducted whereby prevalence of unintended pregnancy was presented in proportions. This was followed by binary logistic regression to investigate correlates associated with unintended pregnancy.

Results: Descriptively, unintended pregnancies were high among women aged 15–19 years (69.4%), unmarried women (45.1%) and non-working women (40.0%). Factors found to be associated with the phenomenon were age, parity and level of education. The binary logistic regression revealed that women in middle wealth category were 1.42 times more probable of having unintended pregnancy than poor women whilst rich women were less likely to experience unintended pregnancy [OR = 0.89, CI = 0.35–0.79] as compared to poor women. Again, urban women were more likely to experience unintended pregnancies as compared rural women [OR = 1.39, CI = 0.86–1.95].

Conclusion: The study has indicated that specific interventions must be targeted at different categories of women. The Reproductive and Child Health unit of the Ghana Health Service ought to collaborate with non-governmental organisations to intensify access to well-tailored family planning services among adolescents and young women, women out of marriage and the non-working category.

Keywords: Unintended pregnancy, Women, Prevalence, Ghana, Correlates

Background

The imminent birth of a child occurs within a complex social context with associated implications for the mother, expected child, the family as well as the society at large. When pregnancy takes place unintendedly, the associated complications are more probable to be enormous [1]. Unintended pregnancies are pregnancies that are either mistimed (wanted earlier or later than occurred) or unwanted (not wanted at all) [2]. As of 2008, 75 million unintended pregnancies occurred among women in LMICs with 23% of these occurring in Sub-Saharan Africa [3, 4]. Unintended pregnancies although declining, has been substantially high as it stood at 213 million on the global scale in 2012 [1].

Unintended pregnancies sometimes increase levels of stress, adoption of risky behaviours, delayed initiation of prenatal care, unwillingness to seek social support during pregnancy, impacts on women's quality of life in general and threaten households' economic status [5–8]. In spite of international commitment toward improving maternal and child health over the past decades, health implications of unintended pregnancies constitute a major public health concern, especially for women living in developing countries [9, 10]. As noted by the ecosocial theory, pregnancy intentions encompass affective, cognitive, cultural and contextual dimensions. The ecosocial theory further holds that social issues such as one's economic standing

Correspondence: edmeyaw19@gmail.com
Department of Population and Health, University of Cape Coast, Cape Coast, Ghana

and marital status influence health related outcomes in general [11, 12].

As of 2014, the Ghana Demographic and Health Survey indicated that unintended pregnancy stands at 29.8% signifying a relative decline from what had initially been reported [13]. Meanwhile, the phenomenon is still high among some sub-categories, for instance it stands at 69% and 42.8% among women aged 15–19 and 20–24 years respectively. Unintended pregnancies in Ghana and other sub-Saharan Africa might imply limited access to reproductive health services among women in these geographical areas. This manifests in limited access to family planning services, low reproductive health rights and truncated empowerment of women [14]. In order to reverse the prevalence of unintended pregnancies, associated factors are to be explored and understood in order to inform suitable interventions. The current study digresses from what has been explored and contributes to the body of knowledge by investigating national prevalence of unintended pregnancies and factors inducing this phenomenon by dwelling on data from the 2014 Ghana Demographic and Health Survey (GDHS).

Methods

Source of data

The study used women's file from the 2014 Ghana Demographic and Health Survey (2014 GDHS) [13]. The GDHS is a national survey carried out every five years. The survey is conducted by the Ghana Statistical Service and Ghana Health Service with technical support from the ICF International. It principally focuses on maternal and child health conditions among developing countries and as such was adjudged suitable for this study. It specifically covers issues such as unintended pregnancy, family planning, nutrition, fertility, health insurance, prenatal care, choice of place of delivery and postnatal care [13]. The 2014 edition interviewed 9396 women aged 15–49 years from 11,835 households emerging from 427 clusters nationwide. However, 4294 women constituted the sample for this study. The inclusion criteria for this sample was that a woman ought to have birth history within the five year period preceding the survey and must also fall within ages 15 and 49. Considering the prime focus of the survey to generate recent and reliable information on fertility, family planning and related issues, five year period is considered suitable to achieve this objective. The survey had a response rate of 97% and it was conducted with an updated frame from the 2010 Population and Housing Census (PHC). The dataset was requested from Measure DHS website. Access to the dataset was granted following approval of the request to use the data [13].

Description of variables

The dependent variable was unintended pregnancy. During the survey, respondents were asked "When you got pregnant, did you want to get pregnant at that time?" The responses to this question were either "Yes" = 1 or "No" = 2. In all, ten independent variables were selected and these independent variables were not chosen arbitrary but based on two main reasons. First, the choice of these variables was premised on the proposition of the underlying theory guiding this study (ecosocial theory) which posits that some societal structures (such as religious affiliation, marital status and educational attainment) induce women's perception about intendedness of pregnancies and secondly by varied conclusions by some previous studies [14, 15]. Following this, the ten independent variables selected were age, wealth status, educational level, religion, marital status, residential status, occupation, parity, contraceptive use and intention as well as decision maker for contraceptive use. Some of these variables were re-coded to fit the purpose of the study. These were wealth status re-coded as poor = 0, middle = 1, rich = 2 whereby women in the least wealth category were referred to as the "poor"; those who are above the least wealth category but not up to those in the high category were categorised as middle whilst those in the high wealth category were considered as rich. Parity was recoded as "between one (1) and four (4)"=0 and "more than four (4+)"=1 taking into cognisance Ghana's current total fertility rate of 4.2 [13]. With respect to occupation, someone was considered as not working if the person was not engaging in any income generating venture; primary occupation was considered as any occupation focusing on extraction of raw materials including all forms of agriculture; secondary occupation referred to the production industry which adds value to raw materials extracted through primary occupation whilst tertiary occupation involved provision of services.

Analytical approach

First of all, descriptive statistics were conducted whereby prevalence of unintended pregnancy was presented in proportions. This was followed by binary logistic regression since the principal outcome variable was dichotomous. With this, multivariate binary logistic regression analysis was carried out and the results displayed in Table 2. The study employed binary logistic regression because this technique permits extrapolation on a combination of continuous and categorical variables. The principal assumption underpinning the binary logistic regression is that the outcome variable must be dichotomous and the data should not have outliers. The data was weighted with the available sample weight factor within the GDHS dataset in order to subside the effect of sampling bias. However, all missing variables were dropped but were not that much to have any significant effect on the outcome.

It is worthy of note that the sample for "decider for contraceptive use" is minimal as a result of the fact that that question was only answered by women who were using contraceptives. The complex design of the survey was also factored whilst STATA version 13 was used for the analysis.

Ethical consideration

The study involved participation of human subjects, however, since the researcher was not directly involved in the data collection no ethical clearance was sought for this particular study. Meanwhile request for the dataset was made from Measuredhs website. Following this, permission for data usage was granted by Measuredhs after accessing the intent for the request of the dataset.

Results

Prevalence of unintended pregnancy

In Table 1, prevalence of unintended pregnancy in Ghana is shown. The overall prevalence of unintended pregnancy stood at 29.8% (data not shown). It was evident from the study that unintended pregnancies were high among 15–19 age cohorts as almost seven out of ten of them had unintended pregnancies (69.4%), which implies that 69.4% of the women interviewed during the survey (aged 15–19) had experienced unintended pregnancies. However, those aged 30–34 had the least share (22.2%). Although a greater share of the women were poor (52.2%), women in the middle wealth status were noted to have relatively high prevalence of unintended pregnancies (39.7%) and similar observation was made among those with secondary/SHS education (36.3%). In addition to the fact that Christians dominated (71.8%), the phenomenon was well pronounced among them (33.3%) than any other religious affiliates.

Married women dominated among the respondents (45.2%). The highest prevalence of unintended pregnancy was recorded among women who had never married (63.6%), whilst widows had the least unintended pregnancies (16.3%). When analysed across residential status, the phenomenon was quite high for both rural (29.5%) and urban residents (29.2%). With regard to occupation, it was realised that a significant proportion of the research participants were engaged in tertiary occupation (38.6%) whilst unintended pregnancy was high among non-working women (40.0%). The least prevalence of unintended pregnancy occurred among those engaged in primary occupation (24.2%). The study further revealed that most research participants had more than four children (72.5%), whilst unintended pregnancy was common among those with one to four children (32.1%) as compared to those with more than four children (28.4%). It was again found that no much variation in unintended pregnancies existed between those using modern contraceptives (32.9%), those using traditional method (31.7%) as well as those who intended to use in the future (32.4%). However, the phenomenon was relatively low among women who do not intend to use contraceptive later (24.2%). Women whose husbands make decision on their contraceptive use had the least prevalence of unintended pregnancy (24.0%).

Correlates of Unintended Pregnancy

Table 2 presents the binary logistic results of correlates of unintended pregnancy. Age, parity and level of education were found to be significantly related with unintended pregnancies. Women in all age categories had less odds of unintended pregnancy as compared to those aged 15–19. Women with higher/tertiary educational qualification were noted to be 2.61 times more likely to have unintended pregnancy than uneducated women (being the reference category) and similar observation was made among those with primary [OR = 1.22, CI = 0.13–0.81] and secondary/SHS education [OR = 1.86, CI = 1.22–2.84].

As compared to Christians, all other religious affiliates were less probable to have unintended pregnancies namely Islam [OR = 0.71, CI = 0.42–0.99], Traditionalists [OR = 0.94, CI = 0.30–0.84] as well as those without any religious affiliation [OR = 0.70, CI = 0.37–2.19]. It was noted that married women had less likelihood of unintended pregnancies as compared to their counterparts who had never married [OR = 0.41, CI = 0.31–0.91]. However, separated women were twice more likely to experience unintended pregnancies as compared with never married women [OR = 2.14, CI = 1.91–3.81]. When the phenomenon was considered across residence, urban women had 1.39 times [CI = 0.86–1.95] likelihood of unintended pregnancies than rural women (reference category). When compared with non-working women, those working in either primary [OR = 1.30, CI = 0.76–1.11], secondary [OR = 1.05, CI = 0.59–1.86] or tertiary [OR = 1.21, CI = 0.75–1.94] sectors were more likely to have unintended pregnancies.

It was additionally revealed that women having more than four children were less probable to have unintended pregnancies [OR = 0.25, CI = 0.16–0.39] as compared to their counterparts with at most four children (being the reference category). On contraceptive use and intention to use, less likelihoods of unintended pregnancies were recorded among traditional method users [OR = 0.82, CI = 0.65–1.06], those intending to use later [OR = 0.98, CI = 0.83–1.15] as well as women who do not intend to use [OR = 0.65, CI = 0.45–2.77] as compared to women using modern contraceptives (reference category). Also, women whose husbands were deciding on contraceptive use were less likely to experience unintended pregnancy [OR = 0.77, CI = 0.45–1.39] than those who were deciding for themselves (reference category), however, in instances where other people were deciding on contraceptive use

Table 1 Prevalence of unintended pregnancy among Ghanaian women by socio-demographic characteristics (*N* = 4294)

Socio-demographic Characteristics	*N*	Percentage (%)	Unintended Pregnancy *n* (%)
Age cohort			
15–19	183	4.3	126 (69.4)
20–24	740	17.2	313 (42.8)
25–29	1058	24.6	263 (25.1)
30–34	968	22.5	211 (22.2)
35–39	789	18.4	177 (22.8)
40–44	409	9.5	118 (29.5)
45–49	147	3.4	36 (24.8)
Wealth status			
Poor	2241	52.2	620 (28.1)
Middle	812	18.9	312 (39.7)
Rich	1241	28.9	312 (25.6)
Highest education level			
No education	1419	33.1	267 (19.0)
Primary/JHS	869	20.2	284 (33.4)
Secondary/SHS	1837	42.8	658 (36.3)
Higher/tertiary	169	3.9	35 (20.9)
Religion			
Christianity	3085	71.8	1011 (33.3)
Islam	885	20.6	156 (17.7)
Traditionalist	154	3.6	25 (16.4)
No Religion	170	4.0	52 (31.1)
Marital status			
Never married	3041	32.4	231 (63.6)
Married	4243	45.2	595 (21.2)
Cohabiting	1213	12.9	336 (40.5)
Separated	370	3.9	77 (50.0)
Divorced	260	2.8	18 (27.3)
Widowed	269	2.9	13 (16.3)
Residential status			
Rural	2516	58.6	733 (29.5)
Urban	1778	41.4	511 (29.2)
Occupation			
Not working	759	17.7	299 (40.0)
Primary	1316	30.7	313 (24.2)
Secondary	557	13.0	147 (26.9)
Tertiary	1654	38.6	483 (29.7)
Parity			
1–4	1183	27.6	373 (32.1)
4+	3111	72.5	871 (28.4)
Contraceptive use and intention			
Using modern method	1101	25.6	362 (32.9)
Using traditional method	145	3.4	46 (31.7)

Table 1 Prevalence of unintended pregnancy among Ghanaian women by socio-demographic characteristics (*N* = 4294) *(Continued)*

Socio-demographic Characteristics	*N*	Percentage (%)	Unintended Pregnancy *n* (%)
Intends to use later	1511	35.2	490 (32.4)
Does not intend to use	1537	35.8	372 (24.2)
Decider for contraceptive use			
Respondent alone	378	26.8	80 (29.3)
Husband alone	151	10.7	25 (24.0)
Joint decision	879	62.3	198 (29.9)
Other	4	0.3	1 (50.0)

Source: Computed from 2014 GDHS dataset

for the women, likelihood of unintended pregnancy was high as compared to women deciding alone [OR = 1.18, CI = 0.06–18.11].

Discussion

The study sought to examine the prevalence and correlates of unintended pregnancy in Ghana with data from the 2014 Ghana Demographic and Health Survey. The findings have revealed high prevalence of unintended pregnancy among women within 15–19 age group than women in all other age categories. This is expected due to the fact that most women aged 15–19 in Ghana are more probable to be in Senior High Schools and as a result pregnancies occurring at that time are unexpected. This might further imply their ignorance or limited depth of knowledge about contraceptives and their reproductive system. Unlike older women, these young ones are more likely to engage in unplanned sexual intercourse without any protection possibly due to peer influence or desire for material gains [16]. The higher prevalence of unintended pregnancy among Ghanaian young women is consistent with an earlier observation [17].

High prevalence of unintended pregnancies were found among women who had never married indicating that most pregnancies occurring outside marriage are unintended in Ghana. Pregnancies occurring outside marriage is unacceptable in most Ghanaian societies and as such it is not surprising that most pregnancies occurring out of marriage were unintended [14]. Similarly, Solomon & Mesganaw [18] found a significant relationship between marital status and unintended pregnancy in Ethiopia whilst similar finding has also been reported in Tanzania [19].

It was realised that unintended pregnancy declines as one's wealth status increases. Unlike the poor, wealthier women are more likely to be highly empowered and have easy access to reproductive health services. This finding corroborates with findings from Iran [20] and other African countries such as the one found at Kenya [21]. Traditionalists, Islam women and those without

Table 2 Binary Logistic Regression Results on Correlates of Unintended Pregnancy

Variable	OR	95% CI	*P*-value
Age cohort			
15–19	1	[1]	–
20–24	0.71***	[0.09–0.56]	0.000
25–29	0.25***	[0.09–0.70]	0.000
30–34	0.21***	[0.07–0.57]	0.000
35–39	0.16***	[0.06–0.47]	0.000
40–44	0.38***	[0.06–0.53]	0.000
45–49	0.14***	[0.04–0.47]	0.000
Wealth status			
Poor	1	[1]	
Middle	1.42*	[0.48–0.91]	0.008
Rich	0.89**	[0.35–0.79]	0.013
Education level			
No education	1	[1]	
Primary/JHS	1.22***	[0.13–0.81]	0.008
Secondary/SHS	1.86*	[1.22–2.84]	0.031
Higher/tertiary	2.61**	[1.24–5.58]	0.024
Religion			
Christianity	1	[1]	
Islam	0.71***	[0.42–0.99]	0.000
Traditionalist	0.94**	[0.30–0.84]	0.011
No religion	0.70	[0.37–2.19]	0.921
Marital status			
Never married	1	[1]	
Married	0.41**	[0.31–0.91]	0.002
Cohabiting	1.19**	[0.51–0.99]	0.001
Separated	2.14	[1.91–3.81]	0.201
Divorced	1.52***	[0.03–0.79]	0.000
Widowed	1.11	[0.62–2.18]	0.491
Residential status			
Rural	1	[1]	
Urban	1.39	[0.86–1.95]	0.069
Occupation			
Not working	1	[1]	
Primary	1.31**	[0.76–1.11]	0.026
Secondary	1.05	[0.59–1.86]	0.084
Tertiary	1.21	[0.75–1.94]	0.298
Parity			
1–4	1	[1]	
4+	0.25***	[0.16–0.39]	0.000
Contraceptive use and intention			
Using modern method	1	[1]	
Using traditional method	0.82	[0.65–1.06]	0.023
Intends to use later	0.98	[0.83–1.15]	0.019
Does not intend to use	0.65	[0.45–2.77]	0.450
Decision maker for contraceptive use			
Respondent alone	1	[1]	
Husband alone	0.77	[0.45–1.39]	0.031
Joint decision	1.01	[0.41–0.99]	0.011
Other	1.18	[0.06–18.11]	0.821

Source: Computed from 2014 GDHS dataset. *OR* Odds Ratio, *CI* Confidence Interval in square brackets; 1 = reference; * $p < 0.05$, ** $p < 0.01$, *** $p < 0.001$

religious affiliations were less likely to experience unintended pregnancies as compared to Christian women. This might be as a result of doctrinal differences among the women along the lines of religion. This observation is in line with the postulation of the ecosocial theory that a strong linkage exists between women's thoughts and behaviour about unanticipated pregnancies [11].

The study revealed that urban residents had relatively high tendency of unintended pregnancies. However, no significant relationship existed between residential status and unintended pregnancy and this is consistent with an earlier study [22]. Generally, pregnancies are appreciated and welcome in rural Ghana than urban settings and this might partly account for the high tendency of unintended pregnancy among urban women [23]. Women in urban settings tend to be much focused on economic activities and their holistic development and as such are more probable to declare pregnancies unintended [15].

Those with more than four children were less probable to have unintended pregnancies. This observation might imply that as women have more children they become more conscious about measures to adopt in order to regulate their fertility rather than becoming pregnant unintendedly. This finding contradicts an earlier study by Denise [15]. The differences in outcome might be as a result of variations in other factors operating at these two different study areas as recognised by the ecosocial theory that various social factors induce health in diverse ways.

Conclusion

Guided by the ecosocial theory, the study has revealed the prevalence of unintended pregnancy in Ghana. The results from this study have highlighted correlates associated with unintended pregnancies in Ghana as age, parity and level of education. This study has contributed substantially to the scanty literature on unintended pregnancy in Ghana by pointing out the prevalence and specific factors contributing to the phenomenon. It has indicated that specific interventions must be targeted at different categories of women. For example, the Reproductive and Child Health unit of the Ghana Health Service in collaboration with non-governmental organisations dedicated to reproductive health ought to intensify access to family planning services among adolescents and young women, women out of marriage more especially separated and divorced women, and the non-working. Expansion in family planning programmes can contribute substantially to reduction in unmet needs for family planning and thereby contribute immensely to combating unintended pregnancies. The study has further indicated that male involvement cannot be overlooked in the quest to curtail unintended pregnancies.

Abbreviations

DALYs: Disability Adjusted Life Years; GDHS: Ghana Demographic and Health Survey; PHC: Population and Housing Census

Acknowledgements

The author is much grateful to Measure DHS for making data accessible for the study.

Author's contributions

EKA conceived, designed and executed the study. He drafted and proofread the manuscript for important intellectual content.

Competing interests

The author declares that he has no competing interests.

References

1. Sedgh G, Singh S, Hussain R. Intended and unintended pregnancies worldwide in 2012 and recent trends. Stud Fam Plan. 2014;45(3):301–14.
2. Guttmacher Institute. The measurement and meaning of unintended pregnancy. Perspect Sex Reprod Health. 2003;35(2):94–101.
3. Singh S, Wulf D, Hussain R, Bankole A, Sedgh G. Abortion worldwide: a decade of uneven progress. New York: Guttmacher Institute; 2009.
4. Guttmacher Institute. In: Singh S, et al., editors. Special analyses. In Adding It Up: The Costs and Benefits of Investing in Family Planning and Maternal and Newborn Health. New York: Guttmacher Institute and United Nations Population Fund; 2009.
5. Sable R, Wilkinson D. Impact of perceived stress, major life events and pregnancy attitudes on low birth weight. Fam Plan Perspect. 2000;32(6): 288–94.
6. Messer C, Dole N, Kaufman S, Savitz A. Pregnancy intendedness, maternal psychosocial factors and preterm birth. Matern Child Health J. 2005;9(4): 403–12.
7. Moreland S, Talbird S. Achieving the millennium development goals: the contribution of fulfilling the unmet need for family planning. USAID: Futures Group; 2006.
8. Shah S, Balkhair T, Ohlsson A, al Beyene JSF e. Intention to become pregnant and low birth weight and preterm birth: a systematic review. Matern Child Health J. 2011;15:205–16.
9. ORC Macro (2007). MEASURE DHS STAT Compiler. Available at http://www.measuredhs.com Accessed on 5 Mar 2018.
10. Gipson JD, Koenig MA, Hindin MJ. The effects of unintended pregnancy on infant, child, and parental health: a review of the literature. Stud Fam Plan. 2008;39(1):18–38.
11. Krieger N, Gruskin S. Frameworks matter: Ecosocial and health and human rights perspectives on disparities in women's health - the case of tuberculosis. J Am Med Wom Assoc. 2001;56(4):137.
12. Bronfenbrenner U. The ecology of human development: experiments by nature and design. Cambridge, MA: Harvard University Press; 1979.
13. Ghana Statistical Service (GSS), Ghana Health Service (GHS), ICF International. Ghana demographic and health survey 2014. Rockville, Maryland: GSS, GHS, and ICF International; 2015.
14. Eliason S, Baiden F, Yankey AB, Awusabo-Asare K. Determinants of unintended pregnancies in rural Ghana. BMC Pregnancy and Childbirth. 2014;14:261.
15. Denise V, et al. Differences between mistimed and unwanted pregnancies among women who have live births. Perspect Sex Reprod Health. 2004; 36(5):192–7.
16. Rahman M. Women's autonomy and unintended pregnancy among currently pregnant women in Bangladesh. Matern Child Health J. 2012;16:1206–14.
17. Exavery A, et al. Predictors of mistimed, and unwanted pregnancies among women of childbearing age in Rufiji, Kilombero, and Ulanga districts of Tanzania. Reproductive Health. 2014;11(63)
18. Solomon W, Mesganaw F. Unintended pregnancy and induced abortion in a town with accessible family planning services: The case of Harare town in eastern Ethiopia. Ethiopia J. Health Dev. 2006;20(2):79–83.
19. Mamboleo, N. (2012). "Unwanted pregnancy and induced abortion among female youths: a case study of Temeke District." Muhimbili University of Health and Allied Science. Muhimbili University of Health and Allied Sciences.
20. Ochako R, Gichuhi W. Pregnancy wantedness, frequency and timing of antenatal care visit among women of childbearing age in Kenya. Reprod Health. 2016;13:51.
21. Mumah J, et al. Unintended Pregnancies in Kenya: A Country Profile, STEP UP Research Report. Nairobi: African Population and Health Research Center; 2014.
22. Buckles KS, Munnich EL. Birth spacing and sibling outcomes. J Hum Resour. 2012;47(3):613–42.
23. Askew, I. (2012). Causes and consequences of unintended pregnancy in developing countries, Population Council.

Low level of knowledge about neonatal danger signs and its associated factors among postnatal mothers attending at Woldia general hospital, Ethiopia

Mekdes Mengesha Jemberia[1], Elsa Tesfa Berhe[1], Hawi Bersisa Mirkena[1], Destaw Molla Gishen[1], Abera Endale Tegegne[1] and Melese Abate Reta[2*]

Abstract

Background: Neonatal mortality has persisted high in Ethiopia in spite of many efforts being applied to decrease this adverse trend. Early detection of neonatal illness is an important step towards improving newborn survival. Toward this end, there is a need for the mothers to be able to identify signs in neonates that signify severe illnesses. The aim of this study was to assess knowledge about neonatal danger signs and its associated factors among postnatal mothers attending at Woldia general hospital, Ethiopian.

Methods: Institutional based cross-sectional study design was conducted from January–May, 2017. The hospital that provides antenatal care (ANC), delivery, and postnatal services was purposively sampled. Structured interviewer managed questionnaire was administered to postnatal mothers attending Woldia general hospital. Frequencies, bivariate and multivariate logistic regression were determined using the SPSS software (Version 20).

Results: During the study period 197 mothers attending postnatal care (PNC) service at Woldia general hospital were interviewed. Information on different neonatal danger signs was not provided to 92(46.7%) postnatal mothers during their antenatal clinic attendance by the healthcare providers. The majority of mothers, 174(88.3%) identified less than six neonatal danger signs. The hotness of the body of neonates was the commonly recognized danger sign by 106(53.8%) postnatal mothers. Of the total mothers, 67(34%), 60(30.5%), 56(28.4%), 44(22.3%) recognized unable to breastfeeding, convulsion, lethargy, difficulty in breathing as newly born danger signs, respectively. Out of 197 mothers, 32(16.2%) were giving birth at home. Mother's age(AOR = 1.33, 95% CI: 1.99–3.08), marital status(AOR = 2.50, 95% CI: 0.29–4.31), mother's education status(AOR = 3.48, 95% CI:1.57–8.72), husband's education(AOR = 4.92, 95% CI: 1.29–12.81), attending ANC (AOR = 2.88, 95% CI: 1.15, 4.85), mother's residence(AOR = 0.78, 95% CI: 0.47–1.65), information about neonatal danger signs(AOR = 3.48, 95% CI 1.40–9.49) had positive association with maternal level of knowledge to identify different neonatal danger signs.

Conclusion: Maternal knowledge level about neonatal danger signs was very low. Therefore, intervention modalities that focus on increasing level of parental education, access to ANC and PNC service are needed.

Keywords: Knowledge, Neonates, Danger signs, Associated factors, Postnatal mothers, Woldia

* Correspondence: melese1985@gmail.com
[2]Department of Medical Laboratory Science, Faculty of Health Science, Woldia University, P.O.Box 400, Woldia, Ethiopia
Full list of author information is available at the end of the article

Background

The neonatal period is the first 4 weeks of life and represents a vulnerable time in an individual's life [1]. Early detection of neonatal illness through identifying neonatal danger signs is an important step towards improving newborn survival [2]. Globally, each year about 4 million children die in the first 28 days of life [3], and this accounts for 40% of the death of children under the age of 5 years globally [4]. Most neonatal death occurs in low-income and middle-income countries, particularly in Sub-Saharan Africa [3]. In Ethiopia, about 120,000 babies died at the first 4 weeks of life [5], and this neonatal mortality rate accounts for 42% of under-5 deaths in the country [5, 6]. The majority of this newborn death occurs at home (outside the formal health system) where only a few mothers and families recognize danger signs of newborn illness [3, 4]. It is terrible that many of newborn die every year especially when their death is preventable. The risk of neonatal death is high in the first 24 h of life [5]. The causes of neonatal mortality are not well documented in Ethiopia, however, some studies reported causes such as sepsis, asphyxia, birth injury, tetanus, preterm birth, congenital malformations and unknown causes [5, 6]. Some of the repeatedly reported neonatal danger signs include unable to breastfeed, the movement only when stimulated, low or high temperature, the respiratory rate over 60 breaths per minute, severe chest in drawing and history of convulsion [3]. Recognizing the occurrence of these signs will result in high overall sensitivity and specificity to predict the need for seeking treatment of the newborn [3, 7, 8]. It is estimated that about 75% of neonatal deaths can be avoided [3, 9]. However, this is only possible if mother's knowledge regarding the neonatal danger signs is good enough to make a decision to seek health care service [3], Because mother's poor knowledge about newborn danger signs delay cares to seek health care service and treatment [2]. According to a report by Nigatu et al., mothers and husbands higher educational achievement, ANC and PNC attendance and access to television for information were positively associated with mother's good knowledge about neonatal danger signs [3]. Okawa et al., reported that potential determinants of neonatal danger signs and factors that would delay for sick newborn treatment were categorized into four domains: maternal factors, family factors, antenatal factors, and delivery factors [10].

For the last era, neonatal deaths have gained attention on the global policy agenda because the Millennium Development Goal (MDG) for child survival cannot be met without substantial reductions in neonatal mortality. It is estimated that reduction of under-5 child mortality by two-thirds by 2015, as called for by the MDG, requires a reduction in neonatal mortality of at least 50% [6].

Different tools to facilitate identification of neonatal health problems and management were introduced into the health programs in several countries like Ethiopia. Integrated Management of Newborn and childhood illness developed by world health organization(WHO) was the one which focused on assessment of neonatal danger signs and applies prompt timely treatment [3, 11]. Similarly, Bhutta et al. report, early identification of newborn danger signs by caregivers with prompt and appropriate referral serves as backbone of the programs aiming at reduction in neonatal mortality [12]. According to a report by Yared et al., in Ethiopia, the neonatal mortality rate declined by 1.9% per annum from 1995 to 2010, logarithmically. The early neonatal mortality rate declined by 0.9% per annum and was where 74% of the neonatal deaths occurred [6]. According to 2016 EDHS report all childhood mortality rates have declined over time; the under-5 mortality rate has declined from 116 deaths per 1000 live births 10–14 years prior to the survey (2002–2006) to 67deaths per 1000 live births in the 0–4 years prior to the survey (2012–2016); and the neonatal mortality rate was 29 deaths per 1000 live births [11].

Generally, reducing neonatal morbidity and mortality requires immediate caregiver's recognition of suggestive danger signs in the neonates and visiting the nearby clinic for early treatment. Trends in Ethiopian society so far recognized mothers as caretakers for the majority of neonates [3, 13]. Therefore, improving maternal knowledge concerning neonatal danger sign is a key entry point [3]. However, studies in the area are limited and inconsistent. Numerous studies have examined the determinants of neonatal mortality, but few have explored maternal levels of knowledge on neonatal danger signs and different danger signs which potentially cause neonatal morbidity [10]. Therefore, the main aim of this study was to explore the maternal level of knowledge on neonatal danger signs and to assess the associated factors among postnatal mothers attending at Woldia general hospital in the study area.

Methods and materials

Study area and period

Woldia town is located at 521 km away from the capital city, Addis Ababa. It is found at 2000 m above sea level with a temperature of 22 °C. According to 2007 Ethiopian National population census [11]; the total population of the town is 75,496 people; among them, 38,167 are males and 37,279 are females. According to 2016 Woldia general hospital annual report; the mothers who had gotten PNC service were 2910. The study was conducted from January–May, 2017. The study employed institutional-based cross-sectional design including all postnatal mothers attending at the hospital during the study period. Mentally and physically incapable postnatal mothers to provide a response during data collection period were excluded.

Study subjects

During the study period, 197 postnatal mothers attending Woldia general hospital for PNC service were interviewed. All eligible postnatal mothers in selected study site were interviewed and neonatal danger signs were assessed through maternal recall.

Data collection and analysis

Pre-tested and interviewer administered questionnaire adopted from previous studies were employed to record mother's knowledge about neonatal danger signs, socio-demographic, and economic factors. The questionnaire was translated into the local language(Amharic) to make data collection process simple and translate back to the English language by translators who are perfect(good in English and Amharic language) to check the content validity of the original version. Three trained BSc degree holder health professionals conducted the data collection process.

The total number of correct spontaneous responses to 12 items (neonatal danger signs) with a minimum score of 0 and maximum of 12 was used to measure knowledge of mothers about neonatal danger signs. Accordingly, two categories were developed for neonatal danger sign. Spontaneous response is respondents naming of neonatal danger signs without giving the option of the respected signs. Mothers who mentioned at least six neonatal danger signs were considered as having good knowledge about neonatal danger signs and mothers who mentioned less than six neonatal danger signs were considered as having poor knowledge.

The completeness and consistency of the data were checked, cleaned and double entered to Epidemiological Information (EPI-INFO) software version 3.5.1 and analyzed by Statistical Package for Social Sciences (SPSS) software version 20. Frequencies, proportions, and summary statistics were used to describe the study population in relation to relevant variables and presented by using tables and graphs. A bivariate logistic regression model was fitted to identify factors, which were significant at $p < 0.2$ and then entered into multivariate logistic regression model to identify independent factors those affected mother's knowledge about neonatal danger signs.

Operational terms

Neonatal danger signs

Are symptoms that complicate the lives of the neonate and happen during the neonatal period.

Postnatal care

Care given to a mother for a period of six weeks from the time of delivery using WHO standards contact time within one hour after birth, at 2–3 days, 6–7 days, and extra contacts for those LBW/mothers living with HIV.

Knowledge

State of awareness of mothers on neonatal danger signs; defined on the basis of the score (mean).

Good knowledgeable

Those mothers who are able to score above the mean of total knowledge based questions.

Poor knowledgeable

Those mothers who are able to score below the mean of total knowledge-based questions.

Ethical considerations

Ethical clearance was obtained from research review and ethical committee of Faculty of Health Science, Woldia University. Communication with the hospital medical director was made through formal letter obtained from Woldia University, Health Science Faculty. After explained the purpose and objective of the study, the researchers obtained written consent of mothers with their age greater than18years. Moreover, written consent was obtained from caretakers on behalf of those with age less than 18 years. Mothers were informed that their participation was on a voluntary basis, and the information obtained from them was kept confidential through no identifier was used.

Results

Social-demographic characteristics of the respondents

A total of 197 mothers were interviewed during data collection; of these, about 141(71.6%) are under 18–35 years old with the mean age of 23.9. Mothers who live in urban accounts 120(60.9%), while 77(39.1%) them were living in rural. Of the total interviewed mothers 163 (82.7%) were married, and the majority 125(63.5%) were the housewife and 50(25.4%) of them can't read and write. About 134 (69.0%) of them are Orthodox Christian followers. Among the total mothers, 106(53.8%) had less than three family size (Table 1).

Antenatal and postnatal care utilizations of mothers

Among 197 mothers, 172(87.3%) of them had ANC follow-up at health institution; and about 13 (6.6%), 38 (19.3%) and 52(26.4%) had 1st visit, 2nd visit, 3rd visit respectively, and 72(36.5%) of them had completed ANC visit. From total participants, only 122(61.9%) had gotten information about PNC followed. The majority of mothers, 99(50.3%) got information from healthcare

Table 1 Socio-demographic characteristics of mothers attending PNC at Woldia General Hospital, January–May, 2017

Attributes		N	%
Age of mother's(years)	< 18	22	11.2
	18–35	141	71.6
	36–45	33	16.8
	> 45	1	0.5
Mother's residence	Urban	120	60.9
	Rural	77	39.1
Mother's marital status	Single	26	13.2
	Married	163	82.7
	Divorced	6	3.0
	Widowed	2	1.0
Mother's occupation	Housewife	125	63.5
	Merchant	20	10.2
	Gov't Employee	31	15.7
	Student	14	7.1
	Others	7	3.6
Family's monthly income(birr)	< 500	76	38.6
	500–1000	46	23.4
	> 1000	75	38.1
Mother's educational status	Can't read and write	50	25.4
	Can read and write	29	14.7
	Grade 1–8	36	18.3
	Grade 9–10	37	18.8
	Grade 11–12	20	10.2
	Diploma & above	25	12.7
Mother's religion	Orthodox Christian	134	68.0
	Muslim	58	29.4
	Protestant	4	2.0
	Catholic	1	0.5
Mother's ethnicity	Amhara	165	83.8
	Tigre	19	9.6
	Afar	12	6.1
	Others	1	0.5
Family size	1–3	106	53.8
	4–6	73	37.1
	> 7	18	9.1
Husband's education status	Can't read and write	28	14.2
	Can read and write	38	19.3
	Grade 1–8	31	15.7
	Grade 9–10	34	17.3
	Grade 11–12	20	10.2
	Diploma & above	46	23.4
Distance to health institution	< 5 km	86	43.7
	5-20 km	63	32.0
	> 20 km	48	24.4

providers. Most of the study participants 127(64.0%) don't know the right postnatal period (PNP) follow-up time. Of the total mothers, 107(54.3%) of them did not know the PNP is a danger time for mothers and neonates. The reason to attend current PNC was 52(26.4%) excessive bleeding, 41(20.8%) neonatal infection, 39(19.8%) unable to breastfeeding. Out of the total respondents, 32(16.2%) delivered their current baby at home (Table 2).

Sources of information for mothers about neonatal danger signs

The study revealed that about 105(53%) of mothers attending PNC at Woldia general hospital had gotten information about neonatal danger sign from health providers, while 33(16.8%) of mothers had gotten information from health extension workers (fig. 1).

Maternal level of knowledge on neonatal danger signs

The scoring of neonatal danger signs was evaluated and scored. For mothers who were able to identify less than six neonatal danger signs were classified as having a low level of knowledge and those who scored more than six were classified as having a good level of knowledge on neonatal danger signs. The majority of mothers, 174(88.3%) had a low level of knowledge. Twenty-three (11.7%) of mothers had good levels of knowledge about neonatal danger sign (95% CI 7.6, 16.3). The most commonly reported source of information was health-care providers (53%) (Fig. 2).

Mother's recognition of neonatal danger signs

The hotness of the body was the commonly recognized neonatal danger sign by 106(53.8%) postnatal mothers. Out of 197 mothers, 67(34%), 60(30.5%), 56(28.4%), 44(22%), 43(21.8%), 40(20.3%), 35(17.8%), 22(11.2%), 21(10.7%), 20(10.2%), 17(8.6%) identified unable to breastfeeding, convulsion, lethargy, difficulty in breathing, persistent vomiting, diarrhea, coldness, umbilical bleeding, abdominal distention, and yellowness of palms and soles as newborn danger signs, respectively(Fig. 3).

Factors associated with maternal level of knowledge about neonatal danger signs

After controlling for socio-demographic, economic, and maternal factors; age of mother's, mother educational status, mothers marital status, Mother's occupation, husband educational status, attending ANC, Mother's residence, Distance to health institution and having neonatal danger signs information to mother were the factors that significantly affect maternal levels of knowledge.

Women whose age 18-35 years were 33%(AOR = 1.33, 95% CI: 1.99–3.08) more likely to be knowledgeable as compared to mothers who are < 18 years old. Women who are widowed had two times less likely (AOR = 2.50, 95% CI: 0.29–4.31) to identify at least six neonatal danger signs. Mothers who are diploma and above

Table 2 Antenatal and postnatal care utilization of mothers attending PNC at Woldia General Hospital, January–May, 2017

Attributes		N	%
Do you know ANC follow up time?	Yes	69	35.0
	No	128	65.0
Did you attend ANC?	Yes	172	87.3
	No	25	12.7
How many ANC visit did you attend?	1 Visit	10	5.1
	2 Visit	38	19.3
	3 Visit	52	26.4
	4 Visit	72	36.5
Did you get information about postnatal service?	Yes	122	61.9
	No	75	38.1
What is your source of information about PNC Service?[a]	Health Provider	99	50.3
	Health Extension workers	17	8.6
	Community Conversation	1	0.5
	Media(TV, Radio)	5	2.5
	Traditional Birth Attendant	0	0
Knowing when PNC starts	On the date of delivery (1-6 h)	41	20.8
	6 h-6 days	18	9.1
	6–7 days	5	2.5
	> 7 days	7	3.6
Knowing PNP is danger time for mothers & neonates	Yes	90	45.7
	No	107	54.3
Do you know danger signs of PNP?	Yes	95	48.2
	No	24	12.2
Types of PNP Danger signs for mothers and neonates[a]	Excessive bleeding	100	50.8
	Neonatal infections	64	32.5
	Unable to breastfeed	68	34.5
	Vomiting	61	31.0
	Others	16	8.1
Reasons to attend current PNC service[a]	Excessive bleeding	41	20.8
	Neonate infections	52	26.4
	Unable to breast feed	39	19.8
	Others	66	33.5
What education did you get during PNC attending time? [a]	Personal hygiene	128	65.0
	Immunization	136	69.0
	Family planning	135	68.5
	Breast feeding	109	55.3
	Neonatal infection	92	46.7
	Care to ill neonates	66	33.5
Did you get the education about your neonate danger signs during PNC?	Yes	105	53.3
	No	92	46.7
What education did you get about your neonate during PNC? [a]	The advantage of breastfeeding	91	46.2
	Cord care	62	31.5
	Eye care	54	27.4
	Thermoregulation	54	27.4
	Different immunization	63	32.0
	About neonatal danger signs	53	26.9
	Others	4	2.0
Where did you deliver your current baby?	Home	32	16.2
	Hospital	149	75.6
	Health Center	16	8.1
How did you deliver?	Spontaneous vertex delivery	132	67.0
	Cesarean section	54	27.4
	Instrumental	11	5.6

[a] Multiple responses of respondents

education level were three times (AOR = 3.48, 95% CI: 1.57–8.72), and more than three times (AOR = 3.05, 95% CI: 1.83–6.90) to be knowledgeable about neonatal danger signs as compared to mothers who can't read and write, respectively. Similarly, mothers whose husbands are preparatory school education(AOR = 4.92, 95% CI:1.29–12.81) were nearly four times more likely to mention at least six neonatal danger signs as compared to husbands who can't read and write. Furthermore, mothers who attended ANC during the last pregnancy were two times more likely to head knowledge (AOR = 2.88, 95% CI 1.15, 4.85) about neonatal danger signs as compared to those who did not follow. Mothers who live in the urban area were 22% more likely to have knowledge (AOR = 0.78, 95% CI: 0.47–1.65) about neonatal danger signs as compared to those living in rural area. Likewise, mothers who had got information about danger signs increased their knowledge about neonatal danger signs by 3 times (AOR = 3.48, 95% CI 1.40–9.49) (Table 3).

Discussion

This institutional based cross-sectional study has assessed the levels of maternal knowledge and the associated factors on neonatal danger signs among mothers attending postnatal care at Woldia general hospital. Reduction of neonatal and infant mortality to an acceptable level is impossible without good maternal knowledge level regarding neonatal danger signs. This is because of

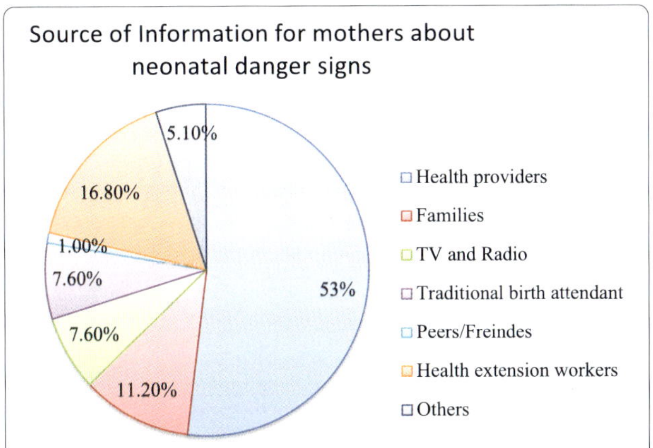

Fig. 1 Source of information for mothers on neonatal danger signs

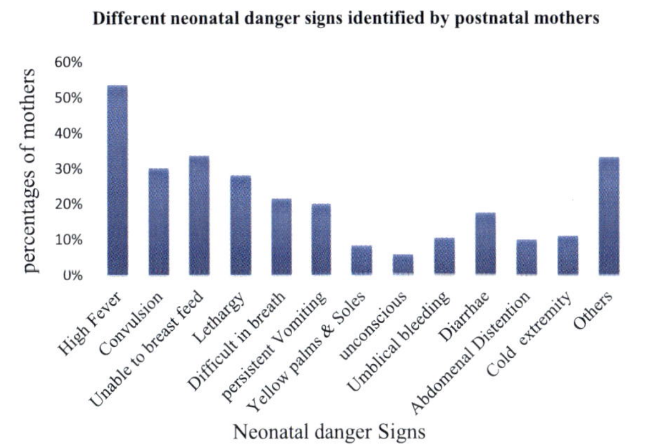

Fig. 3 Different neonatal danger signs identified by postnatal mothers

the fact that, these danger signs are the entry point to provide comprehensive neonatal health care [3].

In this study, the prevalence of mothers' good knowledge (mothers who mentioned at least six and above neonatal danger sign) was found to be 11.67%. The finding reported that most mothers have a very poor level of knowledge 174(88.3%) about neonatal danger signs. This is slightly higher than the finding reported from Kenya that 84.5% of the maternal level of knowledge is poor to identify at least three neonatal danger signs from eight mentioned danger signs [8]. Similarly, low maternal levels of knowledge to identify at least one neonatal danger signs was reported from Southwestern Rural Uganda [2]. This may be due to information on danger sign was not adequately disseminated to mothers both during antenatal and PNC period [8]. From total PNC attending women, 74.7% of respondents had formal education from elementary to higher education. Similarly, a study conducted at Addis Ababa reported that mothers attending PNC (35%) have primary school certificate [14]. Maternal education plays a major role in the understanding of neonatal danger signs. In this study mothers who had diploma certificate and above were three times (AOR = 3.48, 95% CI: 1.57–8.72) more likely to be knowledgeable about neonatal danger signs as compared to mothers who can't read and write. This is in line with neonatal danger signs knowledge level reported from North West of Ethiopia that mothers having secondary and above educational level increased the odds of their knowledge by nearly three times [3]. The possible justification for this could be educated mothers attain knowledge about the neonatal disease and maternal health through their academic life.

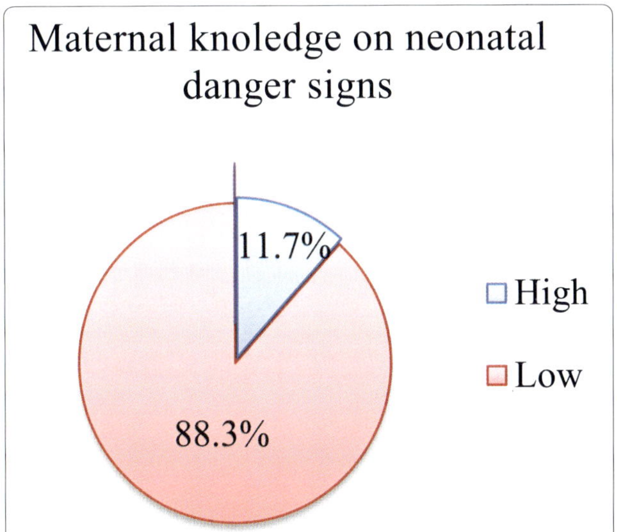

Fig. 2 Maternal level of Knowledge on Neonatal danger signs

The distance of mothers from health institutions can also determine for appropriate ANC and PNC service utilization; our study revealed that 24.4% of mothers travel > 20 km to get PNC service at Woldia general hospital. Mothers who live in the urban area were 22% more likely to have knowledge (AOR = 0.78, 95% CI: 0.47–1.65) about neonatal danger signs as compared to those living in rural area. In contrast to this, the study reported from Southwestern rural Uganda revealed that no association between mothers residence and levels of knowledge on neonatal danger signs [2]. This may be due to those mothers who live far away from health institutions would not have access to ANC and PNC service and would have low access to information about neonatal danger signs.

In our study about 32(16.2%) of women delivered at home (outside the formal health system). In contrast to our report, in India, about 200(70.5%) deliveries take place at home attended by untrained personnel [15]. This difference may be due to study area difference that our study was an institution based whereas Indian study

Table 3 Factors associated with mother's knowledge on neonatal danger signs at Woldia general hospital, January–May, 2017

Characteristics		Knowledge on neonatal danger sign		Crude OR (95% CI)	Adjusted OR (95% CI)
		Good(N)	Poor(N)		
Age of mother's(year)	< 18	1	21	1	1
	18–35	20	121	1.62(1.41–2.96)*	1.50(0.19–2.41)
	36–45	2	31	3.46(2.30–5.71)*	1.33(1.99–3.08)**
	> 45	0	1	0.84(0.41–3.16)*	0.75(0.57–1.95)
Marital status	Married	19	144	1	1
	Single	3	23	1.80(1.54–6.10)	1.60 (0.39–4.32)
	Divorce	0	6	2.88(0.46–4.31) *	1.33 (0.89–4.08)**
	Widowed	1	1	3.94 (0.31–4.26)*	2.50 (0.29–4.31)**
Mother education	Can't read and write	1	49	1	1
	Can read and write	4	25	10.86(2.50–75.43)*	4.50 (2.18–7.51)
	Grade 1–8	2	34	9.83(2.61–55.65)*	5.33 (2.99–6.08)
	Grade 9–10	7	30	4.54 (0.31–5.26)	7.72(1.39–63.46)**
	Grade 11–12	2	18	6.18 (2.42–11.51)	3.05 (1.83–6.90)**
	Diploma & above	7	18	10.2 (5.43–23.01)*	3.48 (1.57–8.72)**
Mother's occupation	Housewife	12	113	1	1
	Merchant	2	18	9.76(3.50–45.23)	4.05 (2.26–8.37)
	Gov't Employee	6	25	10.83(2.61–95.74)*	5.57 (2.82–9.81)**
	Student	2	12	9.83(1.38–83.27)*	3.48 (0.78–5.89)**
	Others	1	6	3.11 (1.26, 8.48)	1.33 (0.28, 7.18)
Husband's education	Can't read and write	1	27	1	1
	Can read and write	3	35	2.52(0.81–4.85)*	1.62(0.91–2.86)
	Grade 1–8	1	30	2.66(1.40–4.81)*	0.96(0.40–1.81)
	Grade 9–10	5	29	2.88(0.37–4.65)	0.78(0.47–1.55)
	Grade 11–12	3	17	9.73 (3.44–27.96)	4.92 (1.29–12.81)**
	Diploma & above	10	36	13.8 (4.12–44.54)*	4.81 (1.43–12.46)
ANC	Yes	22	150	6.71 (4.27–17.49)*	2.88 (1.15, 4.85)**
	No	1	24	1	
Place of delivery	Home	1	31	0.28 (0.23–2.57)	
	Hospital	19	130	2.18 (1.44–3.63)*	
	Health Center	3	13	1	1
Mother's residence	Urban	19	101	2.77 (1.55, 4.93)*	0.78(0.47–1.65)**
	Rural	4	73	1	1
Distance to health institution	< 5 km	14	72	5.66 (2.82–7.82)	2.72(0.46–3.85)
	5-20 km	7	56	1.67 (0.98–2.49)*	0.46(0.30–0.81)**
	> 20 km	2	46	1.33 (0.88–7.89)*	0.78(0.47–1.75)**
Danger signs information to mother	Yes	20	85	7.77 (3.96–16.07)	3.48 (1.40–9.49)**
	No	3	89	1	1

** P-value < 0.2; ** p-value < 0.05*

was community-based. Regarding associated factors; maternal knowledge, mother's age, educational status, marital status, occupation, attending ANC, residence, distance to health institution, danger signs information to the mother, husband educational status were significantly affect maternal levels of knowledge to identify at least six neonatal danger signs in our study. Similarly, the study done in Kenya reported that mother's education level, PNC accompaniment by Spouse, danger signs information to mother were factors positively associated with better knowledge on neonatal danger sign [8].

Conclusion

Investigators agreed that mothers can have a great role in caring new born baby and identifying neonatal danger signs. The findings of our study revealed that there is a poor understanding of neonatal danger signs 174 (88.3%). Even participant's record has the highest number of ANC attendance (87.3%) and institutional deliveries (83.7%), the existing knowledge gap in this key area of neonatal danger signs affect the success of childcare services; this needs to increase educational efforts aimed for all pregnant and delivered women in the hospital as well as in the community.

Abbreviations

ANC: Antenatal care; AOR: Adjusted odds ratio; CI: Confidence interval; EDHS: Ethiopian Demographic and Health Survey; EPI-INFO: Epidemiological Information software; HIV: Human immunodeficiency virus; LBW: Low birth weight; MDG: Millennium Development Goal; PNC: Postnatal care; PNP: Postnatal period; SPSS: Statistical package for social sciences; WHO: World health organization

Acknowledgements

Our sincere gratitude goes to Woldia University, Faculty of Health Science for all supports. We would like to acknowledge the study participants for their participation and without them, the research would not realize.

Competing interests.

The authors declare that they have no competing interests.

Funding

The authors declared that this study has received no financial support.

Authors' contributions.

MMJ, ETB, HBM, DMG, and AET participated in the study design, implementation of the study, and data collections. MAR designed the study, performed the statistical analysis and drafted the manuscript for publication. All authors contributed to the data analysis, read and approved the final manuscript.

Author details

[1]Department of Midwifery, Faculty of Health Science, Woldia University, P.O.Box 400, Woldia, Ethiopia. [2]Department of Medical Laboratory Science, Faculty of Health Science, Woldia University, P.O.Box 400, Woldia, Ethiopia.

References

1. Aijaz N, Huda N, Kausar S. Disease burden of NICU at a tertiary care hospital, Karachi. Journal of the Dow University of Health Sciences Karachi. 2012;6(1):35.
2. Sandberg J, Odberg PK, Asp G, Kabakyenga J, Agardh A. Inadequate knowledge of neonatal danger signs among recently delivered women in southwestern rural Uganda: a community survey. PLoS One. 2014;9(5):e97253.
3. Nigatu GS, Worku GA, Dadi FA. Level of mother's knowledge about neonatal danger signs and associated factors in north west of Ethiopia: a community based study. BMC Res Notes. 2015;8(309)
4. Assefa N, Lakew Y, Belay B, Kedir H, Zelalem D, Baraki N, et al. Neonatal mortality and causes of death in Kersa health and demographic surveillance system (Kersa HDSS), Ethiopia, 2008–2013. *Matern Health, Neonatol, and* Perinatology 2017;2:7.
5. Bogale W, Mulualem G. New born care training participants manual. Addis Ababa,Ethiopia: FMOH; 2012.
6. Mekonnen Y, Tensou B, Telake SD, Degefie T, Bekele A. Neonatal mortality in Ethiopia: trends and determinants. BMC Public Health. 2013;13(483)
7. Joy EL, Kate K, Christabel EL, Simon C, Dip MS. 3.6 Million Neonatal: Deaths—What Is Progressing and What Is Not?Seminar in Perinatology. *Elsevier*. 2010;34:386.
8. Kibaru EG, Otara AM. Knowledge Of neonatal danger signs among mothers attending well baby clinic in Nakuru Central District, Kenya: cross sectional descriptive study. BMC Res Notes. 2016;9(1):481.
9. Mengesha HG, Sahle BW. Cause of neonatal deaths in northern Ethiopia: a prospective cohort study. BMC Public Health. 2017;17(62)
10. Okawa S, Ansah EK, Nanishi K, Enuameh Y, Shibanuma A, Kikuchi K, et al. High incidence of neonatal danger signs and its implications for postnatal Care in Ghana: a cross-sectional study. PLoS One. 2015;10(6):e0130712.
11. Central Statistical Agency[CSA-Ethiopia], and ICF. Ethiopia Demographic and Health Survey : Key Indicators Report. Addis Ababa,Ethiopia, and Rockville, Maryland, USA. CSA and ICF: FEDERAL DEMOCRATIC REPUBLIC OF ETHIOPIA; 2016.
12. Dongre AR, Deshmukh PR, Garg BS. Awareness and health care seeking for newborn danger signs among mothers in peri-urban Wardha. Indian J Pediatr. 2009;76(7):691–3.
13. Choi Y, ETS A, Mannan I, Rahman MS, Bari S, Darmstadt LG, et al. can mothers recognize neonatal illness correctly? Comparison of maternal report and assessment by community health workers in rural angladesh. Trop Med Int Health. 2010;15(6):753.
14. Chewaka L. Preventable causes of neonatal mortality and associated factors among neonates admitted to neonatal intensive care units of Addis Ababa governmental hospitals from 2011–2015 GC: a retrospective study [master]. Addis Ababa: Addis Ababa University; 2016.
15. Shally A, Tuhina V, Monica A. Danger Signs of neonatal illnesses: perceptions of caregivers and health workers in northern India. Bull World Health Organ. 2006;84(10):826.

20

Air displacement plethysmography (pea pod) in full-term and pre-term infants: a comprehensive review of accuracy, reproducibility, and practical challenges

Hajar Mazahery[1], Pamela R. von Hurst[1], Christopher J. D. McKinlay[2,3], Barbara E. Cormack[4] and Cathryn A. Conlon[1*]

Abstract

Air displacement plethysmography (ADP) has been widely utilised to track body composition because it is considered to be practical, reliable, and valid. Pea Pod is the infant version of ADP that accommodates infants up to the age of 6 months and has been widely utilised to assess the body composition of full-term infants, and more recently pre-term infants. The primary goal of this comprehensive review is to 1) discuss the accuracy/reproducibility of Pea Pod in both full- and pre-term infants, 2) highlight and discuss practical challenges and potential sources of measurement errors in relation to Pea Pod operating principles, and 3) make suggestions for future research direction to overcome the identified limitations.

Keywords: Air displacement plethysmography, ADP, Pea pod, Infant, Pre-term, Full-term, Body composition

Background

Early postnatal growth is a major determinant of short- and long-term health outcomes, for both full-term and pre-term infants. The significance of neonatal nutritional management and postnatal growth lies in their effect on infant survival, neurodevelopment and later metabolic function. Postnatal faltering growth is associated with neurodevelopment impairment, especially in preterm infants, and increased risk of cardiometabolic disease, particularly after fetal growth restriction [1, 2]. Rapid postnatal growth is also associated with increased risk of metabolic syndrome or its determinants [3–7]. These complex effects are influenced by differential growth in soft tissue compartments, namely, fat mass (FM) and lean mass (LM). Growth that involves relatively greater gains in LM appears to be protective for brain development [8, 9] and metabolic function [9], whereas accelerated gain in FM, especially centrally and in the first 6 months, is associated with childhood obesity [10]. Preterm infants appear to be particularly susceptible to both postnatal growth failure and central fat deposition [5]. These observations highlight the importance of assessing body composition and not just total mass when monitoring growth in infants.

There are a number of techniques available to measure body composition in infants, including dual energy X-ray absorptiometry (DXA), bioelectrical impedance analysis (BIA), isotope dilution, magnetic resonance imaging (MRI), and air displacement plethysmography (ADP) [11]. Local FM deposits may also be quantified by ultrasound [12]. ADP has gained popularity due to availability, feasibility and acceptability to parents [13]. ADP utilizes the inverse relationship between pressure and volume in two enclosed chambers – employing the gas law of Boyle and Poisson – that allows for the calculation of body density [14]. A two-compartment model is derived assuming a fixed density of fat (0.9007 g/ml) [15] and from age- and sex-specific estimates of fat free mass (FFM) density.

There are two commercially available ADP body composition systems; one for adults (Bod Pod) and one for infants (Pea Pod) (Cosmed, Rome, Italy). While Bod Pod houses both children aged > 2 years old and adults, Pea Pod accommodates infants from birth until approximately 6 months of age (body weight ≤ 10 kg). Recently, Pea Pod

* Correspondence: c.conlon@massey.ac.nz
[1]College of Health, Massey University, Auckland 0745, New Zealand
Full list of author information is available at the end of the article

has also been employed to assess the body composition of pre-term infants from 30 weeks' gestation, and may be a viable method for close monitoring of growth in these infants.

Since the introduction of Pea Pod in 2003 [14, 16, 17] and its validation in 2004 [18], a large number of technical and clinical research papers utilising Pea Pod have been published. Pea Pod has also been included in several recent reviews on body composition, including the utility of ADP technique from infancy to adulthood [19], changes in body composition over the first six months after birth utilising different assessment methods [4, 20], and a comparison of different body composition assessment tools in infancy [11]. However, to our knowledge, no comprehensive review of the use of Pea Pod in both full- and pre-term infants is available.

This review will focus exclusively on studies that have assessed body composition of infants using Pea Pod, including both full- and pre-term infants. We will summarise the published papers, with sections devoted to its accuracy relative to criterion methods, reproducibility, and to practical challenges associated with the use of Pea Pod in clinical settings and studies. From there, we will make suggestions for future research directions to address any identified limitations. At the outset, we present an overview of body composition measures, including assessment of accuracy and reproducibility, following which we describe the results of the review.

Body composition measures

Body composition may be described using two-, three- and four-compartment models. The two-compartment model [21] divides body weight into FM and FFM (with assumptions made regarding the density of FM and FFM) and ignores the interindividual variation in FFM composition. The three-compartment model [22] is based on measurements of body density and total body water, and assumes a constant mineral to protein ratio in the dry FFM and makes no assumptions about the hydration of FFM. The four-compartment model [23] divides the body weight into fat, water, mineral, and protein, and is the most robust and sensitive to interindividual variability in the composition of FFM. Accordingly, the four-compartment model has less error than other models.

Obesity is defined as an excess of body fat that adversely affects health [20]. Body mass index (BMI, kg/m^2) has long been used in clinical practice and epidemiological studies as an indicator of adiposity. However, BMI has been shown to have inconsistent relationship with disease risk and mortality. For example, Nagayama et al. [24] reported an inverse relationship between BMI and cardiometabolic fitness in healthy Japanese adults, whereas Flegal et al. [25] showed that all-cause mortality rate was lower in overweight than normal weight individuals.

This inconsistency may reflect the variable relationship between BMI and adiposity, with the latter being more closely related to disease risk [26]. For example, in a study of 709 adults aged 20–94 years (of both sexes and different ethnicities), Gallagher et al. [26] showed that BMI alone explained only 25% of the between-individual variability in adiposity. Further, Zeng et al. [27] showed that adiposity, but not BMI, was independently associated with cardiovascular risk factors. Even in normal weight individuals, higher adiposity has been shown to be associated with adverse cardiometabolic health outcomes, such as metabolic syndrome, dyslipidemia, hypertension, and cardiovascular disease [28].

In children, increases in BMI can reflect increases in FFM rather than increases in FM due to the rapid growth of musculoskeletal tissues [29]. A recent systematic review and meta-analysis found that BMI had high specificity but low sensitivity for detection of excess adiposity in children, and thus BMI failed to identify > 25% of children with excess FM [30]. Hetherington-Rauth et al. [31] compared indirect measures of adiposity (including BMI) with direct measures (DXA FM% and Fat Mass Index, FMI) in relation to cardiometabolic risk factors in children. Although the authors reported that anthropometric measures performed as well as DXA measures did, addition of direct measures of adiposity to indirect measures may be advantageous for predicting cardiometabolic risk factors such as insulin resistance [31], a finding reported by others [29, 32]. Similarly, in both full-term and pre-term infants, BMI was shown to have a weak association with FM% (defined as FM/weight*100) [33, 34], though the relationships were slightly stronger in full-term infants [35]. Thus, in infants and children, BMI appears to be a poor measure of adiposity, and "normal" BMI may still be associated with excess fat mass for size, particularly if LM is low [36].

Adiposity is often referenced to total mass (e.g, whole-body FM%) but this is statistically problematic given that fat mass is included in both numerator and denominator [37]. As body fat mass increases, FM% does not increase proportionately (depending on relative growth in FFM), resulting in underestimation of adiposity. The growth velocity of the different soft tissue compartments may be variably affected by nutritional interventions and factors such as age, sex, pubertal status, and ethnicity [38]. To overcome these problems, Van-Itallile [39] advocated referencing of FM and FFM to height squared, giving a FM index (FMI) and FFM index (FFMI), which in adults effectively normalises soft tissue mass for height and allows for comparison between individuals of different size.

A similar approach has also been recommended in children [40–42], although second order indices may not render soft tissue mass independent of size [40]. This is particularly important when comparing body composition between infants of differing length, especially in pre-term infants whose lower absolute FFM is partly due to their shorter body length. Two studies have reported centiles for FMI and FFMI in the first 6 months after birth, one using DXA in term and preterm infants [35] and the other using Pea Pod in term infants [43]. However, neither study reported if these indices remained correlated with length, so it is unclear if the measures used adequately accounted for differences in body size. This problem can be overcome with the use of sex-specific FM and FFM z-scores for length [40].

Accuracy and reproducibility

Evaluation of any quantitative assessment technique, including body composition systems, comprises of an examination of its accuracy and reproducibility. Accuracy should be determined against an established criterion method that measures the same physical properties. Hydrostatic weighing is commonly used to validate ADP techniques, but this is not suitable for infants because it requires submerging them in water. Thus, for Pea Pod alternative techniques have been used, including tissue phantoms [17], deuterium dilution [18], DXA [44] and combined techniques with multi-compartment models [45].

Tissue phantoms are constructed from animal tissue using fat and muscle compartments, and the composition is usually determined from chemical analysis. DXA is a non-invasive technique that provides whole-body and regional estimates of three main components: bone mineral, bone-free FFM and FM [46]. DXA relies on the differential absorption of x-rays of two different energies and bone edge detection algorithms to calculate bone area and mineral content, and FM and FFM [46]. Isotope dilution, a standard technique for measuring total body water, involves administration of a known dose of isotope to a subject, allowing the isotope to equilibrate and enrich within the body water compartments (including saliva, urine or blood), and then measuring the isotope amount [47]. Isotope serves as a marker for total body water, from which FFM (using a specific hydration factor) and FM can be calculated [46].

Statistically, accuracy is commonly assessed by Bland-Altman analysis, [48] which relates the differences between two techniques to the mean value of the measures. Bias is the mean difference between the techniques and 95% of limits of agreement indicate the possible range of differences between the techniques. Reproducibility of paired measures can also be assessed by Bland-Altman analysis or for multiple measures of the same subject or phantom, by the coefficient of variation, which is the standard deviation as a percentage of the subject or phantom mean value.

Method

We performed a literature search covering studies published in PubMed from 2003 up to September 2017. Because the first evaluation study of Pea Pod was published in 2003 we limited our search strategy to include papers published after 2003 to September 2017. Key search terms included "air displacement plethysmography" OR "Pea Pod" AND (infant OR infancy). Reviews and non-English papers were excluded. We also excluded papers that included non-human species. However, those studies that used animal species to investigate the accuracy/reproducibility of Pea Pod were included.

Results

Our literature search identified 141 papers, including 13 non-human studies, three non-English papers, and 17 reviews, leaving 108 papers for title and abstract checking. Of these, 26 papers were excluded because they referred to Bod Pod ($n = 7$), reported a study protocol ($n = 5$), or were unrelated to Pea Pod ($n = 14$). Thus 82 papers were included in the final review, two of which were accuracy studies using animal tissues and live animals, four were accuracy/reproducibility studies in full-term infants, two were accuracy/reproducibility studies in pre-term infants, and 74 were clinical studies using Pea Pod to assess the body composition of either full-term infants, pre-term infants or both (Fig. 1). Characteristics of included validation studies are presented in Table 1.

Accuracy and reproducibility of pea pod

Studies using animal tissues and/or live animals

Accuracy As part of the development of Pea Pod, Sainz and colleagues [17] were the first to evaluate the accuracy of Pea Pod against chemical analysis and hydrostatic weighing of 24 bovine tissue phantoms, and to assess its potential use in paediatric body composition assessment. Tissue phantom mass (1.39 to 9.95 kg) and fat content (2.1% to 34.4%) approximated that of infants between birth and six months of age. Compared with chemical analysis, the bias for FM% was – 0.04% and was constant across the FM% range (indicating no systematic bias), and the 95% limits of agreement were – 1.22% to 1.13%. Frondas-Chauty et al. [44] compared Pea Pod measures of FM% with biochemical analysis in 12 piglets at 2 to 21 days of age (weight range 1.03 to 8.49 kg). Bland-Altman analysis showed 95% limits of agreement from – 4% to 3%.

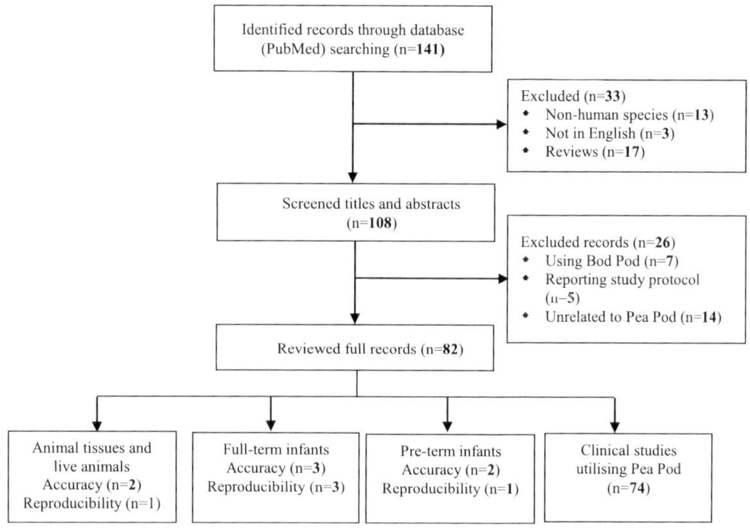

Fig. 1 Flow diagram of study selection process

Reproducibility Frondas-Chauty et al. also evaluated the reproducibility of Pea Pod in piglets (four measurements within one hour) [44]. Reproducibility was limited at low FM% (CV 14% to 32% at mean FM% of 3.7%) but better at higher FM% (CV 4% to 10% at mean FM% of 11.7%).

In summary, these studies suggest that Pea Pod has reasonable accuracy and reproducibility for FM% but reproducibility may be poor with lean body composition.

Studies in full-term infants

The accuracy and reproducibility of Pea Pod was examined in full-term infants by three studies each. All studies included both male and female infants. The accuracy studies included between 49 to 84 infants and the reproducibility studies from 17 to 36. The chronological age ranged from 0.4 to 24.6 weeks. The behavioural states [16, 18] and ethnicity [18, 45] were considered in two studies.

Accuracy Ma et al. [18] examined the accuracy of Pea Pod measures of FM% against deuterium dilution in full-term infants aged 0.4 to 24.4 weeks and weighing 2.7 to 7.4 kg. Limits of agreement (95%) for FM% were relatively wide (– 6.84% to 6.71%). The authors reported that the results were not influenced by infant behavioural state. Ellis et al. [45] evaluated Pea Pod against a four-compartment model in full-term infants at 2 to 17 weeks of age. There was no bias for FM% but the 95% limits of agreement were also wide (– 6.8% to 8.1%). In multiple regression analysis that included protein and hydration fractions, the mineral fraction of FFM was the only significant factor associated with differences in FM% between Pea Pod and the four-compartment reference model (R^2 16%, $P = 0.004$). Fields et al. [49] compared Pea Pod and DXA in 84 full-term infants at 6 months of age. There was bias for FM% of – 4% and 95% limits of agreement of – 8% to 0%. However, the bias was positively related to FM%, suggesting underestimation of FM% in infants with lower fat content.

Reproducibility The reproducibility (within and between days) of Pea Pod was examined in three studies [16, 18, 45]. Yao et al. studied 17 full-term infants aged between 1.4 to 21.7 weeks and reported that reproducibility was not affected by the infants' behavioural state, body weight, urination, defecation, or FM% [16]. The within and between day 95% limits of agreement for FM% were – 2.0 to 1.2 and – 2.2 to 1.7, respectively. Similarly, Ma et al. found that in infants aged between 0.4 to 21.7 weeks, 95% limits of agreement for between day differences in FM% were – 2.9% and 1.9%, and the within subject CV for FM% was 4.9% [18]. Reproducibility was not influenced by infants' behavioural state (awake and active, $N = 147$; crying intensely, $N = 74$; urination during the measurement, $N = 33$) or ethnicity (Asians, $N = 20$; white, $N = 16$). Finally, Ellis et al. [45] reported within day 95% limits of agreement for FM% of – 2.3% to 3.1% in 31 infants at a mean age of 6 weeks.

In summary, Pea Pod has reasonable reproducibility for FM% in full-term infants but only modest accuracy, with overestimation or underestimation of FM% by 6% to 8%. Although one DXA study suggested that Pea Pod systematically underestimates FM%, this not seen when referenced to other criterion measures. Studies included very few infants in the first week of life, so accuracy and reproducibility of Pea Pod in early neonatal period is unclear. Further, there are no data on the reproducibility

Table 1 Accuracy and reproducibility studies of Pea Pod in full-term and preterm infants

Reference	Country	Comparison methods	Inclusion/ Exclusion	Number (sex)	Number of tests	Age at measurement	Results
Animal and Animal Tissues							
Accuracy studies							
Sainz et al. (2003) [17]	The US	ADP, chemical analysis (CA), hydrostatic weighing	Bovine tissue with wide ranges of mass (1.39–9.95 kg) and FM% (2.08–34.40%)	24 bovine tissue phantoms (NA)	NR	NA	%Fat: ADP: 18.55% CA: 18.59% SD %fat ADP: 0.70% CA: 0.73% 95% LoA: −1.22-1. 13 %Fat
Frondas-Chauty et al. (2012) [44]	France	ADP, chemical analysis	Live piglets with wide ranges of mass (1.03–8.49 kg) and FM% (3.2–16.4%)	34 live piglets	NR	2, 7, and 21 days	%Fat: Pea Pod, 8.01 ± 4.03%; CA, 8.7 ± 4.1% Standard error of the estimate: 1.7% R^2: 0.83
Reproducibility studies							
Frondas-Chauty et al. (2012) [44]	France	ADP within a day	Live piglets (aa above)	34 live piglets	Four times	2, 7, and 21 days	CV: ranging from 2.2 to 44.1% Root mean square CV: 17.9% CV values and median differed by age and %fat assessed using CA, with less variability in piglets with higher %fat
Full-Term Infants							
Accuracy studies							
Ma et al. (2004) [18]	The US & China	ADP, deuterium dilution	Healthy f ull-term infants (mixed ethnicity; white and Chinese)	53 (28F, 25 M)	2 days and 2 tests on first day	5.8 (6.0) (0.4–24.4) wks	%fat Pea Pod: 20.32–6.87%; deuterium: 20.39–6.68 95% LoA: − 6.84-6.71% (not related to body mass)
Ellis et al. (2007) [45]	The US	ADP, 4-CM	Full term healthy infants (mixed ethnic groups; white, African American, Hispanic American)	49 (24F, 25 M)	Twice	8.0 (5.4) wks	%Fat Pea Pod: 16.9 (6.5), 4-CM: 16.3 (7.2) ($P = 0.62$) 95% LoA: − 6.8-8.1%
Fields et al. (2012) [49]	The US	Pea Pod, DXA	Full term singleton infants, average for gestational age and with gestational age > =37, staying in hospital less than 3 days after delivery. nfants with congenital malformation were excluded. (ethnicity nor reported)	84 (47F, 37 M)	NR	6 mo; 168.4 (3.8) days	%Fat Pea Pod: 26.7 (4.7), DXA: 31.3 (3.6), ($P < 0.001$)
Reproducibility studies							
Yao et al. (2003) [16]	The US	ADP within and between-days – data from multiple compartment studies of Butte et al. and Fomon et al	Full term healthy infants with weight ranging between 3.40–7.45 kg and age ranging between 1.40–21.70 weeks (ethnicity not reported)	17 (8F, 9 M)	2 days and 2 tests per only one day	1.40–21.70 weeks (all 3 tests);	%fat: ranging 7.49–32.08% SD %Fat within day: 0.52; between day: 0.60 CV %fat within day: 2.85; between day: 2.95 95% LoA within day: − 2.0-1.2%; between day: − 2.2-1.7% (not a function of behavioural state)
Ma et al. (2004) [18]	The US & China	ADP within and between days	Healthy full-term infants (mixed ethnicity; white and Chinese)	36 (16F, 20 M)	2 days and 2 tests on first day	7.6 (7.2) (0.4–21.7) wks	SD %fat within day: 0.69%; between day: 0.72% CV %fat within day: 4.94; between day: 5.10% 95% LoA within day: − 2.7-3.1%; between day: − 2.9-1.9 (not a function of body f atness)
Ellis et al. (2007) [45]	The US	ADP within day	Full term healthy infants (mixed ethnic groups; white, African American, Hispanic American)	31 (18F, 13 M)	Twice	6.0 (3.3) wks	SD %fat within: 0.7% CV %fat within: 7.9% 95% LoA: − 2.3-3.1%
Pre-Term Infants							
Accuracy studies							
Roggero et al. (2012)	Italy	Pea Pod, deuterium dilution	Preterm singleton infants with gestational age = < 36 weeks were included. Also term infants with gestational age > =37 were	10 (4F, 6 M)	NR	< 1 month	%fat Pea Pod: 5.67 (1.84), deuterium dilution: 5.99 (2.56), $P = 0.53$ 95% LoA: −3.4-2.76%

Table 1 Accuracy and reproducibility studies of Pea Pod in full-term and preterm infants *(Continued)*

Reference	Country	Comparison methods	Inclusion/ Exclusion	Number (sex)	Number of tests	Age at measurement	Results
[50]			included. Infants aged > 1 mo of age, with congenital diseases, chromosomal abnormalities, respiratory distress syndrome, or severe brain, metabolic, cardiac, or gastrointestinal diseases were excluded.				(not a function of mean values)
Forsum et al. (2016) [51]	Sweden	Pea Pod, deuterium dilution	Infants without sepsis or malformations born between 32 and 37 gestational weeks (ethnicity not reported)	14 (4F, 10 M)	NR	3–7 days old	%Fat Pea Pod: 4.2 (3.9), deuterium dilution 3.2 (3.8) ($P > 0.05$) 95% LoA: – 6.8-4.8% FFM density by Pea Pod did not correlate with those of deuterium dilution ($r^2 = 0.04$, $P > 0.05$) Hydration factor: 83%
Reproducibility studies							
Roggero et al. (2012) [50]	Italy	NA	Preterm singleton infants with gestational age = < 36 weeks were included. Also term infants with gestational age > =37 were included. Infants aged > 1 mo of age, with congenital diseases, chromosomal abnormalities, respiratory distress syndrome, or severe brain, metabolic, cardiac, or gastrointestinal diseases were excluded.	Precision: 57 (29F, 28 M) Inter-devise reproducibility: 9 full term and 3 preterm (6F, 6 M)	Twice	< 1 month	%Fat SD: 1.1 95% LoA: – 2.05-2.36% **Inter-device reproducibility:** %fat test 1: 8.97%, test 2: 8.55% 95% LoA: – 1.87-2.71

NA, not applicable; *ADP*, air displacement plethysmography; *CA*, chemical analysis; *SD*, standard deviation; *LoA*, limits of agreement; wks, weeks; *US*, united states; *CV*, coefficient of variation; *4-CM*, 4 compartment model; *DXA*, dual energy X-ray absorptiometry

and accuracy specifically in infants born small, large or appropriate for gestational age.

Studies in pre-term infants

Accuracy Only two studies have specifically evaluated the accuracy of Pea Pod in pre-term infants, both using isotope dilution (Table 1) [50, 51]. Roggero et al. referenced Pea Pod with a two-compartment model and included 10 pre-term infants (≤36 weeks) aged less than one month with mean (SD) weight of 1.83 (0.21) kg [50]. The 95% limits of agreement for FM% were – 3.4% to 2.8% with no bias [50]. Forsum et al. [51] measured 14 pre-term infants at 32 to 35 weeks of gestation in the first week with a mean (SD) weight of 2.04 (0.33) kg. Compared to a three-compartment model, the 95% limits of agreement were relatively wide (– 6.8% to 4.8%) but there was no bias. This study also showed that at higher FFM density, Pea Pod underestimated FFM density.

Reproducibility Roggero et al. [50] performed two consecutive Pea Pod measurements in 57 infants and the 95% limits of agreement were – 2.05% and 2.36%. They also compared measurements in 12 infants (3 preterm) using two Pea Pod devices in the same room and the inter-device 95% limits of agreement were – 1.87% and 2.71%.

In summary, there are few data on the validity of Pea Pod in preterm infants, but performance appears to be similar to full-term infants, that is, reasonable reproducibility but only modest accuracy.

Practical challenges of pea pod

Despite the above concerns about accuracy, Pea Pod has been considered a valuable tool with a broad clinical research application. We identified 74 papers utilising Pea Pod to answer research questions, including studies comparing different clinical groups (pre-term vs. full-term infants, small for gestational age vs. appropriate for gestational age, different ethnicities, different feeding methods and breast milk compositions, and different health status or health indicators) [33, 52–69], assessing growth charts, to cross-validate FM values obtained by other techniques and anthropometric measures (e.g. skinfold) [70–76], monitoring growth patterns [54, 77–80], investigating the relationship between maternal and prenatal factors and health outcomes during infancy [81–86], and others [87]. The majority of these studies ($n = 43$) included only full-term infants [33, 52–54, 56–58, 60, 62, 66, 67, 69–72, 74, 75, 78, 80, 81, 83–86, 88–106], 13 only pre-term infants [9, 68, 73, 77, 79, 107–112], and 17 both full- and pre-term infants [55, 59, 61, 63–65, 76, 82, 87, 113–120]. Although, the use of Pea Pod in both full-term and pre-term infants and in specific clinical risk and ethnic groups is feasible, it might be associated with some practical challenges. Herein, we highlight and discuss potential challenges associated with the use of Pea Pod.

Measuring body composition in Pea Pod involves the simultaneous weighing and measuring of length and body volume. Pea Pod assesses body composition considering an infant's anthropometric and demographic characteristics that are entered in to the Pea Pod system by personnel. As weight changes dramatically during early infancy, this information should be obtained consecutively with the Pea Pod test. Per the manufacturer manual, it is advised to conduct the Pea Pod test in duplicate to potentiate the accuracy. Repeat measures in infants might be associated with practical challenges and might require a third test which increases both researcher and caregiver burden. Out of 73 papers utilising Pea Pod, 13 reported repeated measurements, six of which reported duplicate tests [62, 67, 76, 85, 112, 114], six reported a third test if the results of the first two differed significantly [81, 102, 105, 116, 117, 120], and one reported three tests (performed on all subjects) [115], and the remaining studies that did not duplicate did not provide a rationale.

Furthermore, body moisture, temperature, and hair have been shown to significantly influence FM%, and underestimate it by 2% [121, 122]. Thus, Pea Pod testing should always be conducted at a moisture free and normal body temperature prior to measurement and in a resting state while wearing wig cap or smoothed hair using baby oil. Reproducibility studies have not suggested any effect of infant movement, crying, urination and defecation on the body composition measurements [18, 45], although the data are few.

The calibration process requires the placement of a hollow cylinder with known mass and volume into the Pea Pod. Mass and volume calibration should also be adjusted for any objects attached to the infants, which is mainly true for those remaining in hospital. Objects such as name bracelets and cord clamps affect body mass and volume readings and consequently FM and FFM. Some but not all studies reported adjusting for these objects [53, 58, 72, 76, 80, 89, 90, 98, 108]. Ramel et al. [108] also adjusted for other objects such as nasogastric tube and oximetry monitor.

Assessment of body composition by Pea Pod is not suitable for all infants. For example, Pea Pod is limited to infants weighing from 1 kg to 10 kg and with body volume > 1.85 L [14]. Infants who require oxygen, intravenous fluids and who are unstable also cannot easily undergo Pea Pod measurement. The inclusion/exclusion criteria of a large number of papers are based on these characteristics such as weight [9, 43, 55, 65, 71, 73, 78, 79, 88, 93, 108–111, 113, 114] and health condition [9, 33, 54, 61, 76, 77, 98, 100, 112, 123]).

Pea Pod accommodates infants weighing up to 10 kg (approximately six months of age), but the child and adult version of ADP (Bod Pod) only houses children aged ≥2 years. Unfortunately, use of ADP for the measurement of body composition in children aged 6 to 24 months has been shown to be inaccurate [124]. This leaves a large gap, from 6 months to 2 years, where body composition cannot be determined using ADP method. This is an important consideration for longitudinal research projects and may limit the applicability of ADP.

When infants with very low body fat content are measured in Pea Pod, the system may give errors and even a negative body fat content that is not physiologically plausible. Low body fat or negative body fat errors were reported in three studies [43, 80, 88], two of which were from Ethiopia [42, 76], in which 30 and 14 infants had to be excluded, respectively, and one from Australia [80], in which one infant was excluded. Similarly, spuriously high body fat content has also been reported in two studies [76, 80]. Carrberry et al. [80] reported excluding one infant – whose father was of Tongan ethnicity – due to a very high FM%, and Villar et al. [76] excluded three infants due to high FM% or FFM% (> 3 SD). These findings highlight the importance of considering measurement errors in preliminary sample size calculation by study investigators, particularly if a multiethnic population is under the investigation.

ADP devices operate under changing air temperature; for example, as an individual enters the test chamber the air temperature in the test chamber increases, resulting in different compressibility (adiabatic). However, the air in the thoracic cavity and near the surface of skin is isothermic and thus is more easily compressed (40%) than an equivalent volume of adiabatic air [125], which can affect FM readings. In adult ADP devices, thoracic gas volume is measured directly, but this is impractical in infants and young children. Thus, the thoracic gas volume is predicted based on infant weight, length and age. The prediction equation has been validated in full-term infants [126, 127], but its accuracy in pre-term infants and those with lung disease is unknown. Accordingly, Pea Pod measurements in infants with lung disease should be interpreted with caution because of altered thoracic gas volume.

To account for the skin surface artefact, the system software applies a correction factor based on body surface area. Body surface estimates are less accurate at the extremes of body size [128]. This might have implications for studies involving pre-term and growth restricted infants, and those born large for gestational age, such as with maternal diabetes.

The Pea Pod system calculates FM from body weight, volume and the density of FM and FFM. It is well documented that the density of fat mass is constant at 0. 9007 g/ml, though the density of FFM varies with age and physiological state. The FFM density estimates use in Pea Pod are derived from full-term infants [129]. Fomon et al. based their model on the measurements of protein, minerals and water in FFM [129], and Butte et al. on the measurements of body weight, body protein, bone minerals, and body water [130]. An important difference between these two models is the estimated amount of water (hydration factor) in FFM, which is lower in the Fomon model, specifically in the neonatal period (80.6% for both boys and girls at birth; 82.7% for boys and 83.1% for girls at two weeks, respectively) [129, 130]. Thus the Fomon model may produce FM values that are greater than those obtained using the Butte model. For example, Eriksson [91] reported a greater increase in FM% between one and 12 weeks of age when using the Butte model than the Fomon model. Consideration of the FFM model is important in longitudinal research i and when comparing results from different studies.

The hydration factor of FFM changes considerably during early infancy (particularly in pre-term infants) and can affect estimates of FFM and FM [131]. The Pea Pod system has algorithms to account the fluctuation in hydration in this period of life [51]. However, Forsum et al. [51] found that when compared to a three compartment model using isotope dilution, Pea Pod gave biased values for predicted FFM density in moderately pre-term infants (lower by 0.0019 ± 0.0058 g/ml). Biological variability in hydration factors may lead to variations in FFM density and consequently inaccurate body composition readings.

Conclusion and future lines of research

Pea Pod is a convenient a way to measure body composition in infants and may be useful for monitoring groups of infants but appears to have only modest accuracy in individual subjects. Multiple factors may affect accuracy, including body moisture and temperature, objects attached to infants, extremes of body size, thoracic gas prediction equations, FFM density, and fluctuations in FFM hydration factor. There are few data on the accuracy of Pea Pod in preterm infants and a reference body composition for pre-term infants is lacking. Further, the validity of Pea Pod in different clinical risk groups and ethnicities is unknown. Given these gaps in the current literature, the following are suggested as future lines of research:

1) Further validate pea pod in infants against the gold standard four compartment model, especially in pre-term infants and in more diverse populations.
2) Investigate the accuracy/reproducibility of Pea Pod in different birth weight for gestational age categories.
3) Investigate the impact of FFM hydration level and density in Pea Pod measurements.
4) Develop and validate specific prediction equations to estimate thoracic cavity gas in pre-term infants and more diverse infant populations.
5) Investigate the impact of body movement, urination, defecation, and lung disease on Pea Pod measurements.
6) Develop and design equipment working on the ADP principles that could accommodate children aged 6–24 months to support longitudinal research.
7) Develop a set of recommendations for complete and transparent reporting of study procedures when using Pea Pod.
8) Investigate the best body composition measure(s) that accurately predicts growth, nutritional status, obesity and health outcomes.
9) Establish body composition reference data or curves for both full-term and pre-term infants, such as FM/FFM for length z-scores.

Abbreviations

4-CM: 4 Compartment Model; ADP: Air displacement plethysmography; BIA: Bioelectrical Impedance Analysis; BMI: Body Mass Index; CR: Chemical Analysis; CV: Coefficient of variation; DXA: Dual Energy X-ray Absorptiometry; FFM: Fat Free Mass; FFMI: Fat Free Mass Index; FM: Fat Mass; FMI: Fat Mass Index; LM: Lean Mass; LoA: Limits of Agreement; MRI: Magnetic Resonance Imaging; NA: Not Applicable; NR: Not Reported; SD: Standard Deviation; US: United States

Acknowledgements

Not applicable.

Funding

Not applicable.

Authors' contributions

CAC and HM conceived the manuscript idea, HM researched and drafted the manuscript, CJDM, PRvH, BEC, and CAC reviewed and approved the final manuscript.

Competing interests

The authors declare that they have no competing interests.

Author details

[1]College of Health, Massey University, Auckland 0745, New Zealand. [2]Kidz First Neonatal Care, Counties Manukau Health, Auckland, New Zealand. [3]Liggins Institute and Department of Paediatrics: Child and Youth Health, University of Auckland, Auckland, New Zealand. [4]Starship Children's Hospital, Auckland District Health Board, Auckland, New Zealand.

References

1. Eriksson JG, Osmond C, Kajantie E, Forsen TJ, Barker DJ. Patterns of growth among children who later develop type 2 diabetes or its risk factors. Diabetologia. 2006;49(12):2853–8.
2. Osmond C, Barker DJ, Winter PD, Fall CH, Simmonds SJ. Early growth and death from cardiovascular disease in women. BMJ. 1993;307(6918):1519–24.
3. Franz AR, Pohlandt F, Bode H, Mihatsch WA, Sander S, Kron M, et al. Intrauterine, early neonatal, and postdischarge growth and neurodevelopmental outcome at 5.4 years in extremely preterm infants after intensive neonatal nutritional support. Pediatrics. 2009;123(1):e101–9.
4. Corpeleijn WE, Kouwenhoven SM, van Goudoever JB. Optimal growth of preterm infants. World Rev Nutr Diet. 2013;106:149–55.
5. Hemachandra AH, Howards PP, Furth SL, Klebanoff MA. Birth weight, postnatal growth, and risk for high blood pressure at 7 years of age: results from the collaborative perinatal project. Pediatrics. 2007;119(6):e1264–70.
6. Kerkhof GF, Willemsen RH, Leunissen RW, Breukhoven PE, Hokken-Koelega AC. Health profile of young adults born preterm: negative effects of rapid weight gain in early life. J Clin Endocrinol Metab. 2012;97(12):4498–506.
7. Ong KK, Kennedy K, Castaneda-Gutierrez E, Forsyth S, Godfrey KM, Koletzko B, et al. Postnatal growth in preterm infants and later health outcomes: a systematic review. Acta Paediatr. 2015;104(10):974–86.
8. Ramel SE, Gray HL, Christiansen E, Boys C, Georgieff MK, Demerath EW. Greater early gains in fat-free mass, but not fat mass, are associated with improved neurodevelopment at 1 year corrected age for prematurity in very low birth weight preterm infants. J Pediatr. 2016;173:108–15.
9. Pfister KM, Gray HL, Miller NC, Demerath EW, Georgieff MK, Ramel SE. Exploratory study of the relationship of fat-free mass to speed of brain processing in preterm infants. Pediatr Res. 2013;74(5):576–83.
10. Ay L, Hokken-Koelega AC, Mook-Kanamori DO, Hofman A, Moll HA, Mackenbach JP, et al. Tracking and determinants of subcutaneous fat mass in early childhood: the generation R study. Int J Obes. 2008;32(7):1050–9.
11. Demerath EW, Fields DA. Body composition assessment in the infant. Am J Hum Biol. 2014;26(3):291–304.
12. De Lucia Rolfe E, Modi N, Uthaya S, Hughes IA, Dunger DB, Acerini C, et al. Ultrasound estimates of visceral and subcutaneous-abdominal adipose tissues in infancy. J Obes. 2013;2013:9.
13. Lingwood BE. Bioelectrical impedance analysis for assessment of fluid status and body composition in neonates–the good, the bad and the unknown. Eur J Clin Nutr. 2013;67(Suppl 1):S28–33.
14. Urlando A, Dempster P, Aitkens S. A new air displacement plethysmograph for the measurement of body composition in infants. Pediatr Res. 2003;53(3):486–92.
15. Fidanza F, Keys A, Anderson JT. Density of body fat in man and other mammals. J Appl Physiol. 1953;6(4):252–6.
16. Yao M, Nommsen-Rivers L, Dewey K, Urlando A. Preliminary evaluation of a new pediatric air displacement plethysmograph for body composition assessment in infants. Acta Diabetol. 2003;40(Suppl 1):S55–8.
17. Sainz RD, Urlando A. Evaluation of a new pediatric air-displacement plethysmograph for body-composition assessment by means of chemical analysis of bovine tissue phantoms. Am J Clin Nutr. 2003;77(2):364–70.
18. Ma G, Yao M, Liu Y, Lin A, Zou H, Urlando A, et al. Validation of a new pediatric air-displacement plethysmograph for assessing body composition in infants. Am J Clin Nutr. 2004;79(4):653–60.
19. Fields DA, Gunatilake R, Kalaitzoglou E. Air displacement plethysmography: cradle to grave. Nutr Clin Pract. 2015;30(2):219–26.
20. Gianni ML, Roggero P, Orsi A, Piemontese P, Garbarino F, Bracco B, et al. Body composition changes in the first 6 months of life according to method of feeding. J Hum Lact. 2014;30(2):148–55.
21. Brozek J, Grande F, Anderson JT, Keys A. Densitometric analysis of body composition: revision of some quantitative assumptions. Ann N Y Acad Sci. 1963;110:113–40.
22. Withers RT, Laforgia J, Heymsfield SB. Critical appraisal of the estimation of body composition via two-, three-, and four-compartment models. Am J Hum Biol. 1999;11(2):175–85.
23. Fuller NJ, Jebb SA, Laskey MA, Coward WA, Elia M. Four-component model for the assessment of body composition in humans: comparison with alternative methods, and evaluation of the density and hydration of fat-free mass. Clin Sci (Lond). 1992;82(6):687–93.
24. Nagayama D, Imamura H, Sato Y, Yamaguchi T, Ban N, Kawana H, et al. Inverse relationship of cardioankle vascular index with BMI in healthy Japanese subjects: a cross-sectional study. Vasc Health Risk Manag. 2017;13: 1–9.
25. Flegal KM, Kit BK, Orpana H, Graubard BI. Association of all-cause mortality with overweight and obesity using standard body mass index categories: a systematic review and meta-analysis. JAMA. 2013;309(1):71–82.
26. Gallagher D, Visser M, Sepulveda D, Pierson RN, Harris T, Heymsfield SB. How useful is body mass index for comparison of body fatness across age, sex, and ethnic groups? Am J Epidemiol. 1996;143(3):228–39.
27. Zeng Q, Dong S-Y, Sun X-N, Xie J, Cui Y. Percent body fat is a better predictor of cardiovascular risk factors than body mass index. Braz J Med Biol Res. 2012;45(7):591–600.
28. Romero-Corral A, Somers VK, Sierra-Johnson J, Korenfeld Y, Boarin S, Korinek J, et al. Normal weight obesity: a risk factor for cardiometabolic dysregulation and cardiovascular mortality. Eur Heart J. 2010;31(6):737–46.
29. Lawlor DA, Benfield L, Logue J, Tilling K, Howe LD, Fraser A, et al. Association between general and central adiposity in childhood, and change in these, with cardiovascular risk factors in adolescence: prospective cohort study. BMJ. 2010;341:c6224.
30. Javed A, Jumean M, Murad MH, Okorodudu D, Kumar S, Somers VK, et al. Diagnostic performance of body mass index to identify obesity as defined by body adiposity in children and adolescents: a systematic review and meta-analysis. Pediatr Obes. 2015;10(3):234–44.
31. Hetherington-Rauth M, Bea JW, Lee VR, Blew RM, Funk J, Lohman TG, et al. Comparison of direct measures of adiposity with indirect measures for assessing cardiometabolic risk factors in preadolescent girls. Nutr J. 2017;16:15.
32. Addo OY, Himes JH. Are field measures of adiposity sufficient to establish fatness-related linkages with metabolic outcomes in adolescents? Eur J Clin Nutr. 2014;68(6):671–6.
33. De Cunto A, Paviotti G, Ronfani L, Travan L, Bua J, Cont G, et al. Can body mass index accurately predict adiposity in newborns? Arch Dis Child Fetal Neonatal Ed. 2014;99(3):F238–9.
34. Cooke RJ, Griffin I. Altered body composition in preterm infants at hospital discharge. Acta Paediatr. 2009;98(8):1269–73.
35. Goswami I, Rochow N, Fusch G, Liu K, Marrin ML, Heckmann M, et al. Length normalized indices for fat mass and fat-free mass in preterm and term infants during the first six months of life. Nutrients. 2016;8(7):417.
36. Wells JC. A critique of the expression of paediatric body composition data. Arch Dis Child. 2001;85(1):67–72.
37. Wells JCK. Toward body composition reference data for infants, children, and adolescents. Adv Nutr. 2014;5(3):320S–9S.
38. Weber DR, Moore RH, Leonard MB, Zemel BS. Fat and lean BMI reference curves in children and adolescents and their utility in identifying excess adiposity compared with BMI and percentage body fat. Am J Clin Nutr. 2013;98(1):49–56.
39. VanItallie TB, Yang MU, Heymsfield SB, Funk RC, Boileau RA. Height-normalized indices of the body's fat-free mass and fat mass: potentially useful indicators of nutritional status. Am J Clin Nutr. 1990;52(6):953–9.
40. Wells JC, Cole TJ. Adjustment of fat-free mass and fat mass for height in children aged 8 y. Int J Obes Relat Metab Disord. 2002;26(7):947–52.
41. Liu P, Ma F, Lou H, Liu Y. The utility of fat mass index vs. body mass index and percentage of body fat in the screening of metabolic syndrome. BMC Public Health. 2013;13:629.
42. Peltz G, Aguirre MT, Sanderson M, Fadden MK. The role of fat mass index in determining obesity. Am J Hum Biol. 2010;22(5):639–47.
43. Andersen GS, Girma T, Wells JC, Kaestel P, Leventi M, Hother AL, et al. Body composition from birth to 6 mo of age in Ethiopian infants: reference data obtained by air-displacement plethysmography. Am J Clin Nutr. 2013;98(4):885–94.
44. Frondas-Chauty A, Louveau I, Le Huerou-Luron I, Roze JC, Darmaun D. Air-displacement plethysmography for determining body composition in neonates: validation using live piglets. Pediatr Res. 2012;72(1):26–31.
45. Ellis KJ, Yao M, Shypailo RJ, Urlando A, Wong WW, Heird WC. Body-composition assessment in infancy: air-displacement plethysmography compared with a reference 4-compartment model. Am J Clin Nutr. 2007;85(1):90–5.
46. Wells JCK, Fewtrell MS. Measuring body composition. Arch Dis Child. 2006; 91(7):612–7.
47. Davies PS, Wells JC. Calculation of total body water in infancy. Eur J Clin Nutr. 1994;48(7):490–5.
48. Bland JM, Altman DG. Statistical methods for assessing agreement between two methods of clinical measurement. Lancet. 1986;1(8476):307–10.

49. Fields DA, Demerath EW, Pietrobelli A, Chandler-Laney PC. Body composition at 6 months of life: comparison of air displacement plethysmography and dual-energy X-ray absorptiometry. Obesity (Silver Spring). 2012;20(11):2302–6.
50. Roggero P, Gianni ML, Amato O, Piemontese P, Morniroli D, Wong WW, et al. Evaluation of air-displacement plethysmography for body composition assessment in preterm infants. Pediatr Res. 2012;72(3):316–20.
51. Forsum E, Olhager E, Törnqvist C. An evaluation of the pea pod system for assessing body composition of moderately premature infants. Nutrients. 2016;8(4):238.
52. Au CP, Raynes-Greenow CH, Turner RM, Carberry AE, Jeffery HE. Body composition is normal in term infants born to mothers with well-controlled gestational diabetes mellitus. Diabetes Care. 2013;36(3):562–4.
53. Donnelley EL, Raynes-Greenow CH, Turner RM, Carberry AE, Jeffery HE. Antenatal predictors and body composition of large-for-gestational-age newborns: perinatal health outcomes. J Perinatol. 2014;34(9):698–704.
54. Gianni ML, Roggero P, Morlacchi L, Garavaglia E, Piemontese P, Mosca F. Formula-fed infants have significantly higher fat-free mass content in their bodies than breastfed babies. Acta Paediatr. 2014;103(7):e277–81.
55. Gianni ML, Roggero P, Taroni F, Liotto N, Piemontese P, Mosca F. Adiposity in small for gestational age preterm infants assessed at term equivalent age. Arch Dis Child Fetal Neonatal Ed. 2009;94(5): F368–72.
56. Hull HR, Dinger MK, Knehans AW, Thompson DM, Fields DA. Impact of maternal body mass index on neonate birthweight and body composition. Am J Obstet Gynecol. 2008;198(4):416 e1–6.
57. Josefson JL, Zeiss DM, Rademaker AW, Metzger BE. Maternal leptin predicts adiposity of the neonate. Horm Res Paediatr. 2014;81(1):13–9.
58. Lampl M, Lee W, Koo W, Frongillo EA, Barker DJ, Romero R. Ethnic differences in the accumulation of fat and lean mass in late gestation. Am J Hum Biol. 2012;24(5):640–7.
59. Law TL, Korte JE, Katikaneni LD, Wagner CL, Ebeling MD, Newman RB. Ultrasound assessment of intrauterine growth restriction: relationship to neonatal body composition. Am J Obstet Gynecol. 2011;205(3):255 e1–6.
60. Lee W, Balasubramaniam M, Deter RL, Hassan SS, Gotsch F, Kusanovic JP, et al. Fetal growth parameters and birth weight: their relationship to neonatal body composition. Ultrasound Obstet Gynecol. 2009;33(4):441–6.
61. Paviotti G, De Cunto A, Travan L, Bua J, Cont G, Demarini S. Longitudinal growth and body composition of twins versus singletons in the first month of life. Sci World J. 2013;2013:108189.
62. Stanfield KM, Wells JC, Fewtrell MS, Frost C, Leon DA. Differences in body composition between infants of south Asian and European ancestry: the London mother and baby study. Int J Epidemiol. 2012;41(5):1409–18.
63. De Cunto A, Paviotti G, Travan L, Bua J, Cont G, Demarini S. Impact of surgery for neonatal gastrointestinal diseases on weight and fat mass. J Pediatr. 2015;167(3):568–71.
64. Roggero P, Gianni ML, Forzenigo L, Tondolo T, Taroni F, Liotto N, et al. No relative increase in intra-abdominal adipose tissue in healthy unstressed preterm infants at term. Neonatology. 2015;107(1):14–9.
65. Ramel SE, Gray HL, Ode KL, Younge N, Georgieff MK, Demerath EW. Body composition changes in preterm infants following hospital discharge: comparison with term infants. J Pediatr Gastroenterol Nutr. 2011;53(3):333–8.
66. Bartok CJ. Babies fed breastmilk by breast versus by bottle: a pilot study evaluating early growth patterns. Breastfeed Med. 2011;6(3):117–24.
67. Rudolph MC, Young BE, Lemas DJ, Palmer CE, Hernandez TL, Barbour LA, et al. Early infant adipose deposition is positively associated with the n-6 to n-3 fatty acid ratio in human milk independent of maternal BMI. Int J Obes (2005). 2017;41(4):510–7.
68. Gianni ML, Consonni D, Liotto N, Roggero P, Morlacchi L, Piemontese P, et al. Does human milk modulate body composition in late preterm infants at term-corrected age? Nutrients. 2016;8(10):664.
69. Breij LM, Mulder MT, van Vark-van der Zee LC, Hokken-Koelega ACS. Appetite-regulating hormones in early life and relationships with type of feeding and body composition in healthy term infants. Eur J Nutr. 2017;56(4):1725–32.
70. Andres A, Gomez-Acevedo H, Badger TM. Quantitative nuclear magnetic resonance to measure fat mass in infants and children. Obesity (Silver Spring). 2011;19(10):2089–95.
71. Aris IM, Soh SE, Tint MT, Liang S, Chinnadurai A, Saw SM, et al. Body fat in Singaporean infants: development of body fat prediction equations in Asian newborns. Eur J Clin Nutr. 2013;67(9):922–7.
72. Carberry AE, Raynes-Greenow CH, Turner RM, Jeffery HE. Customized versus population-based birth weight charts for the detection of neonatal growth and perinatal morbidity in a cross-sectional study of term neonates. Am J Epidemiol. 2013;178(8):1301–8.
73. Law TL, Katikaneni LD, Taylor SN, Korte JE, Ebeling MD, Wagner CL, et al. Customized versus population-based growth curves: prediction of low body fat percent at term corrected gestational age following preterm birth. J Matern Fetal Neonatal Med. 2012;25(7):1142–7.
74. Lingwood BE, Storm Van Leeuwen AM, Carberry AE, Fitzgerald EC, Callaway LK, Colditz PB, et al. Prediction of fat-free mass and percentage of body fat in neonates using bioelectrical impedance analysis and anthropometric measures: validation against the PEA POD. Br J Nutr. 2012;107(10):1545–52.
75. Cauble JS, Dewi M, Hull HR. Validity of anthropometric equations to estimate infant fat mass at birth and in early infancy. BMC Pediatr. 2017;17:88.
76. Villar J, Puglia FA, Fenton TR, Cheikh Ismail L, Staines-Urias E, Giuliani F, et al. Body composition at birth and its relationship with neonatal anthropometric ratios: the newborn body composition study of the INTERGROWTH-21(st) project. Pediatr Res. 2017;82(2):305–16.
77. Gianni ML, Roggero P, Liotto N, Amato O, Piemontese P, Morniroli D, et al. Postnatal catch-up fat after late preterm birth. Pediatr Res. 2012;72(6):637–40.
78. Roggero P, Gianni ML, Orsi A, Piemontese P, Amato O, Moioli C, et al. Neonatal period: body composition changes in breast-fed full-term newborns. Neonatology. 2010;97(2):139–43.
79. Roggero P, Gianni ML, Liotto N, Taroni F, Orsi A, Amato O, et al. Rapid recovery of fat mass in small for gestational age preterm infants after term. PLoS One. 2011;6(1):e14489.
80. Carberry AE, Colditz PB, Lingwood BE. Body composition from birth to 4.5 months in infants born to non-obese women. Pediatr Res. 2010;68(1):84–8.
81. Shapiro ALB, Boyle KE, Dabelea D, Patinkin ZW, De la Houssaye B, Ringham BM, et al. Nicotinamide promotes Adipogenesis in umbilical cord-derived mesenchymal stem cells and is associated with neonatal adiposity: the healthy start BabyBUMP project. PLoS One. 2016;11(7): e0159575.
82. Shapiro ALB, Kaar JL, Crume TL, Starling AP, Siega-Riz AM, Ringham BM, et al. Maternal diet quality in pregnancy and neonatal adiposity: the healthy start study. Inter J Obes (2005). 2016;40(7):1056–62.
83. Kizirian NV, Markovic TP, Muirhead R, Brodie S, Garnett SP, Louie JCY, et al. Macronutrient balance and dietary glycemic index in pregnancy predict neonatal body composition. Nutrients. 2016;8(5):270.
84. Castro NP, Euclydes VV, Simões FA, Vaz-de-Lima LRA, De Brito CA, Luzia LA, et al. The relationship between maternal plasma leptin and adiponectin concentrations and newborn adiposity. Nutrients. 2017;9(3):182.
85. Lemas DJ, Young BE, Baker PR, Tomczik AC, Soderborg TK, Hernandez TL, et al. Alterations in human milk leptin and insulin are associated with early changes in the infant intestinal microbiome. Am J Clin Nutr. 2016;103(5):1291–300.
86. MacDonald TM, Hui L, Tong S, Robinson AJ, Dane KM, Middleton AL, et al. Reduced growth velocity across the third trimester is associated with placental insufficiency in fetuses born at a normal birthweight: a prospective cohort study. BMC Med. 2017;15:164.
87. Piyasena C, Cartier J, Provençal N, Wiechmann T, Khulan B, Sunderasan R, et al. Dynamic changes in dna methylation occur during the first year of life in preterm infants. Front Endocrinol. 2016;7:158.
88. Andersen GS, Girma T, Wells JC, Kaestel P, Michaelsen KF, Friis H. Fat and fat-free mass at birth: air displacement plethysmography measurements on 350 Ethiopian newborns. Pediatr Res. 2011;70(5):501–6.
89. Au CP, Raynes-Greenow CH, Turner RM, Carberry AE, Jeffery H. Fetal and maternal factors associated with neonatal adiposity as measured by air displacement plethysmography: a large cross-sectional study. Early Hum Dev. 2013;89(10):839–43.
90. Carberry AE, Raynes-Greenow CH, Turner RM, Askie LM, Jeffery HE. Is body fat percentage a better measure of undernutrition in newborns than birth weight percentiles? Pediatr Res. 2013;74(6):730–6.
91. Eriksson B, Lof M, Forsum E. Body composition in full-term healthy infants measured with air displacement plethysmography at 1 and 12 weeks of age. Acta Paediatr. 2010;99(4):563–8.
92. Estampador AC, Pomeroy J, Renstrom F, Nelson SM, Mogren I, Persson M, et al. Infant body composition and adipokine concentrations in relation to maternal gestational weight gain. Diabetes Care. 2014;37(5):1432–8.
93. Fields DA, Gilchrist JM, Catalano PM, Gianni ML, Roggero PM, Mosca F. Longitudinal body composition data in exclusively breast-fed infants: a multicenter study. Obesity (Silver Spring). 2011;19(9):1887–91.

94. Henriksson P, Lof M, Forsum E. Glucose homeostasis variables in pregnancy versus maternal and infant body composition. Nutrients. 2015;7(7):5615–27.
95. Henriksson P, Lof M, Forsum E. Parental fat-free mass is related to the fat-free mass of infants and maternal fat mass is related to the fat mass of infant girls. Acta Paediatr. 2015;104(5):491–7.
96. Josefson JL, Feinglass J, Rademaker AW, Metzger BE, Zeiss DM, Price HE, et al. Maternal obesity and vitamin D sufficiency are associated with cord blood vitamin D insufficiency. J Clin Endocrinol Metab. 2013;98(1):114–9.
97. Josefson JL, Hoffmann JA, Metzger BE. Excessive weight gain in women with a normal pre-pregnancy BMI is associated with increased neonatal adiposity. Pediatr Obes. 2013;8(2):e33–6.
98. Lee W, Riggs T, Koo W, Deter RL, Yeo L, Romero R. The relationship of newborn adiposity to fetal growth outcome based on birth weight or the modified neonatal growth assessment score. J Matern Fetal Neonatal Med. 2012;25(10):1933–40.
99. Moyer-Mileur LJ, Slater H, Thomson JA, Mihalopoulos N, Byrne J, Varner MW. Newborn adiposity measured by plethysmography is not predicted by late gestation two-dimensional ultrasound measures of fetal growth. J Nutr. 2009;139(9):1772–8.
100. Ode KL, Gray HL, Ramel SE, Georgieff MK, Demerath EW. Decelerated early growth in infants of overweight and obese mothers. J Pediatr. 2012;161(6):1028–34.
101. Hawkes CP, Hourihane JOB, Kenny LC, Irvine AD, Kiely M, Murray DM. Gender- and gestational age–specific body fat percentage at birth. Pediatrics. 2011;128(3):e645–51.
102. Starling AP, Brinton JT, Glueck DH, Shapiro AL, Harrod CS, Lynch AM, et al. Associations of maternal BMI and gestational weight gain with neonatal adiposity in the healthy start study. Am J Clin Nutr. 2015;101(2):302–9.
103. Pereira-da-Silva L, Cabo C, Moreira AC, Virella D, Guerra T, Camoes T, et al. The adjusted effect of maternal body mass index, energy and macronutrient intakes during pregnancy, and gestational weight gain on body composition of full-term neonates. Am J Perinatol. 2014;31(10):875–82.
104. Pereira-da-Silva L, Cabo C, Moreira AC, Papoila AL, Virella D, Neves R, et al. The effect of long-chain polyunsaturated fatty acids intake during pregnancy on adiposity of healthy full-term offspring at birth. J Perinatol. 2015;35(3):177–80.
105. Sauder KA, Koeppen HJ, Shapiro ALB, Kalata KE, Stamatoiu AV, Ringham BM, et al. Prenatal vitamin d intake, cord blood 25-hydroxyvitamin d, and offspring body composition: the healthy start study. Nutrients. 2017;9(7):790.
106. Josefson JL, Simons H, Zeiss DM, Metzger BE. Excessive gestational weight gain in the first trimester among women with normal glucose tolerance and resulting neonatal adiposity. J Perinatol. 2016;36(12):1034–8.
107. Meyers JM, Greecher CP, Shaffer ML, Shenberger JS. Potential influence of total parenteral nutrition on body composition at discharge in preterm infants. J Matern Fetal Neonatal Med. 2013;26(15):1548–53.
108. Ramel SE, Gray HL, Davern BA, Demerath EW. Body composition at birth in preterm infants between 30 and 36 weeks gestation. Pediatr Obes. 2015; 10(1):45–51.
109. Roggero P, Gianni ML, Amato O, Liotto N, Morlacchi L, Orsi A, et al. Growth and fat-free mass gain in preterm infants after discharge: a randomized controlled trial. Pediatrics. 2012;130(5):e1215–21.
110. Roggero P, Gianni ML, Amato O, Orsi A, Piemontese P, Puricelli V, et al. Influence of protein and energy intakes on body composition of formula-fed preterm infants after term. J Pediatr Gastroenterol Nutr. 2008;47(3):375–8.
111. Roggero P, Gianni ML, Orsi A, Amato O, Piemontese P, Liotto N, et al. Implementation of nutritional strategies decreases postnatal growth restriction in preterm infants. PLoS One. 2012;7(12):e51166.
112. Simon L, Frondas-Chauty A, Senterre T, Flamant C, Darmaun D, Roze JC. Determinants of body composition in preterm infants at the time of hospital discharge. Am J Clin Nutr. 2014;100(1):98–104.
113. Olhager E, Tornqvist C. Body composition in late preterm infants in the first 10 days of life and at full term. Acta Paediatr. 2014;103(7):737–43.
114. Simon L, Borrego P, Darmaun D, Legrand A, Roze JC, Chauty-Frondas A. Effect of sex and gestational age on neonatal body composition. Br J Nutr. 2013;109(6):1105–8.
115. Crume TL, Shapiro AL, Brinton JT, Glueck DH, Martinez M, Kohn M, et al. Maternal fuels and metabolic measures during pregnancy and neonatal body composition: the healthy start study. J Clin Endocrinol Metab. 2015; 100(4):1672–80.
116. Harrod CS, Fingerlin TE, Chasan-Taber L, Reynolds RM, Glueck DH, Dabelea D. Exposure to prenatal smoking and early-life body composition: the healthy start study. Obesity (Silver Spring). 2015;23(1):234–41.
117. Harrod CS, Reynolds RM, Chasan-Taber L, Fingerlin TE, Glueck DH, Brinton JT, et al. Quantity and timing of maternal prenatal smoking on neonatal body composition: the healthy start study. J Pediatr. 2014;165(4):707–12.
118. Henriksson P, Lof M, Soderkvist P, Forsum E. Variation in the fat mass and obesity-related (FTO) genotype is not associated with body fatness in infants, but possibly with their length. Pediatr Obes. 2014;9(5):e112–5.
119. O'Donovan SM, Murray DM, Hourihane JOB, Kenny LC, Irvine AD, Kiely M. Cohort profile: the Cork BASELINE birth cohort study: babies after SCOPE: evaluating the longitudinal impact on neurological and nutritional endpoints. Inter J Epidemiol. 2015;44(3):764–75.
120. Starling AP, Shapiro ALB, Sauder KA, Kaar JL, Ringham BM, Glueck DH, et al. Blood pressure during pregnancy, neonatal size and altered body composition: the healthy start study. J Perinatol. 2017;37(5):502–6.
121. Fields DA, Higgins PB, Hunter GR. Assessment of body composition by air-displacement plethysmography: influence of body temperature and moisture. Dyn Med. 2004;3(1):3.
122. Higgins PB, Fields DA, Hunter GR, Gower BA. Effect of scalp and facial hair on air displacement plethysmography estimates of percentage of body fat. Obes Res. 2001;9(5):326–30.
123. Gianni ML, Roggero P, Piemontese P, Morlacchi L, Bracco B, Taroni F, et al. Boys who are born preterm show a relative lack of fat-free mass at 5 years of age compared to their peers. Acta Paediatr. 2015;104(3):e119–23.
124. Rosendale RP, Bartok CJ. Air-displacement plethysmography for the measurement of body composition in children aged 6-48 months. Pediatr Res. 2012;71(3):299–304.
125. Dempster P, Aitkens S. A new air displacement method for the determination of human body composition. Med Sci Sports Exerc. 1995; 27(12):1692–7.
126. Higgins PB, Silva AM, Sardinha LB, Hull HR, Goran MI, Gower BA, et al. Validity of new child-specific thoracic gas volume prediction equations for air-displacement plethysmography. BMC Pediatr. 2006;6(1):1–8.
127. Fields DA, Hull HR, Cheline AJ, Yao M, Higgins PB. Child-specific thoracic gas volume prediction equations for air-displacement plethysmography. Obes Res. 2004;12(11):1797–804.
128. Collins AL, McCarthy HD. Evaluation of factors determining the precision of body composition measurements by air displacement plethysmography. Eur J Clin Nutr. 2003;57(6):770–6.
129. Fomon SJ, Haschke F, Ziegler EE, Nelson SE. Body composition of reference children from birth to age 10 years. Am J Clin Nutr. 1982;35(5 Suppl):1169–75.
130. Butte NF, Hopkinson JM, Wong WW, Smith EO, Ellis KJ. Body composition during the first 2 years of life: an updated reference. Pediatr Res. 2000;47(5): 578–85.
131. Rodriguez G, Ventura P, Samper MP, Moreno L, Sarria A, Perez-Gonzalez JM. Changes in body composition during the initial hours of life in breast-fed healthy term newborns. Biol Neonate. 2000;77(1):12–6.

Determinants of choice of skilled antenatal care service providers in Ghana: analysis of demographic and health survey

Kwamena Sekyi Dickson[1*], Eugene Kofuor Maafo Darteh[1], Akwasi Kumi-Kyereme[1] and Bright Opoku Ahinkorah[2]

Abstract

Background: The International Safe Motherhood initiative provides a focus for programmes and research to improve maternal health in low – income countries. Antenatal care is one of the key pillars of the initiative. This study sought to examine the association between background characteristics and choice of skilled providers of antenatal care services in Ghana.

Methods: The study used data from the six rounds of the Ghana Demographic and Health Survey (GDHS). Binary logistic regression models were applied to analyse the data.

Results: Results show that the proportion of women who received antenatal care (ANC) services from skilled providers improved over the period. Also, women with secondary education (OR = 1.42, CI = 1.07–1.88), richest wealth status (OR = 5.10, CI = 2.28–11.85) were more likely to utilise antenatal care services from skilled providers. Whereas women from rural areas (OR = 0.55, CI = 0.41–0.74), with four births or more (OR = 0.55, CI = 0.36–0.85) and from the northern ethnic group were less likely to utilise antenatal care services from skilled providers.

Conclusion: Choice of skilled providers of antenatal care services were predicted by some predisposing factors including education, ethnicity, and ecological zone. Also enabling factors such as wealth status, residence and the need for care factor, parity predicted choice of skilled providers of antenatal care services. Women with secondary or higher education, those within richer and richest wealth status, those from forest zone are more likely to utilise the services of skilled providers during their antenatal care visits. Whereas women from rural areas, those with four births or more and those with the northern ethnic group were more likely to utilise ANC service from unskilled providers. The Ghana Health Service and Ministry of Health should encourage women in rural areas to utilise antenatal care services from skilled providers through social and behaviour change communication campaigns.

Keywords: Skilled providers, Antenatal care services, Utilisation, Women, Ghana

Background

Pregnancy is potentially risky for all women worldwide and millions of women who survive this, experience a form of illness and/or disability related to pregnancy and childbirth [1]. Around the world, complications due to pregnancy and childbearing result in about 830 deaths among women every day and about 303,000 women died during and after pregnancy and childbirth between 1990 and 2015 [2]. In developing countries, maternal mortality ratio in 2015 was 239 per 100,000 live births compared to 12 per 100,000 live births in developed countries [2]. In Africa, dying from complications from pregnancy-related causes during a woman's' lifetime is 1 in 40 compared to 1 in 3300 in Europe and 1 in 190 globally [3]. Ninety-nine percent of these deaths occur in developing countries which can be avoided; as the necessary interventions already exist [4]. In sub-Saharan Africa, several countries halved their maternal mortality rates since 1990 [4]. In other regions like Asia and North Africa, the rates of maternal mortality are even much lower, resulting in a 2.3% decline in the global maternal mortality

* Correspondence: nadicx@gmail.com
[1]Department of Population and Health, University of Cape Coast, Cape Coast, Ghana
Full list of author information is available at the end of the article

ratio [5]. However, in Ghana, maternal mortality ratio increased from 173 in 2011 [6] to 380 in 2014 [4].

The health of women during pregnancy became an immense concern in the early 1980s due to the high maternal mortality ratios [7]. This is because the care given to women during pregnancy provides interventions that enhance maternal health and survival during the period immediately before and after childbirth [8]. This led to the commencement of the safe motherhood programme. The International Safe Motherhood initiation was launched in Nairobi, Kenya in 1987 and provided a focus for programmes and research concerned with the improvement of maternal health in low – income countries. The safe motherhood programme provides awareness, educational support for the women on screening programs and identifies the problems that make the pregnancy high risk [9]. Antenatal care was one of the key pillars of the safe motherhood [7].

Antenatal Care (ANC) Service has been identified by the World Health Organisation (WHO) as an indicator of maternal health that could be used to help reduce maternal mortality ratios [10]. It is a type of preventative care with the aim of providing regular check-ups that offer doctors or midwives the opportunity to treat and prevent potential health problems throughout the course of the pregnancy while promoting healthy lifestyles that benefit both mother and child [11]. It provides pregnant women and their families with advice and information on health promotion, and preventive health services including the management of a healthy pregnancy, safe childbirth, nutritional support, early exclusive breastfeeding and encouraging assisted delivery [12, 13]. The ultimate aim of ANC is to achieve healthy babies and healthy mothers at the end of pregnancy [14].

The World Health Organisation (WHO) as part of its principles underlying antenatal care advocates that antenatal care should be provided by a health care provider - a skilled attendant. A skilled attendant is explained by WHO as a qualified health professional such as a midwife, doctor or nurse who is trained and educated with expertise to manage normal pregnancies and identify and provide referral for complex problems in women and newborn [15]. Globally, nine out of every ten pregnant women access antenatal care from skilled personnel at least once, only six out of ten access at least four antenatal visits from a skilled provider. In regions where the rates of maternal mortality are high, such as sub–Saharan Africa even fewer women obtain at least four antenatal visits from skilled providers - 49% which is less than the global average [16]. There is also evidence that some pregnant women do not utilise antenatal care services from any provider [17–22]. What factors influence pregnant women to utilise antenatal care from skilled providers?

Using the health care service utilisation model, the current study examines the factors that influence antenatal care services utilisation from skilled providers in Ghana over the period from 1988 to 2014. It contributes to the discourse on skilled providers of antenatal care services in Ghana by examining the factors that influence the use of skilled providers in antenatal care services in Ghana.

Conceptual framework

The Health Care Services Utilisation Model is a behavioural model proposed by Anderson in the 1960s to explain the conditions that either promote or hinder the utilisation of health care services [23]. This model identified three main conditions or factors that influence an individual to or not use a health care service as in Fig. 1. These factors are the predisposing factors; enabling factors and need for care factors.

Predisposing factors refer to the demographic, social structure and health belief characteristics of an individual. The demographic characteristics of the individual affect an individual's decision to use or not use a health care service. The characteristics may include the sex of the individual, the age, and the marital status of the individual. Social Structure consists of education, ethnicity and occupation and health belief factors consist of values, attitudes of health care service providers, and knowledge about health.

Enabling factors are the resources or means that are available to an individual to seek health care services. Enabling factors are measured at the household level

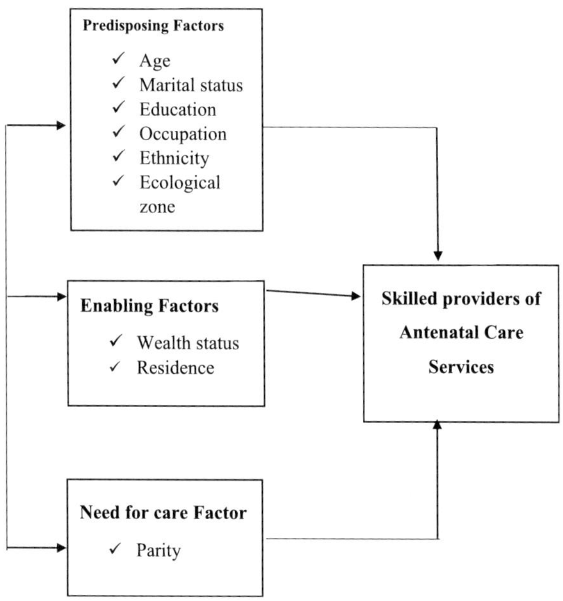

Fig. 1 Health service utilisation model. Predisposing factors, enabling factors, need for care factors, Skilled providers of antenatal care

and include the availability of income and the community level they include the availability and location of health care facilities in the community. Need for care factors refer to how an individual's perceive their own general health and functional condition, as well as their familiarity with the signs and symptoms of ill health, agony and concerns about their health [24].

The strength of the model lies in the fact that it looks at the direct factors that lead to the utilisation of health care services. Specifically, it looks at the individual characteristics and the resources or means available to seek health care services. Amid the strength of the health care service utilisation model is that the model embraces both material and structural factors which are scarcely taken into consideration in the social psychological model [25]. The model has been used to compare childhood morbidity and health service utilisation across six countries using the Demographic and Health Survey [26].

The variables used as predisposing factors for the study were age, marital status, education, occupation, ethnicity and ecological zone. Wealth status and residence were also used as enabling factors and parity was used as need for care factor.

Methods

Data sources

The Ghana Demographic and Health Survey (GDHS) 1988, 1993, 1998, 2003, 2008, and 2014 used standard DHS model questionnaire developed by the Measure DHS programme [27–32]. The Ghana Demographic and Health Survey is a nationwide survey which covers all ten regions and is conducted every 5 years. The survey is done by the Ghana Statistical Service and the Ghana Health Service with ICF International giving technical support for the survey through MEASURE DHS. The GDHS concentrates on child and maternal health and is designed to offer adequate data to monitor the population and health situation in Ghana. The survey gathers data on various demographic and health issues including fertility, contraceptive use, child health, nutrition, malaria, HIV and AIDS, family planning, health insurance and maternal health; antenatal care, delivery care and post-natal care. For the purpose of the study women with birth history were currently pregnant or has given birth up to 5 years before the survey, thus, 4294 women in 2014, 2131 women in 2008, 2734 women in 2003, 2374 women in 1998, 1974 women in 1998 and 2701 women in 1988 [27–32]. Permission to use the data set was given by the MEASURE DHS following the assessment of a concept note.

Description and definition of variables

The study used skilled providers of antenatal care (ANC) services as the outcome variable. The outcome variable was derived from the response to the question "did you see anyone for antenatal care for this pregnancy? If YES: whom did you see?" Responses were categorised under Health Personnel and Other Person. Health Personnel included Doctor, Nurse, Nurse/Midwife, Auxiliary Midwife, Community Health Nurse/Officer. Other Person also consisted of Traditional Birth Attendant (TBA), Traditional Health Volunteer, Village Health Volunteer, Other. For the purpose of the study, skilled providers were services provided by: Doctor, Nurse, Auxiliary Midwife, Nurse/Midwife.

The study made use of nine independent variables, these were; maternal age, marital status, educational Level, residence, wealth status, ethnicity, occupation, parity (Birth order), Ecological zone. Maternal Age was categorized into 7 age groups, thus, 15–19, 20–24, 25–29, 30–34, 35–39, 40–44, 45–49. Marital status was originally captured as Never married, Married, Living together, Widowed, Divorced and Not living together but was recoded as Single (Never married, Widowed, Divorced, Not living together), Married and Cohabitation (Living together). Educational Level was classified into four categories: No education, Primary education, Secondary education and Higher education. Type of Residence coded as Urban or Rural. Wealth Quintile was categorised in Poorest, Poorer, Middle, Richer and Richest.

Ethnicity was recoded as Akan (Asante, Akwapim, Fante, and other Akan), Ga– Adangbe, Ewe, Northern Ethnic Groups (guan, Mole–Dagbani, grussi, gruma, hausa, dagarti) and Other. Occupation was captured as not working and working. Parity (birth order) was captioned from a question that measured if respondents have ever given birth. Responses were categorised as Zero (prior to current pregnancy) one birth, two births, three births and four births or more.

The ecological zone was originally coded as Western, Central, Greater Accra, Volta, Eastern, Ashanti, Brong–Ahafo, Northern, Upper East, and Upper west. Region of residence were re–coded to capture the general ecological zones as follows: Northern, Upper East and Upper West regions were re - coded as the 'Savannah zone'; the Brong–Ahafo, Ashanti and Eastern regions were designated as the 'Forest zone'; while the Western, Central, Greater Accra and Volta regions were coded as the 'Coastal zone'.

Data analysis

The statistical software STATA version 13 was used to process the data. Some variables were recoded and renamed so that they would be consistent across all the rounds and all results were weighted. Univariate and multivariate were carried out. The outcome variable, skilled providers, were coded 0 = No and 1 = Yes. A discrete choice model was employed to show how the independent variables are related to the dependent variable. Precisely, the binary logistic regression was employed given that the model is best fit for dichotomous variables and its ability to predict on a mixture of continuous and categorical variables. The binary logistic regression is based on the assumption that the dependent variable should be dichotomous in nature and the data should not have any outlier.

Results

Utilisation of the services of skilled ANC provider increased from 45% in 1988 to 88% in 2014.The age of respondents ranged from 15 to 49 years. The mean age of the respondents was 28.6 years in 1988, and about 30 years in 2014. Respondents were predominantly aged 20–29 years. For instance, in 1988, about 40% of the sampled women were in the 20–24 age group and about 41% in 25–29 age group years (see Table 1). The highest proportion of the respondents were from the coastal zone in all the years with the exception of 2003 and 2008, where most of the respondents were predominantly from the forest zone. Majority of the urban respondents used the services of skilled ANC provider- about 75% in 1988 and 96% in 2014 respectively.

The level of education of the respondents who predominantly utilised the services of a skilled ANC provider for the years under review were with higher education. For instance, 59% in 1988; and about 98% in 2014 (see Table 1). Majority of the respondent within the richest wealth status used the services of a skilled provider during their ANC visits over the years under review (see Table 1). The highest proportion of women with one birth utilized the services of skilled providers during their ANC visits over the years under review. For instance, about 69% in 1993, 78% in 1998, 94% in 2003, 91% in 2008 and 94% in 2014 (see Table 1). With the exception of 1988 and 2003, single women dominated among those who use the services of a skilled ANC provider during their ANC visits over the years under review. The highest proportion of the respondents from the Ga/Dangme ethnic group utilised the services of a skilled ANC provider in all the year with the exception of 2003, 2008 and 2014) which was dominated by the women from the Akan ethnic group (see Table 1).

The results suggest that women from the forest zone (OR = 2.78, CI = 2.02–3.83) were more likely to use the ANC services from skilled providers during antenatal care services as compared to those from the coastal zone (see Table 2). While women from Northern ethnic group (OR = 0.63, CI = 0.44–0.92) were less likely to utilise antenatal care services from skilled providers during antenatal care as compared to Akan women.

There was a significant relationship between education and utilisation of ANC services received from skilled providers varied. For instance, women with secondary education (OR = 1.34, CI = 1.07–1.88) were more likely to utilise the services of a skilled provider during antenatal care compared to women with no education. With reference to residence, it was observed that women from rural areas (OR = 0.55, CI = 0.41–0.74) were less likely to use the services of a skilled provider during antenatal care as compared to those from the urban areas (see Table 2).

Also, the likelihood of skilled providers providing antenatal care services varied by wealth status and parity. For instance, women with the richest wealth status were more likely to utilise the services of skilled providers (OR = 5.19, CI = 2.28–11.88) (see Table 2) during antenatal care services as compared to women within the poorest wealth status, whiles women with four births or more (OR = 0.55, CI = 0.36–0.85) were also less likely to utilise the services of skilled providers during antenatal care than those with one birth (see Table 2). The likelihood of women receiving antenatal care service from a skilled provider varied from survey wave years (see Table 2). For instance, it was observed that the use of ANC from skilled providers increased in survey wave year 1993 (OR = 5.98, CI = 5.21–6.87); 1998 (OR = 6.13, CI = 5.39–6.99); 2003 (OR = 10.54, CI = 9.12–12.19). Even though the odds decreased in 2008(OR = 7.79, CI = 6.73–9.01), it increased again in 2014 (OR = 30.41, CI = 25.39–36.43).

Discussion

Using the Health Care Service Utilisation model, the study sought to examine the predictors of skilled providers of antenatal care services in Ghana over the period 1988 to 2014. Predisposing factors such as education, ethnicity and ecological zones had significant relationship with skilled providers of antenatal care services. Also, enabling factors such as residence and wealth status had similar associations. Need for change factor, parity, had significance relationship with skilled providers of antenatal care services.

The study observed that women with secondary or higher education are more likely to receive antenatal care services from skilled providers compared with those with no education. This finding is consistent with findings of other studies [17, 19, 33–35]. The possible explanation for the findings is that women with secondary or higher education may have more awareness about the danger signs and complications of pregnancy and may know the need to receive ANC services from a skilled provider.

As expected, wealth status was found to have a significant relationship with skilled providers of antenatal care services. Women within the middle, richer and richest wealth status were more likely to utilise antenatal care services from skilled providers compared to women within the poorest wealth status. This is in line with the

Table 1 Background Characteristics and choice of skilled providers of ANC

Background characteristic	Years					
	1988	1993	1998	2003	2008	2014
	n = 2701	*n* = 1974	*n* = 2374	*n* = 2743	*n* = 2131	*n* = 4294
National	45.0	60.6	68.7	90.8	84.9	87.7
Age						
15–19	38.9	62.8	74.5	91.9	81.0	94.0
20–24	40.4	63.3	73.7	93.9	84.2	89.2
25–29	41.3	61.9	72.9	92.4	90.2	91.3
30–34	50.3	61.4	71.2	91.5	88.2	91.5
35–39	48.7	57.7	69.4	92.2	87.8	91.2
40–44	53.1	53.9	63.9	88.4	81.5	89.6
45–49	49.1	37.5	51.9	89.9	82.8	77.3
Ecological Zone						
Coastal Zone	48.9	66.6	75.4	93.6	87.1	91.7
Forest Zone	38.1	62.0	70.1	94.6	93.5	95.6
Savannah zone	52.3	47.9	59.2	84.7	74.5	77.9
Place of Residence						
Urban	43.1	75.4	83.1	97.6	94.1	95.7
Rural	45.7	54.7	66.4	88.8	81.9	86.0
Level of Education						
No education	48.8	50.8	63.2	86.2	77.7	81.4
Primary	41.3	65.1	75.8	92.3	85.9	89.7
Secondary	47.6	85.7	74.6	97.4	93.1	94.9
Higher	58.8	93.3	84.8	100.0	99.3	98.8
Wealth Status						
Poorest	–	64.3	66.7	83.4	71.9	78.2
Poorer	–	57.9	70.9	91.3	83.4	88.0
Middle	–	58.0	70.1	94.9	92.1	93.0
Richer	–	59.5	71.1	95.1	94.1	96.1
Richest	–	62.8	72.8	98.7	97.5	98.7
Marital Status						
Single	53.8	57.6	71.7	91.1	87.7	92.0
Married	43.3	60.9	70.6	91.8	86.7	90.8
Cohabitation	51.2	60.7	71.1	94.6	86.4	88.7
Parity						
One birth	42.7	68.8	78.0	94.7	90.5	94.1
Two births	42.0	62.7	72.5	94.0	88.5	92.6
Three births	44.7	63.1	72.8	92.4	88.4	91.4
Four or more births	47.1	54.9	65.5	89.5	83.2	87.0
Ethnicity						
Akan	41.5	63.0	73.9	94.7	93.1	94.3
Ga/Dangme	54.0	80.5	79.9	93.9	92.3	93.5
Ewe	43.7	62.1	73.5	92.6	81.7	92.8
Northern Ethnic Group	48.5	51.5	60.1	86.5	79.2	83.1
Other	52.1	62.5	61.2	90.6	82.1	91.9

Table 1 Background Characteristics and choice of skilled providers of ANC *(Continued)*

Background characteristic	Years					
	1988	1993	1998	2003	2008	2014
	$n = 2701$	$n = 1974$	$n = 2374$	$n = 2743$	$n = 2131$	$n = 4294$
Occupation						
Not working	44.1	63.2	66.0	90.5	89.4	91.4
Working	45.8	59.9	71.5	92.2	86.5	90.4

Source: Computed from GDHS 1988, 1993, 1998, 2003, 2008 and 2014

findings of Atunah - Jay, Pettingell, Ohene, Oakes, & Borowsky [20], Ganle et al. [19] and Wang, Alva, Wang and Fort [35] found that women with richest wealth status were more likely to receive ANC services from skilled personnel compared to those from poorest wealth status who utilised ANC services from traditional birth attendants.

Furthermore, women from rural areas were less likely to utilise the services of skilled providers. This is consistent with the findings by Dickson, Darteh and Kumi-Kyereme [17], who also found that women in rural areas were less likely to receive ANC services from doctors and nurses compared to those in urban areas. One reason for the findings could be the urban-rural gap in the distribution of health resources, where those in urban areas are more likely to have access to tertiary health centres compared to those in rural areas. Others reasons could be that women in rural areas prefer home delivery because of lack of health facility near home and being more comfortable at home. A study by [36] also found that reasons for low utilization of ANC services by women in rural areas include walking long distances to access health facilities, lack of midwives, lack of or insufficient items to be used during delivery, long stay and rude health personnel.

The study established that women from the northern ethnic groups were less likely to utilise antenatal care services from skilled providers compared to women from the Akan ethnic group. Cultural beliefs and morals are believed to shape the lives and behaviours of people and this can have influences in their choices of health care provider [37]. Women from minority ethnic group were found not to utilise antenatal care services from skilled provider compared to women from majority ethnic group [38, 39]. Like rural-urban disparity in healthcare utilization by pregnant women in Ghana, the country also experiences differences in access and use of healthcare resources in terms of north-south divide where people in the northern part of the country have low access to healthcare resources including skilled personnel compared to those in the southern part of the country. The inadequate access to healthcare resources could explain why from the northern ethnic groups were less likely to utilise antenatal care services from skilled providers compared to women from the Akan ethnic group, who predominantly live in the southern part of the country.

Our study also observed that parity was associated with receiving antenatal care services from skilled providers. Women with four births or more were less likely to receive ANC services from skilled providers compared to women with parity one. This could be as a result of the experiences and knowledge gained from their previous births hence they may not be willing to go to a skilled provider for antenatal care services. This finding is consistent with Shrestha, Bell and Marais [40], 19Ganle et al. [19] and Wang et al. [35]. Finally, women from forest zone were more likely to utilise ANC services from skilled providers compared to women from the coastal zone. Similar findings were obtained in a study by Dickson, Darteh and Kumi-Kyereme [17], who also found that women from forest zone were more likely to utilise ANC services from nurses compared to those in the coastal zone. The reason for this finding is that the forest zone is mostly made up of more urban than rural communities and most communities in the forest zone have more access to healthcare resources, explaining why the utilization of ANC services in high in those areas.

Conclusion

The study investigated the factors influencing the choice of skilled providers during antenatal care visits among women in Ghana over the period from 1988 to 2014 using the Health Service Utilisation Model. Choice of skilled providers of antenatal care services were predicted by some predisposing factors including education, ethnicity, and ecological zone. Also enabling factors such as wealth status, residence and the need for care factor, parity. Women with secondary or higher education, those within richer and richest wealth status, those from forest zone are more likely to utilise the services of skilled providers during their antenatal care visits. The Ghana Health Service and Ministry of Health should encourage women in rural areas to utilise antenatal care services from skilled providers through social and behaviour change communication campaigns. This can be achieved by government through providing healthcare resources such as skilled health personnel as well as

Table 2 Logistic Regression on Choice of Antenatal Care Services Provided by Skilled Providers from 1988 to 2014

Variable	Odds ratio (OR)	Confidence Interval (CI)
Age		
15–19	1.41	0.77–2.59
20–24	Ref	Ref
25–29	1.24	0.89–1.73
30–34	1.31	0.83–1.82
35–39	1.31	0.86–2.02
40–44	1.12	0.70–1.80
45–49	0.83	0.48–1.45
Ecological Zone		
Coastal zone	Ref	Ref
Forest zone	2.78***	2.02–3.83
Savannah zone	1.15	0.79–1.67
Ethnicity		
Akan	Ref	Ref
Ga/Dangme	0.85	0.48–1.53
Ewe	1.06	0.72–1.57
Northern ethnic group	0.63*	0.44–0.92
Other	1.38	0.52–3.66
Level of Education		
No education	Ref	Ref
Primary	1.37*	1.04–1.80
Secondary	1.42*	1.07–1.88
Higher	3.41	0.52–3.66
Occupation		
Not working	Ref	Ref
Working	1.15	0.87–1.50
Marital status		
Single	Ref	Ref
Married	1.28	0.93–1.76
Cohabitation	0.78	0.55–1.11
Wealth status		
Poorest	Ref	Ref
Poorer	1.33*	1.01–1.76
Middle	1.83**	1.27–2.65
Richer	2.03**	1.26–3.26
Richest	5.19***	2.28–11.85
Place of Residence		
Urban	Ref	Ref
Rural	0.55***	0.41–0.74
Parity		
One birth	Ref	Ref
Two births	0.79	0.54–1.16
Three births	0.67*	0.44–1.00
Four births or more	0.55**	0.36–0.85
Survey wave years		
1988	Ref	Ref
1993	5.98***	5.21–6.87
1998	6.13***	5.39–6.99
2003	10.54***	9.12–12.19
2008	7.79***	6.73–9.01
2014	30.4***	25.39–36.43

Source: computed from GDHS 1988, 1993, 1998, 2003, 2008 and 2014
Ref reference, *OR* Odds Ratio
$^{*}p < 0.10$ $^{**}p < 0.05$ $^{***}p < 0.001$

materials and equipment in health facilities in rural areas that will make pregnant women feel more comfortable accessing antenatal care.

Data limitations

The Ghana Demographic and Health Survey uses a repeated cross-sectional design and the sample that were used were not carried to all the rounds, chances could be that different set respondents were used for the survey in all the different rounds. Changes in the sample over time may have effects on the results due to inherent characteristics. There is also the limitation that comes with self-reporting made by the mothers' interview. Questions were based on birth history; women were asked questions about themselves three to 5 years before the round of the survey. This may be affected by recall bias or deliberate misreporting.

Acknowledgements

We acknowledge Measure DHS for providing us with the data upon which the findings of this study were based.

Funding

The design of questionnaires and data collection was funded by measure DHS and the government of Ghana. This research, the analysis, and interpretation of data and in writing the manuscript received no specific grant from any funding agency in the public, commercial or non – for – profit sectors.

Authors' contributions

KSD conceived the study designed the first draft of the manuscript. EKMD, AKK, KSD and BOA revised the manuscript for intellectual content and gave consent for the version to be published. All authors have read and approved final manuscript.

Competing interests
The authors declare that they have no competing interests.

Author details
[1]Department of Population and Health, University of Cape Coast, Cape Coast, Ghana. [2]Department of Health, Physical Education and Recreation, University of Cape Coast, Cape Coast, Ghana.

References
1. Abosse Z, Woldie M, Ololo S. Factors influencing antenatal care service utilization in hadiya zone. Ethiop J Health Sci. 2010;20(2):75–82.
2. WHO. Maternal mortality: factsheet. 2016. Retrieved from: http://www.who.int/mediacentre/factsheets/fs348/en/.
3. World Health Organisation. World health statistics. Geneva: World Health Organisation; 2014.
4. World Health Organisation. World health statistics 2015. Geneva: World Health Organisation; 2015.
5. World Health Organisation. Maternal mortality: to improve maternal health, barriers that limit access to quality maternal health services must be identified and addressed at all levels of the health system: fact sheet. Geneva: WHO; 2014.
6. Ghana Health Service. Ghana health service 2011 annual report. Accra: Ghana Health Service; 2011.
7. United State Agency for International Development. Maternal and neonatal health technical update. Number 3. New York: USAID; 2006.
8. World Health Organization/AFRO. Framework for monitoring and evaluation of integrated child survival interventions. WHO: Geneva; 2006.
9. Myer L, Harrison A. Why do women seek antenatal care late? Perspectives from rural South Africa. J Midwifery Womens Health. 2003;48(4):268–72.
10. World Health Organization. The world health report 2006: working together for health. World Health Organization; 2006.
11. Begum N, Rahman M, Rahman MM, Nayan SK, Zinia SN, Khan SZ. Utilization of antenatal care services in a selected rural area in Bangladesh. North Int Med Coll J. 2015;6(1):25–8.
12. Lincetto O, Monthebesoane-Andoh, Gomez P, Munjanja S. Antenatal care. Opportunities for Africa's newborns: practical data, policy and programmatic support for newborn care in Africa; 2006. p. 55–62.
13. Abou-Zahr CL, Wardlaw TM, WHO. Antenatal care in developing countries: promises, achievements and missed opportunities: an analysis of trends, levels and differentials, 1990–2001. 2003.
14. AbouZahr C. Safe motherhood: a brief history of the global movement 1947–2002. Br Med Bull. 2003;67(1):13–25.
15. World Health Organization. WHO antenatal care randomized trial: manual for the implementation of the new model. Geneva: World Health Organization; 2002.
16. UNICEF. Global database on DHS, MICs and other nationally representative sources. UNICEF: Geneva; 2016.
17. Dickson KS, Darteh EKM, Kumi-Kyereme A. Providers of antenatal care services in Ghana: evidence from Ghana demographic and health surveys 1988–2014. BMC Health Serv Res. 2017;17(1):203.
18. Asamoah BO, Agardh A, Pettersson KO, Östergren PO. Magnitude and trends of inequalities in antenatal care and delivery under skilled care among different socio-demographic groups in Ghana from 1988–2008. BMC Pregnancy Childbirth. 2014;14(1):295.
19. Ganle JK, Parker M, Fitzpatrick R, Otupiri E. Inequities in accessibility to and utilisation of maternal health services in Ghana after user-fee exemption: a descriptive study. Int J Equity Health. 2014;13(1):89.
20. Atunah-Jay S, Pettingell S, Ohene SA, Michael Oakes J, Borowsky I. The relationship between antenatal provider type and maternal care in rural Ghana: a cross-sectional study. Tropical Med Int Health. 2013;18(6):678–86.
21. Dixon J, Tenkorang EY, Luginaah IN, Kuuire VZ, Boateng GO. National health insurance scheme enrolment and antenatal care among women in Ghana: is there any relationship? Tropical Med Int Health. 2014;19(1):98–106.
22. Owoo NS, Lambon-Quayefio MP. National health insurance, social influence and antenatal care use in Ghana. Heal Econ Rev. 2013;3(1):19.
23. Andersen R, Newman JF. Societal and individual determinants of medical care utilization in the United States. Milbank Mem Fund Q Health Soc. 1973;51:95–124.
24. Andersen RM. Revisiting the behavioral model and access to medical care: does it matter? J Health Soc Behav. 1995;36:1–10.
25. Hausmann-Muela S, Ribera JM, Nyamong I. DCPP working paper no. 14. Health-seeking behaviour and the health system response. 2003.
26. Fosu GB. Childhood morbidity and health services utilization: cross-national comparisons of user-related factors from DHS data. Soc Sci Med. 1994;38(9):1209–20.
27. Ghana Statistical Service, Ghana Health Service and ICF Macro. Ghana demographic and health survey 2014: key indicators. Accra: GSS, GHS and ICF Macro; 2015.
28. Ghana Statistical Service (GSS), Ghana Health (GHS), ICF Macro. Ghana demographic and health survey. Accra: GSS, GHS, and ICF Macro; 2009.
29. Ghana Statistical Services, Noguchi Memorial Institue for Medical Research, ORC Macro. Ghana demographic and health survey 2003. Calverton, Maryland: GSS, NNMR, and ORC Macro; 2004.
30. Ghana Statistical Service, Macro International. Ghana demographic and health survey 1998. Calverton, Maryland: GSS and MI; 1999.
31. Ghana Statistical Service and Macro International. Ghana demographic and health survey 1993. Calverton, Maryland: GSS, MI; 1994.
32. Ghana Statistical Service and Macro International. Ghana demographic and health survey 1988. Maryland: GSS and MI; 1989.
33. Le Meur N, Gao F, Bayat S. Mining care trajectories using health administrative information systems: the use of state sequence analysis to assess disparities in prenatal care consumption. BMC Health Serv Res. 2015;15(1):200.
34. Mekonnen Y, Mekonnen A. Utilization of maternal health care services in Ethiopia. 2002.
35. Wang W, Alva S, Wang S, Fort A. Levels and trends in the use of maternal health services in developing countries. 2011.
36. Kambala C, Morse T, Masangwi S, Mitunda P. Barriers to maternal health service use in Chikhwawa, Southern Malawi. Malawi Med J. 2011;23(1):1–5.
37. Dako-Gyeke P, Aikins M, Aryeetey R, Mccough L, Adongo PB. The influence of socio-cultural interpretations of pregnancy threats on health-seeking behavior among pregnant women in urban Accra, Ghana. BMC Pregnancy Childbirth. 2013;13(1):211.
38. Ha BT, Tac PV, Duc DM, Duong DT, Thi LM. Factors associated with four or more antenatal care services among pregnant women: a cross-sectional survey in eight south central coast provinces of Vietnam. Int J Womens Health. 2015;7:699.
39. Islam MR, Islam MA, Banowary B. Antenatal and postnatal care seeking behavior in a matrilineal society: a study on the Garo tribe of Bangladesh. J Fam Welf. 2009;55(1):62–9.
40. Shrestha S, Bell JS, Marais D. An analysis of factors linked to the decline in maternal mortality in Nepal. PLoS One. 2014;9(4):e93029.

22

Nuchal cord and its implications

Morarji Peesay

Abstract

Nuchal cord occurs when the umbilical cord becomes wrapped around the fetal neck 360 degrees. Nuchal cords occur in about 10–29% of fetuses and the incidence increases with advancing gestation age. Most are not associated with perinatal morbidity and mortality, but a few studies have shown that nuchal cord can affect the outcome of delivery with possible long-term effects on the infants. Nuchal cords are more likely to cause problems when the cord is tightly wrapped around the neck, with effects of a tight nuchal cord conceptually similar to strangulation. Umbilical cord compression due to tight nuchal cords may cause obstruction of blood flow in thin walled umbilical vein, while infant's blood continues to be pumped out of the baby through the thicker walled umbilical arteries causing hypovolemia, acidosis and anemia. Some of these infants have physical features secondary to tight nuchal cords that are distinct from those seen with birth asphyxia. The purpose of this article is to review the pathophysiology of tight nuchal cords and explore gaps in knowledge and research areas.

Keywords: Nuchal cords, Tight Nuchal cord around the neck syndrome (tCAN syndrome), Partial prolonged asphyxia, Adult strangulation

Background

In 1962, J. Selwyn Crawford [1] defined nuchal cord "360 degrees around the fetal neck." Historical interest in nuchal cords has waxed and waned. In 1770, the first edition of the Encyclopedia Britannica (P.421), there were 20 pages written about Umbilical cord pathology including drawings of umbilical cord entanglement. In a book published in 1896, Gould [2] referred to a statement by Hippocrates (460 BC –ca. 370 BC) on nuchal cord as one of the dangers of the eighth month, stating that a nuchal cord persisting until the term, "will cause suffering to the mother and either perish or born difficulties to the fetus." A chapter in Williams Obstetrics (16th Edition, 1980) states, "Coils (nuchal cords) occur in about 25% of cases and ordinarily do no harm, but occasionally they may be so tight that constriction of the umbilical vessels and consequent hypoxic result". The implications of nuchal cords are controversial. Several studies have noted an association between nuchal cords and adverse perinatal outcome. In addition umbilical cord compression due to tight nuchal cords could be an incidental finding that is seldom associated with perinatal morbidity.

Correspondence: Morarji.R.Peesay@gunet.georgetown.edu
Department of Pediatrics Division of Neonatal Perinatal Medicine, MedStar Georgetown University Hospital, 3800 Reservoir Rd, NW; Suite M3400, Washington, DC 20007, USA

Incidence

Larson JD et al. [3] reported that the overall incidence of nuchal cords was 6% at 20 wks GA and 29% at 42 weeks of gestation. Presence of two or more loops of nuchal cords is estimated to affect between 2.4% to 8.3% of all pregnancies. These entanglements may form early in gestation, although definitive evidence is lacking about exact time of its formation. Clapp, et al. [4] also showed increased incidence of nuchal cords with advancing gestational age irrespective of whether the entanglement involved single or multiple loops but without persistence (Figs. 1 and 2). This apparent inconsistency of increased incidence without persistence that Clapp noted was probably related to widely space ultrasonographic evaluations (3–6 weeks) and limited sampling times (5–10 min). In a large multicenter retrospective study, Henry, et al. [5] observed incidence of tight nuchal cord around by 6.6% and 21.6% loose nuchal cord. In his retrospective study Miser et al. [6] showed no influence of maternal age, race, parity on the incidence of nuchal cords but more common in male infants [6].

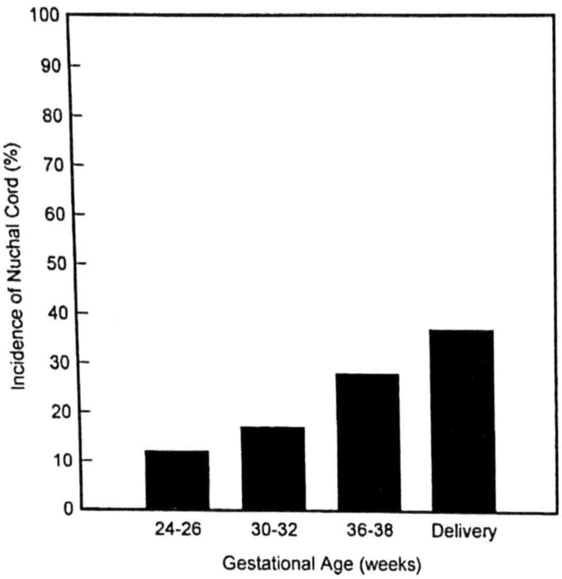

Fig. 1 The incidence of nuchal cords at the four time points studied (Courtesy from Elsevier, with permission)

Biomechanics of umbilical cord

There is limited literature on mechanics of umbilical cords. Ferguson, et al. [7] described bioengineering aspects of the umbilical cord emphasizing that "the umbilical cord is an extension of the fetal cardiovascular system with a great potential for use in studying changes within the fetal vascular tissues." The constituent tissues of umbilical cord include outer layer of amnion and inner porous Wharton's jelly, two umbilical arteries and one umbilical vein. The outer amnion layer seems to regulate fluid pressure within the umbilical cord. Wharton's Jelly is a porous structure with poroelastic behavior and has proteoglycans and hyalauronic acid. It is supposed to protect against constriction due to fetal grasping, labor contractions, knots, kinks, or loops. On average, umbilical cords are 45–55 cm long, diameter of 1–2 cm and 11 helices, but diameters up to 3 cm and helices of as many as 380 per cord have been described [8]. Krakowiak, et al. [9] defines short cords as less than 40 cms and occur in approximately 6% of pregnancies. He notes that when short cord are around the neck, they are more likely to wrap tightly and are more often associated with decreased fetal movements, risk of cord compression, constriction and rupture. Presence of short cords seems to double and triple predictive values of low Apgar scores, low IQ values, neurologic abnormalities and stillbirths. Naeye, et al. [10] showed that long cords (defined as >70 cm length) have poor fetal outcome, higher fetal entanglements, true knots (sometimes multiple) and they are prone for torsion.

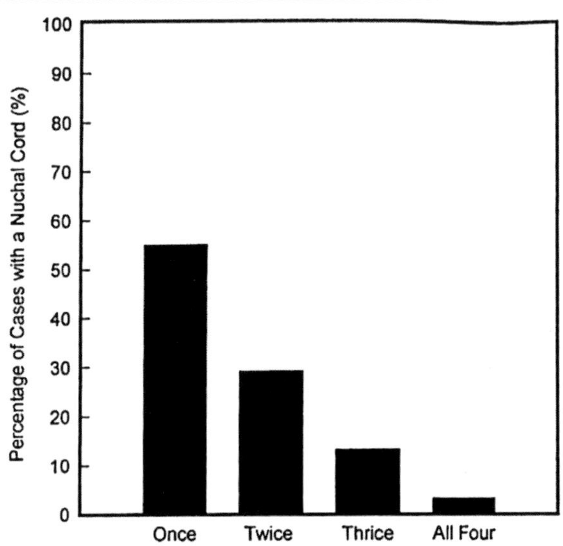

Fig. 2 The frequency of occurrence in individual fetuses who had nuchal cord indentified during the four evaluations (Courtesy from Elsevier, with permission)

The biometrics patterns of uterine, fetal, umbilical cord lengths coupled with placental and amniotic fluid volumes could possibly be playing a role in formation of nuchal cords. Umbilical cords have elastic stretch up to 12.5% of its length [11]. Most cord ruptures happen within 12 in. of the fetus; 22% of the time ruptures occur at the placental end of umbilical cord. Studies have shown that traction forces of 8 lbs. usually separate the placenta from the uterus. Tensile strength of umbilical cord indicates that the average load required to break the cord is around 10–14 lbs. [11]. Majority of umbilical cords coil to the left in anticlockwise at ratio of 7 to 1 [12]. Mechanism of coiling includes intrinsic properties such as growth of vessels, differential blood flow within arteries and fetal movements. While exact causes for left twists are unknown, one of possible mechanisms seem to be that right umbilical artery is usually larger than left, which creates differential flow patterns resulting in left twist of umbilical cord. During embryonic development, physiological gut herniation occurs around 6–8 weeks of gestational age and subsequent reentry of herniated gut is usually anticlockwise and suspected to be another possible mechanism for common left twists of umbilical cords. Gupta et al. [13] defined hypocoiling, defined as <1 coil/5 cm and showed that it is associated with fetal distress, oligohydramnios, preterm delivery, intrauterine growth retardation, meconium stained amniotic fluid, fetal heart rate (FHR) alterations and low cord pH. Horn et al. [14], found association between hyper coiling (more than 1 coil/5 cm) and thinning with consecutive constriction of the umbilical vessels (thin cord syndrome; TCS) and intrauterine fetal death (IUFD). Noncoiled [15] umbilical cords are considered as risk factor for poor perinatal outcome and stillbirth.

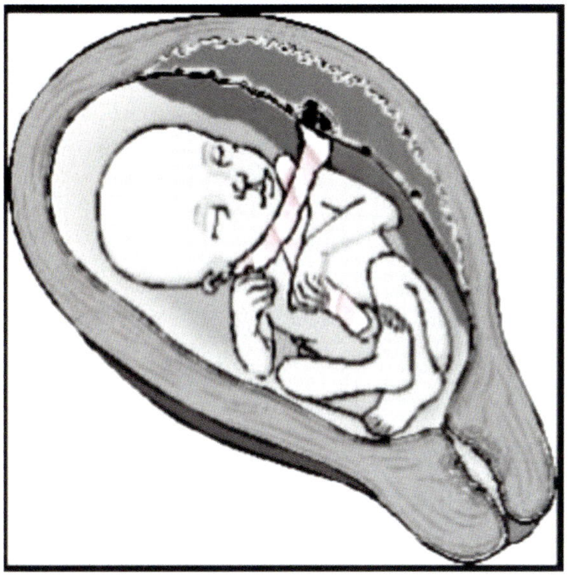

Fig. 3 Nuchal Cord - Free sliding pattern: (Courtesy Philippe Jeanty et al., with permission)

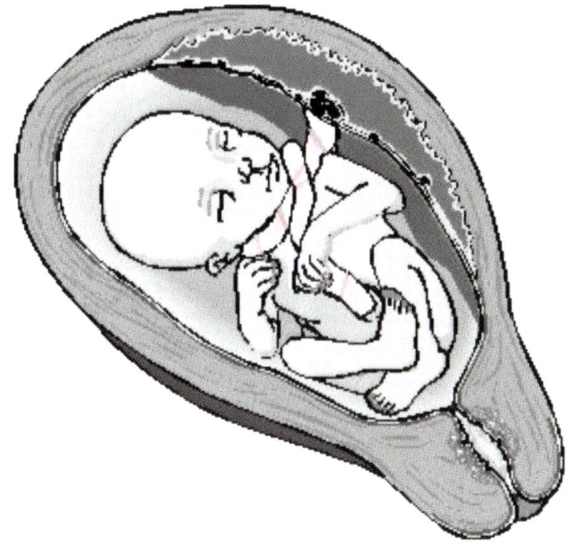

Fig. 4 Nuchal Cord - Locked pattern (Courtesy from Philippe Jeanty et al., with permission)

Pathophysiology

Nuchal cords can be single or multiple loops, and loose or tightly wrapped around the neck. Giacomello, et al. [16] recognized two types of nuchals: Type A- a freely sliding pattern which can undo itself (Fig. 3), and Type B - nuchal loop that encircles the neck in a locked pattern and cannot undo itself (Fig. 4). Very rarely a locked loop can be unlocked spontaneously by fetus that seems to be one of the mechanisms of true knot formation. Knots can be single or multiple (Fig. 5). If there is a nuchal cord at the onset of labor, it is very unlikely to correct itself. If there is no nuchal cord during prelabor, it is unlikely to occur during labor. Nuchal cords, especially when tightly wrapped, seem to have some similar physical features as those seen in strangulations. They include duskiness of face, facial petechiae, and conjunctival hemorrhage. A review article by Stapczynski et al. [17] on strangulations, describes presence of facial petechiae as a hallmark of jugular vein occlusion (lateral neck compression).When the jugular vein is occluded for ~15–30 s, facial petechiae seem to appear. Vagal collapse results from pressure to the carotid sinuses and increased parasympathetic tone. Other described findings of strangulation include retinal hemorrhages, hemotympanum and hyoid bone fractures (considered as pathognomonic of strangulation). The term compression asphyxia is used in adult Forensic Medicine, when strangulated victim torso is compressed by the perpetrator, suffers mechanically limiting expansion of the lungs interfering with breathing. As in normal delivery of newborns, nuchal cord babies' chest is subjected to undue pressure during passage of vaginal canal and may suffer similar thoracic compression mechanically limiting expansion of the lungs. Long term effects of strangulations in adults include stroke and visual deficits. Nuchal cord may be considered worse than strangulation, since in nuchal cord, umbilical cord itself acts as a noose while carrying blood supply and the oxygen and umbilical vein being more vulnerable to collapse. Many of infants with nuchal cord pass meconium, which is probably an indication of vagal collapse. Based on pathophysiological findings mentioned above, author recommends developing grading system of tight nuchal cords as Grade 1: Conjunctival hemorrhage and petechiae. Grade 2: Duskiness of face, facial suffusion and pallor. Grade 3: Respiratory distress, stupor and hypotonia requiring resuscitation.

Pathology

Pathology specimens speak volumes about the rare lethal effects of tight nuchal cords (Fig. 6) leading to stillbirth. Baergen, et al. [18] found that as much as 20% of

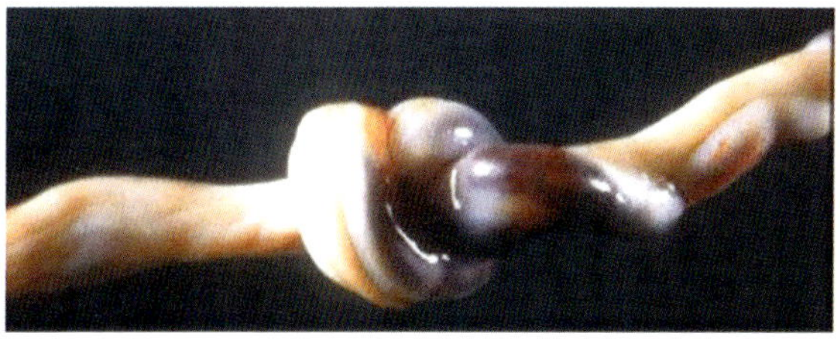

Fig. 5 Umbilical Cord Knot. Notice the area of congestion to the right. The congested side is always the side between the knot and the placenta (Courtesy from University of Mo. Department of Pathology, with permission)

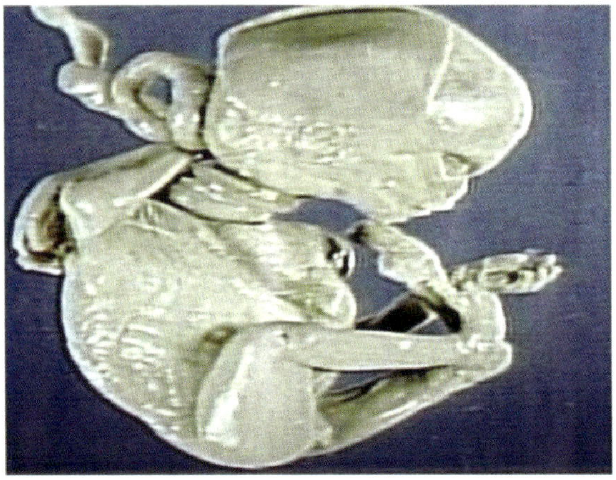

Fig. 6 Pathology specimen of fetus with multiple nuchal cords (Courtesy from Peter Anderson PEIR Digital Library, with permission)

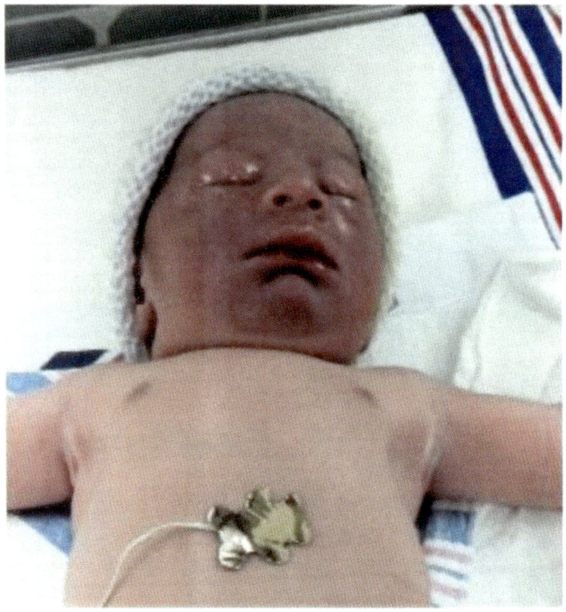

Fig. 7 Facial Duskiness due to tight Nuchal cord

stillbirths at autopsy are due to fatal compromise of umbilical circulation. Parast, et al., [19] for the first time established evidence of placental histologic criteria for umbilical blood flow restriction (cord accident) in unexplained stillborns. Placental slides from 62 cases of third trimester unexplained stillbirths reviewed to define criteria and estimate the frequency of cord accident as cause of stillbirth. By correlating clinical and autopsy information with placental gross and histologic findings from a series of index cases with a strong presumptive evidence of cord accident, minimal histologic criteria for cord accident were established. "Minimal histologic criteria" suggestive of cord accident were defined as vascular ectasia and thrombosis within the umbilical cord, chorionic plate, and/or stem villi. Of 27 stillbirth cases (out of 62 cases reviewed) who had a cause of death determined to be other than cord accident only 3(11%) met all histologic criteria for cord accident(specificity of 89%). In contrast of remaining 25 stillbirth cases with an unknown cause of death, a significantly larger subset (13 cases or 52%) met the criteria for cord accident ($p = 0.0038$). All stillbirth fetuses and placentas that met the histologic criteria for cord accidents exhibited marked normoblastemia, reflecting possible subacute to chronic hypoxic stress prior to demise. Although normoblastemia is by no means specific for cord accident it is a constant finding in nonacute fatal restriction of umbilical blood flow (cord accident).

Clinical features

Infants with a tight nuchal cord may develop signs and symptoms such as hypovolemia, hypotension, decreased perfusion and mild respiratory distress. Other findings occasionally noted may include facial duskiness (Fig. 7), facial petechiae (Fig. 8), subconjuntival hemorrhage (Fig. 9), facial suffusion (Fig. 10), or skin abrasion around the neck (Fig. 11) due to tight nuchal cords. Rarely, infants become neurologically depressed or hypotonic with depressed neonatal reflexes. Based on cardio-respiratory and neurological signs and symptoms associated with a tight nuchal cord, one can group the common findings together into a possible syndrome called tight Cord Around the Neck syndrome, or 'tCAN syndrome. We propose this term as "a cluster of cardio-respiratory and neurological signs and symptoms associated with unique physical features that occurs secondary to tight cord-round-the-neck" [20]. Rarely, there can be significant blood loss, acidosis, and anemia. A few small studies and case reports show nuchal cord as a cause of neonatal

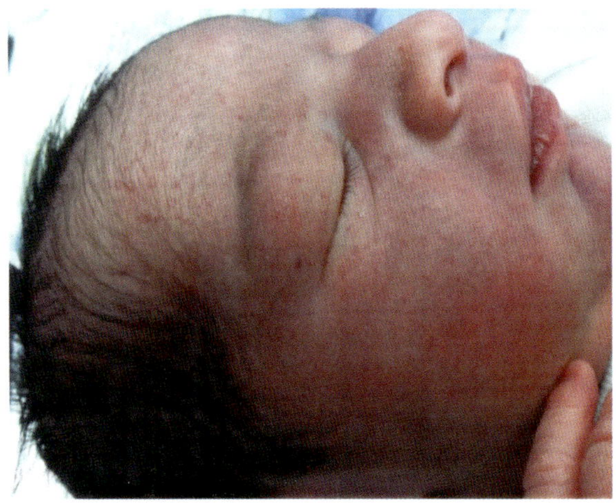

Fig. 8 Petechiae on face due to tight nuchal cord

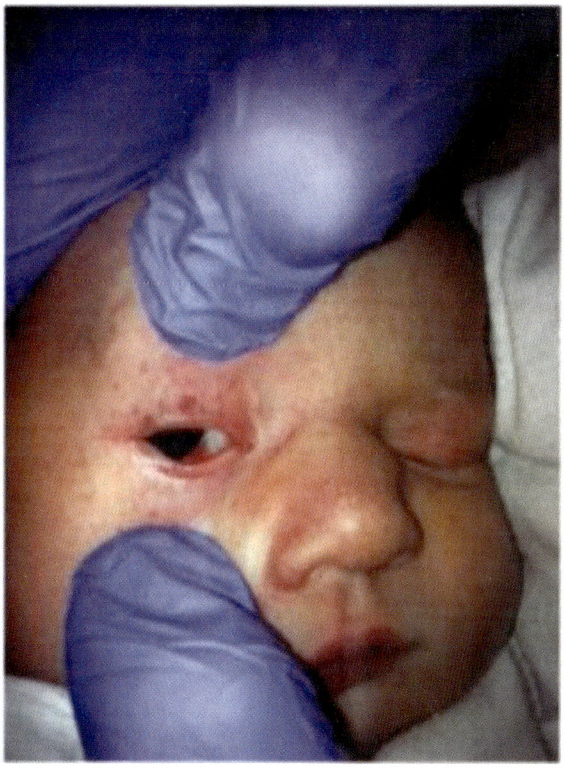

Fig. 9 Facial Petechiae and Subconjuntival hemorrhage due to tight Nuchal cord

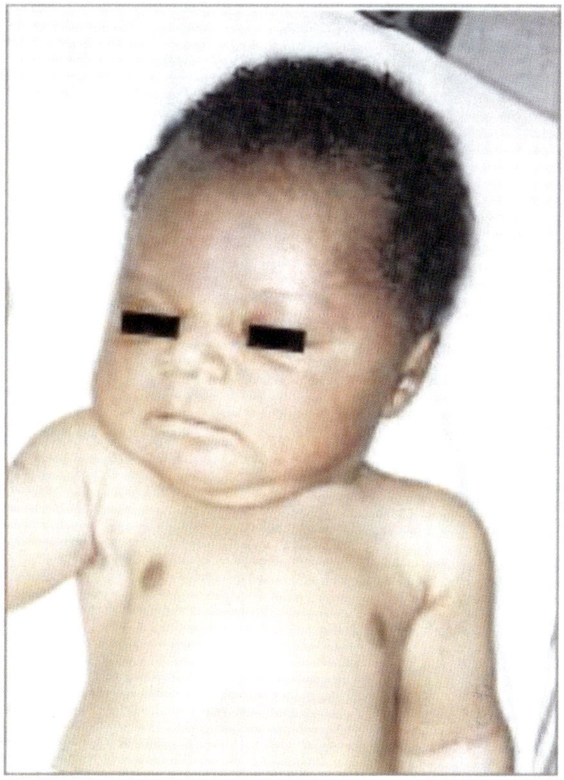

Fig. 10 Suffusion of the face and head due to tight nuchal cord. (From Arnold J. Rudolph, M.D. Atlas of the Newborn, B.C Decker Inc., with permission)

anemia. Shepherd, et al. [21] reported anemia in 5 out of 27 (19%) infants with tight nuchal cord. Three infants had hypotension requiring blood transfusion. Asymptomatic anemia as a complication of loose nuchal cords was also described. Vanhaesebroudk, et al. [22] published a case report of two neonates with acute hypovolemic shock requiring blood transfusion, low APGAR scores and umbilical arterial acidosis after tight nuchal cord. The author also noted from personal experience that if the finding in babies with a history of a loose nuchal cord include one or all of the findings such as facial petechiae and a dusky face, subconjuntival hemorrhage and low umbilical arterial cord pH, it is probably a tight nuchal cord at variable period of time prior to delivery. It is also authors' personal observation that infants with hypermagnesemia due to maternal magnesium sulfate treatment with history of tight nuchal cord show increased risk of apneas and desaturations, possibly due to their combined effect on central nervous system. As of now, there is no scientific evidence supporting these personal experiences.

Diagnosis

One of the causes of variable decelerations in antenatal fetal heart rate monitoring is nuchal cord. Nuchal cords can be diagnosed antenatally by ultrasonography (Figs. 12

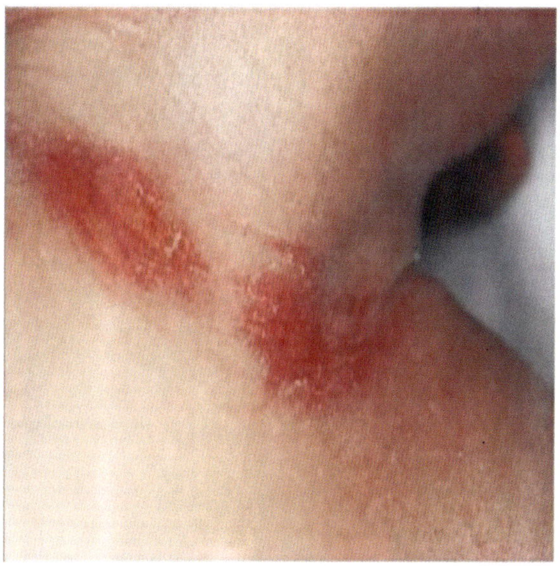

Fig. 11 Nuchal Cord with Skin abrasion of neck - Cord Around the Neck times three. (From Arnold J. Rudolph, M.D. Atlas of the Newborn, B.C Decker Inc., with permission)

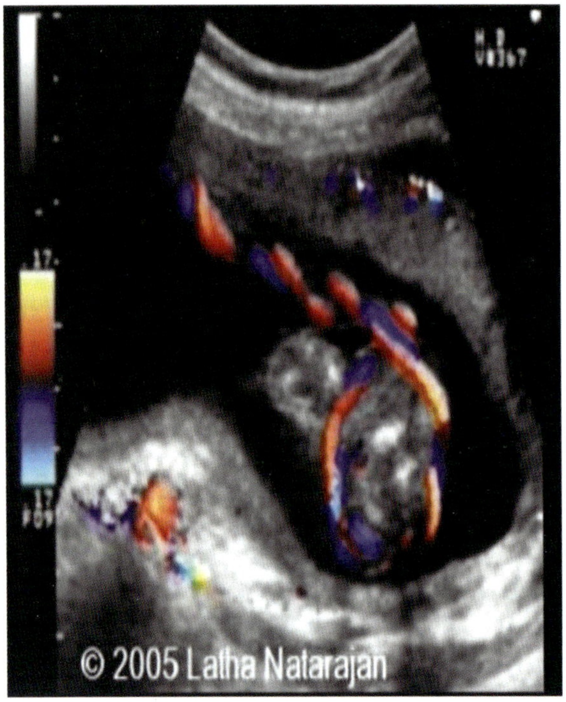

Fig. 12 Fetal Ultra sound color doppler scan of Nuchal Cord (Courtesy from Dr. Latha Natarajan, with permission)

and 13). Jauniaux, et al. [23] showed ultrasonography to be the gold the standard when combined with color Doppler imaging. This seems to correctly identify 72% of single and 94% of multiple nuchal cords, with greatest sensitivity after 36 weeks (93% vs. 67%). Ultrasonographers can look for a "divot" sign on high-resolution ultrasound

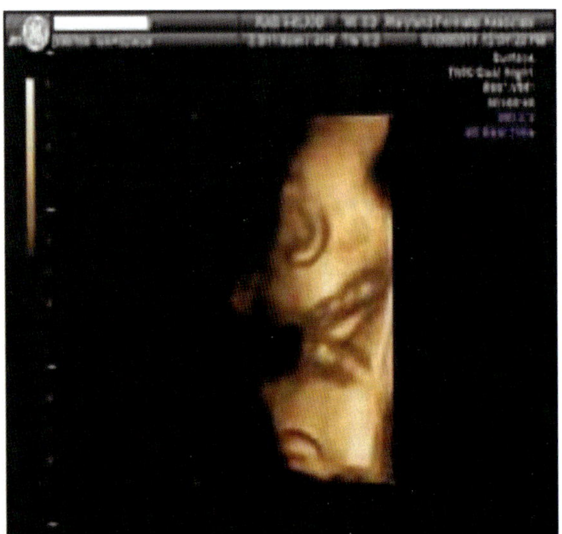

Fig. 13 Fetal Ultra Sound scan - 3D image of double nuchal cord (Courtesy from Maryland Perinatal Associates, with permission)

[24], a circular indentation of the fetal nuchal skin; but care should be exercised not to confuse this finding with posterior cystic masses, folds of skin, or amniotic fluid pockets. Prior to delivery, obstetricians can assess presence of nuchal cords clinically by a test that involves transabdominal manual compression of the fetal neck. If compression of fetal neck elicits fetal heart rate decelerations (FHR), the test is considered positive. This indicates impending risk of cord compression and is an indication for close FHR monitoring. Mendez-Bauer, et al. [25] showed in his study that this noninvasive test has sensitivity of 82.3% and specificity 89.1%. These results were statistically significant in both late pregnancy and labor. A positive test is an indication for close electronic fetal monitoring, particularly during labor. Study concluded that routine use of this test can contribute to decreasing perinatal morbidity and mortality by diminishing the impact of cord problems. One can also diagnose presence of nuchal cords noninvasively prior to delivery, by using vibroacoustic stimulation (electronic artificial larynx) which at particular frequencies of vibrations seem to elicit fetal heart rate decelerations. Anyaegbunam, et al. [26] used vibroacoustic stimulation during second stage of labor eliciting accelerations, decelerations, and acceleration followed by decelerations. The incidence of nuchal cord was significantly higher for the group with a response pattern of fetal heart rate acceleration followed by deceleration than for the acceleration or no-response groups (39.2% versus 10.5% versus 11.1%; $P < .05$).

Fetal hypoxia

Nuchal cords can cause cord compression, leading to obstruction of blood flow in the thin walled umbilical vein, while blood continues to be pumped out through the thicker walled umbilical arteries causing hypovolemia, hypotension and fetal hypoxia [22]. There are only few studies that have focused on tight nuchals causing fetal hypoxia. Xu, et al. [27] investigated the value of middle cerebral artery (MCA) and umbilical artery (UA) resistance index in predicting fetal hypoxia in fetuses with umbilical cord around the neck in late pregnancy. Included in this study are measurements of MCA and UA pulsatility index (PI), resistance index (RI), peak systolic and diastolic (S/D) ratios, and resistance index ratios (RIR). RIR showed no significant difference between the no nuchal cord and the 1-loop nuchal cord group ($P > 0.05$). However, significant differences were noted between the no nuchal cords group and the multiple nuchals group ($P < 0.01$), and between the ≥2-loops nuchal cord group and the 1-loop nuchal cord group ($P < 0.05$). One of the conclusions of study is that MCA/UA RIR compared to PI, RI, S/D ratios is a better indicator for predicting fetal hypoxia in nuchal cord infants. Hashimoto, et al. [28] investigated evidence of fetal hypoxia by studying levels of erythropoietin (EPO) in umbilical cord blood and amniotic fluid. Tissue hypoxia is the major stimulus of erythropoietin (EPO) synthesis in fetuses and adults. Previous studies have shown that EPO does not cross the placenta [29], and that plasma EPO levels correlate with the intensity of hypoxia [30]. Cord blood EPO levels increase in acute fetal hypoxia, and amniotic fluid (AF) EPO levels increase in chronic fetal hypoxia. Hashimoto, et al., showed that in the absence of ante/intra partum complications, higher levels of AF-EPO at birth were more predictive of nuchal cord whereas cord blood EPO levels were not found to have any correlation with nuchal cord. Tightness of the nuchal cord did not affect AF or cord blood EPO concentrations. This study concluded that nuchal cords may not significantly increase the risk of acute or labor-associated fetal hypoxia, but are an independent risk factor of mild, chronic, prelabor fetal hypoxia.

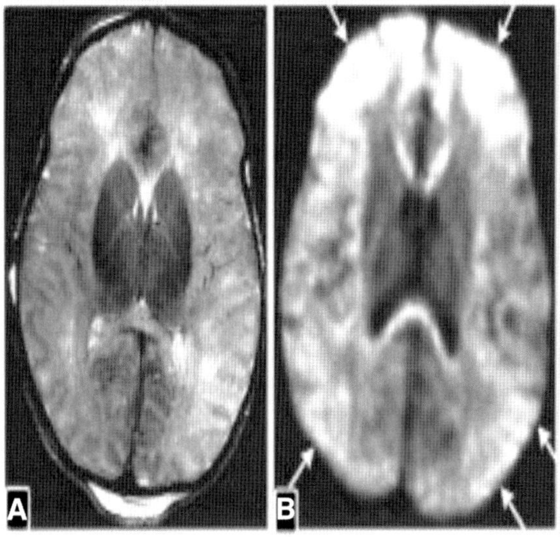

Fig. 14 MRI scans of severe Partial Prolonged Asphyxia: A 4-day-old infant owing to tight cord around neck. A) Axial T2- weighted imaging shows abnormal cortical and subcortical bilateral cerebral increased T2 signal intensity. B) Axial diffusion weighted imaging shows extensive gray and white matter injury (arrows) of both cerebral hemispheres – From KN V: Cerebral Palsy and Early Stimulation. New Delhi, India: Jaypee Brothers. Medical Publishers (P) Ltd., 2014, with permission

Prolonged partial asphyxia evidence

Severe prolonged partial asphyxia could be one of the rare complications of tight nuchal cords [31]. Causes of prolonged partial asphyxia (PPA) include nuchal cord, placental failure and tetanic uterine contractions. In prolonged partial asphyxia there is gradual reduction in blood flow and oxygen over several hours to the brain, probably due to occlusion of intramyometrial segment of uterine and or umbilical artery, while cardiac pumping is generally preserved. Brain injury in PPA primarily affects the cerebral cortex and is associated with severe brain swelling in the watershed areas (especially in the parasagittal region). The vascular watershed zones (anterior–middle cerebral artery and posterior–middle cerebral artery) are involved, thereby affecting white matter (Fig. 14). PPA could be one of the rare complications of tight nuchal cords.

Nuchal cords and birth asphyxia

One of several attempts to distinguish and delineate the effects of nuchal cords from birth asphyxia was done by Martin, et al. [32] in a study on umbilical cord gas acidosis comparing newborns with and without nuchal cords that had normal APGAR scores. They found that while umbilical venous (UV) pH, pCO2, and oxygen content were not statistically different between the two groups, infants with nuchal cord had significantly lower pH, lower oxygen content, and higher PCO2 levels in their arterial cord gases. The Veno-Arterial (VA) differences in pH and PCO2 of the infants with nuchal cord were greater than that of the infants with no nuchal cords. The study concurred with other studies that Apgar score is not a sensitive indicator of acid-base changes in nuchal cord infants. Umbilical venous blood gases can be misleading in these infants, and therefore umbilical arterial blood must be sampled to detect hypercapnia and diminished oxygen content resulting from a nuchal cord. A significant umbilical arterial acidosis can occur in nuchal cord infants even in the setting of normal or near normal APGAR scores. Belai, et al. [33] showed that APGAR scores correlate very weakly with cord pH when the pH is greater than 7.0. We speculate that the physical features of tCAN syndrome may distinguish perinatal depression due to nuchal cords from other causes of birth asphyxia. Miriam Martinez-Biarge et al. [34] in 2013 in their retrospective analysis to determine whether antepartum factors alone, intrapartum factors alone, or both in combinations, are associated with term neonatal hypoxic-ischemic encephalopathy (HIE). A total of 405 infants >35 weeks' gestation with early encephalopathy, were compared with 239 neurologically normal infants newborns. All cases met criteria for perinatal asphyxia, had neuroimaging findings consistent with acute hypoxia-ischemia, and had no evidence for a non–hypoxic-ischemic cause of their encephalopathy. On logistic regression analysis only 1 antepartum factor (gestation > 41 weeks) and 7 intrapartum factors (prolonged membrane rupture, abnormal cardiotocography, thick meconium, sentinel event, shoulder dystocia, tight nuchal cord, failed vacuum) remained independently associated with HIE (area under the curve 0.88; confidence interval 0.85–0.91; P, .001). Tight nuchal cord was noted in 45/396 cases and 15/237 in control group with odds ratio of 1.89 (1.03–3.5). Their results do not support HIE is attributable to antepartum factors alone, but they strongly point to the intrapartum period as the necessary factor in the development of this condition. It is our speculation that the established terminology 'Compression Asphyxia' in forensic medicine [35] could be applied to these infants with tight nuchal cords because of the similarities in their patho-physiological mechanisms and clinical findings. This may help in distinguishing birth asphyxia from infant with the effects of a tight nuchal cord.

Prognosis

Several animal studies have been conducted in order to simulate the effects of nuchal cords. Rocha, et al. [36] examined the effect of intermittent umbilical cord occlusion during brain development in preterm and near-term ovine fetuses. The purpose of this study was to determine the immunoreactivity of selected structural proteins in the preterm and near-term ovine fetal brain and the response to intermittent umbilical cord occlusion as a measure of altered cellular growth. The intermediate filament proteins nestin, vimentin, and glial fibrillary acidic protein was used as markers for astroglial maturation and astrogliosis, and myelin basic protein as a marker for oligodendrocytes and myelin formation. Fetal sheep (control and experimental groups at 0.75 and 0.90 of gestation) were studied over 4 days; umbilical cord occlusion was performed in the experimental group by complete inflation of an occluder cuff for 90 s every 30 min for 3 to 5 h each day. Animals were then euthanized, and the fetal brain was perfusion fixed and processed for immunohistologic examination of the gray and white matter. In both preterm and near-term animal groups, umbilical cord occlusion caused a large decline in arterial Po_2 (to approximately 7 mmHg), a modest decline in pH (to approximately 7.30), and a modest rise in PCo_2 (to approximately 61 mmHg; all $P < .01$), with a return to control values after the occluder release and no cumulative acidosis over each day of study. Vimentin and glial fibrillary acidic protein immunoreactivity showed reciprocal changes, with vimentin decreased and glial fibrillary acidic protein increased in both the gray and white matter of the control group from 0.75 to 0.90 of gestation, which can be attributed to the transition of radial glia into mature astrocytes. Myelin basic protein immunoreactivity increased approximately 3-fold in the white matter of the control group with advancing gestation, which likely reflected active oligodendrocyte differentiation and increased myelination at this time of development. Intermittent umbilical cord occlusion over 4 days resulted in an approximately 60% decrease in nestin, vimentin, and glial fibrillary acidic protein immunoreactivity, which was qualitatively similar for both the gray and white matter and likely indicative of altered protein synthesis and/or degradation, but only in the preterm group and with no change in myelin basic protein immunoreactivity. The results showed that intermittent umbilical cord occlusion as studied with minimal evidence for necrotic cell injury appears capable of altering selected protein synthesis/degradation, more so in younger animals when protein turnover is higher, which might then impact on the brain's development. Due to its common occurrence, mostly benign nature, multifactorial causality, and lack of clear guidance towards management, the long-term neurological injury secondary to nuchal cords has been debated. Some studies published on neonatal outcome include fetal demise and neurological impairments, while the vast majority of studies have shown no long term neurodevelopmental impairment. Yet a very small, but significant, percentage of infants with tight nuchal cords seem to face devastating effects as evidenced in pathophysiological features in tCAN syndrome. In a retrospective study of normal birth weight infants with spastic cerebral palsy, Nelson, et al. [37] showed an association between tight nuchal cords and quadriplegia. In this observational study, none of the infants with diplegia or hemiplegia had potentially asphyxiating conditions. In their study on asphyxia-related risk factors and their timing in spastic cerebral palsy (CP), Neilson, et al. [38] noted a threefold increase in risk of spastic CP in infants with tight nuchal cords. Clapp, et al. [39] performed a prospective study examining neurodevelopmental performance at 1 year of age in infants who had nuchal cords at delivery. Infants of 190 women with clinically normal antenatal courses were evaluated within 1 month of their first birthday by a blinded observer using the Bayley Scales of Infant Development. The cases were grouped based on the presence of a symptomatic nuchal cord (defined as an abnormal fetal heart rate patterns or meconium) during labor and fetuses with symptomatic nuchal cord presentations with one or more additional anatomic findings suggesting increased risk were identified as a symptomatic-complicated subgroup. The additional anatomic findings included the following: nuchal cords that were identified initially as an incidental ultrasound finding 4 or more weeks before labor, which presumably persisted until the time of birth, multiple loops around the neck at birth, an associated true knot or an excessively tight nuchal cord at the time of birth. At 1 year of age scores on both Bayley scales were slightly but significantly ($P < .01$) lower in the offspring delivered with a symptomatic nuchal cord. The mental index was 116 +/− 9 versus 120 +/− 7, and the psychomotor index was 101 +/− 11 versus 107 +/− 9. These differences were accentuated ($P = .09$) when the symptomatic cases complicated by extreme tightness, multiple loops, or antenatal detection were compared to symptomatic cases without these additional complications (overall index 110 +/− 8 versus 105 +/− 10). The differences are not statistically significant, suggesting that this may be largely due to the performance of the offspring born with a symptomatic presentation that was complicated also by additional anatomic findings. There were no between group differences in multiple potential confounding obstetric or demographic variables. These data suggest that symptomatic nuchal cords, which are identified before labor as being extremely tight or having multiple loops, may be associated with a subclinical deficit in neurodevelopmental performance at 1 year of age. There was marked reduction in birth weights seen in about ~25% of fetuses with persistent nuchal cord associated with low middle cerebral artery systolic and diastolic ratios, this is suggestive of a chronic hypoxic state. In contrast, Greenwood, et al. [40] showed that reported associations of nuchal cord with cerebral palsy (CP) were influenced by recording bias. There were 68 cases with cerebral palsy and 157 controls (singleton term infants matched for gestational age and hospital of birth). CP was associated with tight nuchal cord overall (OR = 2.8, 95% CI 1.1–6.8). Where cord around the neck is recorded at the discretion of the accoucheur (37 cases, 97 controls), there was an association between tight nuchal cord and CP (OR = 5.4, 95% CI 1.4–20.4) and, apparent association between nuchal cords and Apgar score < 7 at 1 min (OR = 16.9, 95% CI1.4–456.3). In the hospital where records included a tick box for nuchal cord (31 cases, 60 controls), an association between CP and tight nuchal cord could not be demonstrated (OR = 1.4, 95% CI 0.4–4.9) nor was there an apparent association between nuchal cord and Apgar score < 7 at 1 min (OR = 2.6, 95% CI 0.4–15.9) in controls. Thus showing that an association of CP with nuchal cord is not evident where documentation is systematic. In a retrospective study, Sheiner, et al. [41] concurs with nuchal cord not being associated with adverse perinatal outcomes. In a large multicenter retrospective study, Henry, et al. [5] observed no difference in outcomes following tight nuchal cords. Using electronic data of 219,337 live births over 6-year period (2005 to 2010) in a multihospital healthcare system in the Western United States, they reported an incidence of tight nuchal cord of 6.6% and an incidence of loose nuchal cords of 21.1%. Neonates with tight nuchal cords were slightly more likely to be admitted to a NICU (6.6% vs. 5.9% admission rate, p 0.000). In this study, no difference in outcome was seen in very low birth weight (VLBW) infants with tight nuchal cords. In a retrospective analysis of a perinatal database including 11,748 vaginal deliveries, Schaffer, et al. [42] noted significantly more male than female infants in the nuchal cord group, 52.9% in all nuchal cords ($p < 0.5$) and 54.5% in multiple nuchal cords (p < 0.5). The rates of vaginal operative deliveries or deliveries by cesarean were not significantly increased in any nuchal cord group in term and post term deliveries. Schaffer also noted that there was significantly lower birth weights were found in all nuchal cord groups suggesting potentially prolonged chronic mild fetal hypoxia caused by nuchal cord. This effect was especially pronounced in multiple cords, with a decrease of 93 g in term and 180 g in posterm multiple nuchal cords ($p < 0.05$). Zhang, et al. [43] used a questionnaire to examine possible prenatal and perinatal risk factors for autism in a case control study in Hans Province, China. One hundred and ninety children with autism were recruited from public special education schools, with controls from regular public schools in the same region. Nuchal cord occurred with a higher frequency among children with autism (23.2%) than among the controls (6.3%) ($p = 0.002$).

Obstetrical management

The obstetrical challenge of the clinical management of nuchal cords depends upon number of involved nuchal loops, the amniotic fluid index, the gestational age, and the fetal growth, among other factors. Induction of labor considered as independent risk factor for nuchal cords. A prolonged persistent nuchal cord with poor fetal growth deserves close monitoring and delivery as appropriate. Some obstetricians opt to deliver early when multiple nuchal cord loops are noted on fetal scans. Presence of variable decelerations during fetal heart rate monitoring is indicative of possible presence of nuchal cord.

Conclusions

Nuchal cords are a potential cause for perinatal distress and a rarely significant risk factor for long-term neurodevelopmental consequences in the developing fetus. A renewed interest is needed in diagnosing nuchal cords by judicious use of ultrasound with color Doppler, MCA and UA resistance index ratios, amniotic EPO levels, and possibly the use of manual abdomen compression or vibroacoustic stimulation tests. Examining placenta and cord pathology in cases of tight nuchal cords could also be informative. We speculate that 'Compressional Asphyxia' would be more appropriate terminology for neonates who are asphyxiated secondary to tight nuchal cords. Prospective analysis is needed by neonatologists to report the signs of tight nuchal cord as described in tCAN syndrome. Close follow-up in developmental clinics would help in predicting the outcomes. Studies exploring possible role of fundoscopy, otoscopy, and EEG may expand and help fill the knowledge gaps. Better understanding of bioengineering aspect of umbilical cord especially on mechanism of nuchal cord formation may shed light on management. There needs to be a focus on neuropathology to examine stillborn fetus brains histologic findings that might be unique to tight nuchals. Obstetricians may look for placental histological changes secondary to tCANs in infants born alive. Further study by pathologist on stillborn with tCANs may include fundoscopy for retinal hemorrhages, otoscopy to rule out hemotympanum, and X-ray of hyoid bone to rule out fractures. This would help clarify possible lethal aspects of tCANs.

The enormous anxieties mothers go through when their fetuses have locked pattern of nuchal cords continue to challenge obstetricians. From the perspective of neonatologists, who see evidence of tight nuchals as in tCAN syndrome and pathologists who witness during autopsy, tight nuchal cord as a cause stillbirth, nuchal cords do not seem to be benign.

Abbreviations

(S/D) ratios: Peak Systolic and Diastolic ratios; AF: Amniotic fluid; CP: Cerebral Palsy; EPO: Erythropoietin; FHR: Fetal Heart Rate; FTV: Fetal Thrombotic Vasculopathy; IUFD: Intra Uterine Fetal Death; MCA: Middle Cerebral Artery; PI: Pulsatility index; PPA: Prolonged Partial Asphyxia; RI: Resistance index; RIR: Resistance Index Ratios; tCAN: tight Cord Around the Neck syndrome; TCS: Thin Cord Syndrome; UA: Umbilical artery; UV: Umbilical Venous; VA: Veno-Arterial; VLBW: Very Low Birth Weight

Acknowledgements

Not Applicable.

Funding

No Funding.

Authors' contributions

One author: Morarji Peesay, MD FAAP.

Competing interests

The authors declare that they have no competing interests.

References

1. Gould GM, Pyle WL. Prenatal anomalies. Anomalies and curiosities of medicine. New York: The Julian Press, Inc.; 1896. p. 95.
2. Crawford S. Cord round the neck. Incidence and squeal. Acta Pediátrica. 1962;51:594–603. Version of Record online: 21 JAN 2008.
3. Larson JD, Rayburn WF, Crosby S, Thurnau GR. Multiple nuchal cord entanglements and intrapartum complications. Am J Obstet Gynecol. 1995;173:1228.
4. Clapp JF, Stepanchak W, Hashimoto K, Ehrenberg H, Lopez B. The natural history of antenatal nuchal cords. Am J Obstet Gynecol. 2003;189:488–93.
5. Henry E, Andres RL, Christensen RD. Neonatal outcomes following a tight nuchal cord. J Perinatol. 2013;33:231.
6. Miser W. Outcome of infants born with nuchal cords. J Fam Pract. 1992;34: 441–5.
7. Ferguson Virginia L, et al. Bioengineering aspects of the umbilical cord. European Journal of Obstetrics and Gynecology and Reproductive Biology. 144:S108–13.
8. Heifetz SA. The umbilical cord: obstetrically important lesions. Clin Obstet Gynecol. 1996;39(3):571–87.
9. Krakowiak P, Smith EN, de Bruyn G, et al. Risk factors and outcomes associated with a short umbilical cord. Obstet Gynecol. 2004;103:119–27.
10. Naeye RL, et al. Umbilical cord length: clinical significance. J Pediatr. 1985;107(2):278–81.
11. Crichon JL. Tensile strength of the umbilical cord. Am J Obstet Gynecol. 1973;115:77–80.
12. Lacro RV, Jones KL, Benirschke K. The umblical cord twist: origin, direction and relevance. Am J Obstet Gynecol. 1987;157(4 Pt 1):833–08.
13. Gupta S, Faridi MMA, Krishnan J. Umbilical coiling Indes. J Obstet Gynecol India. 2006;56:315–9.
14. Horn LC, Faber R, Stepan H, Simon E, Robel R, Wittekind C. Umbilical cord hypercoiling and thinning: a rare cause of intrauterine death in the second trimester of pregnancy. Pediatr Dev Pathol. 2006 Jan-Feb;9(1):20–4. Epub 2006 Apr 4
15. Strong TH Jr, Elliott JP, Radin TG. Non-coiled umbilical blood vessels: a new marker for the fetus at risk. Obstet Gynecol. 1993;81(3):409–11.
16. Giacomello F. Ultrasound determination of nuchal cord breech presentation. Am J Obstet Gynecol. 1988;159:531–2.
17. Stapczynski JS, Dietrich AM. Theories of strangulation injuries. Emergency Medicine Reports, A Practical Journal for Emergency Physicians. 2010; 31(Number 17):195–6. emreports.com
18. Baergen RN. Cord abnormalities, structural lesions, and cord "accidents". Semin Diagn Pathol. 2007;24:23–32.
19. Parast MM, Crum CP, Boyd TK. Placental histologic criteria for umbilical blood flow restriction in unexplained stillbirth. Hum Pathol. 2008;39:948–53.
20. Peesay M, Nitin M. Cord around the neck syndrome. Neonatology Today. 2011;6(2):11–2.
21. Shepherd AJ, Richardson CJ, Brown JP. Nuchal cord as a cause of neonatal anemia. Am J Dis Child. 1985;139(1):71–3.
22. Vanhaesebroudk P, Vanneste K, de Praester C, Van Trappen Y, Thiery M. Tight nuchal cord and neonatal hypovolemic shock. Arch Dis Child. 1987;62:1276–7.
23. Jauniaux E, Mawissa C, Peellaerts C, Rodesch F. Nuchal cord in normal third-trimester pregnancy: a color Doppler imaging study. Ultrasound Obstet Gynecol. 1992;2:417.
24. Ranzini AC, Walters CA, Vintzileos AM. Ultrasound diagnosis of nuchal cord: the gray-scale divot sign. Obstet Gynecol. 1999;93:854.
25. Mendez-Bauer C, Troxell RM, Roberts JE, Firman SM, Dubois JF, Menendez A, Freese UE. A clinical test for diagnosing nuchal cords. J Reprod Med. 1987;32:924–7.
26. Anyaegbunam AM, Ditchik A, Stoessel R, Mikhail MS. Vibroacoustic stimulation of the fetus entering the second stage of labor. Obstet Gynecol. 1994 Jun;83(6):963–6.
27. Xu H, Dai WP, Wang CJ, Tian LX, Tang HM, Sun FQ. Prediction of fetal hypoxia by measuring middle cerebral and umbilical artery resistance index in fetuses with umbilical cord around the neck in late pregnancy. Nan Fang Yi Ke Da Xue Bao. 2008;28(12):2207–9.
28. Hashimoto K, Clapp JF. The effect of nuchal cord on amniotic fluid and cord blood erythropoietin at delivery. J Soc Gynecol Investig. 2003;10:406–11.
29. Malek A, Sager R, Eckardt KU, Bauer C, Schneider H. Lack of transport of erythropoietin across the human placenta as studied by an in vitro perfusion system. Pflugers Arch. 1994 May;427(1–2):157–61.
30. Maier RF, Böhme K, Dudenhausen JW, Obladen M. Cord blood erythropoietin in relation to different markers of fetal hypoxia. Obstet Gynecol. 1993 Apr;81(4):575–80.
31. Vykuntaraju KN. Cerebral palsy and early stimulation. Chapter 9. Contributor Veena Karla. JP Medical Ltd; 2014. p. 76–7. ISBN: 9350903016, 9789350903018.
32. Martin GC, Green RS, Holzman IR. Acidosis in newborns with Nuchal cords and normal Apgar scores. J Perinatol. 2005;25:162–5.
33. Belai Y, Goodwin TM, Durand M, et al. Umbilical arteriovenous PO2 and PCO2 differences and neonatal morbidity in term infants with severe acidosis. Am J Obstet Gynecol. 1998;178(1Pt 1):13–9.
34. Martinez-Biarge M, Diez-Sebastian J, Wusthoff CJ, Mercuri E, Cowan FM. Antepartum and Intrapartum factors preceding neonatal hypoxic-ischemic encephalopathy. Pediatrics Volume 132, Number 4, October 2013; page e955.
35. Sauvageau A, Boghossian E. Classification of asphyxia: the need for standardization. J Forensic Sci. 2010;55:1259–67.
36. Rocha E, Totten S, Hammond R, Han V, Richardson B. Structural proteins during brain development in the preterm and near-term ovine fetus and the effect of intermittent umbilical cord occlusion. Am J Obstet Gynecol. 2004;191(2):497–506.
37. Nelson KB, Grether JK. Potentially asphyxiating conditions and spastic cerebral palsy in infants of normal birth weight. Am J Obstet Gynecol. 1998;179:507–13.
38. Nielsen L, Schendel D, Grove J, Hvidtjørn D, Jacobsson B, Josiassen T, Vestergaard M, Uldall P, Thorsen P. Asphyxia-related risk factors and their timing in spastic cerebral palsy. BJOG Int J Obstet Gynaecol. 2008; 115:1518–28.
39. Clapp JF, Lopez B, Simonean S. Nuchal cord and neurodevelopmental performance at 1 year. J Soc Gynecol Investig. 1999;6(5):268–72.
40. Greenwood C, Impey L. The association of nuchal cord with cerebral palsy is influenced by recording bias. Early Hum Dev. 2002 Jun;68(1):15–9.
41. Sheiner E, Abramowicz JS, Levy A, Silberstein T, Mazor M, Hershkovitz R. Nuchal cord is not associated with adverse perinatal outcome. Arch Gynecol Obstet. 2006 May;274(2):81–3. Epub 2005 Dec

Undernutrition and its association with socio-demographic, anemia and intestinal parasitic infection among pregnant women attending antenatal care at the University of Gondar Hospital, Northwest Ethiopia

Gemechu Kumera[1*], Dereje Gedle[1], Animut Alebel[2], Fetuma Feyera[2] and Setegn Eshetie[3]

Abstract

Background: Under nutrition is a worldwide public health problem affecting the well-being of millions of pregnant women in the developing world. Only limited research has been conducted on the prevalence and determinants of maternal nutritional status in Ethiopia. Particularly, data on the nutritional status of pregnant women are lacking. The aim of this study was to assess the prevalence and determinants of undernutrition among pregnant women attending antenatal care at the University of Gondar Hospital, Northwest Ethiopia.

Methods: An institution based cross-sectional study was conducted in January and February 2016. Randomly selected 409 pregnant women were included in the study. Nutritional status was estimated using mid-upper-arm circumference. Data on potential determinants of undernutrition were gathered using a structured questionnaire. The blood sample was collected to analyze hemoglobin. The stool sample was collected to identify intestinal parasitic infections. Statistical analysis was done using logistic regression. *P*-value < 0.05 at 95% confidence interval was considered as statistically significant.

Results: The prevalence of undernutrition among pregnant women was 16.2% (95% CI: 12.4–20.1%). Using a logistic regression model, factors significantly associated with the undernutrition were living in rural areas (AOR = 2.26), low educational status [no formal education (AOR = 2.91), primary education (AOR = 2.69)], history of too many births (AOR = 2.55), anemia (AOR = 2.01), and intestinal parasitic infection (AOR = 2.73).

Conclusion: The study findings provide evidence for the public health significance of under nutrition among pregnant women in the study area. The problem must be combated through rural livelihood promotion, socioeconomic empowerment of women, sustained nutrition education and expansion of family-planning services in the area.

Keywords: Undernutrition, Pregnant women, Northwest Ethiopia

* Correspondence: gemechisfreedom@gmail.com
[1]Department of Public Health, College of Medicine and Health Science, Debre Markos University, Debre Markos, Ethiopia
Full list of author information is available at the end of the article

Background

Undernutrition and poor health from preventable causes disproportionately affect the well-being of millions of people in the developing world [1]. Maternal undernutrition is a worldwide public health problem affecting a high proportion of women in developing countries [2]. Women and young children are the most affected [3]. More than 3.5 million women and children under age five in developing countries die each year due to the underlying cause of undernutrition [4]. Women in sub-Saharan Africa, south-central and southeastern Asia are the most affected [3].

Ethiopia faces one of the world's highest rates of maternal undernutrition. The analysis of Ethiopian Demographic Health Surveys (EDHS) 2000, 2005 and 2011 data revealed 30.5, 26.9, 27% of women in Ethiopia are undernourished respectively [5–7]. Based on recently conducted DHS country surveys, the proportion of undernourished women in sub-Saharan African countries ranges from 7 to 37%, indicating that maternal undernutrition in Ethiopia is higher than the level for many African countries [8].

Maternal prenatal undernutrition has a major impact on their own health as well as their children's health. Increased perinatal and neonatal mortality, a higher risk of low birth weight and stunted babies, intrauterine growth restriction, stillbirths, and miscarriage are some of the consequences of undernutrition in women, which further undermines the human capital development of the family and society, and continues the cycle of poverty and malnutrition [9–15].

Undernutrition is a serious problem in Ethiopia. One of every four (27%) women in Ethiopia are undernourished [7]. Although the government and nongovernmental organizations have been perpetually working to improve the nutritional status of the women, the outcome of these efforts has not yet knocked mitigating effect on the prevalence of undernutrition among women in Ethiopia.

Only limited research has been conducted on the prevalence and determinants of maternal nutritional status in Ethiopia. Particularly, data on the nutritional status of pregnant women are lacking. Information on the nutritional status and associated factors among pregnant women are needed for prioritizing, designing and initiating intervention programs aimed at improving maternal nutrition. In addition, such data can be employed in programmes that are aimed to reduce maternal and child morbidity and mortality. Thus, this study was carried out to provide information regarding the prevalence and factors associated with undernutrition during pregnancy.

Methods

Study design, area and population

An institution based cross-sectional study was conducted at the University of Gondar Hospital in January and February 2016. The University of Gondar Hospital is a tertiary-level service-rendering institution that provides health service to over 4 million people in Gondar town and surrounding area. The Gondar town lies in the average at 2000 m above sea level and over 370,000 population reside in this administrative town [16]. The study populations were all pregnant women in Gondar town and surrounding area who attend antenatal care (ANC) at the University of Gondar Hospital.

Sample size and sampling technique

A sample size of 409 was computed using single population proportion sample size calculation formula with inputs of 95% confidence level, 4% margin of error, 19.1% expected prevalence of undernutrition [17] and 10% non-response rate. A systematic random sampling technique was used to select the study subjects. According to the Hospital report, on average, 35–45 pregnant women visit the ANC daily, and 1241 pregnant women have been enrolled in ANC. Since the sample size was determined as 409, a sampling interval of 3 was used to select study participants. Of the first three pregnant women, one woman was randomly selected by using lottery method (The pregnant women is assigned to unique number (1, 2 and 3), putting it on a piece of paper. The pieces of paper are placed in the container and thoroughly mixed. Then, a blind folded researcher picks a number. Number three (3) was selected.). Accordingly, every 3rd pregnant women were selected to participate in the study until the required sample size of 409 pregnant women was obtained.

Data collection methods

Questionnaire

A structured and pre-tested questionnaire was used for assessing potential determinants of undernutrition. The parts of the questionnaire on dietary diversity were adopted from Food and Nutrition Technical Assistance (FANTA) indicator guideline [18]. Other parts of the questionnaire were developed by the principal investigators. The questionnaire was administered in a local language(Amharic). The English version of the questionnaire was translated into local language and back to English by an expert to ensure its consistency. The translated Amharic version (local language) was pre-tested prior to the actual survey and modifications were made accordingly. The content validity of the tool was checked against the conceptual framework of the study by relevant professionals. Reliability of the tool was checked using a test-retest method. Questions with less than 0.7 kappa or Pearson coefficient values were removed or revised. Five data collectors (three midwives and two laboratory technicians) and one supervisor were recruited. Training was given for data collectors and supervisor by the principal investigator to have consensus and the same understanding of what is intended to be measured by each question in the questionnaire. The data collection process was followed daily by the supervisor and principal investigator. The dietary diversity (DD) level was assessed using 24-h recall method. Respondents were asked whether they had taken any food from predefined 12 food categories on a preceding day. Accordingly, the level of Dietary Diversity Score (DDS) was computed out of 12. According to the recommendation of Food and Agriculture Organization (FAO) of the United Nations, DD was classified into low (DDS ≤3), medium (DDS of 4 or 5), or high (DDS ≥6) [19]. Pregnant women from all trimesters (first, second and third) were included in the study.

Mid upper arm circumference (MUAC) measurement

Mid upper arm circumference was measured halfway between the tip of the shoulder (olecranon process) and the tip of the elbow (acromion process) to the nearest 0.1 cm. An insertion type MUAC tape that is non-elastic and non-stretchable was used to take the measurement. The measurement was taken at the mid-point on the relaxed left arm, without any clothing and with optimal tape tension (not too loose or not too tight) following the standard instructions and steps [20]. Recently published paper based on a review of evidence revealed that MUAC is a preferred anthropometric measurement during pregnancy [21] and also not affected by non-nutritional changes [22]. Undernutrition was defined as MUAC less than 22 cm [23].

Laboratory analysis

Hemoglobin level determination

Venous blood was collected from each pregnant woman, using sterile blood collection tubes following standard procedures. Hemoglobin level was determined using hematological analyzer (Cell Dyn 1800, PD, USA) machine. Anemia was defined as a hemoglobin level of less than 11.0 g/dl during the first or third trimester or less than 10.5 g/dl during the second trimester [24]. According to the formula recommended by Center for Disease Prevention and Control, hemoglobin values were adjusted for altitude [25].

Stool specimen collection and examination

Stool samples were collected from participants using clean, dry and leak-proof cupped plastic container following standard procedures. The stool samples were masked, coded, and processed for parasitological examination. Different stool examinations were used for efficacy in detecting parasites. These were direct wet-mount and formaldehyde-ether sedimentation method [26, 27]. The WHO guide for diagnosis of intestinal parasitosis was used as an identification reference [28].

Data processing and analysis

Data were entered using EPI-INFO version 7 software. The analysis was carried out using SPSS version 20 statistical program. Wealth index (poor, middle and rich) were computed using principal component analysis as a composite indicator of living standard. In this study, undernutrition (MUAC < 22 cm) was an outcome variable. Bivariate and multivariable logistic regression analysis was used to assess the association between the dependent and independent variables and to control confounders. Independent variables significantly associated with the dependent variable in bivariate regression models were exported to multivariable regression models for adjustment. The collinearity effect was tested using the Variance Inflation Factor (VIF) for all independent variables. Model fitness was assessed using the Hosmer-Lemeshow statistic test. *P*-value < 0.05 at 95% CI was considered statistically significant.

Ethical cosideration

The study was conducted in confirmation of national and international ethical guidelines for biomedical research involving human subjects. Ethical clearance was obtained from an ethical review committee of the University of Gondar. Written informed consent was obtained from each study participants prior to participation in the study after the nature of the study was fully explained to the study participants. Women who had intestinal parasites and anemia were treated accordingly. Those women identified as undernourished were referred to ANC clinicians for treatment. Nutrition education was given to all study participants. Those participants identified as undernourished were given nutritional counseling and Ready Use Therapeutic Food (RUTF) in collaboration with the clinicians working in an ART clinic at Hospital.

Results

Socio-demographic characteristics of the study participants

Table 1 summarizes socio-demographic characteristics of the study participants. Of the total 409 pregnant women, initially planned for the study, 402 were volunteered to take part in the study, with a response rate of 98.3%. The vast majority of the respondents were Amhara in ethnicity (94.8%) and orthodox (88.6%) in religion. The majority of participants (62.4%) were in the age group 25–34 years with the mean and standard deviation of 26.6 (± 4.7) years. Nearly One-fourth of study subjects, 92(22.9%) had no formal education and more than half, 221 (55.0%) were housewives. The majority,

Table 1 Socio-demographic characteristics of the study participants, Northwest Ethiopia, 2016 ($n = 402$)

Characteristics		Frequency (n)	Percent (%)
Age(years)	15–24	120	29.9
	25–34	251	62.4
	≥ 35	31	7.7
Residence	Urban	303	75.4
	Rural	99	24.6
Marital status	Married	386	96
	Single	7	1.7
	Divorced	2	0.5
	Separated	6	1.5
	Widowed	1	0.2
Religion	Orthodox	356	88.6
	Muslim	37	9.2
	Protestant	9	2.2
Ethnicity	Amhara	381	94.8
	Tigre	15	3.7
	Oromo	2	0.5
	Other	4	1.0
Educational status	No formal education	92	22.9
	Primary education	84	20.9
	High school education	112	27.9
	Certificate and above	114	28.4
Occupation	House wife	221	55.0
	Farmer	13	3.2
	Merchant	51	12.7
	Government employee	94	23.4
	Daily laborer	11	2.7
	Student	12	3.0
Family size	≤ 3	285	70.9
	4–6	90	22.4
	> 6	27	6.7
Wealth Index	Low	134	33.3
	Middle	134	33.3
	High	134	33.3

303 (75.4%), of the respondents, were urban dwellers. The average household size was 3.2 (± 1.6). The median monthly household income was 2000 Ethiopian birr.

Environmental and sanitation factors

Table 2 summarizes environmental and sanitation characteristics of the study participants. Source of drinking water for the greater number, 368(91.5%) of study subjects was tap water. The majority of study participants, 383(95.3%) had toilet facilities. The large proportion of participants, 283(73.9%) use pit latrine.

Table 2 Environmental and sanitation characteristics of pregnant women attending antenatal care, Northwest Ethiopia, 2016

Characteristics		Frequency (n)	Percent (%)
Source of drinking water	Tab	368	91.5
	Well	11	2.7
	Spring	23	5.7
Possession of toilet facility	Yes	383	95.3
	No	19	4.7
Types of latrine	Pit latrine	283	73.9
	Water flush	97	25.3
	Public	3	0.8

Reproductive health factors

Table 3 summarizes reproductive health factors of study participants. More than half, 224 (55.7%) of the participants were in the third trimester, 117(29.1%) in the second and 61(15.2%) in the first trimester. The results revealed a greater majority of the participants, 198(49.3%) had a first pregnancy at a time of data collection. In 33 (8.2%) of the study participants, the birth interval was less than the recommended 24 months. The mean parity was 1.1 (± 1.6), ranging between 0 and 7 pregnancies. The mean MUAC for nulliparas was 24.7 (+/− 2.6) cm. The corresponding value for parity categories of 1–3 and 4 or more was 25.2 (+/− 3.1) cm and 23.5 (+/− 2.8) cm, respectively.

Dietary intakes of the study participants

Table 4 summarizes dietary intakes of the study participants. The vast majority of the study subjects consumed cereal-based foods (made of teff) (Fig. 1). The commonly and frequently consumed foods were a starchy staple, 100% and legumes, 273(67.9%). Only one-fourth, 86(21.4%) of study subjects were consumed vitamin A rich fruits and vegetables in the reference period. Two hundred forty-six, (61.2%) of the study participants

Table 3 Reproductive health factors among pregnant women attending antenatal care, Northwest Ethiopia, 2016

Characteristics		Frequency (n)	Percent (%)
Trimester of pregnancy	First	61	15.2
	Second	117	29.1
	Third	224	55.7
Parity	0	198	49.3
	1–3	155	38.6
	≥ 4	49	12.2
Birth interval	0(No birth)	198	49.3
	< 2 yr	33	8.2
	≥ 2 yr	171	42.5

Table 4 Dietary intakes of pregnant women attending antenatal care, Northwest Ethiopia, 2016

Characteristics		Frequency (n)	Percent (%)
Number of meals/day	< 3	46	11.4
	3	282	70.1
	> 3	74	18.4
Family food source	Grow their own	70	17.4
	Buy/purchase	330	82.1
	Subsidies/food aid	2	0.5
Dietary diversity	Low	267	66.4
	Medium	123	30.6
	High	12	3.0
Home gardening	Yes	31	7.7
	No	371	92.3
Animal food source	Yes	128	31.8
	No	274	68.2
Coffee intake	Yes	246	61.2
	No	156	38.8
Number of cup of coffee per day	≤ 3	190	77.2
	> 3	56	22.8

reported that they consumed coffee. A small proportion, 128 (31.8%) of study participants reported that they consumed a diet of animal origin prior to the survey. Among animal products, flesh meat was consumed by 94 (23.4%) of the study subjects, whereas egg, milk and milk products and organ meat were consumed by 20 (5%), 25 (6.2%) and 2 (0.5%), respectively. The mean DDS was 3.33 (± 0.77), ranging between 1 and 7. The majority of study participants, 267 (66.4%) had low DDS (≤3 food groups). The meal frequency was three times a day for the majority of the study participants 282(70.1%).

Anemia, HIV and diarrhea among the study participants

Of all study participants, 17(4.2%) were positive for HIV. Among 21 study participants who were positive for HIV, 6(28.6%) were undernourished. The mean MUAC for HIV positive and negative were 23.1(± 3.8) and 24.8(± 2.8) cm, respectively. A small proportion, 26(6.5%) of the pregnant women had diarrhea; of whom nearly one-fourth, 6(23.1%) were undernourished. Overall, the prevalence of anemia was 132(32.8%), and was more evident in undernourished pregnant women (25%) than in normal pregnant women(MUAC≥ 22 cm).

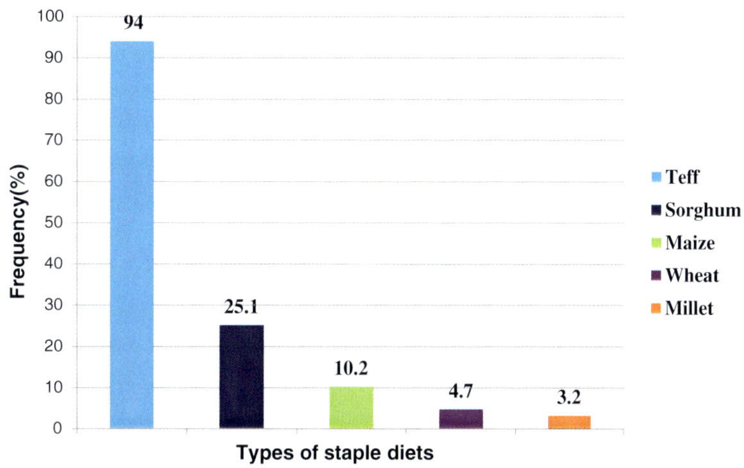

Fig. 1 Staple diets of pregnant women attending antenatal care, Northwest Ethiopia, 2016

Prevalence and type of intestinal parasites among the study participants

Figure 2 summarizes prevalence and type of intestinal parasitic infection among the study participants. One hundred twenty-six, (31.3%) of study participants were infected with one or more intestinal parasites. Of whom, 35(27.8%) were undernourished. The most common single and mixed parasites observed were *Entamoeba histolytica* 48(38.1%) and Ascaris lumbricoides 31(24.6%). Intestinal parasitic infection tends increase among rural dwellers and pregnant women who used other sources of drinking water other than tap water. Of 99 rural dwellers pregnant women, 41(41.4%) were infected with one or more intestinal parasites. Among 11 pregnant women who consumed well water, 7(63.6%) were infected with one or more intestinal parasites. Similarly, among 23 pregnant women who consumed spring water, 12(52.2%) were infected with one or more intestinal parasites.

Prevalence of under nutrition

Undernutrition (MUAC < 22 cm) was observed in 65 of 402 pregnant women studied, yielding a prevalence of 16.2% (95% CI: 12.4–20.1%). The mean MUAC (±SD) of the study participants was 24.8 cm (± 2.9). The value ranged from 18 to 37 cm. The prevalence of undernutrition during the first, second and third trimesters were, 14.8, 16.2 and 16.5%, respectively. The mean MUAC(±SD) for the first, second and third trimesters were, 24.8 (± 3.2), 24.8(± 2.8) and 24.7 (± 2.7) g/dl, respectively.

Factors associated with undernutrition

Table 5 summarizes factors associated with undernutrition among pregnant women. A multivariable analysis in a form of logistic regression was employed to identify the risk factors of undernutrition among pregnant women. The analyses rest on two outcomes of nutritional status of pregnant women: whether they are undernourished (MUAC< 22 cm) or not (MUAC≥ 22 cm). In the bivariate analysis, undernutrition was significantly associated with age, residence, wealth index, educational status, source of drinking water, parity, animal source food, HIV, anemia and intestinal parasite. The multivariable logistic regression analysis revealed that residence, maternal educational status, parity, anemia and intestinal parasite were predictors of undernutrition.

Place of residence was significantly associated with nutritional status of pregnant women ($P = 0.03$). The risk of undernutrition was two times, [AOR = 2.26; 95% CI (1.06, 4.81)] higher among rural pregnant women than their urban counterparts.

The study also witnessed significant association between educational level and maternal nutritional status. The risk of undernutrition for pregnant women with no formal education and primary education was 2.91 and 2.69 times higher, respectively as compared to pregnant women with higher education (certificate and above) [AOR = 2.91; 95% CI (1.11, 7.56)], [AOR = 2.69; 95% CI (1.09, 6.64)].

Significant associations were also observed between nutritional status and parity. The risk of undernutrition for pregnant women with grand multiparas was two and half times higher as compared to pregnant women with no parity [AOR = 2.55; 95% (1.04, 6.26)].

Anemia was found to be significantly associated with undernutrition. Pregnant women who were anemic were

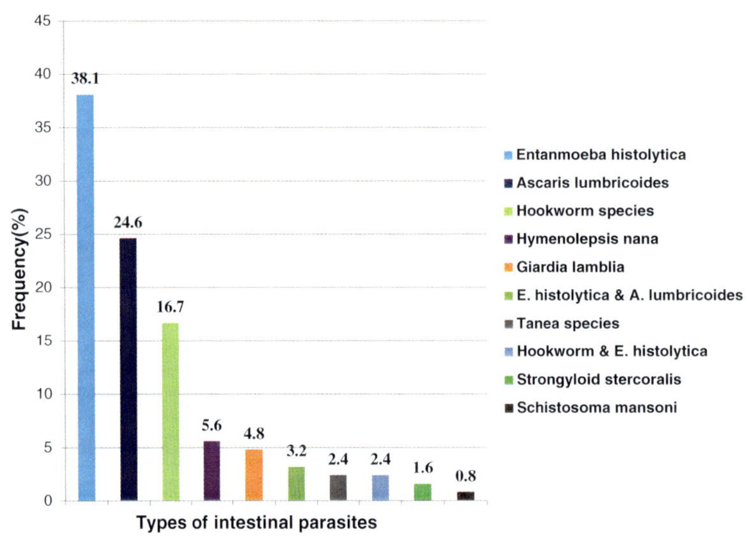

Fig. 2 Prevalence and types of intestinal parasites among pregnant women attending antenatal care, Northwest Ethiopia, 2016

Table 5 Factors associated with the undernutrition among pregnant women

Predictors	Under nutrition		COR (95%CI)	AOR (95% CI)	P-values
	Yes	No			
Age					
15–24	34	86	2.36(1.01, 5.53)		
25–34	28	223	2.17 (0.87, 5.44)		
≥ 35	3	28	1		
Residence					
Rural	32	67	3.91(2.24, 6.81)	2.26 (1.06, 4.81)	0.03*
Urban	33	270	1	1	
Wealth index					
Low	36	98	4.54 (2.13, 9.70)		
Middle	19	115	2.05(1.12, 3.75)		
High	11	123	1		
Educational status					
No formal education	31	61	5.18(2.37, 11.31)	2.91 (1.11, 7.56)	0.02*
Primary education	12	72	4.32(2.06, 9.03)	2.69 (1.09, 6.64)	0.03*
Secondary education	10	102	3.04(1.44, 6.44)		
Certificate and above	12	102	1	1	
Source of drinking water					
Spring	8	15	2.54 (1.00, 6.47)		
Well	3	8	2.16 (0.86, 5.48)		
Tab	54	314	1		
Parity					
No birth	23	175	1		
1–3	24	131	3.63 (1.76, 7.51)		
≥ 4	19	30	4.82 (2.34, 9.91)	2.55 (1.04, 6.26)	0.04*
Animal source food					
Yes	13	115	1		
No	52	222	2.07 (1.08, 3.96)		
HIV					
No	60	325	1		
Yes	5	12	2.38 (1.01, 5.95)		
Anemia					
No	32	238	1	1	
Yes	33	99	2.48 (1.45, 4.25)	2.01 (1.16, 3.79)	0.01**
Intestinal parasite					
Absent	30	246	1	1	
Present	35	91	3.15 (1.83, 5.43)	2.73 (1.48, 5.03)	0.001**

*P-value is significant at < 0.05, **P-value is significant at ≤ 0.01

two times more likely to be undernourished than those with normal hemoglobin level [AOR = 2.01; 95% (1.16, 3.79)].

The intestinal parasite was also found to be significantly associated with undernutrition. Pregnant women who had one or more intestinal parasitic infection were three times more likely to be malnourished as compared to those who had no intestinal parasitic infection [AOR = 2.73; 95% CI (1.48, 5.03)].

In this study, nutritional status did not show any statistical association with regard to dietary diversity, family size, occupation, latrine availability, number of meals per day, coffee intake, staple diets, home gardening and family food source.

Discussion

This study assessed the prevalence and determinants of undernutrition among pregnant women attending antenatal care. The current study witnessed the public health significance of undernutrition in the study area. Findings of the study showed that, 16.2% of pregnant women were undernourished. In Ethiopia, few studies determined the prevalence of undernutrition in pregnant women and came up with figures 9.2% [29], 19.1% [17], 31.4% [30] and 34.0% [31]. The studies consistently witnessed the public health significance of undernutrition in the country. The current study showed that prevalence of undernutrition among pregnant in the country is decreasing as compared to earlier studies. The probable reason for this variation could be the interventions on nutrition, maternal health and other women empowering programs by the government and other non-governmental organizations in the country. Moreover, the variation may be due to geographical variation, smaller land holding, the recurrent food insecurity and the seasonal difference in data collection. Further, the prevalence may have overestimated in earlier studies as only adolescent pregnant women were included in the study.

Women living in rural areas are more undernourished than their urban counterparts. Similar results have been reported from earlier studies [3, 6, 32, 33]. The disparity may be due to less developed infrastructures, low nutritional awareness, low access to health care, safe water, and sanitation facilities, traditional ways of farming as only means of surviving and cultural and religious influences in rural areas. In addition, lower nutritional status among rural pregnant women could be explained partly by the fact that in rural areas women are more vulnerable to early marriage and childbearing than women in urban areas [6]. Hence, in addition to their own health needs, they need an adequate dietary intake for pregnancy and child growth. Further, the higher levels of labor or workload among rural pregnant women may contribute to poor nutritional status among pregnant women in rural areas, as overexertion is a predisposing factor to maternal nutritional depletion [34].

The study findings indicate a negative relationship between the educational status of the pregnant women and undernutrition, with decreasing educational levels from certificate and above to no formal education, the level of undernutrition tends to increase. Previous studies also have documented similar findings [30–32, 35]. The probable reason could be pregnant women who are literate may have more exposure to media, which influence their behaviour in matters related to their own feeding and health [36]. Unawareness of illiterate women about their own health and nutritional status could be another reason associated with their poor nutritional status. Moreover, the low educational level of women could be associated with little or no decision-making power in the household about food distribution, purchase of household consumption items and financial issues which may contribute to their low nutritional status. However, in a study conducted in Iran, there was no statistically significant association between pregnant women's education level and nutritional status [37]. The variation can be due to the difference in socioeconomic status and nutritional care prior to and during pregnancy.

Another finding that affects pregnant women's nutritional status is parity. The odds of undernutrition were observed to rise as parity advances. Previous studies also reported the same [29, 31, 32]. The study witnessed the deleterious effect of too many births on nutritional status. The finding is consistent with the knowledge that repeated reproductive cycles deplete maternal nutrition store. Moreover, higher-level parity obligates women to take care of their children rather than protecting their own health and nutritional status, given limited household resources.

The current study finding witnessed a significant positive association between anemia and undernutrition. The proportion of undernutrition was significantly more among anemic pregnant women compared to normal hemoglobin level pregnant women. This finding is in line with studies conducted in Ethiopia [38], Kenya [39] and India [40], which indicated that the risk of anemia tends to increase among undernourished pregnant women. This might be due to the fact that undernourished pregnant women have a higher risk of being deficient in micronutrients and therefore more likely to be anemic. As the study is cross-sectional, it is not viable to exclude "the chicken or the egg" causality dilemma. However, as protein is known to take part in multiple metabolic pathways, it might have a causal role in anemia. This relation between undernutrition and anemia might be due alterations in spleen and bone marrow erythropoiesis, reduction in reticulocyte as a result of a protein-energy deficiency in undernourished pregnant women [41].

In the present study, intestinal parasitic infection was found to be one of the determinant predictors of risk of undernutrition. Pregnant women who had one or more intestinal parasitic infection were at greater risk of being undernourished as compared to pregnant women with no intestinal parasites. Intestinal parasitic infections may affect nutritional status by reducing appetite and dietary intake. It also affects by increasing nutrient losses due to vomiting, diarrhea, poor digestion and absorption. Further, the nutrient demand of parasite itself and intestinal bleeding caused by the parasite may contribute to poor nutritional status [42–44].

Major strength of this study was the random selection of the study participants. The major limitation was the cross-sectional nature of its design as we can't establish causal relationships between the independent variables and nutritional status of the pregnant women. Secondly, the study was institution based and the study subjects may not represent the general population. Third, the last date of the menstrual period and/or fundal height with a subsequent urine test, were used to diagnose pregnancy, which may not accurately confirm pregnancy.

Recommendation

A national level study should be conducted in Ethiopia. The problem must be combated through an implementation of strategies like rural livelihood promotion, socio-economic empowerment of women and expansion of women's education, particularly in rural areas. Nutritional care should be integrated into maternity services. We also suggest sustained nutrition education to enhance good nutritional awareness and practice of pregnant women. Expansion of family planning services will also have affirmative input. Prevention and control of intestinal parasite infection through improving access to safe and adequate water supply; sanitation and hygiene practices should be considered. Screening of pregnant women for intestinal parasitic infections, universal deworming programs, and expansion of prenatal iron-folate supplementation should also be looked for.

Conclusion

The study findings provide evidence for the public health significance of undernutrition among pregnant in the study area. The important risk factors/ predictors of undernutrition (MUAC < 22 cm) were living in rural areas, low educational status, history of too many births, anemia and intestinal parasitic infection.

Abbreviations

ANC: Antenatal care; DD: Dietary diversity; DDS: Dietary diversity score; EDHS: Ethiopian Demographic and Health Survey; FANTA: Food and Nutrition Technical Assistance; FAO: Food and Agriculture Organization of the United Nations; MUAC: Mid upper arm circumference; SD: Standard deviation

Acknowledgements

We would like to thank the University of Gondar Hospital staffs for their full cooperation and vital assistance during data collection and conducting the laboratory analysis. Special thanks go to entire study subjects for their full participation in the study. We acknowledge University of Gondar and Save the children for funding the study.

Funding

This study was supported by the University of Gondar and Save the children for data collection material and reagents. However, the they had no role in a decision to publish or preparation of the manuscript.

Authors' contributions

GK participated in study protocol development, data collection, analysis, write-up and drafting of the manuscript. AA, FF, and SE assisted in data collection and reviewing papers. All authors read and approved the final manuscript.

Competing interests

We, the authors, have no any competing interests.

Author details

[1]Department of Public Health, College of Medicine and Health Science, Debre Markos University, Debre Markos, Ethiopia. [2]Department of Nursing, College of Medicine and Health Science, Debre Markos University, Debre Markos, Ethiopia. [3]School of Biomedical and Laboratory Sciences, College of Medicine and Health Science, University of Gondar, Gondar, Ethiopia.

References

1. Piot P, Semba R and Bloem M. Nutrition and health in developing countries. Totowa: Springer Science and Business Media; 2008.
2. Adebowale S, Adepoju O, Okareh T. Social epidemiology of adverse nutritional status outcomes among women in Nigeria: NDHS, 2008. Pak J Nutr. 2011;10(9):888–98.
3. Uthman O, Aremu O. Malnutrition among women in sub-Saharan Africa: rural-urban disparity. Rural Remote Health. 2008;8(2):931.
4. Black R, Allen L, Bhutta Z, Caulfield L, Onis M. Maternal and child undernutrition: global and regional exposures and health consequences. Lancet. 2008;371(9608):243–60.
5. Central Statistical Agency (Ethiopia) and ORC Macro. Ethiopia Demographic and Health Survey. Addis Ababa and Calverton: Central Statistical Agency and ORC Macro; 2001.
6. Central Statistical Agency (Ethiopia) and ORC Macro. Ethiopia Demographic and Health Survey. Addis Ababa and Calverton: Central Statistical Agency and ORC Macro; 2006.
7. Central Statistical Agency (Ethiopia) and ICF International. Ethiopia Demographic and Health Survey. Addis Ababa and Calverton: Central Statistical Agency (Ethiopia) and ICF International; 2012.
8. Macro International. Ethiopia Atlas of Key Demographic and Health Indicators. Calverton: Macro International; 2008.
9. Landis S, Lokomba V, Ananth C. Impact of maternal malaria and under-nutrition on intrauterine growth restriction: a prospective ultrasound study in Democratic Republic of Congo. Epidemiol Infection. 2009;137(02):294-304.
10. Goyal R, Mudey A, Banginwar A. Intra-uterine growth restriction (IUGR) among teenage and elderly pregnant women in Vidharba region of Maharashtra, India. Int J Cur Bio Med Sci. 2012;2(1):199–202.
11. Blössner M, Onis M, Prüss-Üstün A. Quantifying the health impact at national and local levels. Geneva: WHO; 2005.
12. Teller C and Yimer G. Levels and determinants of malnutrition in adolescent and adult women in Southern Ethiopia. Ethiop J Health Develop. 2015;14(1):57–66.
13. Girma W, Genebo T. Determinants of nutritional status of women and children in Ethiopia. 2002.
14. Myatt M, Duffield A, Seal A, Pasteur F. The effect of body shape on weight-for-height and mid-upper arm circumference based case definitions of acute malnutrition in Ethiopian children. Ann Human Biol. 2009;36(1):5–20.
15. Garza C, Rasmussen KM. Pregnancy and lactation. In: Garrow JS, James WPT, Ralph A, editors. Human Nutrition and Dietetics. Edinburgh: Churchill Livingstone, London. 2000: p. 437-48.
16. Information and Statistics Office. Information and statistics office. Gondar: University of Gondar Hospital; 2015.
17. Kedir H, Berhane Y, Worku A. Magnitude and determinants of malnutrition among pregnant women in eastern Ethiopia: evidence from rural, community-based setting. Matern Child Nutrit. 2016;12(1):51-63.
18. Swindale A and Bilinsky P. Household dietary diversity score (HDDS) for measurement of household food access: indicator guide. Washington, DC: Food and Nutrition Technical Assistance Project, Academy for Educational Development; 2006.

19. Kennedy G, Ballard T, Dop MC. Guidelines for measuring household and individual dietary diversity. Rome: FAO; 2011.
20. Cogill B. Anthropometric indicators measurement guide. 2003.
21. Ververs M, Antierens A, Sackl A. Which anthropometric indicators identify a pregnant woman as acutely malnourished and predict adverse birth outcomes in the humanitarian context? PLOS Currents Disasters; 2013.
22. López L, Calvo E, Poy M. Changes in skinfolds and mid-upper arm circumference during pregnancy in Argentine women. Matern Child Nutrit. 2011;7(3):253–62.
23. Ferro-Luzzi A, James W. Adult malnutrition: simple assessment techniques for use in emergencies. Brit J Nutrit. 1996;75(1):3–10.
24. Woteki CE, and R Earl. Iron deficiency anemia: recommended guidelines for the prevention, detection, and management among US children and women of childbearing age. Washington, D.C.: National Academies Press;1994.
25. Nestel P. Adjusting hemoglobin values in program surveys. Washington, DC: International Nutritional Anemia Consultative Group, International Life Sciences Institute; 2002.
26. Ridley D, Hawgood B. The value of formol-ether concentration of faecal cysts and ova. J Clin Pathol. 1956;9(1):74.
27. Casemore D, Armstrong M, Sands R. Laboratory diagnosis of cryptosporidiosis. J Clin Pathol. 1985;38(12):1337–41.
28. World Health Organization. Bench aids for the diagnosis of intestinal parasites. Geneva: World Health Organization; 1994.
29. Kuche D, Singh P, Moges D, Belachew T. Nutritional Status and Associated Factors among Pregnant Women in Wondo Genet District, Southern Ethiopia. JFSE. 2015;5:85-94.
30. Regassa N, Stoecker BJ. Contextual risk factors for maternal malnutrition in a food-insecure zone in southern Ethiopia. J Biosoc Sci. 2012;44(5):537–48.
31. Belete Y, Negga B, Firehiwot M. Under nutrition and associated factors among adolescent pregnant women in Shashemenne District, West Arsi Zone, Ethiopia: a community-based. J Nutrit Food Sci. 2016;6(1):1-7.
32. Okwu GN, Ukoha AI, Nwachukwu N, Agha NC. Studies on the Predisposing Factors of Protein Energy Malnutrition Among Pregnant Women in a Nigerian Community. Online J Health Allied Scs. 2008;6(3):1–9.
33. Bitew, F.H. and D.S. Telake, Undernutrition among women in Ethiopia: rural-urban disparity. 2010.
34. Winikoff B, Castle M. Defining maternal depletion syndrome. Am J Public Health. 1993;83(7):1052.
35. Nucci LB, et al. Nutritional status of pregnant women: prevalence and associated pregnancy outcomes. Rev Saude Publica. 2001;35(6):502–7.
36. Begum S, Sen B. Maternal Health, Child Well-Being and chronic poverty: does Women's agency matter? The Bangladesh Development Studies; 2009. p. 69–93.
37. Abasizadeh S, Hemati Z, Deres F. Prevalence of malnutrition during pregnancy and associated factors in women of Ardal County in 2012–2013. Int J Epidemiol Res. 2016;3(1):19–25.
38. Gedefaw L, Ayele A, Asres Y, Mossie A. Anaemia and associated factors among pregnant women attending antenatal care clinic in Walayita Sodo town, Southern Ethiopia. Ethiop J Health Sci. 2015;25(2):155-64.
39. Okubatsion Tekeste Okube* WM, Odhiambo E, Wakasiaka Sabina MH. Prevalence and factors associated with Anaemia among pregnant women attending antenatal Clinic in the Second and Third Trimesters at Pumwani maternity hospital, Kenya. Open J Obstet Gynecol. 2016;6:16–27.
40. Mondal B, Tripathy V, Gupta R. Risk factors of Anemia during pregnancy among the Garo of Meghalaya, India. J Hum Ecol. 2006;14:27-32.
41. Borelli P, et al. Reduction of erythroid progenitors in protein–energy malnutrition. Br J Nutr. 2007;97(2):307–14.
42. Arimond M, Daelmans B, Dewey K, Morris S. Maternal and Child Undernutrition 5 Effective international action against undernutrition: why has it proven so difficult and what can be done to accelerate progress? Commentary. Lancet. 2008;371(9612):608–21.
43. Crompton D, et al. Hookworm infection, nutritional status and productivity. In: Hookworm disease-current status and new directions; 1990. p. 231–64.
44. Jardim-Botelho A, et al. Age patterns in undernutrition and helminth infection in a rural area of Brazil: associations with ascariasis and hookworm. Tropical Med Int Health. 2008;13(4):458–67.

24

Facilitators and barriers to birth preparedness and complication readiness in rural Rwanda among community health workers and community members: a qualitative study

Richard Kalisa[1,2*], Patrick Smeele[3], Marianne van Elteren[3], Thomas van den Akker[4] and Jos van Roosmalen[2,4]

Abstract

Background: Birth preparedness and complication readiness (BP/CR) comprise a strategy to make women plan for birth and encourage them to seek professional care in order to reduce poor pregnancy outcome. We aimed to understand the facilitators and barriers to BP/CR among community health workers (CHWs) and community members in rural Rwanda.

Methods: Eight focus group discussions were conducted with 88 participants comprising of CHWs, elderly women aged 45–68 and men aged 18–59, as well as two key informant interviews in Musanze district, Rwanda, between November and December 2015. Qualitative data were digitally recorded, transcribed verbatim and analysed using content analysis.

Results: Participants perceived the importance of family assistance, medical insurance and attending antenatal care (ANC) to facilitate BP/CR and enhance professional care at birth. CHWs reinforced BP/CR messages by SMS alerts and during community gatherings. 'Ubudehe (collective action to combat poverty)' was known as a tool to identify the poorest families in need of government aid to pay for medical care. Disrespect and abuse of women during labor by health workers were perceived as important barriers to access professional care, as well as conflicting health policies such as user fees for ANC and family planning services, and imposing fines on women giving birth outside health facilities.

Conclusion: CHWs, ANC and medical insurance are perceived to be important facilitators of BP/CR. Respectful care is paramount for improved maternal health. There is a need for addressing inconsistent health policies hindering the intention to access professional care.

Keywords: Pregnancy, facility delivery, birth preparedness, Perceptions, Respectful maternity care

* Correspondence: kalichard@gmail.com
[1]Department of Obstetrics and Gynecology, Ruhengeri Hospital, Musanze, Rwanda
[2]Athena Institute, VU University, Amsterdam, The Netherlands
Full list of author information is available at the end of the article

Background

Access to maternal and newborn health services may be hampered by cultural, socioeconomic, and demographic factors [1]. Receiving care from skilled birth attendants [2–4] and birth preparedness and complication readiness (BP/CR) to encourage such attendance of professional care continue to be key components in programs to reach the Sustainable Development Goals (SDGs) for improved maternal and neonatal survival [5, 6].

BP/CR was previously shown to promote active preparation and decision making for birth among pregnant women and their families [2, 6–8]. Recommendations for birth planning include identifying a birth attendant and the closest appropriate care facility; saving funds for birth and emergency expenses; making arrangements for transport; and looking for compatible blood donors [5].

In 2003, Rwanda adopted BP/CR as part of focused antenatal care to increase facility births [9]. This may have contributed to the reduction of the maternal mortality ratio by roughly two-thirds from 750 in 2005 to 210 per 100,000 live births in 2015 and an increase in skilled birth attendance rate from 28% to 91% in this same time frame [10, 11]. This study aimed to understand the facilitators and barriers to BP/CR among community health workers (CHWs) and community members in rural Rwanda.

Methods

We used a qualitative content analysis [12] to explore perceptions held by CHWs and community members' about BP/CR. The study was conducted in Musanze district, northern Rwanda, with a population of 368,267 inhabitants and a skilled birth attendance rate of 66% [11]. In addition, there is access to one provincial referral hospital for high-risk obstetric cases from 12 health centers and other district hospitals in the northern province. It is also supported by CHWs and a SMS-based system which was developed to improve maternal and child health (MCH) using RapidSMS® that enables communication between CHWs at community level, and the rest of the health system (ambulance, health facility staff, district hospital and RapidSMS-MCH system) through mobile phones [13]. The CHWs referred to throughout this paper were responsible for MCH activities and covered a catchment area of 100–150 households. Medical services offered are paid for using community-based health insurance (commonly known as mutuelles de santé), with an annual fee of RWF 3000 (US$ 4), plus a 10% copayment for each episode of illness.

Sampling and recruitment procedures

Different sampling strategies were used for different groups of participants. We applied purposeful sampling to recruit CHWs, elderly women aged 45–68 and men aged 18–59. First, we used the existing list of all active CHWs covering the entire district and then randomly selected four CHWs to represent one health centre (HC) , and continued the same process to enrol other CHWs from the remaining eleven HCs. The selected representative CHWs from one HC were joined with two additional groups of CHWs from other HCs to make up one focus group discussion (FGD), which was held at an agreed nearby location where privacy was ensured. While elderly women and men were selected with assistance from CHWs after introducing the aim of the study to them. CHWs were asked to select those elderly women who had daughters or daughters-in-law and men who had a female partner, daughters or daughters-in-law, who delivered within the last two years assuming that these elderly women and men had some knowledge of BP/CR.

Data collection

Data collection took place in November and December 2015 using pretested FGDs and key informant interviews (KIIs) guides which were developed in English and translated in Kinyarwanda. Topics covered in the discussion guide were: steps taken to prepare for birth and potential complications during birth in the community, cultural and social issues surrounding BP/CR, recognition of maternal and newborn danger signs, access towards skilled care and challenges at community level. We conducted a total of 8 focus group discussions, with a total of 88 participants from the following groups: CHWs (four groups), elderly women (two groups) and men (two groups). Each discussion included 8 to 12 members. We used two KIIs based on their position to inform policy with regards to maternal health within the district; one with the nurse-in-charge from the district hospital and the head of CHWs at district level respectively. Two other participants for the planned KIIs refused to take part after several attempts to meet them for interview.

The interviews were carried out in Kinyarwanda, the national language. In FGDs, we encouraged all participants to contribute and each session took approximately 60 to 90 min. Interviewers briefed participants on study aims and that the conversation would be audio-recorded and verbal consent obtained at the beginning of the FGDs and KIIs. One researcher with experience in conducting qualitative studies (RK) who is fluent in the local language assisted by second author (moderator/ note taker) conducted all the FGDs and KIIs. The KIIs were held at the district hospital. All participants received Rwandan Francs 4000 (US$ 5) to compensate for their time, which was consistent with the standard payment dispensed by nongovernmental organizations active in the sites.

Data analysis

All FGDs and KIIs were transcribed verbatim in Kinyarwanda and then translated into English by the first author and a research assistant increasing their familiarity with the data. The transcripts were then entered into the NVivo 10 software package to aid in the coding of the data and analysis was then conducted using qualitative content analysis [12, 14]. The first author and a qualitative research assistant independent read and reread the transcripts, and coded the transcripts line by line to identify meaning units. Similar meaning units were grouped into condensed meaning units. Further coding was performed to expound on the condensed meaning units and then grouped together through an inductive and deductive process to develop categories. Categories were further checked with the data to ensure they reflect the content of the transcripts and constant comparison done between categories to develop the final themes.

Results

During the analysis, two categories emerged from the FGDs and KIIs, related to BP/CR, which we labelled 'Pathway' and 'Modifying factors', with each subdivided into several subcategories. Quotes are given to illuminate views of participants.

Pathway

Financial savings

Families tried to save money during pregnancy to ensure access to labor supplies, transport and medical insurance prior to labor.

"During our home visits to pregnant women we do motivate men to provide financial support for their wives... However, in cases of unwanted or teenage pregnancies from poor families this is not always the case. So you find women struggle on their own and for those who cannot afford it (insurance), *it becomes a challenge to access medical care so they give birth at home."* (CHWs FGD 1).

Linkage to care

CHWs identify pregnant women and were often the first to be consulted for questions with regard to pregnancy. CHWs were seen to provide advise with regard to HIV testing and counseling, birth planning, personal hygiene and medical insurance, vaccines and nutritional supplements.

"After you have been told that there is a pregnant woman in your village, you visit her at their home where you will inquire if it's true she is pregnant. And if she isn't sure then escort her to the health center for pregnancy test first. After it's confirmed, I will register her in my book and send a Rapid SMS to Ministry of Health system (Rapid SMS-MCH System) which continues to send me reminders about her next ANC visit..." (CHW FGD 3).

CHWs provide postpartum care including surveillance of severe vaginal bleeding, abdominal pain and dizziness/anemia. Newborns are checked for abnormal body temperature, heart rate, weight, discharge and yellowness until one month of age.

"They (CHWs) will visit the mother-baby pair to verify if both are in good health which will be followed by sending a Rapid SMS system confirming that, then continue with consecutive postnatal checkups on 3rd, 7th and 28th days" (KIIs; In-charge CHW at District level).

Social/emotional support

Participants reported it was the responsibility of family members to support pregnant women in house chores such as cooking, washing clothes, fetching water and firewood collection. At community level, 'family meetings' were organized by village chiefs in order to create a dialogue as to how to solve socio-economic problems in the community. These meetings are known as 'umuganda (gathering of the people of each neighborhood for community work once a month)' or 'umugoroba w'ababyeyi (parents' evening forums)' in which parents at the village level meet to discuss financial security, health and social issues, including intimate partner violence among pregnant women.

"During these meetings, he (village chief) calls for community members who discuss on to why the family has delayed to pay their medical insurance contributions. If they find them (family) to lie within 'poorest group' using ubudehe (collective action to combat poverty) *categories then a letter will be written to the sector administrator who communicates to the social affairs at district level... While those families categorized above 'poorest' they confiscate their property until they have paid..."* (FGD 4 CHW).

Modifying factors

Social factors

Participants reported that some couples refused to seek ANC services out of fear to be chased away for not coming with their spouses, since this is a requirement for being tested for HIV. Teenagers and single women were said to hide their pregnancies even up to term, avoiding to be asked about the father of the baby during ANC visits or labor. Others were ashamed to attend in old clothes or for not having baby layettes to show at the clinic. Multiparous women felt embarrassed to seek health care for being 'laughed at' as 'family planning failures'.

"I think too the requirement of a man attending ANC should be stopped. A woman might need to go for ANC when the husband is not around. If you take my case as

an example, I work from upcountry and it is that job I make a living out of..., may want to come but my employer refuses to give me permission...Meaning my wife may miss out completely on her appointments." (Men FGDs 1).

Women perceived hospital costs as prohibitively high, especially for those without medical insurance barring unintended consequences to those women from poor backgrounds. Single or teenage women in most cases were not in stable relationships and not financially supported. Participants highlighted reasons for delayed enrolment into medical insurance programs, such as the need for everyone in the family to sign up and pay immediately upon enrolment or while other women enrolled towards term not knowing the insurance sometimes takes a month or longer to be functional.

"... when labor starts, they will first attempt to be delivered at home and after failing come to the health center thus exposing them to severe obstetric complications. Nevertheless, we have done a lot of sensitization either through media or during CHWs home visits on the importance of health insurance which many families have adhered too..." (KII; Nurse-in-charge at district hospital).

Structural factors

Reasons cited for women not using health facilities include difficult terrain hindering access, rapid progress of labor and most health centers did not have ready available ambulance to transport women during emergencies.

"...we were escorting a woman to give birth at the health center, she reached a point and couldn't walk anymore; so she squat and delivered. We still had 2 Km to reach the health center, so I called at the health center to send us an ambulance only to be told it had been sent elsewhere. Then requested that same midwife to come and assist me to cut the baby's cord, instead she replied me to come and collect the kits myself... Finally, what I did was to organize with the local traditional stretcher 'ingobyi' team from the area she had delivered from and they assisted me to carry her...By the time we reached, baby appeared white and very cold but thank God they both survived". (CHWs FGD 2).

Participants expressed abandonment by health workers, dirty maternity units and rudeness of healthcare staff, particularly the midwives. When women go to a health facility they should be treated like human beings, with respect and not shouted at as they are brought in.

"...some tell of sad stories about their deliveries and they even think that they should not give birth anymore because of the abuse and mistreatment that they receive. (Men FGDs 1) *I remember way back when I had gone to deliver my baby instead of being assisted, the nurses kept insulting me (you enjoyed doing it, why are you screaming now), don't try and scream here. Nurses are just there not helping; you wonder if it's a health facility you were brought to?"* (Elderly women FGDs 2).

Inconsistent health policies factors

Most participants were supportive of women giving birth at the health facility, but they questioned inconsistent health policies regarding fee charges upon each ANC or family planning visit, which had previously been free. Also, fines imposed on women who had given birth *en* route or at home were perceived to be counterproductive.

"Since the introduction of user fees upon each ANC visit, we are most likely to go back to those old days when women delivered at home. Even I told the in-charge of CHWs at district level that if nothing is done, our job as CHWs is coming to an end because women have started lying to us even their last menstrual period so that they can go for ANC once (towards term) in order to save money from the prior ANC visits to be able to buy baby clothes. Therefore, we propose that these fees should be removed so that women can attend ANC freely as it was previously." (CHWs FGD group 3).

Discussion

Participants perceived the importance of family assistance, medical insurance and attending ANC, to facilitate BP/CR and enhance professional care at birth. Community health workers reinforced BP/CR messages by SMS alerts and during community gatherings. Disrespect and abuse of women during labor by health workers were perceived as important barriers to access professional care, as well as conflicting health policies such as user fees for ANC and family planning services, and imposing fines on women giving birth outside health facilities.

It has been well documented that in sub-Saharan Africa, as in other settings, BP/CR entails saving money for buying birth items and transport to health facilities [7, 8, 15]. In Rwanda, this was possible through CHW activities where they engaged with women/families on a one-to-one basis prior to delivery about birth preparedness [16]. In addition, community members saved money to comply with medical insurance but costs were still a barrier and even some challenged the threats associated with failure to comply with the guidelines and regulations used to pay premiums for medical insurance [17].

Our findings are consistent with other studies were CHWs aided skilled birth attendance [16, 18, 19]. In addition, they were the final decision makers in case of emergency obstetric care contrary to what other studies have reported that approval was needed first directly or indirectly from the husband or a family member respectively [20, 21]. This could be explained by a high level of trust and respect expectant mothers from rural Rwanda have for CHWs, whom they called on their mobile phones to offer assistance thus reducing delays in seeking care [13, 16].

This study has demonstrated how integration of mobile phone technology ensured that mother or neonate were timely transferred for emergency obstetric and neonatal care [13]. In addition, it has been suggested to be used as a continuing professional development tool to enhance clinical decision making in emergency obstetric care in low-resource settings [22, 23]. Other strategies were use of community gatherings *'umuganda'* and *'umugoroba w'ababyeyi'* as a platform where issues and plans are discussed inclusive about the importance of BP/CR [17]. While *ubudehe* categorization identified families from poorest communities who benefited from free health care paid for by either government or development partners [24].

Our study has found barriers to utilization of ANC services such as fear of being tested for HIV, contrary to other authors [25, 26], women being chased away and asked to return with their partner to access care similarly to another study from urban Rwanda, but in that particular study women opted to pay a man who is not necessarily the partner – in order to access care [27]. Others were ashamed to attend in old clothes or for not having baby layettes to show at the clinic [8], and teenage/single mothers who hid their pregnancies even up to term after being rejected by the baby's father, making them to go live with their mothers whom in most cases due to poor socio-economic status were more likely to face complex decision-making patterns [28]. Special attention must be paid to improve the interactions with this group and with their mothers as decision-makers.

Most studies have indicated that distance to health facility, rapid progress of labor and lack of preparation for transport hindered health seeking behavior and access to care, hence resulting in pregnant women deliver en route or at home [8, 28, 29]. Therefore, preventive strategies are of utmost importance, such as establishment of maternity waiting homes [30] in communities where it is difficult to access emergency obstetric care, when required.

Studies have, similarly to ours, reported abandonment and rudeness by midwives to women when they come to health facilities for delivery. The latter were described as unwelcoming and negatively affected the integrity of women seeking obstetric emergency care [31, 32]. Thus, a need exists to improve communication to make services appealing and trustworthy to women and their social networks [33] and recognize continuous support for respectful maternity care especially in our labor rooms [31–33].

Delivery in health facilities was reported to be mandatory. Our findings, however, reported inconsistent health policies which were perceived to be conflicting with BP/CR in a community which still reveals socio-cultural barriers towards women's access to ANC and contraception services [34, 35], posing threats and should be addressed. In addition, caution should therefore be taken when introducing any financing reforms to ensure that the needs of the poor and vulnerable are protected and that they are implemented within the context of universal coverage [36].

The strength of this study is that we used both FGDs and KIIs to explore community perceptions of how BP/CR is discussed and used. In addition, we included different participants in terms of age, and gender because they provided different perspectives related to the topic of discussion. The limitation of our study is the social desirability bias rather than a genuine reflection. This could have occurred because the moderators and note-takers were of a medical background, and hence participants may have had a desire to show preference for the use of skilled care. In addition, the moderators were all male and this could have caused women to be shy and reserved. However, we believe this did not happen, as the participants were all vibrant and participated in dynamic discussions.

Conclusions

In this community, perceptions regarding BP/CR were in favour of skilled care. Community health workers reinforced BP/CR messages by SMS alerts and during community gatherings (*umuganda or umugoroba w'ababyeyi*). Disrespect and abuse of women mentioned during labor by midwives together with some health policies such as user fees for ANC and family planning services, and imposing fines on women giving birth outside health facilities were perceived as important barriers to access professional care.

There is a need for addressing inconsistent health policies hindering the intention to access professional care. Additionally, to continue emergency preparedness in education to women and their spouses during ANC, key family members—mothers, mother in laws as well as other women in the community to address some barriers to making preparations or delivering in health facilities. We recommend further studies to understand more dimensions regarding disrespectful maternity care in Rwanda.

Abbreviations

ANC: Antenatal Care; BP: Birth Preparedness; CHWs: Community Health Workers; CR: Complication Readiness; FGDs: Focus Group Discussions; HCs: Health centers; KIIs: Key informant interviews; NGO: Non-governmental Organization; SBA: Skilled Birth Attendant

Acknowledgements

We are grateful to all participants and the data collection team who took part in this study; special gratitude goes out to Anqeligue Nyirasafari for organizing CHWs who participated in this study, Ken O'donye for data treatment and analysis.

Funding
No funding received for this study.

Authors' contributions
Contribution of the authors is as follows; RK and PS designed the study and wrote the protocol. RK, PS collected data, RK worked on the data analysis and drafted the manuscript. MvE, TvdA and JvR critically revised the draft manuscript. All authors read and approved the final manuscript.

Competing interests
The authors declare that they have no competing interests.

Author details
[1]Department of Obstetrics and Gynecology, Ruhengeri Hospital, Musanze, Rwanda. [2]Athena Institute, VU University, Amsterdam, The Netherlands. [3]Department of Medical Humanities, VU University Medical Center, Amsterdam, The Netherlands. [4]Department of Obstetrics, Leiden University Medical Center, Leiden, The Netherlands.

References
1. Ayele DZ, Belayihun B, Teji K, Ayana DA. Factors affecting utilization of maternal health care services in Kombolcha District, eastern Hararghe zone, Oromia regional state, eastern Ethiopia. Int Sch Res Not. 2014;2014:7.
2. Tura G, Afework M, Yalew AW. The effect of birth preparedness and complication readiness on skilled care use: a prospective follow-up study in Southwest Ethiopia. Reprod Health. 2014;11:60.
3. Lee AC, Cousens S, Darmstadt GL, Blencowe H, Pattinson R, Moran NF, et al. Care during labor and birth for the prevention of intrapartum-related neonatal deaths: a systematic review and Delphi estimation of mortality effect. BMC Public Health. 2011;11(Suppl 3):S10.
4. Holmer H, Oyerinde K, Meara JG, Gillies R, Liljestrand J, Hagander L. The global met need for emergency obstetric care: a systematic review. BJOG. 2015;122(2):183–9.
5. JHPIEGO/Maternal and Neonatal Health Program. Birth Preparedness and Complication Readiness: A matrix of shared responsibility. Baltimore,MD; 2001.
6. Solnes Miltenburg A, Roggeveen Y, Shields L, van Elteren M, van Roosmalen J, Stekelenburg J, et al. Impact of birth preparedness and complication readiness interventions on birth with a skilled attendant: a systematic review. PLoS One. 2015;10(11):e0143382.
7. Gebre M, Gebremariam A, Abebe TA. Birth preparedness and complication readiness among pregnant women in Duguna Fango District, Wolayta zone, Ethiopia. PLoS One. 2015;10(9):e0137570.
8. August F, Pembe AB, Kayombo E, Mbekenga C, Axemo P, Darj E. Birth preparedness and complication readiness- a qualitative study among community members in rural Tanzania. Glob Health Action. 2015;8:26922.
9. Ministry of Health. National Reproductive Health Policy. Kigali, Rwanda. 2013.
10. Rwanda Demographic and Health Survey 2005. Rwanda, Rwanda National Statistical Institute, and Calverton, MD, USA, ORC Macro, 2006.
11. National Institute of Statistics of Rwanda. Rwanda demographic and health survey 2014–15. Calverton: Ministry of Health; 2014.
12. Graneheim UH, Lundman B. Qualitative content analysis in nursing research: concepts, procedures and measures to achieve trustworthiness. Nurs Educ Today. 2004;24(2):105–12.
13. Ngabo F, Nguimfack J, Nwaigwe F, Mugeni C, Muhoza D, Wilson DR, et al. Every death counts: use of maternal death audit data for decision making to save the lives of mothers in Rwanda. Pan Africa Medical Journal. 2012;13:31.
14. Krippendorff K. Content analysis: an introduction to its methodology. In the sage Comm text series. London: Sage; 1980.
15. Kabakyenga J, Ostergren P-O, Turyakira E, Pettersson K. Knowledge of obstetric danger signs and birth preparedness practices among women in rural Uganda. Reprod Health. 2011;8:33.
16. Condo J, Mugeni C, Naughton B, Hall K, Tuazon MA, Omwega A, et al. Rwanda's evolving community health worker system: a qualitative assessment of client and provider perspectives. Hum Resour Health. 2014;12:71.
17. Gaynor N. "A nation in a hurry": the costs of local governance reforms in Rwanda. Rev Afr Polit Econ. 2014;41(sup1):S49–63.
18. Gilmore B, McAuliffe E. Effectiveness of community health workers delivering preventive interventions for maternal and child health in low- and middle-income countries: a systematic review. BMC Public Health. 2013; 13:847.
19. Aboubaker S, Qazi S, Wolfheim C, Oyegoke A, Bahl R. Community health workers: a crucial role in newborn health care and survival. J Glob Health. 2014;2(4):1–5.
20. Kakaire O, Kaye DK, Osinde MO. Male involvement in birth preparedness and complication readiness for emergency obstetric referrals in rural Uganda. Reprod Health. 2011;8:12.
21. August F, Pembe AB, Mpembeni R, Axemo P, Darj E. Community health workers can improve male involvement in maternal health: evidence from rural Tanzania. Glob Health Action. 2016;9:30064.
22. Nyamtema A, Mwakatundu N, Sunday D, Kasanga M, Jamadini F, Maokola K, et al. Introducing eHealth strategies to enhance maternal and perinatal health care in rural Tanzania. Matern Health Neonatol Perinatol. 2017;3:3.
23. Obasola OI, Mabawonku I, Lagunju I. A review of e-health interventions for maternal and child health in sub-Sahara Africa. Matern Child Health J. 2015; 19(8):1813–24.
24. Niringiye A, Ayebale C. Impact evaluation of the Ubudehe Programme in Rwanda: an examination of the sustainability of the Ubudehe Programme. J Sus Dev Afr. 2012;14:3.
25. Kayigamba FR, Bakker M, Lammers J, Mugisha V, Bagiruwigize E, Asiimwe A, et al. Provider-initiated HIV testing and Counselling in Rwanda: acceptability among clinic attendees and workers, reasons for testing and predictors of testing. PLoS One. 2013;9(4):e95459.
26. Kelley AL, Karita E, Sullivan PS, Katangulia F, Chomba E, Carael M, et al. Knowledge and perceptions of Couples' voluntary counseling and testing in urban Rwanda and Zambia: a cross-sectional household survey. PLoS One. 2011;6(5):e19573.
27. Påfs J, Musafili A, Binder-Finnema P, Klingberg-Allvin M, Rulisa S, Essén B. 'They would never receive you without a husband': paradoxical barriers to antenatal care scale-up in Rwanda. Midwifery. 2015;31(12):1149–56.
28. Munguambe K, Boene H, Vidler M, Bique C, Sawchuck D, Firoz T, et al. Barriers and facilitators to health care seeking behaviours in pregnancy in rural communities of southern Mozambique. Reprod Health. 2016;13(Suppl 1):31.
29. Påfs J, Musafili A, Binder-Finnema P, Klingberg-Allvin M, Rulisa S, Essén B. Beyond the numbers of maternal near-miss in Rwanda – a qualitative study on women's perspectives on access and experiences of care in early and late stage of pregnancy. BMC Pregnancy and Childbirth. 2016;16:257.
30. van Lonkhuijzen L, Stekelenburg J, van Roosmalen J. Maternity waiting facilities for improving maternal and neonatal outcome in low-resource countries. Cochrane Database Syst Rev. 2012;10:CD006759.
31. Warren CE, Njue R, Ndwiga C, Abuya T. Manifestations and drivers of mistreatment of women during childbirth in Kenya: implications for measurement and developing interventions. BMC Pregnancy and Childbirth. 2017;17:102.
32. McMahon S, George A, Chebet JJ, Mosha IH, Mpembeni RN, Winch PJ. Experiences of and responses to disrespectful maternity care and abuse during childbirth; a qualitative study with women and men in Morogoro region, Tanzania. BMC Pregnancy Childbirth. 2014;14:268.
33. Østergaard LR. Trust matters: a narrative literature review of the role of trust in health care systems in sub-Saharan Africa. Glob Public Health. 2015;10(9): 1046–59.
34. Farmer DB, Berman L, Ryan G, Habumugisha L, Basinga P, Nutt C, et al. Motivations and constraints to family planning: a qualitative study in Rwanda's southern Kayonza District. Glob Health Sci Pract. 2015;3(2):242–54.
35. Brunie A, Tolley EE, Ngabo F, Wesson J, Chen M. Getting to 70%: barriers to modern contraceptive use for women in Rwanda. Int J Gynecol Obstet. 2013;123(suppl 1):e11–5.
36. Tangcharoensathien V, Patcharanarumol W, Ir P, Aljunid SM, Mukti AG, Akkhavong K, et al. Health-financing reforms in Southeast Asia: challenges in achieving universal coverage. Lancet. 2011;377(9768):863–73.

25

The fortification method relying on assumed human milk composition overestimates the actual energy and macronutrient intakes in very preterm infants

Israel Macedo[1*], Luis Pereira-da-Silva[2,3] and Manuela Cardoso[4]

Abstract

Background: To achieve recommended nutrient intakes in preterm infants, the target fortification method of human milk (HM) was proposed as an alternative to standard fortification method. We aimed to compare assumed energy and macronutrient intakes based on standard fortified HM with actual intakes relying on measured composition of human milk (HM), in a cohort of HM-fed very preterm infants.

Methods: This study is a secondary retrospective analysis, in which assumed energy and macronutrient contents of daily pools of own mother's milk (OMM) from 33 mothers and donated HM (DHM) delivered to infants were compared with the measured values using a mid-infrared HM analyzer. A fortification method consisting of modular protein and/or fat supplements added to standard fortified HM was used to provide the minimum recommended daily intakes of energy 110 Kcal/kg and protein up to 4.0 g/kg. Assumed nutrient intakes were compared with actual nutrient intakes from full enteral feeding to 35 weeks plus 6 days postmenstrual age, using the Wilcoxon matched-pairs signed ranks test.

Results: The composition of 1181 samples of daily pools of HM were measured. For 90.2% of study days, infants were exclusively fed OMM and in remaining days fed OMM *plus* DHM. Comparing with reported preterm OMM composition, measured protein concentration was significantly lower, and energy and other macronutrient concentrations were lower only from the second to third postnatal week. Using fortified HM, the actual median daily intakes of energy, protein, and fat were significantly lower (113.3 vs. 120.7 Kcal/kg, 4.45 vs. 4.73 g/kg, and 4.96 vs. 5.35 g/kg, respectively) and the actual protein-to-energy ratio (PER) significantly higher than what was assumed (4.2 vs. 4.0), without differences in carbohydrate intake.

Conclusions: When fortifying the HM, we used conservative target intakes trying not to exceed the osmolarity recommended for infant feeds. Actual energy, protein and fat intakes in OMM were significantly lower than assumed. This resulted in inadequate intake using our fortification method, that did not compensate the suboptimal measured energy and macronutrient contents of OMM delivered. Further studies comparing assumed with the gold standard target fortification are needed to determine safe upper limits of assumed fortification.

Keywords: Human milk composition, Human milk fortification, Nutrient intake, Target fortification, Very preterm infants

* Correspondence: israeljmacedo@gmail.com
[1]NICU, Maternidade Dr Alfredo da Costa, Centro Hospitalar de Lisboa Central, Rua Viriato, n° 1, 1050-010 Lisbon, Portugal
Full list of author information is available at the end of the article

Background

The American Academy of Pediatrics [1] and the European Society for Paediatric Gastroenterology, Hepatology, and Nutrition [2] recommend human milk (HM) as the first choice for feeding very preterm infants, provided it is fortified with nutrients necessary to meet requirements [2]. To provide adequate care for this infant population, strategies to prevent severe in-hospital nutrient deficits encompass the multicomponent fortification of HM [3]. However, the widely used standard fortification method, in which a fixed dose of nutrients is added independently of HM composition, rarely meets the recommended intake of protein for preterm infants [2], with inherent risks of growth faltering and neurocognitive impairment [3–6]. As an alternative, the targeted fortification method was proposed to tailor the individual infant's needs, based on previous analyses of HM energy and macronutrients [7]. However, this method is time consuming and labor intensive, and analyzers are commonly unavailable [8, 9]. Other fortification methods of HM have been described, including the addition of modular protein and fat to fortified HM [10–13].

Some authors have compared fortification methods based on assumed HM composition with methods relying on measured HM composition [8, 11, 13, 14]. In these studies, differences between assumed and measured HM composition [8], assumed and actual intakes provided by fortified HM [8, 13], and growth [8, 11, 14] were assessed. Results from similar strategies have not been consistent, probably due to differences in methods of fortification and different characteristics of studied infants.

In our unit, logistical constraints related with reduction of health personnel precluded targeted fortification during a certain period of time, but samples of HM delivered to infants were stored frozen for later composition analysis. An alternative method of fortification was used, based on the assumed variable HM composition [3, 15]. Specifically, modular protein and fat supplements were added to standard fortified HM [11] to achieve recommended intakes [2].

In this study, we aimed to compare retrospectively the assumed energy and macronutrient intakes with the correspondent actual values relying on measured HM composition, in a cohort of HM-fed very preterm infants.

Methods

This single-center study is a secondary retrospective analysis that used data from a birth cohort study aimed to determine the associations between macronutrient intake, body composition, and neurodevelopmental outcome in exclusively or predominantly HM-fed very preterm infants [7, 15]. The cohort study was performed in the neonatal intensive care unit (NICU) of Maternidade Dr. Alfredo da Costa, Centro Hospitalar de Lisboa Central, Lisbon, Portugal. The study was registered with the International Standard Randomized Controlled Trial Number (ISRCTN) registry (ID: 27916681) and approved by the Hospital Ethics Committee (ID 116/2012). Parents or guardians of all infants gave their informed consent before inclusion in the study, and the study was conducted in accordance with the tenets of the Declaration of Helsinki.

The characteristics of the 33 infants included are described elsewhere [6]. In brief, they were born at a mean (standard deviation [SD]) gestational age of 30 (1.8) weeks, with a median (interquartile range [IQR]) weight of 1175 (1010–1408) g. Infants were exclusively or predominantly HM-fed (formula-feeding < 12.5% enteral volume intake). Human milk fortification was initiated when enteral daily intake reached 100 mL/kg at a median (IQR) of 12 (11–14) postnatal days; full enteral feeding was achieved approximately at the same age, at a median (IQR) of 11 (8–16) postnatal days.

Mothers of studied infants were advised to sequentially collect milk every 3 h, either in the hospital or at home, and to record date and hour of each collection. The own mother's milk (OMM) was stored frozen at – 25 °C in the maternity milk bank. For each infant, a daily pool of sequentially collected OMM batches, roughly representing the composition of OMM collected within a day, was thawed at 37 °C and mechanically homogenized to deliver to infants. A 3-mL sample from this pool was collected and again frozen for later analysis. Donated human milk (DHM) from mothers of term infants was frozen at home, transported frozen to the maternity milk bank, and stored at – 25 °C in the maternity milk bank. After negative screening for transmissible infectious diseases according to National Institute for Health and Care Excellence (NICE) guidelines [16], milk of each donor was thawed, pooled for microbiological control and macronutrient analysis, pasteurized using the Holder method [17], and frozen again. When DHM was necessary to complete the daily amount of prescribed HM, a pool of DHM was thawed using the aforementioned method.

A mid-infrared HM analyzer (Miris AB, Uppsala, Sweden) was used to measure the content of total protein, fat, carbohydrates, and energy of OMM. This is reported to be an accurate method to measure HM composition, validated and calibrated against chemical analysis for nitrogen and fat [13, 18]. Before analysis, samples of native OMM and DHM were thawed by warming to 40 °C and ultrasonically homogenized. As almost all infants were breastfed (unknown volume intake and composition) by 35 weeks plus 6 days postmenstrual age (PMA), the OMM analysis was suspended at this age.

Following the nutrition protocol used in our unit, we assumed in preterm OMM averages of 1.1 g/100 mL of protein in the first 3 postnatal weeks and 0.8 g/ 100 thereafter; in DHM, we assumed 0.8 g/ 100 mL of protein, and 67 kcal/ 100 mL of energy in both OMM and DHM. A fortification method consisting of modular protein and fat supplements added to standard fortified HM was used to provide the minimum recommended daily intakes according to body weight, as follows: energy 110 kcal/kg; protein (g/kg) 4.0 if < 1000 g, 3.7 if < 1200 g, 3.6 if < 1800 g, and 3.4 if > 1800 g; and protein-to-energy ratio (PER) of 3.6 if < 1000 g, 3.2 if < 1800 g, and 2.6 if > 1800 g [2, 3, 19]. The composition of the HM fortifier (Aptamil FMS®; Milupa/Danone GmbH, Friedrichsdorf, Germany), modular protein (Aptamil Protein Supplement powder®; Milupa/Danone GmbH, Friedrichsdorf, Germany), and medium-chain triglycerides (MCT OIL; SHS Nutricia/Danone®, GmbH, Friedrichsdorf, Germany) are shown in Table 1.

For each infant, the study period was from full enteral feeding to 35 weeks plus 6 days PMA, or to the PMA at which the infant became breastfed and the OMM analysis suspended. For the whole sample, the mean (SD) study period was of 29 (8) days.

The measured composition of OMM was retrospectively compared with recent longitudinal data from a meta-analysis on preterm OMM composition [15] and measured composition of DHM was compared with reported composition of pooled DHM [12], using the t test. The actual energy and macronutrient intakes were calculated based on measured OMM and DHM compositions *plus* compositions provided by the manufacturers of the HM fortifier, modular protein and modular fat. As OMM composition measurements were not always possible in this study, mixed models were used for imputation of missing values. These models used logarithmic transformations of preterm OMM energy and macronutrient measured concentrations (as non-linear dependent variables), the postnatal days as the fixed effect and each case as a random effect. The composition of delivered DHM has always been measured. The assumed energy and macronutrient intakes were calculated based on the aforementioned reported compositions of preterm OMM [15] and pooled DHM [12] *plus* the compositions of HM fortifier, modular protein, and fat. The actual energy and macronutrient intakes were compared with the assumed intakes using the Wilcoxon matched-pairs signed ranks test.

Table 1 Energy and nutrient contents of the human milk fortifier (Aptamil FMS®), modular protein hydrolysate (Aptamil Protein Supplement®) and modular medium-chain triglycerides (MCT OIL SHS®) used

Product	Energy (kcal)	Protein (g)	Fat (g)
Aptamil FMS® (*per* 100 g)	347	25.2	0
Aptamil Protein Supplement ® (*per* 100 g)	328.4	82.1	0
MCT OIL SHS® (*per* 100 mL)	855	0	95

Results are expressed as median (interquartile range - IQR) and significance was considered as $p < 0.05$. Statistical analysis was performed using SPSS (version 13, SPSS Inc., Chicago, IL).

Results

One thousand one hundred eighty-one daily pools of HM have been individually delivered to infants, and the composition of 1021 (86.5%) of these pools (905 OMM and 116 DHM) has been analyzed. Concerning HM with analyzed composition, in 99.4% of study days, infants were exclusively OMM fed, in 4.3% OMM *plus* DHM fed, and in 0.3% exclusively DHM fed.

When compared with reported longitudinal OMM composition [15], measured protein content was always significantly lower, energy and carbohydrate contents significantly lower only from the second postnatal week, and fat content significantly lower only from the third postnatal week (Table 2).

Compared with reported pooled DHM composition [12], measured energy and fat contents were significantly lower and carbohydrate significantly higher, without differences in protein content (Table 3).

The actual energy, protein, and fat intakes were significantly lower than the assumed intakes (Figs. 1, 2 and 3), without significant differences in carbohydrate intake (Fig. 4); the actual PER was significantly higher than the assumed value (Table 4).

Discussion

In this study, energy and macronutrient intakes were mainly influenced by OMM composition, since infants received DHM in a very small percentage of the days. Compared with recently reported values [15], measured OMM protein content was significantly lower, and energy and other macronutrients became significantly lower from the second or third postnatal week. When fortifying the HM, we targeted the minimum recommended intakes, concerned to not exceed the recommended threshold of 400 mOsm/L for infant feeds, which could easily occur with the addition of both fortifier and modular protein to HM [20]. The fortification method was guided by our unit protocol that inappropriately assumed lower energy and protein contents than reported in literature. In consequence, the HM fortification did not compensate the low measured OMM energy and macronutrient contents, and our fortification method resulted in actual energy, protein, and fat intakes significantly lower than the assumed values. Particularly, the actual energy intake was relatively lower than the

Table 2 Comparison between measured composition of OMM and data from a meta-analysis [15]

Postnatal day	Measured energy (Kcal/100 mL)	Reporte denergy (Kcal/100 mL)	Measured protein (g/100 mL)	Reported protein (g/100 mL)	Measured fat (g/100 mL)	Reported fat (g/100 mL)	Measured carbohydrate (g/100 mL)	Reported carbohydrate (g/100 mL)
Day 1–3	*N* = 73	*N* = 143	N = 73	*N* = 163	N = 73	*N* = 173	N = 73	N = 143
Mean (SD)	61.0 (14.00)	58.80 (7.91)	1.84** (0.53)	2.57 (1.44)	3.01* (1.15)	2.52 (0.98)	6.25 (1.52)	6.2 (0.92)
Day 4–7	*N* = 96	N = 96	N = 96	*N* = 44	N = 96	*N* = 110	N = 96	*N* = 87
Mean (SD)	64.5 (10.49)	67.9 (14.1)	1.89* (0.49)	2.11 (0.44)	3.34 (1.11)	3.31 (1.27)	6.34 (1.54)	6.17 (0.49)
Week 2	*N* = 157	*N* = 417	N = 157	*N* = 383	N = 157	*N* = 426	N = 157	*N* = 389
Mean (SD)	62.0** (11.75)	69.1 (10.1)	1.70** (0.50)	1.98 (0.68)	3.19 (1.00)	3.19 (1.04)	6.32** (1.93)	6.72 (0.46)
Week 3–4	*N* = 203	*N* = 481	N = 203	*N* = 528	N = 203	*N* = 485	N = 203	*N* = 464
Mean (SD)	63.9** (9.62)	70.87 (9.34)	1.61 (0.46)	1.6 (0.5)	3.32** (0.87)	3.83 (1.01)	6.53** (1.26)	7.05 (0.51)
Week 5–6	*N* = 84	*N* = 354	N = 84	*N* = 330	N = 84	*N* = 371	N = 84	N = 354
Mean (SD)	67.6** (7.92)	73.97 (9.1)	1.55* (0.60)	1.43 (0.25)	3.63* (1.00)	4.04 (0.91)	6.71** (1.42)	7.14 (0.36)
Week 7–9	N = 42	*N* = 239	N = 42	*N* = 223	N = 42	*N* = 236	N = 42	*N* = 235
Mean (SD)	64.4** (9.81)	74.24 (8.77)	1.18** (0.23)	1.34 (0.2)	3.63* (0.85)	4.21 (0.92)	6.40** (1.16)	7.13 (0.38)

t test; * $p < 0.001$; ** $p < 0.0001$ Abbreviations: *OMM* own mother's milk

Table 3 Comparison between measured composition of DHM and reported pooled DHM [12]

	Measured Samples = 116		Reported Samples = 179		p ‡
	Mean	SD	Mean	SD	
Energy (kcal/dL)	60.0	3.6	66.0	12.0	< 0.0001
Protein (g/dL)	0.9	0.2	0.9	0.4	NS
Fat (g/dL)	2.8	0.3	4.0	1.4	< 0.0001
Carbohydrates	7.1	0.4	6.6	0.7	< 0.0001

‡ t test Abbreviations: *DHM* donated human milk

low actual protein intake, reflected by a higher actual PER compared with the assumed PER.

In a previous study on the same infants [6], it was found that minimum recommended intakes were achieved only in 63.6% of infants for protein, 15.2% for energy, and 93.9% for PER; this was associated with a low weight gain velocity (mean 10.1 g/kg/day) compared with that described in similar populations [21].

In surveys, enteral nutritional practices used for preterm infants were found to be quite heterogeneous [22, 23]. Moreover, varied methods of HM fortification have been used [10]. This may explain different results on energy and nutrient intakes [8, 13] and growth [8, 11, 14] reported in studies that have compared fortification methods based on assumed HM composition with those relying on measured HM composition.

de Halleux et al. (2013) compared energy and nutrient intakes between individualized fortification relying on measured HM composition and standard fortification based on assumed HM composition [13]. The individualized fortification resulted in actual energy and fat intakes higher than the assumed values and actual protein intake and PER lower than the assumed values. This seems contrary to our results and may be explained by different fortification methods used. In standard fortification, de Halleux et al. [13] added to HM a fixed recommended amount of fortifier; the individualized fortification was performed after analysis of HM and its fat content was first adjusted up to 4.0 g/100 mL using modular fat; subsequently, HM fortifier was added to achieve a protein intake of 4.3 g/kg/d. This method resulted in actual mean intakes of 140 Kcal/kg/d of energy and 4.25 g/kg/d of protein. In our study, modular protein and fat supplements were added to standard fortified HM to achieve intakes of 4.0 g/kg/d of protein and 110 Kcal/kg/d of energy. Compared with de Halleux et al. data [13], our nutritional strategy resulted in a lower actual mean energy intake (113 Kcal/kg/d), but slightly higher actual mean protein intake (4.45 g/kg/d). This might be explained by excessive protein added to reach the minimum targeted intake according to our unit protocol that inappropriately assumed a lower protein concentration than described for preterm OMM [15].

McLeod et al. (2016) [8], in a trial including 40 very preterm infants, compared routine fortification based on assumed HM composition with targeted fortification relying on measured HM composition. Human milk fortifier, modular protein and carbohydrate plus fat supplement were used for HM fortification.

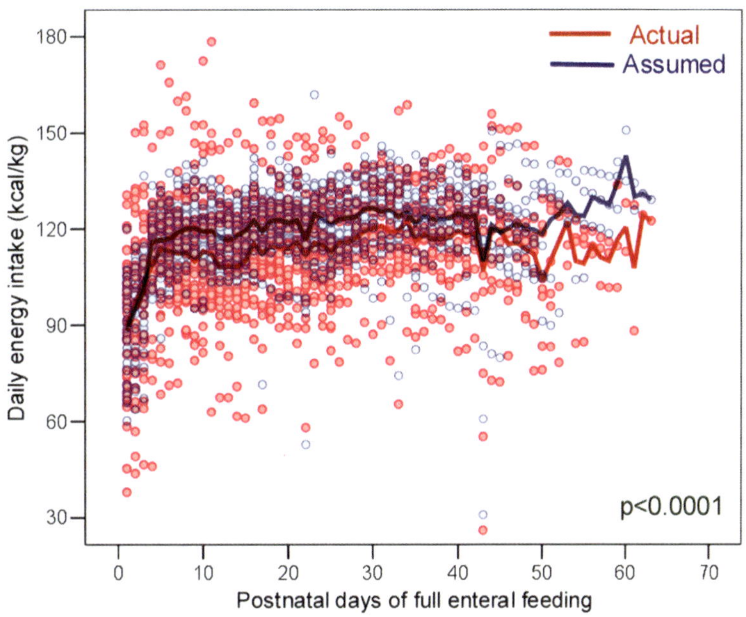

Fig. 1 The actual daily total energy intake provided by exclusive enteral feeding was significantly lower than the assumed energy intake, during the study period

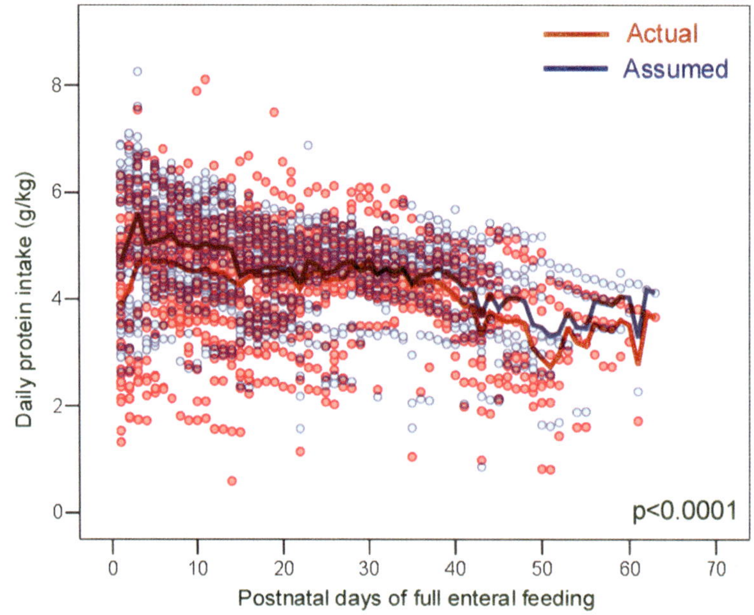

Fig. 2 The actual daily protein intake provided by exclusive enteral feeding was significantly lower than the assumed protein intake, during the study period

In HM, mean measured protein content (1.6 g/100 mL) was higher than the assumed value (1.4 g/100 mL), which is contrary to our result. Despite differences in measured and assumed protein content, neither significant differences in energy and macronutrient intakes, nor in weight gain velocity were found between groups. Compared with our study, McLeod et al. (2016) targeted the intakes to upper daily values of protein (3.8–4.4 g/kg) and energy (130–150 Kcal/kg) [8].

Limitations of our study should be acknowledged. First, for 19.4% of the study days, OMM with unknown composition was delivered to infants, potentially affecting the calculation of nutrient intakes. To mitigate this inconvenience, mixed models for imputation of missing nutrient values of OMM were used. In a previous study,

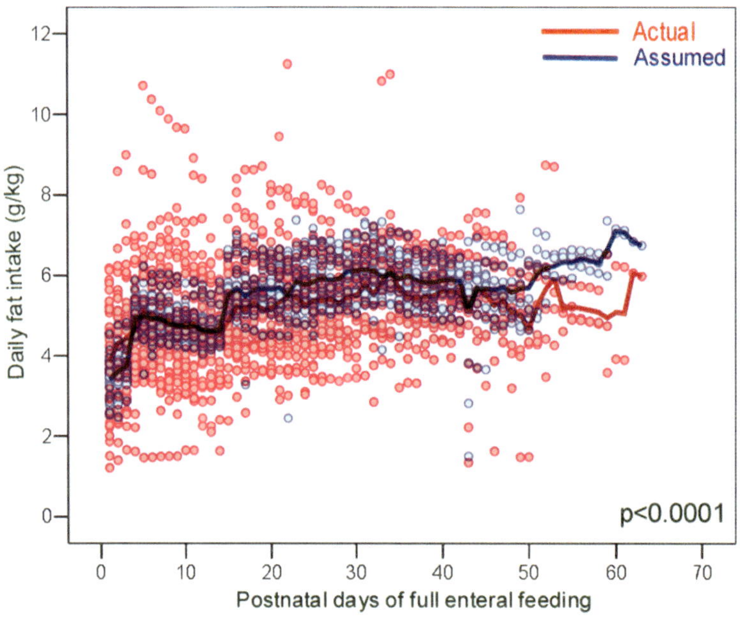

Fig. 3 The actual daily fat intake provided by exclusive enteral feeding was significantly lower than the assumed fat intake, during the study period

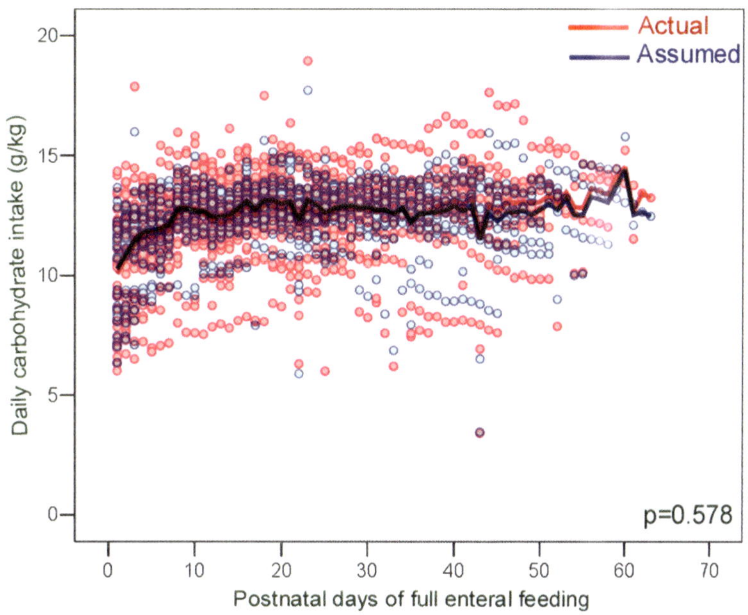

Fig. 4 The actual daily carbohydrate intake provided by exclusive enteral feeding did not differ from the assumed carbohydrate intake, during the study period

we found good agreement between curves obtained with model-predicted data and those from a meta-analysis on preterm OMM composition [6]. Second, processes of freezing, thawing, and homogenization may have caused a reduction in fat and protein concentrations [24]. Nevertheless, processing of HM in our study was also used in studies whose results we compared [8, 12, 13].

Conclusion

In this study we compared assumed with actual macronutrient intakes in a cohort of very preterm infants fed HM, predominantly fed OMM. When fortifying the HM, we chose conservative targeted nutrient intakes hoping not to exceed the osmolarity recommended for infant feeds. Actual energy, protein and fat intakes in OMM were significantly lower than assumed. This resulted in inadequate intake using our fortification method, that did not compensate the suboptimal measured energy and macronutrient contents of OMM delivered.

Further studies comparing assumed with target fortification are needed to determine safe upper limits of assumed fortification to guide clinicians in their fortification practice [8]. Meanwhile, the target fortification tailored to the infant's needs is the reference to achieve the recommended nutrient intakes, although this method is time consuming, laborious and HM analyzers are commonly unavailable.

Table 4 Comparison between actual and assumed daily intakes during the study period

Nutrients	Actual daily intake median (IQR)	Assumed daily intake median (IQR)	*p* ‡
Energy (kcal/kg)	113.3 (102.8–123.7)	120.7 (113.6–127.3)	< 0.0001
Protein (g/kg)	4.45 (3.70–5.07)	4.73 (4.09–5.26)	< 0.0001
PER (protein g/100 kcal)	4.2 (3.6–4.7)	4.0 (3.5–4.6)	0.011
Fat (g/kg)	4.96 (4.19–6.00)	5.35 (4.76–5.93)	< 0.0001
Carbohydrates (g/kg)	12.64 (11.63–13.55)	12.71 (12.05–13.29)	0.578

Abbreviations *IQR* interquartile range, *PER* protein-to-energy ratio ‡ Wilcoxon signed rank test

Abbreviations

DHM: Donated human milk; HM: Human milk; NICE: National Institute for Health and Care Excellence; OMM: Own mother's milk; PER: Protein to energy ratio; PMA: Postmenstrual age

Acknowledgments

This study is part of a Ph.D. thesis in Medicine – Pediatrics. One of the authors (I.M) is supervised by one of the other authors (L.P.d.S.) from NOVA Medical School, Universidade NOVA de Lisboa, Lisbon, Portugal.

Funding

This study was partially supported by the "Milupa 2011" grant for perinatal and neonatal research, provided by the Portuguese Neonatal Society.

Authors' contributions

I.M. designed and conducted the study, performed the analyses of human milk composition, the statistical analyses, and drafted the manuscript; L.P.d.S. contributed to the study design and drafting the manuscript; M.C. contributed to the collection of data. All the authors reviewed and approved the final version of the manuscript prior to submission.

Competing interests
The authors declare no conflict of interest. The funding sponsors had no role in the design of the study, in the collection, analyses, or interpretation of data, in the writing of the manuscript and in the decision to publish the findings.

Author details
[1]NICU, Maternidade Dr Alfredo da Costa, Centro Hospitalar de Lisboa Central, Rua Viriato, n° 1, 1050-010 Lisbon, Portugal. [2]Medicine of Woman, Childhood and Adolescence, NOVA Medical School, Universidade NOVA de Lisboa, Lisbon, Portugal. [3]NICU, Hospital Dona Estefânia, Centro Hospitalar de Lisboa Central, Lisbon, Portugal. [4]Dietetics Unit, Maternidade Dr Alfredo da Costa, Centro Hospitalar de Lisboa Central, Lisbon, Portugal.

References

1. Eidelman AI. The aap's 2012 Breastfeeding policy statement: is there anything new? Breastfeed Med. 2012;7:203–4. https://doi.org/10.1089/bfm.2012.9989.
2. Agostoni C, Buonocore G, Carnielli VP, De Curtis M, Darmaun D, Decsi T, Domellof M, Embleton ND, Fusch C, Genzel-Boroviczeny O, et al. Enteral nutrient supply for preterm infants: commentary from the european society of paediatric gastroenterology, hepatology and nutrition committee on nutrition. J Pediatr Gastroenterol Nutr. 2010;50:85–91. https://doi.org/10.1097/MPG.0b013e3181adaee0.
3. Ziegler EE. Meeting the nutritional needs of the low-birth-weight infant. Ann Nutr Metab. 2011;*58*(Suppl 1):8–18. https://doi.org/10.1159/000323381.
4. Nutritional composition of breast milk produced by mothers of preterm infants. Nutr Rev. 1980;38:312–3.
5. Corvaglia L, Aceti A, Paoletti V, Mariani E, Patrono D, Ancora G, Capretti MG, Faldella G. Standard fortification of preterm human milk fails to meet recommended protein intake: bedside evaluation by near-infrared-reflectance-analysis. Early Hum Dev. 2010;86:237–40. https://doi.org/10.1016/j.earlhumdev.2010.04.001.
6. Macedo I, Pereira-da-Silva L, Cardoso M. Associations of measured protein and energy intakes with growth and adiposity in human milk-fed preterm infants at term postmenstrual age: a cohort study. Am J Perinatol. 2018;35:882–91. https://doi.org/10.1055/s-0038-1626717.
7. Polberger S. III. Individualized fortification of human milk: Targeted fortification. J Pediatr Gastroenterol Nutr. 2015;*61*(Suppl 1):S3–4. https://doi.org/10.1097/01.mpg.0000471451.55494.e4.
8. McLeod G, Sherriff J, Hartmann PE, Nathan E, Geddes D, Simmer K. Comparing different methods of human breast milk fortification using measured v. Assumed macronutrient composition to target reference growth: a randomised controlled trial. Br J Nutr. 2016;115:431–9. https://doi.org/10.1017/S0007114515004614.
9. Rochow N, Fusch G, Zapanta B, Ali A, Barui S, Fusch C. Target fortification of breast milk: how often should milk analysis be done? Nutrients. 2015;7:2297–310. https://doi.org/10.3390/nu7042297.
10. Kemp JE, Wenhold FA. Human milk fortification strategies for improved in-hospital growth of preterm infants. S Afr J Clin Nutr. 2016;29:8. https://doi.org/10.1080/16070658.2016.1217646.
11. Rochow N, Fusch G, Choi A, Chessell L, Elliott L, McDonald K, Kuiper E, Purcha M, Turner S, Chan E, et al. Target fortification of breast milk with fat, protein, and carbohydrates for preterm infants. J Pediatr. 2013;163:1001–7. https://doi.org/10.1016/j.jpeds.2013.04.052.
12. Cooper AR, Barnett D, Gentles E, Cairns L, Simpson JH. Macronutrient content of donor human breast milk. Arch Dis Child Fetal Neonatal Ed. 2013;98:F539–41. https://doi.org/10.1136/archdischild-2013-304422.
13. de Halleux V, Rigo J. Variability in human milk composition: benefit of individualized fortification in very-low-birth-weight infants. Am J Clin Nutr. 2013;98:529S–35S. https://doi.org/10.3945/ajcn.112.042689.
14. Morlacchi L, Mallardi D, Gianni ML, Roggero P, Amato O, Piemontese P, Consonni D, Mosca F. Is targeted fortification of human breast milk an optimal nutrition strategy for preterm infants? An interventional study. J Transl Med. 2016;14:195. https://doi.org/10.1186/s12967-016-0957-y.
15. Mimouni FB, Lubetzky R, Yochpaz S, Mandel D. Preterm human milk macronutrient and energy composition: a systematic review and meta-analysis. Clin Perinatol. 2017;44:165–72. https://doi.org/10.1016/j.clp.2016.11.010.
16. Drummond M, A.G., Arkley C, Gillen D. Donor milk banks: Service operation, clinical guidelines. In NICE clinical guidelines, NICE: London, 2010; p 35.
17. Peila C, Moro GE, Bertino E, Cavallarin L, Giribaldi M, Giuliani F, Cresi F, Coscia A. The effect of holder pasteurization on nutrients and biologically-active components in donor human milk: a review. Nutrients. 2016;8 https://doi.org/10.3390/nu8080477.
18. Polberger S, Raiha NC, Juvonen P, Moro GE, Minoli I, Warm A. Individualized protein fortification of human milk for preterm infants: comparison of ultrafiltrated human milk protein and a bovine whey fortifier. J Pediatr Gastroenterol Nutr. 1999;29:332–8.
19. Nutrition Committee, C.P.S. Nutrient needs and feeding of premature infants. CMAJ. 1995;152:1765–85.
20. Kreissl A, Zwiauer V, Repa A, Binder C, Haninger N, Jilma B, Berger A, Haiden N. Effect of fortifiers and additional protein on the osmolarity of human milk: is it still safe for the premature infant? J Pediatr Gastroenterol Nutr. 2013;57:432–7. https://doi.org/10.1097/MPG.0b013e3182a208c7.
21. Roggero P, Gianni ML, Amato O, Orsi A, Piemontese P, Morlacchi L, Mosca F. Is term newborn body composition being achieved postnatally in preterm infants? Early Hum Dev. 2009;85:349–52. https://doi.org/10.1016/j.earlhumdev.2008.12.011.
22. Cormack BE, Bloomfield FH. Increased protein intake decreases postnatal growth faltering in elbw babies. Arch Dis Child Fetal Neonatal Ed. 2013;98:F399–404. https://doi.org/10.1136/archdischild-2012-302868.
23. Valla FV, Gaillard-Le Roux B, Ford-Chessel C, De Monte M, Tume L, Letois F, Mura T, Choueiry E, Rooze S, Moullet C, et al. A nursing survey on nutritional care practices in french-speaking pediatric intensive care units: Nutrirea-ped 2014. J Pediatr Gastroenterol Nutr. 2016;62:174–9. https://doi.org/10.1097/MPG.0000000000000930.
24. Vieira AA, Soares FV, Pimenta HP, Abranches AD, Moreira ME. Analysis of the influence of pasteurization, freezing/thawing, and offer processes on human milk's macronutrient concentrations. Early Hum Dev. 2011;87:577–80. https://doi.org/10.1016/j.earlhumdev.2011.04.016.

26

Implementing the World Health Organization safe childbirth checklist in a district Hospital in Rwanda: a pre- and post-intervention study

Eugene Tuyishime[1,2*], Paul H. Park[3,4,5,6], Dominique Rouleau[5], Patricia Livingston[1,7], Paulin Ruhato Banguti[1,8] and Rex Wong[5,9]

Abstract

Background: Worldwide maternal mortality remains high, with approximately 830 maternal deaths occurring each day. About 90% of these deaths occur in low-income countries. Evidenced-based essential birth practices administered during routine obstetrical care and childbirth are key to reducing maternal and neonatal deaths. The WHO Safe Childbirth Checklist (SCC) is a low-cost tool designed to ensure birth attendants perform 29 essential birth practices (EBP) at four critical periods in the birth continuum. This study aimed to evaluate compliance with EBP in Masaka District Hospital both before and after the implementation of the WHO-SCC.

Methods: This quality improvement project took place in the Masaka District Hospital in Rwanda. Observations of the 29 EBPs were done before and after WHO SCC implementation. The implementation process consisted of providing training in the use of the checklist to all clinical staff and posting SCC posters at different locations in the maternity unit.

Results: A total 391 birth events were observed pre-intervention and 389 post-intervention. The overall EBP compliance rate increased from 46% pre-intervention to 56% post-intervention ($P = 0.005$). Significant improvements were seen in 11 out of 29 EBPs.

Conclusion: The implementation of the WHO SCC improved the overall EBP compliance rate in Masaka District Hospital. Determining the root cause of low compliance rate of some EBP may allow for more successful implementation of EBP interventions in the future. After further study, the SCC should be considered for scale up.

Keywords: Quality improvement, Essential birth practice, WHO safe childbirth checklist, Evidence-based, Maternal mortality, Child mortality, Rwanda

Background

Reducing maternal mortality is a major focus worldwide. It was estimated that about 830 maternal deaths occurred every day around the globe in 2015; with 95% of the deaths having occurred in low-income countries and over 60% in Sub Saharan Africa [1]. In the 2000 UN Millennium Summit, many world leaders collaboratively developed eight Millennium Development Goals (MDG) to reduce extreme poverty globally [2]. By 2015, less than half of the countries had achieved MDG 4 - reduce child mortality, and MDG 5 – improve maternal health [3]. The use of evidenced-based essential birth practices (EBPs) for routine prenatal care and management of complications during childbirth is key to achieving high quality of care and reducing maternal and child deaths [4]. Following the success of the surgical safety checklist at reducing surgical complications [5–8], WHO developed the Safe Childbirth Checklist (SCC) in 2009 [9, 10]. The WHO Safe Childbirth Checklist (SCC) includes 29 essential birth practices targeting major causes of maternal deaths, intrapartum-related stillbirths and neonatal

* Correspondence: tuyishime36@gmail.com
[1]Department of Anesthesia, Critical Care and Emergency Medicine, University of Rwanda, Kigali, Rwanda
[2]University Teaching Hospital of Kigali, Kigali, Rwanda
Full list of author information is available at the end of the article

deaths that occur in facilities around the world [1]. This low-cost tool is designed to be accessible to birth attendants to ensure that timely, lifesaving practices are performed for every facility-based birth. The SCC is focused on care delivered for births at term gestation as these represent the overwhelming majority of births. The SCC is designed to address quality of care at four critical periods in the birth continuum: on admission to facility, at the time of pushing (or before cesarean delivery), soon after birth (within 1 h), and at discharge [11]. Previous studies have shown that use of the SCC increases the compliance rate of EBP in low resources settings [12, 13]. The use of the WHO-SCC has also been shown to contribute to the improvement of quality of care through three mechanisms: it serves as a reminder for the essential care practices; it is an advocacy tool for data collection and performance improvement; and it standardizes care so that every patient receives the essential components [13]. A one-center study conducted in India showed an increase in the EBP compliance of 150% after the introduction of SCC [13]. Another study conducted in three hospitals in India showed improvements in 13 EBP [14].

Rwanda has achieved the MDG 4 and MDG 5 and the maternal and neonatal mortality rates have decreased considerably. Between 2000 and 2015 maternal deaths were reduced from 1071 to 210 per 100,000 births, and neonatal death from 42 to 19 per 1000 births ([15]; World Bank, 2015). However, cost effective interventions remain needed in order to reach the Sustainable Development Goals (SDGs) of decreasing the maternal mortality rate to below 70 per 100,000 birth and neonatal mortality rate to below 12 per 1000 births by 2030 [16]. To our knowledge one health facility in Rwanda has implemented the WHO SCC, but its effectiveness for improving EBP compliance had never been evaluated. In response to this need, our study evaluates the effectiveness of implementing the WHO SCC on EBP compliance in one district hospital in Rwanda. The results of this study could inform the scaling up of the SCC in other district hospitals in Rwanda.

Methods

Aim

This study aimed to evaluate the effectiveness of implementing the WHO SCC on EBP compliance in one district hospital in Rwanda.

Setting

The study was conducted in Masaka District Hospital in Rwanda. The hospital has 35 maternity beds and offers both emergency obstetric care and caesarean deliveries. In 2016, the average hospital length of stay was 1 day after vaginal delivery and 3 days after cesarean section. Approximately 500 vaginal deliveries are performed monthly. The maternity unit team includes eight physicians, 20 midwives and three nurses. Despite the large number of deliveries performed, the hospital had not adopted the WHO Safe Childbirth Checklist prior to our intervention.

Study design

This study utilized a pre- and post-intervention design to evaluate the effectiveness of implementing the WHO SCC checklist on the compliance of essential birth practices.

The pre-intervention between January and February 2017 included a baseline assessment of the compliance on 29 EBP in the maternity service of Masaka District Hospital. Data was collected through observation by the data collection team over 14 consecutive day shifts (7 am – 7 pm) and 4 night shifts (7 pm – 7 am). The data collecting team was comprised of the principal investigator, two midwives and two medical students. After receiving a 2-day training, the data collectors were assigned to observe and record the completion of EBP at the four different "pause points": 1) at admission (5 items), 2) before pushing and 1 min after delivery (11 items), 3) within 1 h post-deliver (6 items), and 4) within 1 h before discharge (7 items) (Table 1). Since the primary objective of this study was to observe the health care professionals' behavior toward EBP, not the health outcomes of individual mothers, we conducted four independent cross sectional sampling on different women at the four pause points. The same observations were repeated between March and April 2017 to collect data post-implementation of the WHO SCC. To ensure data quality, the principal investigator performed random observations and data collections 2 days per week and compared the results to those collected by data collectors. Feedback was provided to data collectors when needed.

Sample

Women who were present at Masaka District Hospital maternity ward during the four pause points were included in the study. Mothers were excluded from the study if they declined or were unable to provide consent. Patients who had seizures, cardiac arrest, severe respiratory distress, hemodynamic instability, severe bleeding, and mental disorders were also excluded from this study.

Intervention

In February 2017, the principal investigator provided a 2-day training session on the implementation of SCC to all clinical staff and administrators at the maternity unit. The principle investigator also provided clear and open communication with staff so that they understood the

Table 1 Pre- and post-intervention essential birth practice compliance rate

EBP	pre-intervention	post-intervention	*P*-value
Pause point 1. "On admission"			
Observations (n)	106	95	–
1. Appropriate referral	100 (100%)	100 (100%)	1.000
2. Maternal temperature **	75 (70.8%)	51 (53.7%)	0.014**
3. Maternal blood pressure	90 (84.9%)	81 (85.3%)	1.000
4. Partograph started	59 (55.7%)	45 (47.4%)	0.26
5. Birth companion **	1 (0.9%)	7 (7.4%)	0.028**
Average	65 (61%)	56.8 (60%)	0.848
Pause point 2. "Before pushing and within 1 min after delivery"			
Observations (n)	92	98	
6. Water used to clean hands	22 (22.4%)	18 (18.2%)	0.483
7. Soap used to clean hands	18 (18.4%)	17 (17.2%)	0.854
8. Alcohol rub used	2 (2%)	3 (3%)	1.000
9. Clean towel **	63 (64.3%)	84 (85.7%)	0.001**
10. Clean gloves used	100(100%)	100(100%)	1.000
11. Clean scissors/ blade	88 (89.8%)	84 (84.8%)	0.392
12. Clean cord ligature/tie **	58 (59.2%)	89 (90.8%)	< 0.001**
13. Aspiration bulb or Mucus extractor	66 (67.3%)	70 (70.7%)	0.646
14. Clean pads for mother **	43 (43.9%)	61 (61.6%)	0.015**
15. Oxytocin	76 (77.6%)	84 (84.8%)	0.206
16. Birth companion present **	0 (0%)	10 (10.2%)	0.002**
Average	48.7 (53%)	56.4 (58%)	0.591
Pause point 3. "Within 1 h after delivery"			
Observation (n)	92	98	
17. Newborn weight taken**	76 (77.6%)	94 (94.9%)	< 0.001**
18. Newborn temperature	5 (5.1%)	4 (4.1%)	1.000
19. Neonatal bag and mask prepared	69 (70.4%)	69 (69.7%)	1.000
20. Baby placed skin-to-skin**	48 (49.0%)	89 (89.9%)	< 0.001**
21. baby still skin-to-skin at 1 h	2 (2.0%)	6 (6.1%)	0.279
22. Breastfeeding initiated**	32 (32.7%)	47 (47.5%)	0.042**
Average	38.7 (42%)	51.5 (53%)	0.161
Pause point 4. "Before discharge"			
Observation (n)	101	98	
23. Maternal blood pressure obtained**	14 (13.9%)	58 (58.6%)	< 0.001**
24. Mother's temperature **	3 (3.0%)	54 (54.5%)	< 0.001**
25. Baby's temperature	1 (1.0%)	5 (5.1%)	0.115
26. Baby's respiratory rate	1 (1.0%)	5 (5.1%)	0.115
27. Baby's feeding	89 (88.1%)	84 (84.8%)	0.54
28. Family planning options discussed	94 (93.1%)	88 (88.9%)	0.333
29. Danger signs explained **	1 (1.0%)	66 (66.7%)	< 0.001**
Average **	29 (29%)	51.4 (52%)	0.001**
Overall compliance			
Observation (n)	391	389	
Overall average **	46%	56%	0.005**

**Statistically significant at $P = 0.05$

importance and objective of this project. Regular feedback was provided to the staff to ensure both timely positive reinforcement and corrective actions. All necessary equipment, included documentations and thermometers, was available for the maternity unit to promote compliance. SCC posters were posted on the walls around the delivery wards as reminders to clinicians of the EBPs and their importance. Staff coaching was also provided during implementation and training.

Data analysis

The overall compliance rates of EBP at the four pause points, and for each of the 29 EBP items, were compiled and compared before and after the intervention. Chi-Square tests were used for the analyses, using SPSS v.20 with *P*-value set at 0.05.

Results

All hospital staff involved in childbirth agreed to participate in the study. In total, 590 patients gave their informed consent to participate in the study, 299 before and 291 after the implementation. All patients from pause point II were also followed for pause point III using the same informed consent.

For all four IV pause points, a total of 391 childbirth EBP events were observed pre-intervention and 389 post-intervention.

The overall compliance rate of EBP practices significantly increased from 46% pre-intervention to 56% post-intervention ($p = 0.005$). Three pause points (pause points II, III, and IV) had shown improvement on the compliance of EBP; particularly for pause point IV – before discharge, which significantly increased from 29% pre-intervention to 52% post-intervention ($p = 0.001$). The average compliance rate of EBP during admission (pause point I) showed slight decreased from 61% pre-intervention to 60% post-intervention, although statistically not significant ($p = 0.848$) (Table 1).

Out of the 29 EBPs, 11 (38%) showed statistically significant increase in compliance rates and 1 (3.4%) showed a statistically significant decrease post-intervention. Among the 11 EBPs showing significant improvement, 1 out of 5 was from pause point I, 4 out of 11 from pause point II, 3 out of 6 from pause point III and 3 out of 7 from pause point IV.

The improved EBP from pause point I was 1) birth companion presence on admission ($P = 0.028$); from pause point II were 2) clean towel use ($P = 0.001$), 3) clean cord ligature/tie use ($P < 0.001$), 4) clean pad for the mother use ($P = 0.015$), 5) birth companion presence before pushing and within 1 min after delivery ($P = 0.002$); from pause point III were 6) newborn weight ($P < 0.001$), 7) breastfeeding initiation ($P < 0.001$), 8) initiation of baby's skin to skin at 1 min ($P = 0.042$); and from pause point IV were 9) maternal blood pressure check before discharge ($P < 0.001$), 10) maternal temperature check before discharge ($P < 0.001$), and 11) danger signs explanation ($P < 0.001$) (Table 1). The EBP with significant decrease from pause point I was maternal temperature on admission ($P = 0.014$) (Table 1).

Discussion

The implementation of the WHO SCC was associated with an overall increase in compliance with EBP by the staff in the maternity ward of Masaka District Hospital, suggesting the feasibility of using the SCC to potentially improve maternal and perinatal care. Our result was consistent with other previous studies although the magnitude of improvement of our study was not as substantial as in other studies [13, 14]. The study conducted in India showed the EBP compliance rate increase as high as 150% after the introduction of SCC over a period of 3 months evaluation [13]. In contrast, our study post-intervention evaluation was only 3 weeks, much shorter than the other study. Such longer evaluation period also may have allowed the involved health care professionals to enhance their competency and familiarity of the EBP using the checklist. Longer-term follow up evaluation in the future may show more comparable changes. The highest increase in EBP was at pause point IV (before discharge), which also had the lowest pre-intervention compliance rate (29%). We speculate that the medical needs of the patients who were ready to be discharged may have been considered relatively less urgent, and thus received less attention and prioritization compared to those of patients at earlier stages of their delivery, particularly if there was a shortage of staff. Measuring the blood pressure and temperature of mother, or explaining the danger signs to the family before discharge could easily be missed or conducted but not properly documented. The introduction of SCC reminded the staff to perform these EBP despite their busy workload. Furthermore, the EBPs at this pause point mostly focus on patient education and prevention of complications after discharge; this kind of tasks requires relatively less human resources and equipment, thus should be easier to accomplish once reminded by the SCC.

The only EBP that showed statistical significant decrease from pre-intervention to post-intervention was taking maternal temperature at pause point I. During the implementation period, there was one staff on leave and the workload was distributed to other staff. From our discussion with them, many staff believed taking the temperature upon admission was relatively less important compared to the other EBP practices during active labor. Thus when the workload is high, the seemingly less important practices is more likely to be missed by the staff. However further investigation on this is required.

The keys to the success of the project was the application of many quality improvement principles during training and coaching including strategic problem solving skills, internal ownership, regular monitoring and evaluation, and engagement of leadership [17–19]. The implementation was taken on using a team approach. The team included the researchers, the clinical director, the head of maternity unit, and the head of post-delivery unit, who all worked collaboratively in the preparation, assessment, implementation, and evaluation. The team not only measured the baseline practices but also assessed the working situation to identify and understand the barriers to proper EBP performance. Feedback was provided to the staff regularly to ensure timely positive reinforcement and corrective actions.

The support from the hospital senior management team and the relevant staff was vital. Clear directives from management allowed the staff to understand the importance of this project. Involving the staff in the maternity ward from the planning stage of the project allowed them to take ownership of it and fostered early buy-in. We identified some highly motivated staff who were eager to improve the performance of their department and volunteered to coach during the implementation period. The early and continuous engagement of key actors helped to build a culture of teamwork and promote sustainability. With the support from the hospital administration and quality improvement team, the WHO Safe Childbirth Checklist has become part of the hospital protocol. All new staff working in the maternity unit will receive an orientation to the checklist. Such support from the hospital could increase the sustainability of the continuous use of the WHO SCC despite the end of this study.

Similar to what was described in other studies [20, 21], the implementation of the SCC, including its planning and training activities created an extra workload for the already small staff in the post-delivery unit.

This study has several limitations. Firstly, we could not eliminate Hawthorne effect; we could not control whether or not the staff changed their behavior due to their being observed. However, because the same approach was used both at baseline and post-intervention observations, we believe the Hawthrone effect should be similar in both pre- and post-intervention data collections. Secondly, our study was conducted in only one district hospital and the results and conclusions may not be applicable to other hospital settings. Thirdly, the patient numbers in our studied was small during the relatively short follow-up period (3 weeks) compared to some other similar studies, for example, 3 months evaluation in India [13] despite we detected statistical significance. Also, the clinical improvement was small, however as staff become more familiar with the SCC, the learning effect will probably increase the compliance rate. Longer term follow-up is needed to understand the sustainability and, naturally, larger study will be needed before any scale up of the project. Lastly, we acknowledge that there is a risk of bias in our study design. By excluding women with pregnancy complications, the study design could have potentially inflated the uptake at pause points 2, 3 and 4. After considerable discussion among hospital management team and project team, we have decided when pregnancy complication occurs, all staff should focus on saving lives rather than worrying about observing behavior and collecting data. By not having an observer in the already limited space room could ensure the health care professionals to be more efficient and not worrying about being observed and thus causing extra stress.

Conclusion

The implementation of the WHO SCC improved the overall EBP compliance rate in Masaka District Hospital. Determining the root cause of low compliance rate of some EBP may allow for more successful implementation of EBP interventions in the future. After further study, the SCC should be considered for scale up.

Abbreviations

EBP: Essential birth practices; MDG: Millennium development goal; SCC: Safe childbirth checklist; SDG: Sustainable development goals; SPSS: Statistical package for the social sciences; WHO: World Health Organization

Acknowledgements

The authors would like to thank Nyiramuhire Claudine and Dusabimana Raban for their contribution in data collection, and Uwizeye Marcel, Director of Masaka District Hospital, for supporting the implementation of this project.

Funding

All data collection and training costs were covered by Ariadne Labs.

Authors' contributions

ET and RW led the study design, protocol development, data analysis and manuscript writing. PP, DR, PI and PRB contributed to study design, protocol development and results interpretation. ET led and supervised data collection and led data cleaning. All authors critically reviewed and approved the final manuscript.

Competing interests

The authors declare that they have no competing interests.

Author details
[1]Department of Anesthesia, Critical Care and Emergency Medicine, University of Rwanda, Kigali, Rwanda. [2]University Teaching Hospital of Kigali, Kigali, Rwanda. [3]Partners In Health - Inshuti Mu Buzima, Rwinkwavu, Kayonza, Rwanda. [4]Brigham and Women's Hospital, Boston, MA, USA. [5]University of Global Health Equity, Kigali, Rwanda. [6]Harvard Medical School, Harvard University, Cambridge, USA. [7]Dalhousie University, Halifax, Canada. [8]King Faisal Hospital, Kigali, Rwanda. [9]Yale Global Health Leadership Institute, Yale University, New Haven, CT, USA.

References

1. WHO. Global Health Observatory data : Maternal mortality. 2015. http://www.who.int/gho/maternal_health/mortality/maternal_mortality_text/en/, Accessed on 16 Feb 2016.
2. UN. Millennium Project. http://www.unmillenniumproject.org/goals/, Accessed on 20 July 2017.
3. Victora CG, Requejo JH, Barros AJ, Berman P, Bhutta Z, Boerma T, Chopra M, de Francisco A, Daelmans B, Hazel E, Lawn J. Countdown to 2015: a decade of tracking progress for maternal, newborn, and child survival. Lancet. 2016; 387(10032):2049–59.
4. Tunçalp Ö, Were WM, MacLennan C, et al. Quality of care for pregnant women and newborns-the WHO vision. BJOG. 2015;122(8):1045–9. https://doi.org/10.1111/1471-0528.13451.
5. Haynes AB, Weiser TG, Berry WR, et al. Safe surgery saves lives study group. A surgical safety checklist to reduce morbidity and mortality in a global population. N Engl J Med. 2009;360(5):491–9. Available at: http://data.wordbank.org/indicators/SH.DYN.NMRT?start=2000 Accessed on 22 July 2017.
6. Kim R, Kwakye G, Kwok A, Baltaga R, Ciobanu G, Merry A, et al. Sustainability and Long-term Effectiveness of the WHO Surgical Safety Checklist Combined With Pulse Oximetry in a Resource-Limited Setting: Two-Year Update From Moldova. *JAMA Surg*. 2015;*150*(5):473–9. https://doi.org/10.1001/jamasurg.2014.3848 Accessed on 13 Mar 2016
7. Pronovost P, Needham D, Berenholtz S, et al. An intervention to decrease catheter-related bloodstream infections in the ICU. N Engl J Med. 2006; 355(26):2725–32.
8. Treadwell JR, Lucas S, Tsou AY. Surgical checklists: a systematic review of impacts and implementation. BMJ Qual Saf. 2014;23(4):299–318. https://doi.org/10.1136/bmjqs-2012-001797
9. Spector JM, Lashoher A, Agrawal P, et al. Designing the WHO safe childbirth checklist program to improve quality of care at childbirth. Int J Gynaecol Obstet. 2013;122(2):164–8.
10. World Health Organization (WHO). WHO Safe Childbirth Checklist Implementation Guide: Improving the Quality of Facility-Based Delivery for Mothers and Newborns. Geneva: WHO; 2015. http://apps.who.int/iris/bitstream/10665/199177/1/9789241549455_eng.pdf Accessed June 2017
11. Semrau KEA, Hirschhorn LR, Kodkany B, et al. Effectiveness of the WHO safe childbirth checklist program in reducing severe maternal, fetal, and newborn harm in Uttar Pradesh, India: study protocol for a matched-pair, cluster-randomized controlled trial. Trials. 2016;17(1):576.
12. Patabendige M, Senanayake H. Implementation of the WHO safe childbirth checklist program at a tertiary care setting in Sri Lanka: a developing country experience. BMC Pregnancy Childbirth. 2015;15:12. https://doi.org/10.1186/s12884-015-0436-0.
13. Spector, J. M., Agrawal, P., Kodkany, B., Lipsitz, S., Lashoher, A., Dziekan, G., … Gawande, A. Improving quality of care for maternal and newborn health: Prospective pilot study of the who safe childbirth checklist program. *PLoS ONE*, 2012, *7*(5). https://doi.org/10.1371/journal.pone.0035151 Accessed on 6 July 2016.
14. Hirschhorn LR, Semrau K, Kodkany B, Churchill R, Kapoor A, Spector J, et al. Before leaping: integration of an adaptive study design process prior to initiation of BetterBirth, a large-scale randomized controlled trial in Uttar Pradesh, India. Implementation Science : IS. 2015;10:117. https://doi.org/10.1186/s13012-015-0309-y
15. National Institute of Statistics of Rwanda (NISR), Statistical Yearbook, 2016 edition. (SYB2016), 2016, page 4.
16. UN. (2015). Goal 3 : Sustainable development goals, 1–6. Available at: http://www.un.org/sustainabledevelopment/health/. Accessed on 16 Feb 2016.
17. Banaszak-Holl J, Nembhard IME, Taylor L, Bradley EH. Leadership and management: a framework for action. Shortell Kaluzny's Healthc Manag Organ Des Behav. 2011:40–5.
18. Hayes E, Ka K. From the sidelines : coaching as a nurse practitioner strategy for improving health outcomes. J Am Acad Nurse Pract. 2007;*19*(11). https://doi.org/10.1111/j.1745-7599.2007.00264.x) Accessed on 16 Oct 2016
19. Stover K, Tesfaye S, Ah F, Mohammed H, Barry D, Alamineh L, et al. Building district-level capacity for continuous improvement in maternal and newborn health. J Midwifery Womens Health. 2014;12164:S91–S100. https://doi.org/10.1111/jmwh.12164. Accessed on 16 Sept 2016
20. Grimshaw J. From best evidence to best practice : effective implementation of change in patients' care. Lancet. 2003;362(9391) https://doi.org/10.1016/S0140-6736(03)14546-1.
21. Stove Belizán JM, Campbell MK, Ph D, Moss N, Ph D, Hartwell T, et al. A behavioral intervention to improve obstetrical care. NEJM. 2008;358(18): 1929–40.

27

Milrinone in congenital diaphragmatic hernia – a randomized pilot trial: study protocol, review of literature and survey of current practices

Satyan Lakshminrusimha[1], Martin Keszler[2], Haresh Kirpalani[3], Krisa Van Meurs[4], Patricia Chess[5], Namasivayam Ambalavanan[6], Bradley Yoder[7], Maria V. Fraga[3], Holly Hedrick[3], Kevin P. Lally[8], Leif Nelin[9], Michael Cotten[10], Jonathan Klein[11], Stephanie Guilford[1*], Ashley Williams[1], Aasma Chaudhary[3], Marie Gantz[12], Jenna Gabrio[12], Dhuly Chowdhury[12], Kristin Zaterka-Baxter[12], Abhik Das[12] and Rosemary D. Higgins[13]

Abstract

Background: Congenital diaphragmatic hernia (CDH) is commonly associated with pulmonary hypoplasia and pulmonary hypertension (PH). PH associated with CDH (CDH-PH) is frequently resistant to conventional pulmonary vasodilator therapy including inhaled nitric oxide (iNO) possibly due to right and left ventricular dysfunction. Milrinone is an intravenous inotrope and lusitrope with pulmonary vasodilator properties and has been shown anecdotally to improve oxygenation in PH. We developed this pilot study to determine if milrinone infusion would improve oxygenation in neonates ≥36 weeks postmenstrual age (PMA) with CDH.

Methods/design: Data on pulmonary vasodilator management and outcome of CDH patients was collected from 18 university NICUs affiliated with the Neonatal Research Network (NRN) from 2011 to 2012. The proposed pilot will be a masked, placebo–controlled, multicenter, randomized trial of 66 infants with CDH with an oxygenation index (OI) ≥10 or oxygen saturation index (OSI) ≥5. The primary outcome is the oxygenation response, as determined by change in OI at 24 h after initiation of study drug. As secondary outcomes, we will determine oxygenation at 48 h and 72 h post-infusion, right ventricular pressures on echocardiogram and the incidence of systemic hypotension, arrhythmias, intracranial hemorrhage, survival without extracorporeal membrane oxygenation, and chronic lung disease (oxygen need at 28 days postnatal age). Finally, we will evaluate the pulmonary and nutritional status at 4, 8 and 12 months of age using a phone questionnaire.

Results: Three hundred thirty-seven infants with CDH were admitted to NRN NICUs in 2011 and 2012 of which 275 were ≥36 weeks PMA and were exposed to the following pulmonary vasodilators: iNO (39%), sildenafil (17%), milrinone (17%), inhaled epoprostenol (6%), intravenous epoprostenol (3%), and intravenous PGE1 (1%). ECMO was required in 36% of patients. Survival to discharge was 71%.

Discussion: CDH is an orphan disease with high mortality with few randomized trials evaluating postnatal management. Intravenous milrinone is a commonly used medication in neonatal/pediatric intensive care units and is currently used in 17% of patients with CDH within the NRN. This pilot study will provide data and enable further studies evaluating pulmonary vasodilator therapy in CDH.

(Continued on next page)

* Correspondence: sguilford@upa.chob.edu
[1]University at Buffalo, Buffalo, NY, USA
Full list of author information is available at the end of the article

(Continued from previous page)

Keywords: Oxygen, Phosphodiesterase, Pulmonary hypertension, Persistent pulmonary hypertension, Extracorporeal membrane oxygenation

Background

Congenital diaphragmatic hernia (CDH) is one of the common serious congenital anomalies managed in the neonatal intensive care unit (NICU) [1]. Approximately 1600 newborn infants with CDH are born in the United States every year (http://www.cherubs-cdh.org/), and CDH is an orphan disease that is excluded from many trials involving persistent pulmonary hypertension of the newborn (PPHN). Infants with CDH usually have pulmonary hypoplasia (underdeveloped lungs) and pulmonary hypertension (CDH-PH) leading to hypoxemic respiratory failure (HRF). The presence of other anomalies (especially cardiac defects), location of the liver (intraabdominal vs. herniation in part to the thorax), degree of pulmonary hypoplasia and side of the hernia defect (right or left sided) may be associated with a different prognosis [2].

Despite many technological advances over the past two decades, including high frequency ventilation, inhaled nitric oxide (iNO) and extracorporeal membrane oxygenation (ECMO), CDH presenting in the neonatal period continues to be associated with relatively high rates of morbidity and mortality (28–30%) [1, 3]. Survival of infants at tertiary care centers automatically selects for patients who survive birth, resuscitation, and transport from an outside facility, and therefore likely underestimates the true hidden mortality associated with CDH. The major underlying pathophysiology in such infants appears to be a combination of lung immaturity, hypoplasia, and CDH-PH, which may be further aggravated by left ventricular underdevelopment [4–7] (Fig. 1).

Randomized trials in preoperative management of CDH

In spite of such high mortality, a randomized controlled trial targeting iNO use in CDH-PH [the Inhaled nitric oxide and hypoxic respiratory failure in infants with congenital diaphragmatic hernia (NINOS)] [8] and one trial targeting mode of ventilation have been published to date (VICI trial) [9, 10]. The NINOS-CDH study was conducted through the Neonatal Research Network (NRN) and the Canadian Institute of Health Research over 15 years ago. In the past decade following the completion of the NINOS-CDH study, significant changes in mechanical ventilation, such as a 'gentle' approach to ventilation of newborn infants, recognition of oxygen toxicity, tolerance to lower SpO_2 and higher $PaCO_2$ (permissive hypercapnia) and delayed surgical repair have changed the management of CDH. The NINOS-CDH study failed to demonstrate any benefit of iNO; in fact, the need for ECMO was significantly increased in iNO treated infants. Data from the extracorporeal life support organization (ELSO) registry (http://www.elsonet.org/) indicate that CDH, in addition to being the most common indication for neonatal respiratory ECMO (29.8% of cases), is also the diagnosis associated with the highest mortality (50.5% between July 2008 and June 2013) in infants who had undergone ECMO for neonatal respiratory indications. Regrettably, in patients with CDH on ECMO, survival has decreased from 53.4% during 1990–2000 to 45.4% ($p < 0.0001$) during 2001 to 2011 [11]. Survivors with CDH have long-term problems including pulmonary hypertension, reflux disease [12, 13] and chronic lung disease. [14]

A second trial randomized infants with prenatally diagnosed CDH into high frequency oscillation ($n = 80$) versus conventional mechanical ventilation ($n = 91$) as the initial mode of ventilation in Europe [10]. There was no difference in primary outcome of mortality/oxygen need at 28 days postnatal period (referred to as chronic lung disease in the current manuscript). However, patients on conventional ventilation as the initial mode had less use of ECMO, iNO, and sildenafil. The duration of vasoactive drugs was shorter in patients randomized to conventional ventilation. A third trial evaluating the use of sildenafil in chronic pulmonary hypertension associated with CDH was recently terminated at University of California, San Francisco (NCT00133679). The change in clinical practice allowing chronic therapy with sildenafil, incompatible with possibility of placebo is listed as the reason for termination of this study. A trial evaluating IV Treprostinil (Remodulin, NCT02261883) and one evaluating IV sildenafil (NCT01720524) in PPHN are recruiting and include patients with CDH-PH. To our knowledge, there are no other trials currently evaluating milrinone therapy in CDH-PH.

Milrinone is a phosphodiesterase 3 (PDE3) inhibitor and is currently approved for adult patients with heart failure. In addition to its inotropic and lusitropic effects on the heart, it is also a pulmonary vasodilator [15, 16]. It causes systemic vasodilation and reduces afterload in patients with heart failure. Vascular PDE3 breaks down cyclic adenosine monophosphate (cAMP) in arterial smooth muscle cells and the myocardium. By inhibiting PDE3, milrinone increases cAMP levels in cardiac

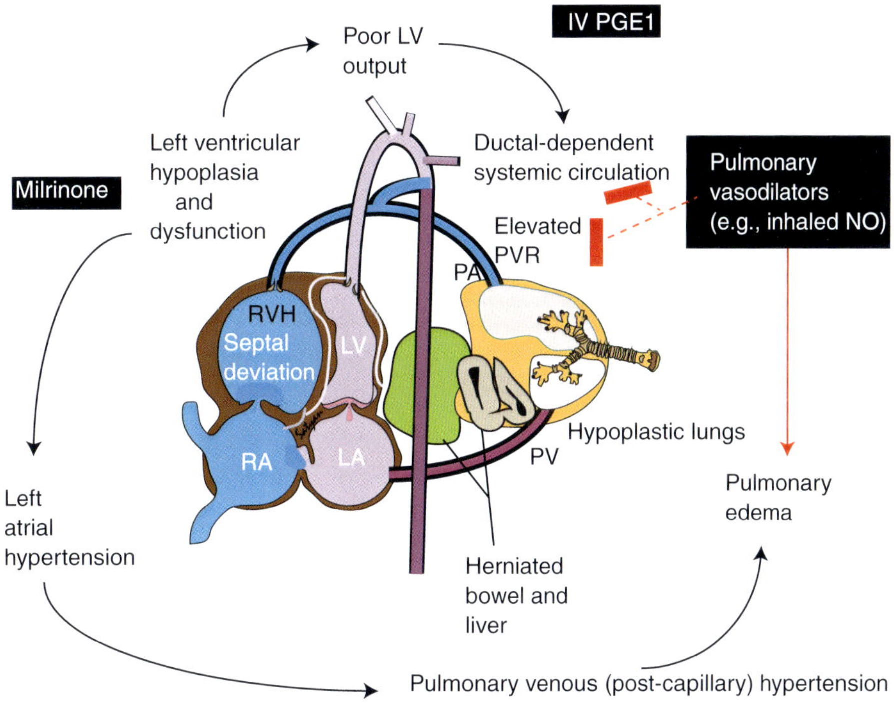

Fig. 1 Patients with left sided CDH may have left ventricular hypoplasia and dysfunction. Such dysfunction may be associated with elevated left atrial pressure, pulmonary venous hypertension and poor LV output. The systemic circulation may be dependent on right to left ductal flow due to elevated PVR. Pulmonary vasodilators such as inhaled NO may result in pulmonary arterial dilation and exacerbate pulmonary edema in the presence of pulmonary venous hypertension and decrease ductal-dependent systemic flow ("ductal steal"). IV PGE1 maintains ductal patency leading to reduced RV afterload and support systemic circulation. Milrinone, by improving left ventricular diastolic and systolic function reduces left atrial pressure and also dilates pulmonary vasculature resulting in improved oxygenation in CDH. The presence of hypoplastic lungs with remodeled pulmonary vasculature and volutrauma, barotrauma and oxygen toxicity contribute to poor response to pulmonary vasodilator therapy. We hypothesize that a combination of milrinone with "gentle" ventilation will improve oxygenation and response to pulmonary vasodilator therapy in CDH. RVH – right ventricular hypertrophy; RA – right atrium; LA – left atrium; LV – left ventricle: PVR – pulmonary vascular resistance; NO – nitric oxide; PA – pulmonary artery; PV – pulmonary vein; IV PGE1 – intravenous prostaglandin E1 (alprostadil)

muscle and vascular cells; it functions as a vasodilator and improves ventricular function directly and by decreasing afterload. Animal models of PPHN demonstrate increased PDE3 expression, which could promote vascular dysfunction [17]. Recent laboratory studies also indicate that hyperoxic ventilation with iNO dramatically increases PDE3 activity [18], suggesting that these therapies may reduce cAMP and paradoxically contribute to vascular dysfunction [19]. Such enhanced PDE 3 levels, in theory, augment the effectiveness of milrinone as a pulmonary vasodilator. Milrinone inhibits PDE3 and enhances cAMP levels and promotes vasodilation of pulmonary arterial rings in animal models of PPHN [20].

Studies evaluating milrinone use in children

The benefits of milrinone therapy in children following surgery for congenital heart disease have been well established in several studies (including the randomized, double-blind Prophylactic intravenous use of milrinone after cardiac operation in pediatrics (PRIMACORP) study, with 238 infants) [21–24]. In the PRIMACORP study among 238 treated patients, 25.9%, 17.5%, and 11.7% in the placebo, low-dose milrinone, and high-dose milrinone groups, respectively, developed low cardiac output syndrome in the first 36 h after cardiac surgery. High-dose milrinone significantly reduced the risk of development of low cardiac output syndrome compared with placebo, with a relative risk reduction of 55% ($P = 0.023$) in 238 treated patients and 64% ($P = 0.007$) in 227 patients without major protocol violations.

Milrinone in PPHN

Anecdotal reports have shown that milrinone can be an effective therapeutic option in PPHN [25, 26]. Three retrospective case reports from two different hospitals in Ontario, Canada evaluated late preterm/term infants [except one infant at 26 weeks postmenstrual age (PMA)] with HRF or PPHN unresponsive to iNO. Bassler et al. reported four infants with PPHN. Some of the infants were "primed" with normal saline (15 ml/kg) and administered a loading dose of milrinone at 50 μg/kg over 30 min followed by a 0.33 μg/kg/min infusion.

None of the infants developed systemic hypotension, and all of them showed consistent improvement in oxygenation. One of the infants was born at 26 weeks PMA and developed bilateral intraventricular hemorrhage (IVH) with moderate dilation of all ventricles. Another term infant developed an IVH. The third infant (39 weeks PMA) showed a small left subependymal hemorrhage. [27] McNamara et al. reported 9 term infants with PPHN and poor response to iNO who received IV milrinone. [25] Because of the potential risk of systemic hypotension, a loading dose was avoided in these patients with PPHN. The infusion was started at 0.33 μg/kg/min and increased in increments of 0.33 μg/kg/min according to clinical response to a maximum of 0.99 μg/kg/min. There was a significant improvement in oxygenation after commencement of milrinone, particularly in the first 24 h of infusion. Tachycardia improved and there was no systemic hypotension. More recently, the same authors performed pharmacokinetic studies in 11 late preterm and term infants with PPHN resistant to iNO with a loading dose of 50 μg/kg over 60 min followed by an infusion of 0.33 to 0.99 μg/kg/min and demonstrated an improvement in oxygenation and cardiac output by echocardiography, as well as a reduction in pulmonary arterial pressure without any associated IVH [28]. Milrinone improves right ventricular function and reduces strain and increases right and left ventricular output in infants with PPHN. [29] The safety and pharmacokinetics of milrinone in preterm infants has been evaluated [30–32]. The available information on the pharmacokinetics of milrinone in different age groups is presented in Table 1.

Rationale for use of milrinone in CDH

The poor oxygenation response to iNO and other vasodilators in infants with CDH may be due to a combination of right and left ventricular dysfunction. Remodeled pulmonary vasculature in CDH results in severe PH that leads to right ventricular dysfunction. An inotropic vasodilator such as milrinone improves right ventricular diastolic function and increases right ventricle systolic velocity in CDH resulting in improved pulmonary blood flow and oxygenation [33]. Recently, a case series from Australia suggested that right ventricular diastolic dysfunction measured by tissue Doppler on day 1 and 2 of life correlates with length of stay and duration of respiratory support [34] in infants with CDH. Compared to other causes of PPHN, infants with left sided CDH have significantly lower left ventricular mass; and it has been noted that infants who required ECMO had a lower left ventricular mass than those who did not require ECMO [7, 35]. We speculate that the reduced left ventricle mass is related to dysfunction, resulting in increased left atrial pressure and pulmonary venous hypertension. This may explain why iNO and other pulmonary arterial dilators are less effective in infants with CDH. [36] These agents can often worsen oxygenation in the presence of pulmonary venous hypertension and/or cardiac dysfunction [37]. Milrinone, an "inodilator" (inotrope with vasodilator properties) [16], may improve left ventricular function and potentially promote pulmonary vasodilation in infants with CDH (Fig. 1).

Methods/design (Fig. 2)

This pilot study is designed as a prospective, randomized, placebo-controlled, multicenter trial with a 1:1 randomization to milrinone or placebo (5% dextrose infusion). All participating centers are part of the Neonatal Research Network (NRN). The NRN is a well-established Eunice Kennedy Shriver National Institute of Child Health and Human Development (NICHD) funded network of 15 universities and affiliated academic hospitals across the US that has collaborated to improve neonatal care.

Outcome measures

The primary outcome is the oxygenation response, as determined by change in oxygenation index (OI = mean airway pressure in cmH_2O X FiO_2 X 100 ÷ PaO_2) at 24 h after initiation of study drug. In patients that require ECMO or die prior to completion of 24 h from the initiation of the study drug, the last OI prior to initiation of ECMO or death will be used for analysis. In subjects without an indwelling arterial line, or access to

Table 1 Pharmacokinetic data on milrinone in various age groups - modified from Lakshminrusimha et al. [43]

Age group	Loading dose	Maintenance dose	Half-life (h)	Total body clearance (mL/kg/min)	Volume of distribution (L/kg)
Adult [44]	12.5 to 75 μg/kg	0.5 μg/kg/min	0.8 ± 0.22	6.1 ± 1.3	0.32 ± 0.08
Child [45]	25 to 75 μg/kg	0.25 to 0.75 μg/kg/min	3.7	2.5 to 10.6 (increases with age)	0.7–0.9
Neonate (post-op CHD) [21]	25 μg /kg over 60 min (low dose) 75 μg /kg (high dose)	0.25 μg /kg/ min (low dose) 0.75 μg /kg/min (high dose)		1.64 ± 0.37	0.523 ± 0.028
Neonate (PPHN) [46] [47]	50 μg /kg over 60 min	0.33 (to 0.99) μg /kg/min	4.1 ± 1.1	1.83 ± 0.17 to 3.05	0.56 ± 0.19
Preterm neonate [32]	0.75 μg /kg/min for 3 h	0.2 μg /kg/min	10.3	0.64	0.576

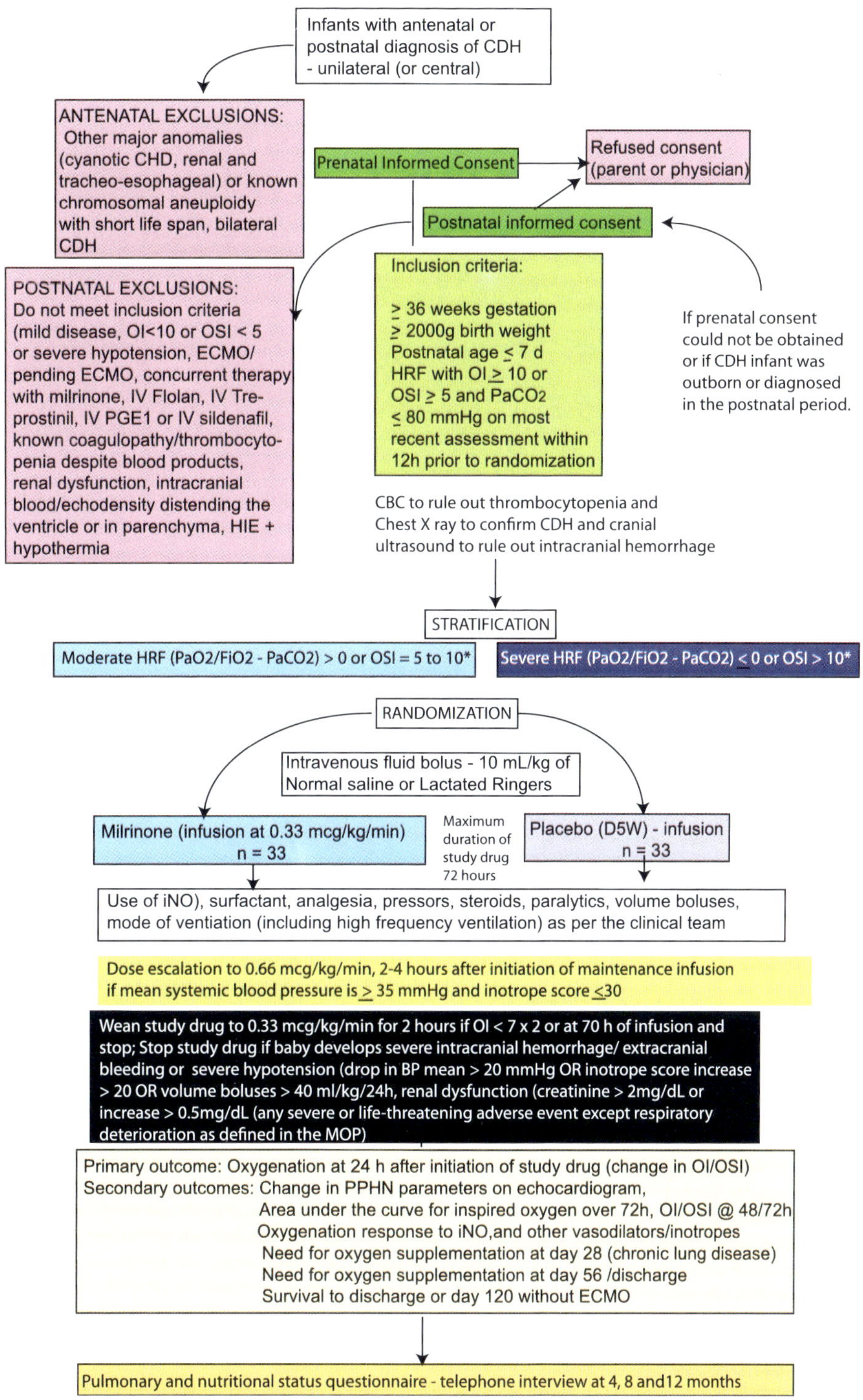

Fig. 2 Study design – please see text for details. * In the presence of an indwelling arterial catheter, or if there is an arterial blood gas drawn by arterial stick, oxygenation index (OI) values are preferred for making decisions regarding study drug therapy over oxygen saturation index (OSI) values

an arterial gas by an arterial stick, oxygen saturation index (OSI = mean airway pressure in cm H_2O X FiO_2 X 100 ÷ preductal systemic oxygen saturation - SpO_2) will be calculated using representative SpO_2 values recorded at protocol-specified time points. In subjects with an arterial line, OSI will be calculated at the time of the ABG sampling. In subjects without an arterial line, the stable pulse oximeter reading (both preductal and post-ductal, if available) closest to the beginning of the 6 h window will be recorded. If the study drug was started at 9 am and the 6–12 h window is from 3 pm to 9 pm, the preductal SpO2 close to 3 pm will be used for this period.

Secondary outcomes include:

(i) Oxygenation response at 24 h after initiation of study drug assigning a minimum OI of 40 or OSI of 20 for subjects that need ECMO or die after initiation of study drug infusion but prior to 24 h of study-drug infusion. In this analysis, if the patient's OI is 30 (or OSI of 15) and the patient is cannulated for ECMO due to hemodynamic instability, he/she will be assigned an OI of 40 (or OSI of 20) for calculating this outcome. However, if the OI prior to ECMO is 47 (i.e., > 40), the higher number (47) will be used for analysis of this secondary outcome. This secondary outcome was added as some infants with CDH are placed on ECMO for hemodynamic instability at a lower OI/OSI.

(ii) Oxygenation index (or OSI) at 48 and 72 h (or OI at the time of initiation of ECMO or death, for infants placed on ECMO or who die before these time points)

(iii) Area under the curve for inspired oxygen after initiation of the study drug (inspired oxygen and ventilator data from 4 time points per day – every 6 h will be recorded to calculate area under the curve)

(iv) Change in echocardiographic findings – velocity of tricuspid regurgitation, left ventricular ejection fraction, position of the interventricular septum and direction of shunt at the PDA and interatrial shunt – prior to and 24–72 h after starting the study medication

(v) Vasoactive Inotrope score (defined as a quantitative assessment of the degree of therapeutic support required by the patient to maintain adequate perfusion and/or blood pressure. The score is calculated as follows: (dose of dopamine in µg/kg/min + dose of dobutamine in µg/kg/min + 100 X epinephrine dose in µg/kg/min + 100 X norepinephrine dose in µg/kg/min + 100 X phenylephrine dose in µg/kg/min + vasopressin dose in U/kg/min × 10,000). We will also evaluate systemic blood pressure changes with the study drug.

(vi) If subsequent to initiation of the study drug, additional inotropes were used (such as dopamine, dobutamine, vasopressin, epinephrine and norepinephrine), an inotrope score will be calculated daily for 3 days from initiation of study drug [38]

(vii) If additional pulmonary vasodilator therapy is used (such as iNO), we will evaluate the oxygenation response to these agents. The OI and PaO_2/FiO_2 ratio prior to and after initiation of the inotrope/vasodilator will be recorded. The change in OI and PaO_2/FiO_2 ratio in response to these agents will be evaluated as a continuous variable and arbitrarily classified into responders, partial responders and non-responders similar to prior trials [39, 40]
   a. complete response is defined as an increase in PaO_2/FiO_2 ratio > 20 mmHg from baseline
   b. partial response is an increase in PaO_2/FiO_2 ratio of 10 to 20 mmHg from baseline
   c. no response is defined as an increase of <10 mmHg (or a decrease) in PaO_2/FiO_2 ratio from baseline
   d. the site of sampling (preductal or postductal) will be recorded
   e. in subjects without arterial access, an OSI will be used to determine response to vasodilators

(viii) Supplemental oxygen at 28 days, and 56 days and at discharge (or day 120, whichever time point is earlier).

(ix) Survival to discharge (or day 120, whichever comes earlier) without ECMO.

(x) Clinical status – pulmonary (use of supplemental oxygen or respiratory medications – pulmonary vasodilators), diuretics, methylxanthines, steroids, inhaled or nebulized steroids or bronchodilators, and nutritional (weight, length, head circumference, use of anti-reflux medications) at 4, 8, and 12 months of age.

(xi) Feasibility to perform definitive trial with the primary outcome of improved survival without ECMO. The following factors will be considered: slow recruitment, length of time for recruitment, number of serious adverse events reported, and interest from non-NRN hospitals or international collaboration in performing a definitive trial.

Inclusion criteria

Infants are eligible if they meet *all* of the following criteria:

- Antenatal or postnatal diagnosis of CDH confirmed with a chest x-ray
- ≥ 36 0/7 weeks postmenstrual age (PMA) by best obstetric estimate and birth weight ≥ 2000 g
- Postnatal age ≤ 7 days
- Invasive mechanical ventilation for HRF secondary to CDH with OI ≥ 10 (or OSI ≥ 5) on the most recent arterial blood gas (ABG) within 12 h prior to randomization
  - An acute reversible mechanical factor such as endotracheal tube obstruction or pneumothorax as a cause of elevated OI or OSI should be ruled out prior to randomization
- At least one blood gas with PCO_2 ≤ 80 mmHg on the most recent blood gas within 12 h prior to randomization

Exclusion criteria

Infants are ineligible if they meet *any* of the following criteria:

- Antenatal or postnatal diagnosis of bilateral CDH
- Known cyanotic congenital heart disease (acyanotic conditions such as patent ductus arteriosus - PDA, atrial septal defect - ASD and ventricular septal defect – VSD are included)
- Hypertrophic cardiomyopathy
- Enrolled in conflicting clinical trials (mothers enrolled in fetal tracheal occlusion studies such as FETO may be enrolled if permitted by investigators of the fetal tracheal occlusion study)
- Associated abnormalities of the trachea or esophagus (e.g., trachea-esophageal fistula, esophageal atresia, laryngeal web, tracheal agenesis)
- Renal anomalies resulting in renal dysfunction or severe oligohydramnios (Amniotic Fluid Index <5) associated with renal dysfunction (with serum creatinine >2 mg/dL, not due to maternal factors)
- Decision is made to provide comfort/palliative care and not full treatment
- Known large intraventricular hemorrhage resulting in distension of the ventricle or intraparenchymal bleed or any intracranial hemorrhage associated with a midline shift
- Thrombocytopenia (platelet count $<80,000/mm^3$) or coagulopathy (INR > 1.7) despite blood product administration on the most recent blood draw
- Hemodynamic instability with severe systemic hypotension (mean blood pressure < 35 mmHg for at least 2 h with a vasoactive inotrope score of >30
- Aneuploidy associated with short life span (such as trisomy 13 or 18)
- Use of milrinone infusion prior to randomization
- Infants on intravenous pulmonary vasodilator therapy (such as sildenafil or prostacyclin analogs including PGE1, epoprostenol, or treprostinil) prior to initiation of study drug
- Therapeutic hypothermia for hypoxic-ischemic encephalopathy
- Subjects already on ECMO or patients who are being actively considered for ECMO
- Attending (neonatal, critical care or surgical) refusal for participation in the trial (including concern about presence of hemodynamic instability)

Statistical analysis

Sample size

In the case series describing the effect of milrinone among neonates with CDH, baseline OI (mean ± SD) was 10.6 ± 5.6, and improved to 7.9 ± 6.2 and 5.1 ± 2.6 at 12–24 h and at 48–72 h, respectively [33]. Assuming that (a) children receiving placebo will have no additional change in OI (mean change in OI = 0 at 24 h), (b) that children receiving milrinone will improve to a mean OI of 6.0 (a mean change in OI of 4.6) at 24 h, and (c) that the standard deviation of the change from baseline OI at 24 h in each group is 6.2, 33 subjects in the control group and 33 subjects in the milrinone group would have 84% power to detect this difference with a two-sided alpha of 0.05. Phrased differently, if both the control and treatment OI's were to change, for any given difference in OI, the sample size would be sufficient to detect an effect size of 0.7 with a power of 84%. The sample size will be sufficient to provide estimates of adverse event rates in the treatment group.

Stratification based on assessment of severity of CDH

There is wide variation in CDH severity and asymmetric distribution of severity between the control arm and a treatment arm of a randomized trial needs to be avoided. Patients will be stratified based on the severity of HRF into two categories at the time of randomization.

(a) Moderate HRF: PaO_2/FiO_2 ratio – $PaCO_2$ value ≥0.

(b) Severe HRF: PaO_2/FiO_2 ratio – $PaCO_2$ value <0 [41]. The overall mortality for CDH in a study evaluating $PaO_2 - PaCO_2$ as a predictor of mortality was 30.7%. If the initial ($PaO_2 - PaCO_2$) value was <0, mortality was 55.3%. [41]

(c) In subjects without an ABG, moderate HRF is defined as a preductal OSI of 5 to 10 and severe HRF is defined as an OSI > 10.

Details of the planned analysis

Baseline data will be collected prior to randomization including gestational age, side of the diaphragmatic hernia, birth weight, mode of delivery and arterial blood gas parameters (oxygenation index-OI) and/or pulse oximetry data (oxygen saturation index-OSI). Data from a baseline clinical echocardiogram is recorded (if performed prior to study drug initiation or first echocardiogram performed after initiation of study drug). During the infusion of study drug, arterial blood gas parameters and hemodynamic data (blood pressure, heart rate and echocardiography results) will be recorded. After completing the study infusion, surgical details, and mortality information will be collected. Among survivors, respiratory and nutritional status at discharge and at 4, 8 and 12 months of age will be collected.

Data will be presented as mean ± SD for normally distributed variables and as median and ranges (with percentiles) for non-normally distributed data. All analysis will be by intention-to-treat. Baseline characteristics will be compared between treatment groups using chi-square and Fisher's exact test for discrete variables and t-test and ANOVA for continuous variables. The primary outcome, difference from baseline OI at 24 h, will be compared between treatment groups using a general linear model adjusted for the stratification factor of HRF severity. Other continuous outcomes will be analyzed similarly. Models for longitudinal outcomes such as oxygenation and vasoactive inotrope scores (short-term) and nutritional and pulmonary outcomes at 12 months (long-term) will include the effect of time, the interaction between time and treatment, and random effects to account for the correlation between measures taken on the same individual over time. Categorical outcomes will be analyzed using analogous generalized linear models. Cox regression models (with adjustment for HRF severity) will be used to plot proportion of responders who survive without ECMO against survival time in hours. Analyses may adjust for clinical site if treatment assignments are severely imbalanced for some sites provided that it is computationally feasible to do so. The potential influence of baseline measures such as time of diagnosis – antenatal vs. postnatal, side of the defect, and gender on pulmonary and nutritional outcome will be explored through the use of additional models similar to those described above.

Sample size limitations

This pilot study is not powered to compare rates of the outcome of death or ECMO between groups. To detect a reduction of 10% (from 40% incidence of death/ECMO in control arm to 30% incidence in the milrinone arm), with a 1:1 ratio of treatment and control subjects, a power of 0.8 and an alpha value of 0.05, we would require 376 subjects in each arm. We intend to obtain preliminary data for a definitive trial with a primary outcome of death/ECMO. The study is not powered to compare a sicker cohort of CDH (OI ~ 40s) patients similar to that evaluated in the CDH NINOS study. The patients in this study had an OI of approximately 45 with standard deviations of 16.3 and 14.5 in control and treatment groups respectively. Such a cohort will require a sample size of 207 patients in each arm.

Arrangements for randomization, allocation concealment and blinding

Central randomization with computer random number generation will be implemented with 1:1 allocation, stratified by severity of HRF. Stratification based on center and side of the defect is ideal. Since this is a relatively small trial, stratification is not possible for these two variables. The allocation will be unknown to the members of the clinical and research teams and all staff at the coordinating center except the pharmacist compounding the medication.

Study procedures

Management of infants with CDH in the study is based on individual center protocols or as per individual physician/provider preference. Suggested guidelines for management are shown in Fig. 3. Mothers with an antenatal diagnosis of fetal CDH and infants admitted to participating NICUs with a postnatal diagnosis of CDH will be approached for screening and consent (Fig. 4). In many institutions, mothers are referred by the Obstetrician and/or Maternal-Fetal Medicine (MFM) specialist for a consult with Pediatric Surgery and Neonatology. This would be an ideal time to obtain consent. Mothers admitted to labor and delivery with an antenatal diagnosis may be approached for consent (if not in active labor or on narcotic analgesia). Infants that are diagnosed postnatally, or born to mothers that could not be consented during the prenatal period or transferred from outside hospitals may be approached in the first 168 h of postnatal life (7 days). Using inclusion and exclusion criterion, study staff will determine if the infant is eligible for randomization. Eligible infants will be stratified based on the severity of HRF into the moderate or severe categories at the time of randomization. Infants will be randomized to either the milrinone arm or the placebo arm using a web-based system in a 1:1 ratio. Once the randomization code is received, the study pharmacist at the center will prepare an infusion of study drug. Infusion is initiated at 0.33 μg/kg/min (19.8 μg/kg/h; about 0.1 ml/kg/h using the premixed bag 200 μg/ml milrinone in 5% dextrose solution) after priming the infusion circuit. An equivalent volume of 5% dextrose will be used for infants randomized to the placebo arm. The premix solution in 5% dextrose has a pH of 3.2 to 4.0.

Dose

Milrinone/placebo will be initiated as an infusion of 0.33 μg/kg/min (Fig. 5). It is recommended that infants receive a fluid bolus (Lactated Ringers solution or 0.9% normal saline 10 mL/kg) *before* initiating study drug to avoid systemic hypotension, unless there is a contraindication. However, this is optional and based on clinical team decision. If after 2–4 h of infusion at this dose, no evidence of hypotension (defined as mean blood pressure ≥ 35 mmHg and a vasoactive inotrope score of ≤30) is observed, the rate of the infusion is increased to 0.66 μg/kg/min. Invasive blood pressure measurements through an indwelling arterial line (if available) are preferred to non-invasive assessment of blood pressure.

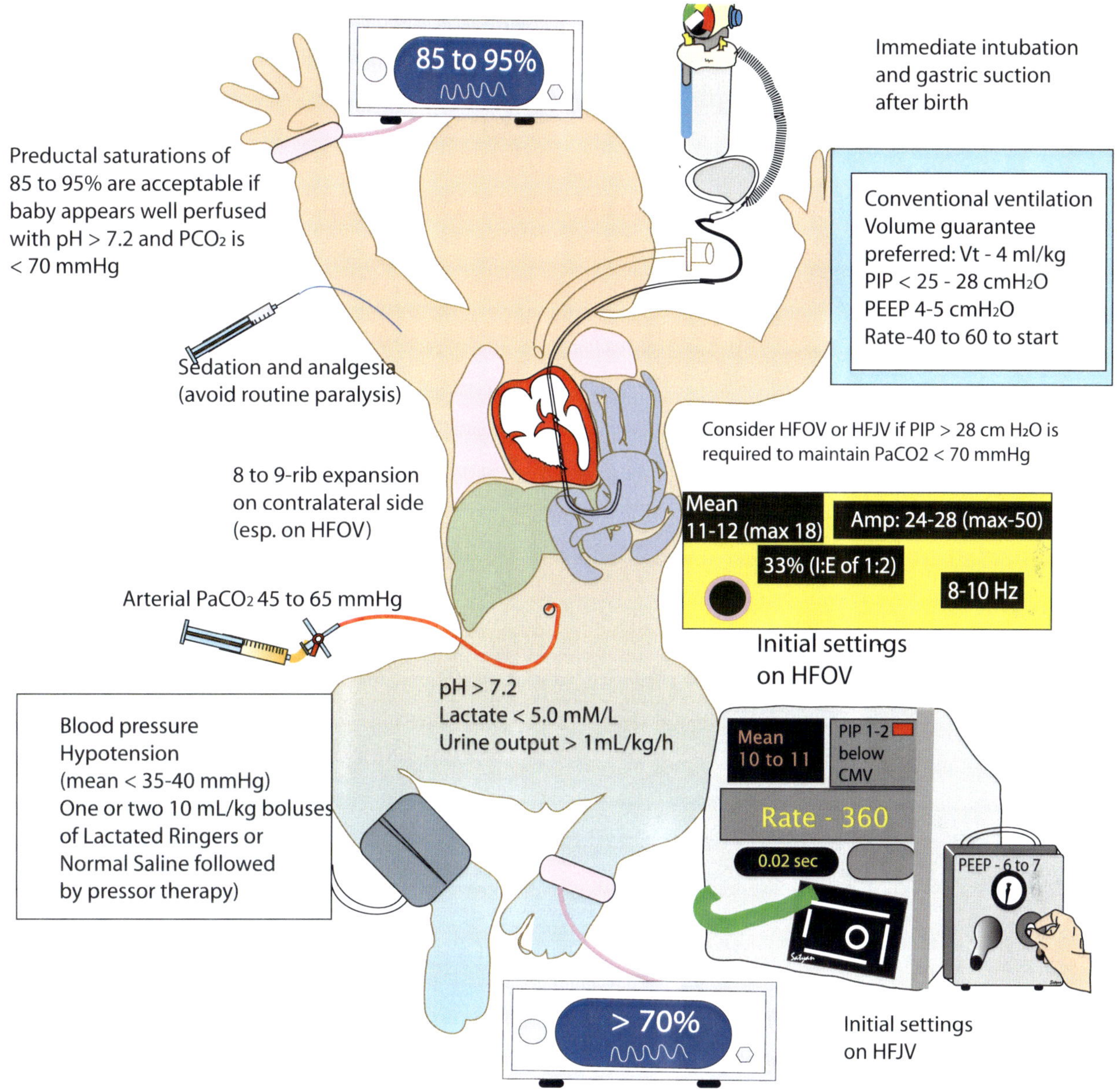

Fig. 3 Optional guidelines for "optimal" management of a neonate with congenital diaphragmatic hernia in the preoperative period. A nasogastric or orogastric suction tube is placed to decompress the stomach in the delivery room. Respiratory management includes intubation and positive pressure ventilation with care to avoid high PIP. The target of respiratory management is to maintain preductal oxygen saturations in the 85–95% range and $PaCO_2$ between 45 and 70 mmHg with a pH > 7.20. If $PaCO_2$ of ≤70 mmHg cannot be achieved with conventional ventilation (maximum PIP of 28 cm H_2O and a maximum rate of 60/min), high frequency ventilation (high frequency oscillator – HFOV or jet ventilator – HFJV) may be required. Blood pressure is maintained to achieve adequate perfusion and avoid lactic acidosis and oliguria. Monitoring chest X-rays to maintain contralateral lung expansion to 8 to 9 ribs may avoid baro/volutrama. A trial of inhaled NO may be considered when oxygenation index exceeds 15 with clinical or echocardiographic evidence of pulmonary hypertension. CMV – conventional mechanical ventilation. Modified from Chandrasekharan et al. [48]

Compatibility

Milrinone is compatible with 5% dextrose, normal saline and Lactated Ringers solution. Milrinone is incompatible with chlorothiazide, furosemide, imipenem/cilastatin and procainamide. Detailed compatibility information is listed in Table 2.

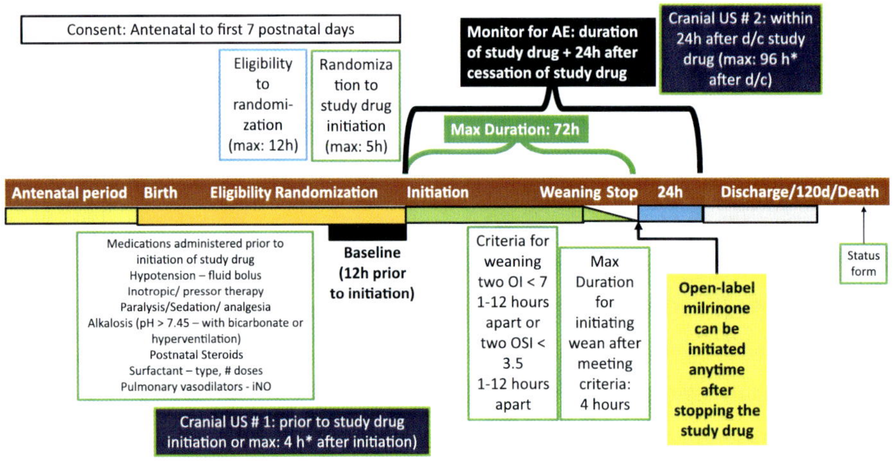

Fig. 4 Protocol for the milrinone CDH study. Parents are approached for consent during either the antenatal period or the first 7 postnatal days. Once eligibility is determined based on presence of hypoxemic respiratory failure and meeting all the inclusion criteria and absence of any of the exclusion criteria, subjects are randomized to milrinone or placebo. Details of other modalities of treatment (alkalosis, surfactant), medications administered (including pulmonary vasodilator therapy, vasopressor therapy and postnatal steroids) are recorded. A baseline cranial ultrasound (#1) is obtained either prior to or within 4 h of study drug initiation. Randomization is performed within 12 h of establishing eligibility. The study drug should be initiated within 5 h of randomization. Maximum duration of study drug therapy is 72 h. Patient is monitored for adverse events (AE) 24 h after cessation of study drug. The criteria for triggering study drug wean/discontinuation are two oxygenation indices (OI) < 7 at least an hour or maximum 12 h apart. If arterial access is not available, oxygen saturation index (OSI) will be used to assess hypoxemia. Once weaning/discontinuation criteria are met, study drug should be weaned within 4 h. Open label milrinone can be initiated any time after completion of the study drug. Status form (including data on surgical details) will be collected at the end of the hospital course or at 120 days of postnatal age or death (whichever is earlier)

Duration of study intervention and study drug discontinuation criteria:

In the absence of complications:

(i) Milrinone/placebo is continued until oxygenation improves and two OIs obtained at least one (up to 12) hour apart are less than 7 (or OSIs less than 3.5), then weaned according to the protocol below, or.

(ii) Milrinone/placebo is weaned and discontinued after a maximum of 3 days of therapy (total maximum duration of therapy = 72 h from the initiation of study drug).

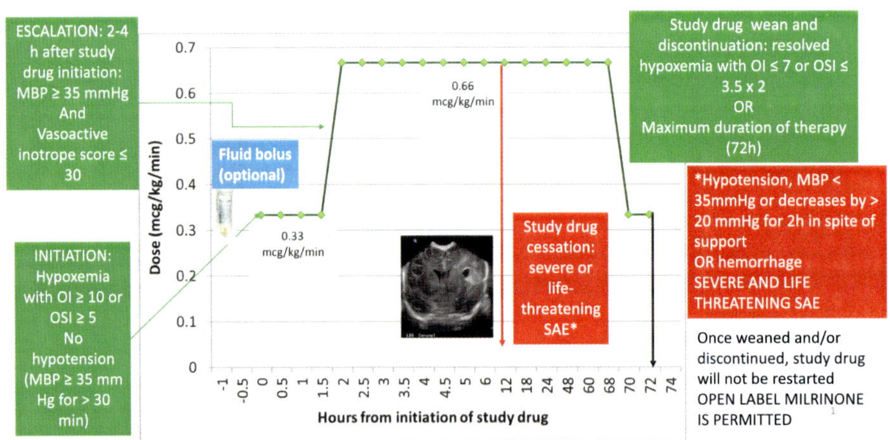

Fig. 5 Protocol for initiation, escalation, weaning and discontinuation of study drug. The study drug (milrinone or placebo – D5W) is initiated after documentation of hypoxemia (oxygenation index – OI ≥ 10 or oxygen saturation index – OSI ≥ 5), in the absence of hypotension and other exclusion criteria. A fluid bolus (10 ml/kg of lactated Ringers solution or normal saline) is recommended prior to study drug initiation. The starting dose is 0.33 μg/kg/min. After 2–4 h of therapy at this dose, study drug is escalated to 0.66 μg/kg/min in the absence of hypotension (mean systemic BP ≥ 35 mmHg and vasoactive inotrope score ≤ 30). The maximum duration of therapy is 72 h. Study drug is weaned to 0.33 μg/kg/min when study discontinuation criteria are met (two OIs < 7 or two OSIs <3.5 at least an hour apart). After 2 h of study drug infusion at 0.33 μg/kg/min, study drug can be discontinued. The presence of any severe and life threatening serious adverse events (SAE) necessitates immediate cessation of study drug. Open label milrinone is permitted after cessation of study drug

Table 2 Terminal site compatibility with Milrinone (Primacor®)

Medication	Trade name	Compatible?
Acyclovir		YES
Albumin		unknown
Ampicillin		YES
Calcium chloride		YES
Calcium gluconate		YES
Ceftriaxone	Rochephin	unknown
Chlorothiazide	Diuril	NO
Cisatracurium	Nimbex	unknown
Clindamycin		YES
Dexamethasone	Decadron	YES
Dexmedetomidine	Precedex	YES
Diazepam	Valium	unknown
DoBUTamine		YES
DoPAMine		YES
Epinephrine		YES
Famotidine	Pepcid	unknown
Fentanyl	Duragesic	YES
Fosphenytoin	Cerebyx	unknown
Furosemide	Lasix	NO
Gentamicin		YES
Heparin		YES
Imipenem/cilastatin		NO
Insulin, regular		YES
Ketamine		unknown
Magnesium sulfate		YES
Meropenem	Merrem	YES
Methylprednisolone	Solu-Medrol	YES
Metronidazole	Flagyl	YES
Midazolam	Versed	YES
Morphine		YES
Nafcillin		unknown
Norepinephrine	Levophed	YES
Phenylephrine	Neo-Synephrine	unknown
Potassium chloride		YES
Procainamide		NO
Ranitidine	Zantac	YES
Sodium bicarbonate		YES
Terbutaline		unknown
TPN + Lipids		YES
Vancomycin		YES
Vasopressin		YES
Vecuronium		YES

Surgery and ECMO:

(i) The study drug can be continued if the patient requires ECMO.
(ii) It is recommended that the study drug be continued through surgery. If the medical service overseeing ECMO treatment or if the surgical team prefers to discontinue the study drug, this indication should be recorded and study drug weaned as per protocol.

If serious, potentially drug-related complications occur, drug should be discontinued immediately (without weaning):

(i) The study drug is discontinued (without weaning) if the patient develops severe or life-threatening hypotension/shock. Severe hypotension is defined as a decrease in mean blood pressure > 20 mmHg compared to baseline OR receiving extensive volume therapy (>40 ml/kg during a 24 h period of the study monitoring period or escalation of vasoactive inotropic score by >20 compared to baseline).
(ii) The study drug is discontinued if the subject is detected to have a severe intracranial hemorrhage on cranial imaging (defined as unilateral or bilateral blood in the ventricles distending the ventricles or a parenchymal hemorrhage associated with a midline shift) or if patient is noted to have clinically significant extracranial bleeding.
(iii) If a significant deterioration of renal function is observed (defined as serum creatinine >2 mg/dL, increase in serum creatinine by >0.5 mg/dl compared to baseline prior to study drug, urine output <0.25 ml/kg/h over 12 h), milrinone/placebo infusion is discontinued immediately without weaning. Milrinone is excreted by the kidney and renal dysfunction can result in accumulation of milrinone.
(iv) Arrhythmias have been reported in adults during milrinone therapy. The study drug is discontinued in the presence of a heart rate rhythm abnormality including persistent bradycardia (heart rate ≤ 70/min) or tachycardia (heart rate > 220). The study drug is also discontinued if the heart rate abnormality is treated with anti-arrhythmic medications, cardioversion or defibrillation or associated with a > 5 mmHg decrease in mean blood pressure from the time prior to the onset of arrhythmia

The study drug can be discontinued (with or without weaning) by the clinical team at any time point if the team is concerned that the study drug poses a risk to the infant. An indication for discontinuation should be recorded.

Weaning of study drug

Once discontinuation criteria are reached, milrinone/placebo is weaned by 0.33 μg/kg/min every two hours and discontinued (total duration of wean 2 h if the patient is on 0.66 μg/kg/min and abrupt cessation of the medication infusion if the patient is on 0.33 μg/kg/min). If the subject is on 0.33 μg/kg/min, no weaning is required and the study drug is stopped at 72 h after initiation.

After the patient has met criteria for study drug discontinuation, study drug is discontinued and cannot be reinitiated even if the indication for initial discontinuation is resolved (for e.g., hypotension is resolved and blood pressure is normal). The clinical team may start open-label milrinone.

Open-label milrinone use

Immediately after completion of study intervention, open-label milrinone is permitted at the discretion of the clinical team.

Clinical criteria for ECMO

The decision to place an infant with CDH on ECMO *is entirely up to the clinical team.* Many centers prefer to use ECMO for preoperative stabilization. [42].

Cranial ultrasounds

An initial cranial ultrasound will be obtained prior to initiation of study drug or within 4 h of commencement of the study drug. A second cranial ultrasound will be obtained preferably within 24 h (maximum - within 96 h) of completion of the study drug. Both these cranial ultrasounds are covered by the study budget. Additional head imaging may be performed based on clinical indications (but are not covered by the study budget).

Echocardiography

Data from clinical echocardiograms will be recorded (maximum 4 studies – one prior to study drug initiation, two during study drug infusion and one after study drug infusion). The echocardiograms will be used to assess if there is shunting at the atrial level (and if present, the direction of the shunt), the presence of PDA (direction and velocity of shunt), position of the interventricular septum, the presence of tricuspid regurgitation (if present the pressure gradient will be recorded), chamber measurements, and any other relevant findings. These echocardiograms are obtained for clinical indications in this pilot trial.

The design of this pilot study includes randomization based on oxygenation status and not on underlying cardiac physiology. For the sake of simplicity, no echocardiograms are mandated prior to randomization. It is possible that subjects with CDH-PH without LV dysfunction and strict pulmonary arterial hypertension respond well to inhaled pulmonary vasodilator such as iNO. Subjects with LV dysfunction may have ductal dependent systemic perfusion and as such have poor outcomes with initiation of iNO. In addition, the presence of increased end diastolic pressure in the subgroup with LV dysfunction may lead to left atrial hypertension and post-capillary (or pulmonary venous) hypertension, leading to pulmonary edema aggravated by pulmonary vasodilators such as iNO. The subset of infants with LV dysfunction may respond better to milrinone and potentially deteriorate with the use of inhaled pulmonary vasodilators such as iNO. Information obtained from echocardiograms will be used to plan a future definitive trial. Echocardiographic evidence of LV dysfunction will be considered as an inclusion criterion for the definitive trial.

Follow-up

The infants will be followed during their inpatient stay; a phone follow up will be performed at 4, 8 and 12 months to evaluate the infant's pulmonary and nutritional status.

Safety reporting

Proposed frequency of analysis, including any interim analysis

An independent data safety and monitoring committee (DSMC) has been appointed and consists of a chair and scientific and methodological experts including a neonatologist, a surgeon, a statistician, and an ethicist. The DSMC is independent of the trial investigators and sponsors. The DSMC will monitor the progress of the trial on a routine basis for futility and review the accruing safety data.

Ethical approval

The protocol and the informed consent forms will be submitted to local institutional review boards (IRB) and ethics committees for review and approval. After initial approval, any updates to the protocol along with safety and progress reports will be submitted for review to the IRB/ethics committee at least annually and within 6 month of study termination or completion. The reports will include summaries of DSMC review of safety and efficacy.

Survey of CDH patients in the network current vasodilator therapy

A brief survey of the NRN centers was conducted in early 2013 (there were 18 centers in the network during that cycle. Following the renewal in 2016, the number of centers was reduced to 15). The number of patients with CDH, survival, ECMO utilization and information on pulmonary vasodilator therapy was collected and is shown in Table 3. Inhaled NO is the most commonly used pulmonary vasodilator in CDH-PH and more than half of CDH patients received iNO during some part of their hospital course in the NICU. Significant center variation was observed in iNO use for CDH-PH (varying from 13 to 100% of patients). Milrinone (IV) was used in 17% of patients (range 0 to 70%) and sildenafil (IV and PO) were used in 17% of CDH-PH patients (range 0 to 73%). The primary physician managing pulmonary vasodilator therapy for CDH-PH also varied from center to center with neonatologists managing this therapy in nearly two-thirds of centers (Table 3).

Variation in practice

There is significant variation in management of CDH-PH among centers participating in the network. The general guidelines for management shown in Fig. 3 are provided to all centers. These guidelines are not mandatory.

a. Preductal oxygen saturation limits of 85 to 95% (unless in 21% oxygen) after immediate postnatal stabilization.
b. Conventional ventilation (preferably in the volume guarantee or a similar mode) is the preferred mode of initial ventilation. If ventilation or oxygenation cannot be maintained on conventional ventilation, the infant may be switched to a high frequency ventilator (either oscillatory ventilation or jet ventilation).
c. Indications for iNO: Inhaled NO may be used for hypoxemic respiratory failure with an OI of at least >15 and clinical and/or echocardiographic evidence of CDH-PH.

Plans for a future definitive trial

This pilot trial is being conducted to collect data on safety, oxygenation and echocardiographic response to milrinone in CDH-PH and to test the feasibility of conducting a large definitive trial. This large trial will need to be a multicenter, international trial where randomization is based on oxygenation status and echocardiographic criteria with a clinically meaningful outcome such as survival without ECMO. The estimated sample size for such a trial is likely to be close to 750–800 patients with CDH-PH.

Conclusion

Infants with CDH continue to have high mortality with high morbidity among survivors. Survival to hospital discharge among tertiary care centers with the NICHD Neonatal Research Network is 68%. Although no evidence-based guidelines are available for pulmonary vasodilator therapy, multiple vasodilators including iNO are commonly used within the network. The primary team managing pulmonary vasodilator therapy is distributed between neonatal and surgical services. Optimal

Table 3 Infants with congenital diaphragmatic hernia in the Neonatal Research Network

	2011	2012	Average	Range among centers
Total CDH admissions	175	162	169	
CDH ≥ 36 0/7 week PMA	142	133	138 (81%)	
Inhaled NO in the preoperative period among CDH ≥ 36 0/7 weeks PMA	53	55	54 (39%)	0–100%
Other medications used in the preoperative period among CDH ≥ 36 0/7 weeks PMA				
Milrinone	17	29	23 (17%)	0–70%
Sildenafil	27	21	24 (17%)	0–73%
Flolan ® (inhaled epoprostenol)	8	9	9 (6%)	0–68% [a]
Flolan ® (intravenous epoprostenol)	6	3	5 (3%)	0–25% [a]
Alprostadil (intravenous PGE1)	6	5	6 (4%)	0–50%
Epinephrine	2	0	1 (1%)	0–25% [a]
ECMO among all CDH	59	56	58 (34%)	8–87%
ECMO among CDH ≥ 36 0/7 weeks PMA	51	48	50 (36%)	9–59%
Survival to discharge				
- All CDH	111	117	114 (68%)	40–100%
- CDH ≥ 36 0/7 weeks PMA	94	101	98 (71%)	53–100%
Concern regarding use of iNO in CDH	Yes – 8; No – 11[b]			
Primary physician managing pulmonary vasodilator therapy Surgeons – 4; Neonatologists – 10; Joint (surgeons + neonatologists – 3); Pediatric Intensivists – 1				

[a] These medications were used in one center only within the Network
[b] One center with two hospitals had a different response at each hospital

management during the preoperative period focusing on gentle ventilation, avoiding oxygen toxicity, baro/volu-trauma to the hypoplastic lung, cardiac support and management of pulmonary hypertension (Fig. 3) may be beneficial. Intravenous milrinone is a commonly used medication in neonatal and pediatric intensive care units and is currently used in 17% of patients with CDH within the NRN. This pilot will provide data and enable further studies evaluating pulmonary vasodilator therapy in CDH.

Abbreviations

ASD: Atrial septal defect; cAMP: Cyclic adenosine monophosphate; CDH: Congenital diaphragmatic hernia; CDH-PH: Pulmonary hypertension associated with CDH; DSMC: Data Safety Monitoring Committee; ECMO: Extracorporeal membrane oxygenation; HRF: Hypoxemic respiratory failure; iNO: Inhaled nitric oxide; IVH: Intraventricular hemorrhage; NICHD: Eunice Kennedy Shriver National Institute of Child Health and Human Development; NICU: Neonatal intensive care unit; NRN: Neonatal research network; OI: Oxygenation index; OSI: Oxygen saturation index; PDA: Patent ductus arteriosus; PDE3: Phosphodiesterase 3; PH: Pulmonary hypertension; PMA: Postmenstrual age; PPHN: Persistent pulmonary hypertension of newborn; VSD: Ventricular septal defect

Acknowledgements

We thank Drs. Matthew Harting, Stephanie Chao, and Gabriel Altit for their review and critique of this manuscript. We thank the NRN Steering Committee, Protocol Review and Publication Subcommittees for their support in the preparation of this protocol and manuscript.

Funding

National Institute of Child Health and Human Development (NICHD).

Authors' contributions

SL, MK, HK, KVM, PC, NA, LN, MC, JK, AC planned the study, wrote the manuscript, edited, reviewed and approved the final version of this manuscript. BY and MF edited, reviewed and approved the final version of this manuscript. HH and KL served as surgical consultants on the subcommittee and edited, reviewed and approved the final version of this manuscript. SG planned the study, wrote the manuscript, edited, reviewed and approved the final version and is the corresponding author of this manuscript. AW wrote the initial draft of the manuscript, edited, reviewed and approved the final version of this manuscript. MG wrote the statistical analysis section of the manuscript, planned the study, edited, reviewed and approved the final version of this manuscript. JG wrote the protocol, edited, reviewed and approved the final version of this manuscript. DC and AD reviewed the statistical section of the manuscript, edited and approved the final version of this manuscript. KZB reviewed the study protocol and adverse events sections of the manuscript, edited, reviewed and approved the final version of this manuscript. RH planned the study, edited, reviewed and approved the final version of this manuscript.

Competing interests

The authors declare that they have no competing interests.

Author details

[1]University at Buffalo, Buffalo, NY, USA. [2]Women and Infants Hospital, Providence, RI, USA. [3]Children's Hospital of Philadelphia, Philadelphia, PA, USA. [4]Stanford University, Palo Alto, CA, USA. [5]University of Rochester, Rochester, NY, USA. [6]University of Alabama at Birmingham, Birmingham, AL, USA. [7]University of Utah, Salt Lake City, UT, USA. [8]University at Texas at Houston, Houston, TX, USA. [9]Nationwide Children's Hospital, Columbus, OH, USA. [10]Duke University, Durham, NC, USA. [11]University of Iowa, Iowa City, IA, USA. [12]RTI, Research Triangle Park, NC, USA. [13]NICHD, Neonatal Research Network, Bethesda, MD, USA.

References

1. Yoder BA, Lally PA, Lally KP. Does a highest pre-ductal O(2) saturation <85% predict non-survival for congenital diaphragmatic hernia? J Perinatol. 2012; 32(12):947–52.
2. Schaible T, Kohl T, Reinshagen K, Brade J, Neff KW, Stressig R, Busing KA. Right- versus left-sided congenital diaphragmatic hernia: postnatal outcome at a specialized tertiary care center. Pediatr Crit Care Med. 2012;13(1):66–71.
3. Keller RL. Management of the infant with congenital diaphragmatic hernia. In: Bancalari E, Polin RA, editors. The newborn lung. 2nd ed. Philadelphia: Elsevier Saunders; 2012. p. 381–406.
4. Aggarwal S, Stockman PT, Klein MD, Natarajan G. The right ventricular systolic to diastolic duration ratio: a simple prognostic marker in congenital diaphragmatic hernia? Acta Paediatr. 2011;100(10):1315–8.
5. Irish MS, Karamanoukian HL, O'Toole SJ, Glick PL. You gotta have heart. J Pediatr. 1996;129(1):175–6. author reply 176-177
6. Menon SC, Tani LY, Weng HY, Lally PA, Lally KP, Yoder BA. Congenital diaphragmatic hernia study group: clinical characteristics and outcomes of patients with cardiac defects and congenital diaphragmatic hernia. J Pediatr. 2013;162(1):114-19.
7. Schwartz SM, Vermilion RP, Hirschl RB. Evaluation of left ventricular mass in children with left-sided congenital diaphragmatic hernia. J Pediatr. 1994; 125(3):447–51.
8. NINOS. Inhaled nitric oxide in full-term and nearly full-term infants with hypoxic respiratory failure. The Neonatal Inhaled Nitric Oxide Study Group. [erratum appears in N Engl J Med 1997 Aug 7;337(6):434]. N Engl J Med. 1997;336(9):597–604.
9. Snoek KG, Capolupo I, van Rosmalen J, Hout Lde J, Vijfhuize S, Greenough A, Wijnen RM, Tibboel D, Reiss IK, Consortium CE. Conventional mechanical ventilation versus high-frequency oscillatory ventilation for congenital diaphragmatic hernia: a randomized clinical trial (the VICI-trial). Ann Surg. 2016;263(5):867–74.
10. van den Hout L, Tibboel D, Vijfhuize S, te Beest H, Hop W, Reiss I, Consortium C-E. The VICI-trial: high frequency oscillation versus conventional mechanical ventilation in newborns with congenital diaphragmatic hernia: an international multicentre randomized controlled trial. BMC Pediatr. 2011;11:98.
11. Paden ML, Conrad SA, Rycus PT, Thiagarajan RR, Registry E. Extracorporeal life support organization registry report 2012. ASAIO J. 2013;59(3):202–10.
12. Peetsold MG, Heij HA, Kneepkens CM, Nagelkerke AF, Huisman J, Gemke RJ. The long-term follow-up of patients with a congenital diaphragmatic hernia: a broad spectrum of morbidity. Pediatr Surg Int. 2009;25(1):1–17.
13. Muratore CS, Kharasch V, Lund DP, Sheils C, Friedman S, Brown C, Utter S, Jaksic T, Wilson JM. Pulmonary morbidity in 100 survivors of congenital diaphragmatic hernia monitored in a multidisciplinary clinic. J Pediatr Surg. 2001;36(1):133–40.
14. Hollinger LE, Harting MT, Lally KP. Long-term follow-up of congenital diaphragmatic hernia. Semin Pediatr Surg. 2017;26(3):178–84.
15. Opie LH. Inodilators. Lancet. 1986;1(8493):1336.
16. Lakshminrusimha S, Steinhorn RH. Inodilators in nitric oxide resistant persistent pulmonary hypertension of the newborn. Pediatr Crit Care Med. 2013;14(1):107–9.
17. Murray F, MacLean MR, Pyne NJ. Increased expression of the cGMP-inhibited cAMP-specific (PDE3) and cGMP binding cGMP-specific (PDE5) phosphodiesterases in models of pulmonary hypertension. Br J Pharmacol. 2002;137(8):1187–94.
18. Chen B, Lakshminrusimha S, Czech L, Groh BS, Gugino SF, Russell JA, Farrow KN, Steinhorn RH. Regulation of phosphodiesterase 3 in the pulmonary arteries during the perinatal period in sheep. Pediatr Res. 2009;66(6):682–7.
19. Thelitz S, Oishi P, Sanchez LS, Bekker JM, Ovadia B, Johengen MJ, Black SM, Fineman JR. Phosphodiesterase-3 inhibition prevents the increase in pulmonary vascular resistance following inhaled nitric oxide withdrawal in lambs. Pediatr Crit Care Med. 2004;5(3):234–9.
20. Lakshminrusimha S, Porta NF, Farrow KN, Chen B, Gugino SF, Kumar VH, Russell JA, Steinhorn RH. Milrinone enhances relaxation to prostacyclin and iloprost in pulmonary arteries isolated from lambs with persistent pulmonary hypertension of the newborn. Pediatr Crit Care Med. 2009;10(1): 106–12.
21. Bailey JM, Miller BE, Lu W, Tosone SR, Kanter KR, Tam VK. The pharmacokinetics of milrinone in pediatric patients after cardiac surgery. Anesthesiology. 1999;90(4):1012–8.

22. Chang AC, Atz AM, Wernovsky G, Burke RP, Wessel DL. Milrinone: systemic and pulmonary hemodynamic effects in neonates after cardiac surgery. Crit Care Med. 1995;23(11):1907–14.
23. Hoffman TM, Wernovsky G, Atz AM, Bailey JM, Akbary A, Kocsis JF, Nelson DP, Chang AC, Kulik TJ, Spray TL, et al. Prophylactic intravenous use of milrinone after cardiac operation in pediatrics (PRIMACORP) study. Prophylactic intravenous use of Milrinone after cardiac operation in pediatrics. Am Heart J. 2002;143(1):15–21.
24. Hoffman TM, Wernovsky G, Atz AM, Kulik TJ, Nelson DP, Chang AC, Bailey JM, Akbary A, Kocsis JF, Kaczmarek R, et al. Efficacy and safety of milrinone in preventing low cardiac output syndrome in Infants and children after corrective surgery for congenital heart disease. Circulation. 2003;107(7):996–1002.
25. McNamara PJ, Laique F, Muang-in S, Whyte HE. Milrinone improves oxygenation in neonates with severe persistent pulmonary hypertension of the newborn. J Crit Care. 2006;21(2):217–22.
26. Bassler D, Kreutzer K, McNamara P, Kirpalani H. Milrinone for persistent pulmonary hypertension of the newborn. The Cochrane database of systematic reviews. 2010;10(11):CD007802.
27. Bassler D, Choong K, McNamara P, Kirpalani H. Neonatal persistent pulmonary hypertension treated with milrinone: four case reports. Biol Neonate. 2006;89(1):1–5.
28. McNamara PJ, Shivananda SP, Sahni M, Freeman D, Taddio A. Pharmacology of Milrinone in neonates with persistent pulmonary hypertension of the newborn and suboptimal response to inhaled nitric oxide. Pediatr Crit Care Med. 2012;
29. James AT, Corcoran JD, McNamara PJ, Franklin O, El-Khuffash AF. The effect of milrinone on right and left ventricular function when used as a rescue therapy for term infants with pulmonary hypertension. Cardiol Young. 2016; 26(1):90–9.
30. Paradisis M, Evans N, Kluckow M, Osborn D. Randomized trial of milrinone versus placebo for prevention of low systemic blood flow in very preterm infants. J Pediatr. 2009;154(2):189–95.
31. Paradisis M, Evans N, Kluckow M, Osborn D, McLachlan AJ. Pilot study of milrinone for low systemic blood flow in very preterm infants. J Pediatr. 2006;148(3):306–13.
32. Paradisis M, Jiang X, McLachlan AJ, Evans N, Kluckow M, Osborn D. Population pharmacokinetics and dosing regimen design of milrinone in preterm infants. Arch Dis Child Fetal Neonatal Ed. 2007;92(3):F204–9.
33. Patel N. Use of milrinone to treat cardiac dysfunction in infants with pulmonary hypertension secondary to congenital diaphragmatic hernia: a review of six patients. Neonatology. 2012;102(2):130–6.
34. Moenkemeyer F, Patel N. Right ventricular diastolic function measured by tissue Doppler imaging predicts early outcome in congenital diaphragmatic hernia. Pediatr Crit Care Med. 2014;15(1):49–55.
35. Siebert JR, Haas JE, Beckwith JB. Left ventricular hypoplasia in congenital diaphragmatic hernia. J Pediatr Surg. 1984;19(5):567–71.
36. Patel N, Kipfmueller F. Cardiac dysfunction in congenital diaphragmatic hernia: pathophysiology, clinical assessment, and management. Semin Pediatr Surg. 2017;26(3):154–8.
37. Lakshminrusimha S. The pulmonary circulation in neonatal respiratory failure. Clin Perinatol. 2012;39(3):655–83.
38. Cruz DN, Antonelli M, Fumagalli R, Foltran F, Brienza N, Donati A, Malcangi V, Petrini F, Volta G, Bobbio Pallavicini FM, et al. Early use of polymyxin B hemoperfusion in abdominal septic shock: the EUPHAS randomized controlled trial. JAMA. 2009;301(23):2445–52.
39. NINOS. Inhaled nitric oxide in full-term and nearly full-term infants with hypoxic respiratory failure. The neonatal inhaled nitric oxide study group. N Engl J Med. 1997;336(9):597–604.
40. The Neonatal Inhaled Nitric Oxide Study Group N. inhaled nitric oxide and hypoxic respiratory failure in infants with congenital diaphragmatic hernia. The neonatal inhaled nitric oxide study group (NINOS). Pediatrics. 1997; 99(6):838–45.
41. Park HW, Lee BS, Lim G, Choi YS, Kim EA, Kim KS. A simplified formula using early blood gas analysis can predict survival outcomes and the requirements for extracorporeal membrane oxygenation in congenital diaphragmatic hernia. J Korean Med Sci. 2013;28(6):924–8.
42. Reiss I, Schaible T, van den Hout L, Capolupo I, Allegaert K, van Heijst A, Gorett Silva M, Greenough A, Tibboel D, Consortium CE. Standardized postnatal management of infants with congenital diaphragmatic hernia in Europe: the CDH EURO consortium consensus. Neonatology. 2010;98(4): 354–64.
43. Lakshminrusimha S, Mathew B, Leach CL. Pharmacologic strategies in neonatal pulmonary hypertension other than nitric oxide. Semin Perinatol. 2016;40(3):160–73.
44. Young RA, Ward A. Milrinone. A preliminary review of its pharmacological properties and therapeutic use. Drugs. 1988;36(2):158–92.
45. Bailey JM, Hoffman TM, Wessel DL, Nelson DP, Atz AM, Chang AC, Kulik TJ, Spray TL, Akbary A, Miller RP, et al. A population pharmacokinetic analysis of milrinone in pediatric patients after cardiac surgery. J Pharmacokinet Pharmacodyn. 2004;31(1):43–59.
46. McNamara PJ, Shivananda SP, Sahni M, Freeman D, Taddio A. Pharmacology of milrinine in neonates with persistent pulmonary hypertension of the newborn (PPHN) and suboptimal response to inhaled nitric oxide. Pediatr Crit Care Med. 2012;
47. Giaccone A, Zuppa AF, Sood B, Cohen MS, O'Byrne ML, Moorthy G, Mathur A, Kirpalani H. Milrinone pharmacokinetics and pharmacodynamics in neonates with persistent pulmonary hypertension of the newborn. Am J Perinatol. 2017;
48. Chandrasekharan PK, Rawat M, Madappa R, Rothstein DH, Lakshminrusimha S. Congenital diaphragmatic hernia - a review. Maternal health, neonatology and perinatology. 2017;3:6.

28

Association between furosemide in premature infants and sensorineural hearing loss and nephrocalcinosis

Wesley Jackson[1*], Genevieve Taylor[1], David Selewski[2], P. Brian Smith[3], Sue Tolleson-Rinehart[1,4] and Matthew M. Laughon[1]

Abstract

Furosemide is a potent loop diuretic commonly and variably used by neonatologists to improve oxygenation and lung compliance in premature infants. There are several safety concerns with use of furosemide in premature infants, specifically the risk of sensorineural hearing loss (SNHL), and nephrocalcinosis/nephrolithiasis (NC/NL). We conducted a systematic review of all trials and observational studies examining the association between these outcomes with exposure to furosemide in premature infants.

We searched MEDLINE, EMBASE, CINAHL, and clinicaltrials.gov. We included studies reporting either SNHL or NC/NL in premature infants (< 37 weeks completed gestational age) who received at least one dose of enteral or intravenous furosemide. Thirty-two studies met full inclusion criteria for the review, including 12 studies examining SNHL and 20 studies examining NC/NL. Only one randomized controlled trial was identified in this review. We found no evidence that furosemide exposure increases the risk of SNHL or NC/NL in premature infants, with varying quality of studies and found the strength of evidence for both outcomes to be low. The most common limitation in these studies was the lack of control for confounding factors.

The evidence for the risk of SNHL and NC/NL in premature infants exposed to furosemide is low. Further randomized controlled trials of furosemide in premature infants are urgently needed to adequately assess the risk of SNHL and NC/NL, provide evidence for improved FDA labeling, and promote safer prescribing practices.

Keywords: Furosemide, Infant, Premature, Sensorineural hearing loss, Nephrocalcinosis, Nephrolithiasis

Background

Furosemide is a potent diuretic that acts in the proximal and distal tubules, as well as the loop of Henle, to inhibit sodium and chloride reabsorption in the kidneys. The use of diuretics such as furosemide may alleviate symptoms associated with volume overload, including pulmonary edema. In premature infants, early pulmonary edema and excessive intravenous fluid administration are associated with an increased risk of bronchopulmonary dysplasia (BPD), also called chronic lung disease of prematurity [1, 2]. Therefore, furosemide may be part of a clinical approach to reducing the risk of BPD in premature infants.

The Food and Drug Administration (FDA) has approved furosemide for the treatment of edema associated with congestive heart failure, cirrhosis, and nephrotic syndrome in children and adults. Furosemide is not approved by the FDA for use in premature infants and, as a result, any use in this population is considered off-label. Specifically, the FDA label for furosemide includes a warning that infants < 31 weeks postmenstrual age receiving doses > 1 mg/kg/day intravenously may develop plasma levels resulting in ototoxicity. The label also notes that renal function monitoring and renal sonography should be considered in premature infants, as furosemide may precipitate nephrocalcinosis.

* Correspondence: wesley.jackson@unchealth.unc.edu
[1]Division of Pediatrics, University of North Carolina at Chapel Hill, UNC Hospitals 101 Manning Dr. 4th Floor, Chapel Hill, NC CB 7596, USA
Full list of author information is available at the end of the article

The primary safety concern of furosemide use in premature infants is sensorineural hearing loss (SNHL). The incidence of SNHL is approximately 0.7–1.5% among infants admitted to the NICU and is more common in infants born prematurely [3, 4]. The association of SNHL and furosemide relies heavily on studies conducted in adults receiving high doses of furosemide. In one study, reversible hearing loss occurred in 50% of adult patients with uremia given a single 1000 mg intravenous dose of furosemide, which is 50 times the usual adult dose [5]. A case series reported transient deafness in 3 adult patients with renal impairment given intravenous doses of 2000–3000 mg [6]. Finally, a trial of 19 adult patients receiving furosemide or placebo resulted in one patient with permanent deafness who had received 14 days of 1000 mg per day. The authors of the trial reported that furosemide levels > 100 μg/mL were associated with ototoxicity [7]. The proposed mechanisms for furosemide-induced ototoxicity include changes in potassium concentrations in the cochlear endolymph and impairment of cellular proliferation [8, 9].

Furosemide use in premature infants has also been implicated in the development of nephrocalcinosis and nephrolithiasis, or renal calcifications and stones, although the etiology in this population is likely to be multifactorial [10, 11]. Nephrocalcinosis is diagnosed by renal ultrasonography and has the appearance of increased echogenicity in the medullary pyramids of the kidney. Renal calculi, or nephrolithiasis, are detected on ultrasound by echogenic foci in the calyces or renal pelvis. Loop diuretics, such as furosemide, reduce renal tubular reabsorption of calcium resulting in hypercalciuria, which is the proposed mechanism for its association with nephrocalcinosis. However, this association is often confounded by concomitant exposure to other therapies, such as dexamethasone, long-term parenteral nutrition, and mechanical ventilation, which have been identified as risk factors for renal calcifications [12, 13].

In the absence of robust data from large, well-powered clinical trials, the best available method for evaluating the safety of furosemide in premature infants includes a thorough review of the limited number of randomized control trials, as well as non-controlled studies such as cohort and case-control studies. This systematic review will synthesize all trials and observational studies in which premature infants were exposed to at least one dose of furosemide and report on the following outcomes: SNHL and nephrocalcinosis/nephrolithiasis (NC/NL). This review differs from Cochrane reviews in its inclusion of observational studies, which comprise the majority of available evidence for furosemide safety in premature infants. The key questions this systematic review will address are the following:

Key Question 1: Does exposure to furosemide in premature infants increase the risk of SNHL?
Key Question 2: Does exposure to furosemide in premature infants increase the risk of NC/NL?

Methods

We reviewed all observational cohort studies or clinical trials in which premature infants (< 37 weeks completed gestational age) were exposed to at least one dose of furosemide while hospitalized in the NICU. We used premature infants without exposure to furosemide, when available, as comparators. The outcomes of interest were SNHL and NC/NL. Table 1 displays the eligibility criteria for this systematic review.

We searched the following databases for the relevant literature published in English: MEDLINE, EMBASE, and CINAHL. We also searched clinicaltrials.gov to include results of unpublished studies. The references of relevant articles within this search were reviewed by the investigators for additional articles of interest. The date of the most recent search was February 3, 2018. The MEDLINE search used the following Medical Subject Heading terms: "furosemide" AND "infant, premature." The final search included the following string of search terms: "furosemide"[MeSH Terms] OR "furosemide"[All Fields] AND "infant, premature"[MeSH Terms] OR ("infant"[All Fields] AND "premature"[All Fields]) OR "premature infant"[All Fields] OR "preterm"[All Fields] AND "infant"[All Fields] OR "preterm infant"[All Fields] OR "neonate"[All Fields]. The EMBASE and CINAHL searches used the following terms: ('premature infant'/exp. OR 'premature infant' OR (('premature'/exp. OR premature) AND ('infant'/exp. OR infant))) AND ('furosemide'/ exp. OR furosemide). The clinicaltrials.gov search used the terms "premature infant" and "furosemide."

We compiled all studies resulting from the preceding search strategy and removed duplicates. Two authors (WJ and GT) reviewed titles and abstracts for relevance using the software program Abstrackr [14]. We screened

Table 1 Eligibility Criteria

Patient/Population	Infant < 37 weeks completed gestational age
Intervention	≥1 dose of furosemide (IV or PO) during hospitalization in the neonatal intensive care unit
Control	Infant < 37 weeks completed gestational age without exposure to furosemide
Outcomes	sensorineural hearing loss; nephrocalcinosis/nephrolithiasis
Study Design	clinical trials, retrospective or prospective cohort studies, case-control studies

full text articles and developed data abstraction forms to determine eligibility of each study. If eligibility criteria were met, we recorded the study design, population characteristics, characteristics of comparison group, outcomes examined, sample size, duration of follow-up, and funding sources. These data abstraction forms were used by the investigators to report on the results (Additional file 1).

We assessed the quality (internal validity) of randomized controlled trials using the Cochrane Collaboration's tool for assessing risk of bias in clinical trials [15]. This tool includes the assessment of randomization procedures, allocation concealment, blinding of participants and investigators, completeness of outcomes data, selective reporting, and the risk of other biases. Each randomized controlled trial included in the systematic review was graded on each of these parameters as high risk of bias, low risk of bias, or unclear risk of bias. We assessed the risk of bias in non-randomized studies using the ROBINS-1 tool, which assesses confounding biases, bias in the selection of participants, classification biases, biases due to deviations from intended interventions, missing data biases, and biases in measurement of outcomes [16]. Bias is rated on a scale of low, moderate, serious, or critical risk of bias, or no information. We then graded the strength of the evidence for each key question using guidance from the Evidence-based Practice Center program of the U.S. Agency for Healthcare Research and Quality [17].

The pre-specified outcome measures were odds ratios and risk ratios, where appropriate, with 95% confidence intervals for the exposure of furosemide in premature infants with each of the outcomes of interest addressed in the key questions. Results of each study were described and only the information pertaining to the outcomes of interest in the key questions were included.

Results

We identified 260 records through MEDLINE, 620 records through EMBASE, 51 records from CINAHL, and 1 study from clinicaltrials.gov. After removing duplicates, we screened 390 records for eligibility. We excluded 224 records due to study design, non-human population, or non-English language. We reviewed the full text of the remaining 166 articles and excluded 139 articles for inappropriate study population or lack of relevant safety outcome. We identified 5 articles in the reference lists of reviewed articles which met the eligibility criteria. These studies did not appear in the original search due to the use of a variation in the drug name: "frusemide", instead of "furosemide." In total, 32 articles were included in the quantitative analysis. See Fig. 1 for the PRISMA flow diagram.

Key question 1: Does exposure to furosemide in premature infants increase the risk of sensorineural hearing loss?

Only one randomized controlled trial of furosemide compared to placebo in premature infants reported on the outcome of SNHL [18]. In this trial, 24 premature infants were randomized to receive either furosemide or placebo for 7 days. The initial dose of furosemide (1 mg/kg IV or 2 mg/kg orally every 12 h) was doubled after 48 h in infants where there was not a 50% increase in urine output over 12 h. In the 17 infants available for analysis (7 infants in treatment group and 10 infants in the control group), no SNHL was detected prior to discharge.

We identified 11 observational studies examining the association of furosemide and SNHL in premature infants: 5 retrospective cohort studies and 6 case-control studies [19–29]. The results of the studies were mixed; however, an association between furosemide and SNHL was found in 8 of the 11 observational studies [19–23, 25, 27, 29]. Two cohort studies and one case-control study did not identify an association with furosemide and SNHL [24, 26, 28]. These negative studies were conducted in single centers and did not consider dose exposure of furosemide.

Table 2 summarizes the population characteristics, sample size, outcome measures, and results from each study. The studies varied considerably in their definitions of SNHL, including the type of auditory testing used and length of follow-up. However, every study included a hearing screen in all infants prior to NICU discharge and every infant classified as having SNHL failed the initial newborn hearing screen. Auditory testing in these studies included either auditory brain stem response (ABR) [19, 20, 22, 28], brainstem auditory evoked response (BAER) [21], otoacoustic emission (OAE) test [23], behavioral audiometry in older children, or some combination of these tests [24–27, 29]. Several studies differentiated auditory neuropathy or auditory neuropathy spectrum disorders, in which there is a defect in the transmission of sound from the inner hair cells of the cochlea to the brain via the auditory nerve, from the broader category of SNHL [25–27]. Infants with auditory neuropathy have an abnormal ABR with preserved OAE testing, while those with SNHL have abnormal results on both tests.

Although a majority of the studies did not consider dosing, three studies described the dose and duration of furosemide and its association with SNHL and each of these studies found a positive association between furosemide and SNHL [20, 22, 27]. One found higher cumulative dose exposure of furosemide in infants with hearing loss than was true in infants without hearing loss (mean +/− standard deviation: 139.1 +/− 130 mg/kg vs. 41.5 +/− 76 mg/kg; $p < 0.001$), in addition to longer duration of furosemide use in the hearing loss group (52.5 +/− 43 days vs. 19 +/− 23 days; $p < 0.001$) [20]. In another study, investigators described higher maximum daily dose of furosemide (3.2 +/− 0.58 mg/kg vs. 2.45 +/− 0.79 mg/kg; $p = 0.05$), longer duration of treatment (17 +/− 8.3 days vs. 3.4 +/− 2.1 days; $p < 0.001$), and higher cumulative dose exposures (26.9 +/− 13.7 mg/kg vs. 6.17 +/− 4 mg/kg; p < 0.001) in infants with SNHL than in infants with normal hearing [22]. A third study reported a longer duration of furosemide treatment in infants with SNHL compared to those with normal hearing (17.5 +/− 10 days vs. 7 +/− 4.9 days; $p = 0.002$) [27].

Quality assessment

We assessed the quality of each study based on the risk of bias in the seven domains of the ROBINS-I tool for non-randomized studies (Table 3). The risk of bias in the McCann study is included in Table 4 using the Cochrane Risk of Bias Tool. The primary determining factor for the assessment of moderate or serious risk of bias was whether an appropriate analysis method was used that controlled for important perinatal factors, such as severity of illness, duration of hospitalization, birth weight, gestational age, and co-morbidities known to be risk factors for hearing loss. We considered two studies to have a critical risk of bias due to grouping furosemide exposure with other medications as a single variable termed "ototoxins" [19, 29]. There was no pattern relating quality to the results of the studies (i.e., both positive and negative studies included a mix of moderate and serious risks of bias).

Strength of evidence

We determined that the strength of evidence for the association of SNHL and furosemide exposure in premature infants is low based on our review of the existing

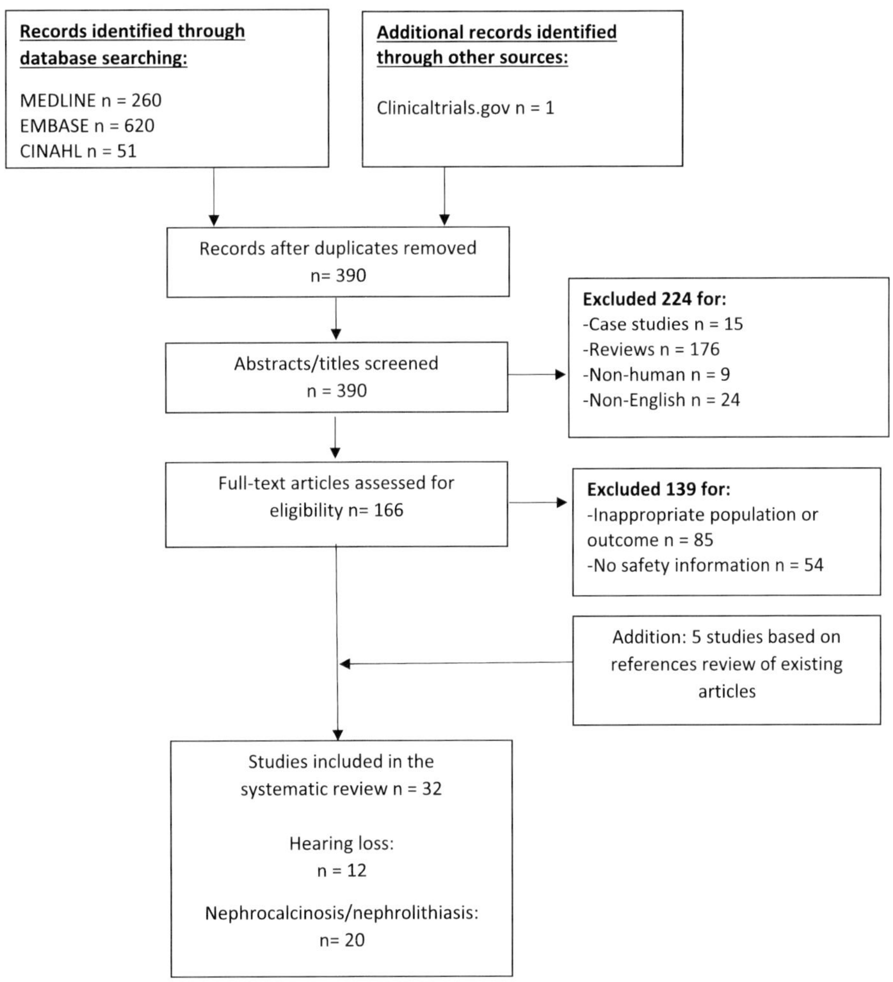

Fig. 1 PRISMA flow diagram for inclusion and exclusion of studies [71]

Table 2 Summary of studies examining risk of hearing loss in premature infants

Study (Year)	Design	Population and Sample Size	Outcome Measure	Results
Mjoen (1982) [19]	cohort	60 high-risk infants 27–44 weeks GA	ABR testing in NICU and follow-up visits	• 4 infants with evidence of SNHL. • 3/4 infants exposed to ototoxic medications (furosemide and/or aminoglycoside).
McCann (1985) [18]	randomized controlled	17 premature infants with BPD (7 infants received furosemide and 10 infants received placebo)	Audiology screen at discharge and follow-up visits	• Normal hearing in all infants.
Salamy (1989) [20]	cohort	GA 24–34 weeks	ABR in NICU and follow-up; behavioral audiometry from 3 months to 4 years	• Infants with SNHL received greater amounts of furosemide for longer durations, in combination with aminoglycoside or vancomycin therapy ($p < 0.001$ for all factors).
Brown (1991) [21]	case-control	35 infants with SNHL and 70 matched hearing-intact controls	BAER testing prior to discharge from NICU	• 17/35 (49%) infants with SNHL and 6/70 (9%) controls were exposed to furosemide ($p < 0.0001$).
Borradori (1997) [22]	case-control	8 children with progressive bilateral deafness born preterm (GA ≤ 34 weeks) with 16 controls matched on GA and BW and 15 controls matched on perinatal complications	ABR at NICU discharge and follow-up	• 8/8 (100%) infants with SNHL and 13/15 (87%) controls received furosemide (NS). • Mean duration ($p < 0.001$), total cumulative dose ($p < 0.001$), and maximum daily dose ($p = 0.05$) were higher in SNHL group.
Ertl (2001) [23]	case-control	22 premature infants with SNHL and 25 controls matched on GA, BW, and perinatal factors associated with hearing loss	OAE test and ABR if failed OAE	• 4/22 (18%) infants with SNHL and 1/25 (4%) controls received furosemide ($p < 0.01$).
Rais-Bahrami (2004) [24]	cohort	57 infants who received furosemide and 207 infants who did not receive furosemide	OAE, ABR, or both prior to NICU discharge	• No difference in abnormal hearing screen in furosemide and non-furosemide groups (16% vs. 16%; $p = 0.95$).
Xoinis (2007) [25]	case-control	71 infants with SNHL, 24 with auditory neuropathy,and 95 controls matched on GA, BW, and birth year	ABR and OAE	• Higher exposure to furosemide in SNHL group (51%) and AN group (96%) compared to control group (32.6%) ($p < 0.05$) for both comparisons.
Coenraad (2011) [26]	case-control	9 infants with hearing loss and 36 controls matched on GA, gender, and birth year	ABR screening prior to NICU discharge and repeat ABR and OAE at follow-up visit for failed screening.	• No differences in furosemide exposure between groups (44% vs. 25%; $p = 0.56$).
Martinez-Cruz (2012) [27]	case-control	6 children with SNHL and 87 normal-hearing controls with birth weights < 750 g	BAER screening and OAE at follow-up visits for failed initial screening	• 6/6 (100%) infants with SNHL and 45/87 (52%) control infants received furosemide ($p = 0.002$). • Longer average duration of furosemide in SNHL infants who received furosemide compared with controls (18 days vs. 7 days).
Rastogi (2013) [28]	cohort	Infants with BW < 1500 g.	ABR prior to NICU discharge; Follow-up at 2 years for failed screening to determine hearing status	• No association with furosemide and hearing loss when adjusting for BW, GA, and other perinatal risk factors (OR 1.18; $p = 0.3$).
Wang (2017) [29]	cohort	Included all infants with BW ≤ 1500 g. 297 infants with normal hearing and 12 infants with hearing loss	OAE before discharge and BAER at 3 months corrected age if failed initial screen	• Exposure to ototoxins (furosemide and/or gentamicin) was associated with hearing loss (OR 3.62; 95% CI 1.67–7.82).

Legend: *GA* Gestational Age, *ABR* Auditory brainstem response, *BPD* Bronchopulmonary dysplasia, *SNHL* Sensorineural hearing loss, *BAER* Brainstem auditory evoked response, *NICU* Neonatal Intensive Care Unit, *BW* Birthweight, *NS* Non-significant, *OAE* Otoacoustic emission, *AN* Auditory neuropathy, *ANSD* Auditory neuropathy spectrum disorder, *OR* Odds ratio, *CI* Confidence Interval

Table 3 Quality assessment of observational studies examining risk of hearing loss in premature infants

Study (Year)	Risk of Bias (Low, Moderate, Serious, Critical, No Information)	Comments
Mjoen (1982) [19]	Critical	Critical risk of bias in classification of interventions domain: ototoxic medications grouped as one variable (i.e., furosemide not identified as a single risk factor).
Salamy (1989) [20]	Moderate	Confounding well-accounted for by assessing "neonatal status" based on duration of hospitalization, days of assisted ventilation, radiography and lab results, etc.
Brown (1991) [21]	Serious	Serious risk of bias in confounding domain: Selection of variables included in the multivariate analyses based solely on results of univariate analyses and did not adequately account for severity of illness in each group.
Borradori (1997) [22]	Moderate	Confounding well-accounted for by the creation of two control groups based on BW/GA and perinatal complications related to risk of ototoxicity.
Ertl (2001) [23]	Serious	Serious risk of bias in confounding domain: infants not matched on severity of illness or co-morbidities associated with hearing loss.
Rais-Bahrami (2004) [24]	Serious	Serious risk of bias in confounding domain: no adjustment for perinatal factors related to hearing loss.
Xoinis (2007) [25]	Serious	Serious risk of bias in confounding domain: infants not matched on severity of illness or co-morbidities associated with hearing loss.
Coenraad (2011) [26]	Serious	Serious risk of bias in confounding domain: infants not matched on severity of illness or co-morbidities associated with hearing loss.
Martinez-Cruz (2012) [27]	Serious	Serious risk of bias in confounding domain: infants not matched on severity of illness or co-morbidities associated with hearing loss.
Rastogi (2013) [28]	Moderate	Confounding well-accounted for in multivariate analyses, which adjusted for GA, BW, and other known perinatal risk factors for hearing loss.
Wang (2017) [29]	Critical	Critical risk of bias in classification of interventions domain: ototoxic medications grouped as one variable (i.e., furosemide not identified as a single risk factor).

Legend: *BW* Birth weight, *GA* Gestational age

literature. This judgement is based on the high risk of bias in the observational studies, which often did not adequately account for the severity of illness in infants exposed to furosemide, and the inconsistency in the results. Furthermore, there is a problem with the directness of comparisons as infants exposed to furosemide are also more likely to receive additional interventions which may increase the risk of SNHL, such as concomitant ototoxic medications and mechanical ventilation. According to the Agency for Healthcare Research and Quality (AHRQ), a low grade indicates "low confidence that the evidence reflects the true effect [and] further research is likely to change the confidence in the estimate of effect and is likely to change the estimate" [17]. It is clear that further clinical trials are needed to adequately assess the risk of SNHL in premature infants exposed to furosemide.

Key question 2: Does exposure to furosemide in premature infants increase the risk of nephrocalcinosis/nephrolithiasis?

No randomized controlled trials of furosemide in premature infants have been performed that include outcome data on the incidence of NC/NL. We identified 20 cohort studies examining the association of furosemide exposure and NC/NL [30–49]. The results of the studies were mixed; however, 12 of the 20 studies found an association between furosemide and NC/NL [30–32, 34–37, 40, 41, 44, 46, 47, 49]. All studies were performed at single centers, except one, which included infants from two centers [40]. Three of the studies resembled case series in that there was no inclusion of adequate control groups without NC: one of these studies found an association of furosemide with NC and two studies did not [30, 38, 42].

Table 4 Risk of bias in trials examining risk of hearing loss in premature infants

Study (Year)	Risk of Bias (High, Low, Unclear)						
	Random Sequence Generation	Allocation Concealment	Blinding of Participants and Personnel	Blinding of Outcome Assessment	Incomplete Outcome Data	Selective Reporting	Other Bias
McCann (1985) [18]	Low	Low	Low	Low	High	Unclear	Low

Table 5 summarizes the population characteristics, sample size, outcome measures, and results from each study. There was considerable variability in the inclusion criteria, the timing of renal ultrasonography, and duration of long-term follow-up. However, all of the reviewed studies included premature infants with sonographic evidence of NC/NL prior to discharge from the NICU. Of the studies that included subsequent ultrasounds after NICU discharge, complete resolution of NC occurred in 44–100% of infants by 2 years of age [31, 33, 35, 36, 38, 39, 42, 46–49]. However, these data on outcomes are incomplete, as they do not include infants with the most severe disease, who expired during their NICU hospitalization, and infants lost to follow-up after discharge.

A dose-response relationship between furosemide and NC/NL was evaluated in 8 studies [33, 34, 38, 39, 41, 42, 44, 46]. Half of these studies found no association between dose and the development of NC/NL. Two studies found no difference in average daily dose or duration of furosemide between infants with NC and infants without NC [33, 34]. Investigators reported no difference in cumulative dose or duration of treatment between infants with resolution of NC compared to those with persistent findings of NC [38]. An additional study found no difference in median total dose of furosemide before detection of NC and in those infants without NC in another study [41]. In contrast, one study found that infants with resolution of NC received lower daily dosages of furosemide than did those with persistent NC ($p < 0.05$) and another determined that mean cumulative doses of furosemide were significantly higher in infants with NC than in those without NC (18.8 mg vs 5.0 mg; p: 0.001) [39, 42]. A single center study found higher cumulative doses of furosemide in infants with development of NC than in those without NC (mean +/− standard deviation: 102.2 +/− 118.2 mg vs 32.3 +/− 81.1 mg; $p = 0.001$) [44]. Investigators identified exposure to furosemide with cumulative dose > 10 mg/kg was the strongest independent risk factor for NC in a multivariable analysis of premature infants (OR 48.1 (95% CI 4.0–585); $p < 0.01$) [46].

Quality assessment

We assessed the quality of each study based on the risk of bias in the seven domains of the ROBINS-I tool for non-randomized studies (Table 6). We determined that one study had a critical risk of bias and resembled a case series in its lack of the use of a control group [30]. The most common reason we considered a study to have a serious risk of bias was the absence of adjustment for severity of illness. Three studies used multivariable analysis to control for the high correlation of cumulative furosemide exposure with birthweight, duration of mechanical ventilation, and severity of BPD, all variables that are independently associated with the development of NC/NL [34, 41, 46]. One study found that furosemide exposure was the strongest independent risk factor for NC, despite controlling for multiple markers of illness severity. However, two studies that considered the temporal relationship between furosemide and NC found no difference in mean dose of furosemide before detection of NC on renal ultrasound in infants who did or did not subsequently develop NC [34, 41]. There was no pattern relating quality to the results of the studies (i.e., both positive and negative studies included a mix of moderate and serious risks of bias).

Strength of evidence

We determined that the strength of evidence for the association of NC/NL and furosemide exposure in premature infants is low based on our review of the existing literature. No clinical trials of furosemide have examined the outcome of NC/NL. There is a high risk of bias in the numerous observational studies reviewed as only a few studies accounted for other renal stone-promoting factors, such as concomitant medication use and supplementation of calcium, phosphorus, and vitamin D to reduce the risk of osteopenia of prematurity. The AHRQ classifies evidence as indirect if "it uses intermediate or surrogate outcomes instead of ultimate health outcomes; one body of evidence links the intervention to intermediate outcomes and another body of evidence links the intermediate to most important (health or ultimate) outcomes." (p. 515) The endpoint of NC/NL is likely a surrogate outcome for chronic kidney disease and cardiovascular disease, which were detected in a minority of infants included in the studies. Although clinical trials are needed to determine the relationship of furosemide and NC/NL, adequate long-term follow-up will also be required to determine any lasting effects of NC/NL on renal and cardiovascular health.

Discussion

We found no evidence that furosemide exposure increases the risk of SNHL or NC/NL in premature infants. We determined that the strength of evidence for the association of these outcomes with furosemide exposure is low. With the exception of one randomized controlled trial including SNHL as an outcome, all reviewed studies were cohort or case-control studies. These studies' observational designs left many important potential confounding variables not well-accounted for, such as severity of illness, duration of mechanical ventilation, and concomitant medication exposures. Some of the included cohort studies were of high quality and used multivariable analyses to account for confounding, but randomized controlled trials of furosemide are

Table 5 Summary of studies examining risk of nephrocalcinosis/nephrolithiasis (NC/NL) in premature infants

Study (Year)	Design	Population and Sample Size	Outcome Measure	Results Summary
Hufnagle (1982) [30]	cohort	10 premature infants with NC	RUS during NICU admission	• All infants received furosemide of at least 2 mg/kg/day for at least 12 days prior to NC.
Woolfield (1988) [31]	cohort	36 infants with BW ≤ 1500 g	RUS at 12 months of age	• 3/32 (9%) infants had NC on RUS and had received chronic furosemide with doses ranging from 2 to 8 mg/kg/day. • NC resolved in 2/3 (67%) cases; 1 died of unrelated causes.
Jacinto (1988) [32]	cohort	31 infants with BW < 1500 g	RUS in third week of life and every 3 week thereafter until NICU discharge	• NC was diagnosed in 20/31 (64%) of infants. • Exposure to furosemide was more common in NC group (65% vs 9%; $p < 0.001$).
Ezzedeen (1988) [33]	cohort	17 premature infants with NC treated with furosemide; 3 premature infants treated with furosemide without NC (control group)	RUS during NICU admission	• No difference in average daily dose or duration of furosemide in NC group compared to control group.
Short (1991) [34]	cohort	79 infants with GA < 32 weeks	Serial RUS	• 21/79 (27%) of infants diagnosed with NC. • No difference in mean total dose of furosemide.
Downing (1991) [35]	cohort	117 infants with BW < 1750 g and BPD treated with furosemide	RUS prior to discharge and in 3–6 month intervals for positive findings of NC/NL	• 20/117 (17%) had evidence of NC/NL on RUS prior to discharge. • Infants maintained on furosemide were more likely to have persistent NC/NL compared to those for whom furosemide was stopped ($p < 0.001$).
Downing (1992) [36]	cohort	27 infants with BW < 1500 g enrolled into 3 groups: 1) not exposed to furosemide ($n = 7$); 2) received furosemide without NC ($n = 10$); and 3) received furosemide with NC ($n = 10$)	RUS and laboratory testing for glomerular and tubular kidney function	• Infants in group 3 had lower creatinine clearance (reduced glomerular function) and higher tubular dysfunction compared to infants in group 1 and 2.
Stafstrom (1992) [37]	cohort	11 premature infants with post-hemorrhagic hydrocephalus treated with furosemide and acetazolamide	Serial RUS	• 5/11 (45%) infants with evidence of NC. • No correlation between duration of treatment, total dosage of medications, and development of renal calculi.
Pope (1996) [38]	cohort	13 premature infants with NC and exposed to furosemide divided into 2 groups: resolution of NC ($n = 6$) and persistent NC ($n = 7$).	Serial RUS	• No difference in duration of or cumulative dose of furosemide in infants with resolution of NC compared to those with persistence of NC.
Saarela (1999) [39]	cohort	129 infants with BW < 1500 g	RUS at 2 weeks, 6 weeks, and 3 months of life	• 26/129 (20%) of infants diagnosed with NC. • The mean cumulative doses of furosemide were significantly higher in infants with NC compared to those without NC (19 mg vs 5 mg; $p < 0.001$).
Schell-Feith (2000) [40]	cohort	215 infants with GA < 32 weeks	RUS at 4 weeks of life and at term	• NC diagnosed in 50/150 (33%) of infants at 4 weeks of life and 83/201 (41%) at term (NS). • At term, furosemide exposure was higher in those with NC (32%) compared to those without NC (18%) ($p < 0.001$).
Narendra (2001) [41]	cohort	101 infants with GA < 32 weeks or BW < 1500 g	RUS at 1 month of age and at term or NICU discharge	• 16/101 (16%) diagnosed with NC. • The median total dose of furosemide was not significantly different before detection of NC on term RUS and in infants without NC ($p = 0.75$).
Hoppe (2002) [42]	cohort	16 infants with GA < 37 weeks and diagnosed with NC	RUS during NICU admission and every 3–6 months following discharge	• NC persisted in 4/12 (33%) infants who received follow-up. • Infants with resolution of NC received lower dosages of furosemide compared to those with persistent NC ($p < 0.05$).

Table 5 Summary of studies examining risk of nephrocalcinosis/nephrolithiasis (NC/NL) in premature infants *(Continued)*

Study (Year)	Design	Population and Sample Size	Outcome Measure	Results Summary
Hein (2004) [43]	cohort	114 infants with BW < 1500 g divided into 2 groups: 1) NC (*n* = 20); 2) without NC (*n* = 94). 20 infants from control group matched to NC group based on BW and GA.	RUS every 2 weeks during NICU admission	• No difference in duration of furosemide therapy between groups.
Ketkeaw (2004) [44]	cohort	36 infants with GA < 32 weeks and BW < 1250 g	RUS prior to NICU discharge	• 14/36 (39%) were diagnosed with NC. • The mean cumulative dose and mean duration of furosemide was higher in infants with NC compared to those without NC (102 mg vs 32 mg; *p* = 0.001 and 39 vs 7 days; p = 0.001).
Cranefield (2004) [45]	cohort	Cohort of infants enrolled in randomized trial of two regimens of dexamethasone for the prevention of BPD.	RUS on study entry, day of life 28, and at discharge or 36 weeks postmenstrual age	• 15/18 (83%) of infants for whom complete data were available were diagnosed with NC prior to discharge or 36 weeks postmenstrual age. • Furosemide was used infrequently in the trial. 7/8 (88%) of the infants who never received furosemide developed NC.
Gimpel (2010) [46]	cohort	55 infants with GA < 32 weeks and BW < 1500 g	RUS obtained after the first month of life	• 15/55 (27%) of infants were diagnosed with NC. • The strongest independent risk factor for NC was furosemide therapy with cumulative dose > 10 mg/kg (OR 48.1 (95% CI 4.0–585); *p* < 0.01).
Chang (2011) [47]	cohort	102 infants with GA < 34 weeks and BW < 1500 g	RUS at term or prior to NICU discharge	• 6/102 (6%) of infants were diagnosed with NC. • Exposure to furosemide was more common in the NC group compared to the group without NC (33% vs 3%; *p* = 0.027).
Lee (2014) [48]	cohort	52 infants with BW < 1500 g	RUS at 4 and 8 weeks of life	• Exposure to furosemide did not differ significantly between infants with NC and those without NC.
Mohamed (2014) [49]	cohort	97 infants with GA ≤ 34 weeks	RUS at first week of life, at term, and at one year corrected age	• Exposure to furosemide was more common in the NC group compared to the group without NC (50% vs 16%; *p* = 0.003).

Legend: *BW* Birth weight, *GA* Gestational age, *OR* Odds ratio, *CI* Confidence interval, *BPD* Bronchopulmonary dysplasia

urgently needed to assess the risks of SNHL and NC/NL in premature infants.

Despite the proposed benefits and biological plausibility of using furosemide to improve respiratory outcomes, the efficacy of furosemide in premature infants has not been established. A Cochrane systematic review examining loop diuretics for preterm infants found no evidence to support an improvement in long-term outcomes, including BPD [50]. However, results from the review indicated that chronic administration of furosemide (i.e., at least 7 days) improves oxygenation and lung compliance in premature infants with established BPD. The review emphasizes the need for randomized clinical trials to assess the effects of furosemide administration on morbidity and mortality.

Notwithstanding the absence of data supporting the efficacy of furosemide, the medication is commonly used by clinicians in the neonatal intensive care unit (NICU) with the intention to improve oxygenation and wean respiratory support in premature infants. A cohort study from more than 300 NICUs in the U.S. found that furosemide was the fifth most common drug used between the years 2005 to 2010 in premature infants with birth weights < 1000 g, with approximately 50% of these infants exposed to at least one dose of furosemide during their initial hospitalization [51]. Although other diuretic medications are used in the NICU for similar indications, furosemide is by far the most commonly used diuretic in the NICU, accounting for 93% of diuretic use [52]. Furosemide is also variably used in the NICU setting. A cohort study of infants with birth weights < 1500 g from more than 200 U.S. NICUs over a 15 year period found considerable variability in the percentage of infants exposed to at least one dose of furosemide at each particular site, with a median exposure by site of 33% and a range of 0 to 75%. The observations from this study emphasize the lack of a universally accepted standard governing when to expose an infant in the NICU to furosemide and indicate that at some centers, no exposure to furosemide is an option [52].

Additional potential adverse outcomes of furosemide use in premature infants include metabolic bone disease (osteopenia) of prematurity and electrolyte abnormalities related to urinary loss of sodium, chloride, and calcium [53–55]. As with other adverse outcomes, the etiology of metabolic bone disease in premature infants likely has many causes, and infants with severe illness often have multiple risk factors such as insufficient phosphorus intake, vitamin D deficiency, prolonged immobilization, mechanical ventilation, and exposure to steroids and antibiotics [56–58]. However, there is a lack of consensus on the definition of metabolic bone disease of prematurity, with some definitions relying on serum mineral levels and others based on radiographical findings [59]. As a result, this review did not focus on metabolic bone disease of prematurity as an outcome of interest in premature infants exposed to furosemide.

Existing safety data on the use of furosemide in adults and children cannot be extrapolated to premature infants due to higher extracellular fluid volume per unit body weight, immature hepatic and renal function, and a more permeable blood-brain barrier in premature infants, variables which can alter the rates of drug absorption, distribution, metabolism, and elimination [60]. Four studies of furosemide pharmacokinetics in premature infants demonstrate significant variability in the volume of distribution, clearance, and half-life of the drug based on gestational age at birth, birth weight, and

Table 6 Quality assessment of observational studies examining risk of nephrocalcinosis/nephrolithiasis (NC/NL) in premature infants

Study (Year)	Risk of Bias (Low, Moderate, Serious, Critical, No Information)	Comments
Hufnagle (1982) [30]	Critical	Critical risk of bias in confounding domain: no statistical tests performed in the analysis to test association of NC and furosemide. Critical risk of bias in selection of participants into the study: All infants were exposed to furosemide and had NC; lack of control group.
Woolfield (1988) [31]	Serious	Serious risk of bias in confounding domain: no statistical tests performed in the analysis to test association of NC and furosemide.
Jacinto (1988) [32]	Serious	Serious risk of bias in confounding domain: Lower BW and GA associated with outcome (NC), along with exposure to furosemide. Did not control for severity of illness.
Ezzedeen (1988) [33]	Serious	Serious risk of bias in confounding domain: no adjustment for severity of illness; small number of infants in control group.
Short (1991) [34]	Moderate	Multivariate analyses controlling for other risk factors for NC. Dose-response relationship evaluated.
Downing (1991) [35]	Moderate	All infants screened for the outcome had a diagnosis of chronic lung disease; high percentage of follow-up imaging obtained.
Downing (1992) [36]	Moderate	Robust comparators; long-term follow-up.
Stafstrom (1992) [37]	Serious	Serious risk of bias in confounding domain: no statistical tests performed in the analysis to test association of NC and furosemide. No reporting of frequency of NC in infants with post-hemorrhagic hydrocephalus not exposed to furosemide.
Pope (1996) [38]	Moderate	Similar severity of illness in each group; long-term follow up with serial ultrasounds. Dose-response relationship evaluated.
Saarela (1999) [39]	Moderate	Dose-response relationship evaluated.
Schell-Feith (2000) [40]	Moderate	Large sample size. Control group without NC included.
Narendra (2001) [41]	Moderate	Multivariate analyses controlling for other risk factors for NC. Dose-response relationship evaluated.
Hoppe (2002) [42]	Serious	Serious risk of bias in confounding domain: Lack of control group without NC.
Hein (2004) [43]	Moderate	Large sample size with appropriate control groups.
Ketkeaw (2004) [44]	Moderate	Appropriate control group included. Dose-response relationship evaluated.
Cranefield (2004) [45]	Moderate	All infants with comparable severity of illness.
Gimpel (2010) [46]	Moderate	Multivariate analyses controlling for other risk factors for NC. Dose-response relationship evaluated.
Chang (2011) [47]	Serious	Serious risk of bias in confounding domain: no adjustment for severity of illness. Low incidence of NC in sample.
Lee (2014) [48]	Serious	Serious risk of bias in confounding domain: no adjustment for severity of illness.
Mohamed (2014) [49]	Serious	Serious risk of bias in confounding domain: no adjustment for severity of illness.

Legend: *BW* Birth weight, *GA* Gestational age

postnatal age [61–64]. The limited available data on pharmacokinetics and safety have led to a growing recognition of the need for clinical trials in premature infants to determine the safety and efficacy of therapeutic agents, such as furosemide [65, 66].

A phase II clinical trial by the Pediatric Trials Network is underway to better understand the safety of furosemide in premature infants at risk of BPD [67]. This trial will enroll premature infants born < 29 weeks' gestation and receiving positive airway pressure or mechanical ventilation on 7–28 days postnatal age. The study design includes a dose escalation schedule with three cohorts randomized to placebo or furosemide. Primary outcomes will include safety information on SNHL (based on BAER prior to discharge) and NC/NL determined by serial renal ultrasounds. Secondary outcomes will assess effectiveness of early furosemide in the prevention of BPD or death. The dose escalation design of the study will allow for evaluation of a dose-response relationship of furosemide and the outcomes of SNHL and NC.

Premature infants, particularly those born small for gestational age, are at an increased risk for cardiovascular and renal disease in later life, likely due to a combination of genetic and environmental factors [68]. It is important to understand whether furosemide exposure, with or without evidence of NC/NL, contributes to the development of chronic kidney disease in these infants. Future studies investigating the safety of furosemide in premature infants will need to consider long-term surveillance of renal disease, particularly in those who develop NC/NL. The study design of trials investigating furosemide in the neonatal population should incorporate serial renal sonography, blood pressure measurements, urinalysis for proteinuria, and serum creatinine, where appropriate, to determine renal function over time.

This systematic review was limited by the inclusion of only one randomized controlled trial. The remaining studies were cohort and case-control studies, which by the nature of their study design are unable to demonstrate a causal role. While many randomized controlled trials of furosemide in premature infants have been performed, very few included data on safety outcomes, which were the subject of this review. In addition, the search strategy was limited to studies published in English may not have included all available studies; for instance, we found that some studies included from our review of reference lists used variable spellings of "furosemide." The field of neonatology has changed dramatically over the past 20 years with the introduction of antenatal steroids, surfactant replacement therapy, and non-invasive ventilation strategies. These practices have resulted in significantly improved survival and reduced morbidities in premature infants [69, 70]. Therefore, results from studies included in this review which were performed decades ago may not be applicable to infants born in the current era. Finally, we were unable to perform a meta-analysis of the included observational studies due to a lack of uniformity in outcome definitions, population characteristics, and length of follow-up.

Conclusions

This systematic review of the safety of furosemide in premature infants focuses on the outcomes of SNHL and NC/NL. Irrespective of the efficacy of furosemide in premature infants, the existing literature on safety outcomes depends almost entirely on observational data. Furthermore, few studies used analytic approaches to control for confounding causes of additional risk of SNHL and NC/NL on premature infants exposed to furosemide. The strength of evidence for the association of SNHL and NC/NL and furosemide is therefore determined to be low. Further randomized controlled trials with robust safety measures, such as the ongoing PTN trial, are urgently needed to assess the safety of furosemide in premature infants.

Abbreviations

ABR: Auditory brain stem response; AHRQ: Agency for Healthcare Research and Quality; BAER: Brainstem auditory evoked response; BPD: Bronchopulmonary dysplasia; FDA: Food and Drug Administration; NC: Nephrocalcinosis; NICU: Neonatal intensive care unit; NL: Nephrolithiasis; OAE: Otoacoustic emission test; PTN: Pediatric Trials Network; SNHL: Sensorineural hearing loss

Acknowledgements

Not applicable.

Funding

No external funding was obtained for this study.

Authors' contributions

WJ and GT conducted the review, DS, PBS, STR and MML were major contributors in development of manuscript. All authors read and approved the final manuscript.

Competing interests

The authors declare that they have no competing interests.

Author details

[1]Division of Pediatrics, University of North Carolina at Chapel Hill, UNC Hospitals 101 Manning Dr. 4th Floor, Chapel Hill, NC CB 7596, USA. [2]Division of Nephrology, Department of Pediatrics and Communicable Diseases, C.S. Mott Children's Hospital, University of Michigan, Ann Arbor, MI, USA. [3]Duke Department of Pediatrics, Duke University Medical Center, Durham, NC, USA. [4]Gillings School of Global Public Health, University of North Carolina at Chapel Hill, Chapel Hill, USA.

References

1. Marshall DD, Kotelchuck M, Young TE, Bose CL, Kruyer L, O'Shea TM. Risk factors for chronic lung disease in the surfactant era: a North Carolina population-based study of very low birth weight infants. North Carolina Neonatologists Association. Pediatrics. 1999;104(6):1345–50.
2. Oh W, Poindexter BB, Perritt R, Lemons JA, Bauer CR, Ehrenkranz RA, Stoll BJ, Poole K, Wright LL. Association between fluid intake and weight loss during the first ten days of life and risk of bronchopulmonary dysplasia in extremely low birth weight infants. J Pediatr. 2005;147(6):786–90.
3. Cristobal R, Oghalai JS. Hearing loss in children with very low birth weight: current review of epidemiology and pathophysiology. Arch Dis Child Fetal Neonatal Ed. 2008;93(6):F462–8.
4. Fawke J. Neurological outcomes following preterm birth. Semin Fetal Neonatal Med. 2007;12(5):374–82.
5. Wigand ME, Heidland A. Ototoxic side-effects of high doses of frusemide in patients with uraemia. Postgrad Med J. 1971;47(Suppl):54–6.
6. Schwartz GH, David DS, Riggio RR, Stenzel KH, Rubin AL. Ototoxicity induced by furosemide. N Engl J Med. 1970;282(25):1413–4.
7. Brown CB, Ogg CS, Cameron JS, Bewick M. High dose frusemide in acute reversible intrinsic renal failure. A preliminary communication. Scott Med J. 1974;19(Suppl 1):35–9.
8. Rybak LP. Furosemide ototoxicity: clinical and experimental aspects. Laryngoscope. 1985;95(9 Pt 2 Suppl 38):1–14.
9. Iwamoto LM, Fujiwara N, Nakamura KT, Wada RK. Na-K-2Cl cotransporter inhibition impairs human lung cellular proliferation. Am J Physiol Lung Cell Mol Physiol. 2004;287(3):L510–4.
10. Myracle MR, McGahan JP, Goetzman BW, Adelman RD. Ultrasound diagnosis of renal calcification in infants on chronic furosemide therapy. J Clin Ultrasound. 1986;14(4):281–7.
11. Schell-Feith EA, Kist-van Holthe JE, van der Heijden AJ. Nephrocalcinosis in preterm neonates. Pediatr Nephrol. 2010;25(2):221–30.
12. Campfield T, Braden G. Urinary oxalate excretion by very low birth weight infants receiving parenteral nutrition. Pediatrics. 1989;84(5):860–3.
13. Kamitsuka MD, Peloquin D. Renal calcification after dexamethasone in infants with bronchopulmonary dysplasia. Lancet. 1991;337(8741):626.
14. Abstrackr. http://abstrackr.cebm.brown.edu. Accessed 3 Oct 2018.
15. Higgins JP, Altman DG, Gotzsche PC, Juni P, Moher D, Oxman AD, Savovic J, Schulz KF, Weeks L, Sterne JA. The Cochrane Collaboration's tool for assessing risk of bias in randomised trials. BMJ. 2011;343:d5928.
16. Sterne JA, Hernan MA, Reeves BC, Savovic J, Berkman ND, Viswanathan M, Henry D, Altman DG, Ansari MT, Boutron I, et al. ROBINS-I: a tool for assessing risk of bias in non-randomised studies of interventions. BMJ. 2016;355:i4919.
17. Owens DK, Lohr KN, Atkins D, Treadwell JR, Reston JT, Bass EB, Chang S, Helfand M. AHRQ series paper 5: grading the strength of a body of evidence when comparing medical interventions--agency for healthcare research and quality and the effective health-care program. J Clin Epidemiol. 2010;63(5):513–23.
18. McCann EM, Lewis K, Deming DD, Donovan MJ, Brady JP. Controlled trial of furosemide therapy in infants with chronic lung disease. J Pediatr. 1985; 106(6):957–62.
19. Mjoen S, Langslet A, Tangsrud SE, Sundby A. Auditory brainstem responses (ABR) in high-risk neonates. Acta Paediatr Scand. 1982;71(5):711–5.
20. Salamy A, Eldredge L, Tooley WH. Neonatal status and hearing loss in high-risk infants. J Pediatr. 1989;114(5):847–52.
21. Brown DR, Watchko JF, Sabo D. Neonatal sensorineural hearing loss associated with furosemide: a case-control study. Dev Med Child Neurol. 1991;33(9):816–23.
22. Borradori C, Fawer CL, Buclin T, Calame A. Risk factors of sensorineural hearing loss in preterm infants. Biol Neonate. 1997;71(1):1–10.
23. Ertl T, Hadzsiev K, Vincze O, Pytel J, Szabo I, Sulyok E. Hyponatremia and sensorineural hearing loss in preterm infants. Biol Neonate. 2001;79(2):109–12.
24. Rais-Bahrami K, Majd M, Veszelovszky E, Short BL. Use of furosemide and hearing loss in neonatal intensive care survivors. Am J Perinatol. 2004;21(6): 329–32.
25. Xoinis K, Weirather Y, Mavoori H, Shaha SH, Iwamoto LM. Extremely low birth weight infants are at high risk for auditory neuropathy. J Perinatol. 2007;27(11):718–23.
26. Coenraad S, Goedegebure A, van Goudoever JB, Hoeve LJ. Risk factors for auditory neuropathy spectrum disorder in NICU infants compared to normal-hearing NICU controls. Laryngoscope. 2011;121(4):852–5.
27. Martinez-Cruz CF, Garcia Alonso-Themann P, Poblano A, Ochoa-Lopez JM. Hearing loss, auditory neuropathy, and neurological co-morbidity in children with birthweight <750 g. Arch Med Res. 2012;43(6):457–63.
28. Rastogi S, Mikhael M, Filipov P, Rastogi D. Effects of ventilation on hearing loss in preterm neonates: nasal continuous positive pressure does not increase the risk of hearing loss in ventilated neonates. Int J Pediatr Otorhinolaryngol. 2013;77(3):402–6.
29. Wang CH, Yang CY, Lien R, Chu SM, Hsu JF, Fu RH, Chiang MC. Prevalence and independent risk factors for hearing impairment among very low birth weight infants. Int J Pediatr Otorhinolaryngol. 2017;93:123–7.
30. Hufnagle KG, Khan SN, Penn D, Cacciarelli A, Williams P. Renal calcifications: a complication of long-term furosemide therapy in preterm infants. Pediatrics. 1982;70(3):360–3.
31. Woolfield N, Haslam R, Le Quesne G, Chambers HM, Hogg R, Jureidini K. Ultrasound diagnosis of nephrocalcinosis in preterm infants. Arch Dis Child. 1988;63(1):86–8.
32. Jacinto JS, Modanlou HD, Crade M, Strauss AA, Bosu SK. Renal calcification incidence in very low birth weight infants. Pediatrics. 1988;81(1):31–5.
33. Ezzedeen F, Adelman RD, Ahlfors CE. Renal calcification in preterm infants: pathophysiology and long-term sequelae. J Pediatr. 1988;113(3):532–9.
34. Short A, Cooke RW: The incidence of renal calcification in preterm infants. Arch Dis Child 1991, 66(4 Spec No):412–417.
35. Downing GJ, Egelhoff JC, Daily DK, Alon U. Furosemide-related renal calcifications in the premature infant. A longitudinal ultrasonographic study. Pediatr Radiol. 1991;21(8):563–5.
36. Downing GJ, Egelhoff JC, Daily DK, Thomas MK, Alon U. Kidney function in very low birth weight infants with furosemide-related renal calcifications at ages 1 to 2 years. J Pediatr. 1992;120(4 Pt 1):599–604.
37. Stafstrom CE, Gilmore HE, Kurtin PS. Nephrocalcinosis complicating medical treatment of posthemorrhagic hydrocephalus. Pediatr Neurol. 1992;8(3):179–82.
38. Pope JC, Trusler LA, Klein AM, Walsh WF, Yared A, Brock JW 3rd. The natural history of nephrocalcinosis in premature infants treated with loop diuretics. J Urol. 1996;156(2 Pt 2):709–12.
39. Saarela T, Vaarala A, Lanning P, Koivisto M. Incidence, ultrasonic patterns and resolution of nephrocalcinosis in very low birthweight infants. Acta Paediatr. 1999;88(6):655–60.
40. Schell-Feith EA, Kist-van Holthe JE, Conneman N, van Zwieten PH, Holscher HC, Zonderland HM, Brand R, van der Heijden BJ. Etiology of nephrocalcinosis in preterm neonates: association of nutritional intake and urinary parameters. Kidney Int. 2000;58(5):2102–10.
41. Narendra A, White MP, Rolton HA, Alloub ZI, Wilkinson G, McColl JH, Beattie J. Nephrocalcinosis in preterm babies. Arch Dis Child Fetal Neonatal Ed. 2001;85(3):F207–13.
42. Hoppe B, Duran I, Martin A, Kribs A, Benz-Bohm G, Michalk DV, Roth B. Nephrocalcinosis in preterm infants: a single center experience. Pediatr Nephrol. 2002;17(4):264–8.
43. Hein G, Richter D, Manz F, Weitzel D, Kalhoff H. Development of nephrocalcinosis in very low birth weight infants. Pediatr Nephrol. 2004;19(6):616–20.
44. Ketkeaw K, Thaithumyanon P, Punnahitananda S. Nephrocalcinosis in very low birth weight infants: a single center experience. J Med Assoc Thail. 2004;87(Suppl 2):S72–7.
45. Cranefield DJ, Odd DE, Harding JE, Teele RL. High incidence of nephrocalcinosis in extremely preterm infants treated with dexamethasone. Pediatr Radiol. 2004;34(2):138–42.
46. Gimpel C, Krause A, Franck P, Krueger M, von Schnakenburg C. Exposure to furosemide as the strongest risk factor for nephrocalcinosis in preterm infants. Pediatr Int. 2010;52(1):51–6.
47. Chang HY, Hsu CH, Tsai JD, Li ST, Hung HY, Kao HA, Chang JH, Chung HY, Wang HK. Renal calcification in very low birth weight infants. Pediatr Neonatol. 2011;52(3):145–9.
48. Lee HS, Sung IK, Kim SJ, Youn YA, Lee JY, Lim GY, Im SA, Ku YM, Lee JH, Kim SY. Risk factors associated with nephrocalcinosis in preterm infants. Am J Perinatol. 2014;31(4):279–86.
49. Mohamed GB, Ibrahiem MA, Abdel Hameed WM. Nephrocalcinosis in pre-term neonates: a study of incidence and risk factors. Saudi J Kidney Dis Transpl. 2014;25(2):326–32.
50. Stewart A, Brion LP. Intravenous or enteral loop diuretics for preterm infants with (or developing) chronic lung disease. Cochrane Database Syst Rev. 2011;(9):Cd001453.

51. Hsieh EM, Hornik CP, Clark RH, Laughon MM, Benjamin DK Jr, Smith PB. Medication use in the neonatal intensive care unit. Am J Perinatol. 2014; 31(9):811–21.
52. Laughon MM, Chantala K, Aliaga S, Herring AH, Hornik CP, Hughes R, Clark RH, Smith PB. Diuretic exposure in premature infants from 1997 to 2011. Am J Perinatol. 2015;32(1):49–56.
53. Viswanathan S, Khasawneh W, McNelis K, Dykstra C, Amstadt R, Super DM, Groh-Wargo S, Kumar D. Metabolic bone disease: a continued challenge in extremely low birth weight infants. JPEN J Parenter Enteral Nutr. 2014;38(8): 982–90.
54. Jensen EA, White AM, Liu P, Yee K, Waber B, Monk HM, Zhang H. Determinants of severe metabolic bone disease in very low-birth-weight infants with severe bronchopulmonary dysplasia admitted to a tertiary referral center. Am J Perinatol. 2016;33(1):107–13.
55. Shankaran S, Liang KC, Ilagan N, Fleischmann L. Mineral excretion following furosemide compared with bumetanide therapy in premature infants. Pediatr Nephrol. 1995;9(2):159–62.
56. Stalnaker KA, Poskey GA. Osteopenia of prematurity: does physical activity improve bone mineralization in preterm infants? Neonatal Netw. 2016;35(2): 95–104.
57. Ukarapong S, Venkatarayappa SKB, Navarrete C, Berkovitz G. Risk factors of metabolic bone disease of prematurity. Early Hum Dev. 2017;112:29–34.
58. Cediel G, Pacheco-Acosta J, CastiUo-Durdn C. Vitamin D deficiency in pediatric clinical practice. Arch Argent Pediatr. 2018;116(1):e75–81.
59. Rustico SE, Calabria AC, Garber SJ. Metabolic bone disease of prematurity. J Clin Transl Endocrinol. 2014;1(3):85–91.
60. Kearns GL, Abdel-Rahman SM, Alander SW, Blowey DL, Leeder JS, Kauffman RE. Developmental pharmacology--drug disposition, action, and therapy in infants and children. N Engl J Med. 2003;349(12):1157–67.
61. Aranda JV, Perez J, Sitar DS, Collinage J, Portuguez-Malavasi A, Duffy B, Dupont C. Pharmacokinetic disposition and protein binding of furosemide in newborn infants. J Pediatr. 1978;93(3):507–11.
62. Peterson RG, Simmons MA, Rumack BH, Levine RL, Brooks JG. Pharmacology of furosemide in the premature newborn infant. J Pediatr. 1980;97(1):139–43.
63. Vert P, Broquaire M, Legagneur M, Morselli PL. Pharmacokinetics of furosemide in neonates. Eur J Clin Pharmacol. 1982;22(1):39–45.
64. Mirochnick MH, Miceli JJ, Kramer PA, Chapron DJ, Raye JR. Furosemide pharmacokinetics in very low birth weight infants. J Pediatr. 1988;112(4): 653–7.
65. Laughon MM, Benjamin DK Jr, Capparelli EV, Kearns GL, Berezny K, Paul IM, Wade K, Barrett J, Smith PB, Cohen-Wolkowiez M. Innovative clinical trial design for pediatric therapeutics. Expert Rev Clin Pharmacol. 2011; 4(5):643–52.
66. Rodriguez W, Selen A, Avant D, Chaurasia C, Crescenzi T, Gieser G, Di Giacinto J, Huang SM, Lee P, Mathis L, et al. Improving pediatric dosing through pediatric initiatives: what we have learned. Pediatrics. 2008;121(3): 530–9.
67. Safety of furosemide in premature infants at risk of bronchopulmonary dysplasia. https://clinicaltrials.gov/ct2/show/NCT02527798. Accessed 21 June 2018.
68. Abitbol CL, Rodriguez MM. The long-term renal and cardiovascular consequences of prematurity. Nat Rev Nephrol. 2012;8(5):265–74.
69. Bixler GM, Powers GC, Clark RH, Walker MW, Tolia VN. Changes in the diagnosis and Management of Patent Ductus Arteriosus from 2006 to 2015 in United States neonatal intensive care units. J Pediatr. 2017;189:105–12.
70. Soll RF, Edwards EM, Badger GJ, Kenny MJ, Morrow KA, Buzas JS, Horbar JD. Obstetric and neonatal care practices for infants 501 to 1500 g from 2000 to 2009. Pediatrics. 2013;132(2):222–8.
71. Liberati A, Altman DG, Tetzlaff J, Mulrow C, Gotzsche PC, Ioannidis JP, Clarke M, Devereaux PJ, Kleijnen J, Moher D. The PRISMA statement for reporting systematic reviews and meta-analyses of studies that evaluate health care interventions: explanation and elaboration. PLoS Med. 2009;6(7):e1000100.

Permissions

All chapters in this book were first published in MHNP, by BioMed Central; hereby published with permission under the Creative Commons Attribution License or equivalent. Every chapter published in this book has been scrutinized by our experts. Their significance has been extensively debated. The topics covered herein carry significant findings which will fuel the growth of the discipline. They may even be implemented as practical applications or may be referred to as a beginning point for another development.

The contributors of this book come from diverse backgrounds, making this book a truly international effort. This book will bring forth new frontiers with its revolutionizing research information and detailed analysis of the nascent developments around the world.

We would like to thank all the contributing authors for lending their expertise to make the book truly unique. They have played a crucial role in the development of this book. Without their invaluable contributions this book wouldn't have been possible. They have made vital efforts to compile up to date information on the varied aspects of this subject to make this book a valuable addition to the collection of many professionals and students.

This book was conceptualized with the vision of imparting up-to-date information and advanced data in this field. To ensure the same, a matchless editorial board was set up. Every individual on the board went through rigorous rounds of assessment to prove their worth. After which they invested a large part of their time researching and compiling the most relevant data for our readers.

The editorial board has been involved in producing this book since its inception. They have spent rigorous hours researching and exploring the diverse topics which have resulted in the successful publishing of this book. They have passed on their knowledge of decades through this book. To expedite this challenging task, the publisher supported the team at every step. A small team of assistant editors was also appointed to further simplify the editing procedure and attain best results for the readers.

Apart from the editorial board, the designing team has also invested a significant amount of their time in understanding the subject and creating the most relevant covers. They scrutinized every image to scout for the most suitable representation of the subject and create an appropriate cover for the book.

The publishing team has been an ardent support to the editorial, designing and production team. Their endless efforts to recruit the best for this project, has resulted in the accomplishment of this book. They are a veteran in the field of academics and their pool of knowledge is as vast as their experience in printing. Their expertise and guidance has proved useful at every step. Their uncompromising quality standards have made this book an exceptional effort. Their encouragement from time to time has been an inspiration for everyone.

The publisher and the editorial board hope that this book will prove to be a valuable piece of knowledge for researchers, students, practitioners and scholars across the globe.

List of Contributors

Vinay Sharma
Department of Pediatrics (Neonatology), Hennepin County Medical Center, 701 Park Avenue, Shapiro Building, Minneapolis, MN 55415, USA

Sara Berkelhamer and Satyan Lakshminrusimha
Department of Pediatrics, Women and Children's Hospital of Buffalo, 219 Bryant St, Buffalo, New York 14222, USA

Naome Nyirahabimana, Joel Mubiligi, Martin Macharia and Theoneste Nkurunziza
Partners In Health, Inshuti Mu Buzima, Kigali 3432 Rwanda

Bethany Hedt-Gauthier
Partners In Health, Inshuti Mu Buzima, Kigali 3432 Rwanda
Department of Global Health and Social Medicine, Harvard Medical School, Boston, USA

Christine Minani Ufashingabire and Stephen Rulisa
College of Medicine and Health Sciences, University of Rwanda, Kigali, Rwanda

Yihan Lin
Department of Global Health and Social Medicine, Harvard Medical School, Boston, USA.
University of Colorado School of Medicine, Colorado, USA

Robert Riviello
Department of Global Health and Social Medicine, Harvard Medical School, Boston, USA
Brigham and Women's Hospital, Boston, USA

Jackline Odhiambo
Partners In Health, Boston, USA

Illuminee Uwicyeza, Patient Ngamije and Fulgence Nkikabahizi
Ministry of Health, Kigali, Rwanda

Lisa M. Tussing-Humphreys and Sarah Olender
Department of Medicine and Cancer Center, University of Illinois at Chicago, 1747 W Roosevelt Road, #416, Chicago, IL 60618, USA

Jessica L. Thomson and Melissa H. Goodman
United States Department of Agriculture, Agricultural Research Service, 141 Experiment Station Road, Stoneville, MS 38776, USA

Tina Lavin and David B. Preen
Centre for Health Services Research, School of Population Health, The University of Western Australia (M431), 35 Stirling Highway, Crawley, WA 6009, Australia

Robert Pattinson
SAMRC Maternal and Infant Health Care Strategies, Department of Obstetrics and Gynaecology, University of Pretoria, Pretoria, South Africa

Praveen Kumar Chandrasekharan, Munmun Rawat and Satyan Lakshminrusimha
Department of Pediatrics, Women and Children's Hospital of Buffalo, Buffalo, NY, USA

Rajeshwari Madappa
SIGMA Hospital, Mysore, India

David H. Rothstein
Department of Pediatric Surgery, Women and Children's Hospital of Buffalo, Buffalo, NY, USA

Oded Langer
Columbia University, New York, USA

Eric Ngabireyimana, Olivier Bigirumwami, Evelyne S. Mukakabano and Fulgence Nkikabahizi
Rwinkwavu District Hospital, Ministry of Health, Rwinkwavu, Rwanda

Catherine M. Kirk
Department of Pediatrics, Partners In Health/Inshuti Mu Buzima, Rwinkwavu, Rwanda

Hema Magge
Department of Pediatrics, Partners In Health/Inshuti Mu Buzima, Rwinkwavu, Rwanda
Division of Global Health Equity, Brigham and Women's Hospital, Boston, USA
Division of General Pediatrics, Boston Children's Hospital, Boston, USA

Christine Mutaganzwa
Department of Pediatrics, Partners In Health/Inshuti Mu Buzima, Rwinkwavu, Rwanda Kigali, Rwanda

Kim Wilson
Division of General Pediatrics, Boston Children's Hospital, Boston, USA
Harvard Medical School, Department of Global Health and Social Medicine, Boston, USA

Ann C. Miller
Harvard Medical School, Department of Global Health and Social Medicine, Boston, USA

Evodia Dushimimana
Division of Clinical Services, Ministry of Health, Kigali, Rwanda

Andrea Dall'Asta
Centre for Fetal Care, Queen Charlotte's and Chelsea Hospital, Imperial College Healthcare NHS Trust, Du Cane Road, London W12 0HS, United Kingdom
Department of Obstetrics and Gynecology, University of Parma, Parma, Italy

Tiziana Frusca
Department of Obstetrics and Gynecology, University of Parma, Parma, Italy

Valentina Brunelli and Federico Prefumo
Department of Obstetrics and Gynaecology, Maternal-Fetal Medicine Unit, University of Brescia, Brescia, Italy

Christoph C Lees
Centre for Fetal Care, Queen Charlotte's and Chelsea Hospital, Imperial College Healthcare NHS Trust, Du Cane Road, London W12 0HS, United Kingdom
Department of Surgery and Cancer, Imperial College London, London, United Kingdom
Department of Development and Regeneration, KU, Leuven, Belgium

Joffre Amim Junior
Maternidade Escola da Universidade Federal do Rio de Janeiro, Rio deJaneiro, RJ, Brazil
Faculdade de Medicina da Universidade Federal do Rio de Janeiro, Rio de Janeiro, RJ, Brazil

Penélope Saldanha Marinho
Maternidade Escola da Universidade Federal do Rio de Janeiro, Rio deJaneiro, RJ, Brazil
Rua das Laranjeiras, 180 - Laranjeiras, Rio de Janeiro CEP: 22240-003, RJ, Brazil

Antonio José Cunha
Faculdade de Medicina da Universidade Federal do Rio de Janeiro, Rio de Janeiro, RJ, Brazil

Arnaldo Prata-Barbosa
Faculdade de Medicina da Universidade Federal do Rio de Janeiro, Rio de Janeiro, RJ, Brazil.
Instituto D'Or de Pesquisa e Ensino - IDOR, Rio de Janeiro, RJ, Brazil

Fiona Broughton Pipkin and Pamela V. Loughna
Division of Child Health, Obstetrics and Gynaecology, School of Medicine, University of Nottingham, Nottingham NG7 2RD, UK

Barrie Hayes-Gill
Electrical Systems and Optics Research Division, University of Nottingham, University Park, Nottingham NG7 2RD, UK

Habiba Kapaya
Department of Oncology and Metabolism, Academic Unit of Reproductive and Developmental Medicine, 4th Floor Jessop Wing, Tree Root Walk, Sheffield S102SF, UK.0

Margo S. Harrison and Robert L. Goldenberg
Department of Obstetrics/Gynecology, Columbia University, New York, NY, USA

Hillary Mabeya
Moi University School of Medicine, Eldoret, Kenya

Elizabeth M. McClure
RTI International, Durham, NC, USA

Kate A. Hodgson
Newborn Research Centre, The Royal Women's Hospital, Locked Bag 300, Flemington Road, Parkville 3052, Melbourne, VIC, Australia

Calum T. Roberts
Newborn Research Centre, The Royal Women's Hospital, Locked Bag 300, Flemington Road, Parkville 3052, Melbourne, VIC, Australia
Department of Obstetrics and Gynaecology, The University of Melbourne, Melbourne, Australia

Kidanemariam Alem Berhie
Department of Statistics, College of Natural and Computational Sciences, University of Gondar, Gondar, Ethiopia

Habtamu Gebremariam Gebresilassie
Department of Statistics, College of Natural and Computational Sciences, Dilla University, Dilla, Ethiopia

Margaret Atuahene
School of Public Health, University of Ghana, Legon, Accra, Ghana

David Mensah
National Malaria Control Programme, Accra, Ghana

Martin Adjuik
INDEPTH Network Secretariat, Accra, Ghana

Daynia E. Ballot, Faustine Agaba, Peter A. Cooper, Victor A. Davies, Tanusha Ramdin, Lea Chirwa, David Rakotsoane and Lethile Madzudzo
Department of Paediatrics and Child Health, University of the Witwatersrand, Private Bag X 39, Johannesburg 2000, South Africa

Sandra E. Juul and Dennis E. Mayock
Department of Pediatrics, Division of Neonatology, University of Washington, 1959 Pacific Ave NE, Box 356320, Seattle, WA 98195-6320, USA

Bryan A. Comstock and Patrick J. Heagerty
Department of Biostatistics, University of Washington, 4333 Brooklyn Avenue NE, Box 359461, Seattle, WA 98195-9461, USA

Stephanie L. Smith
Uniformed Services University of Health Sciences, 4301 Jones Bridge, Bethesda, MD 20814, USA

Christopher A. Rouse
Uniformed Services University of Health Sciences, 4301 Jones Bridge, Bethesda, MD 20814, USA
Walter Reed National Military Medical Center, 8901 Rockville Pike, Bethesda, MD 20814, USA

Edward Kwabena Ameyaw
Department of Population and Health, University of Cape Coast, Cape Coast, Ghana

Mekdes Mengesha Jemberia, Elsa Tesfa Berhe, Hawi Bersisa Mirkena, Destaw Molla Gishen and Abera Endale Tegegne
Department of Midwifery, Faculty of Health Science, Woldia University, P.O.Box 400, Woldia, Ethiopia

Melese Abate Reta
Department of Medical Laboratory Science, Faculty of Health Science, Woldia University, P.O.Box 400, Woldia, Ethiopia

Hajar Mazahery, Pamela R. von Hurst and Cathryn A. Conlon
College of Health, Massey University, Auckland 0745, New Zealand

Christopher J. D. McKinlay
Kidz First Neonatal Care, Counties Manukau Health, Auckland, New Zealand
Liggins Institute and Department of Paediatrics: Child and Youth Health, University of Auckland, Auckland, New Zealand

Barbara E. Cormack
Starship Children's Hospital, Auckland District Health Board, Auckland, New Zealand

Kwamena Sekyi Dickson, Eugene Kofuor Maafo Darteh and Akwasi Kumi-Kyereme
Department of Population and Health, University of Cape Coast, Cape Coast, Ghana

Bright Opoku Ahinkorah
Department of Health, Physical Education and Recreation, University of Cape Coast, Cape Coast, Ghana

Morarji Peesay
Department of Pediatrics Division of Neonatal Perinatal Medicine, MedStar Georgetown University Hospital, 3800 Reservoir Rd, NW; Suite M3400, Washington, DC 20007, USA

Gemechu Kumera and Dereje Gedle
Department of Public Health, College of Medicine and Health Science, Debre Markos University, Debre Markos, Ethiopia

Animut Alebel and Fetuma Feyera
Department of Nursing, College of Medicine and Health Science, Debre Markos University, DebreMarkos, Ethiopia

Setegn Eshetie
School of Biomedical and Laboratory Sciences, College of Medicine and Health Science, University of Gondar, Gondar, Ethiopia

Richard Kalisa
Department of Obstetrics and Gynecology, Ruhengeri Hospital, Musanze, Rwanda
Athena Institute, VU University, Amsterdam, The Netherlands

Jos van Roosmalen
Athena Institute, VU University, Amsterdam, The Netherlands
Department of Obstetrics, Leiden UniversityMedical Center, Leiden, The Netherlands

Patrick Smeele and Marianne van Elteren
Department of Medical Humanities, VU University Medical Center, Amsterdam, The Netherlands

Thomas van den Akker
Department of Obstetrics, Leiden UniversityMedical Center, Leiden, The Netherlands

Israel Macedo
NICU, Maternidade Dr Alfredo da Costa, Centro Hospitalar de Lisboa Central, Rua Viriato, n° 1, 1050-010 Lisbon, Portugal

Luis Pereira-da-Silva
Medicine of Woman, Childhood and Adolescence, NOVA Medical School, Universidade NOVA de Lisboa, Lisbon, Portugal

NICU, Hospital Dona Estefânia, Centro Hospitalar de Lisboa Central, Lisbon, Portugal

Manuela Cardoso
Dietetics Unit, Maternidade Dr Alfredo da Costa, Centro Hospitalar de Lisboa Central, Lisbon, Portugal

Wesley Jackson, Genevieve Taylor and Matthew M. Laughon
Division of Pediatrics, University of North Carolina at Chapel Hill, UNC Hospitals 101 Manning Dr. 4th Floor, Chapel Hill, NC CB 7596, USA

David Selewski
Division of Nephrology, Department of Pediatrics and Communicable Diseases, C.S. Mott Children's Hospital, University of Michigan, Ann Arbor, MI, USA

P. Brian Smith
Duke Department of Pediatrics, Duke University Medical Center, Durham, NC, USA

Sue Tolleson-Rinehart
Division of Pediatrics, University of North Carolina at Chapel Hill, UNC Hospitals 101 Manning Dr. 4th Floor, Chapel Hill, NC CB 7596, USA
Gillings School of Global Public Health, University of North Carolina at Chapel Hill, Chapel Hill, USA

Index